Principles and Labs for Physical Fitness

SIXTH EDITION

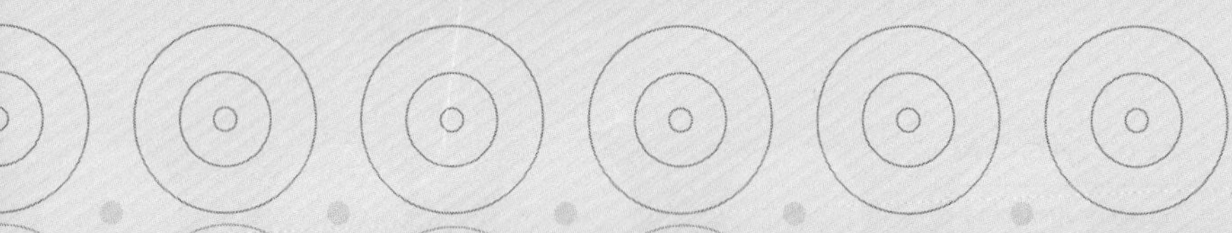

Principles and Labs for Physical Fitness

SIXTH EDITION

WERNER W.K. HOEGER
Boise State University

SHARON A. HOEGER
Fitness & Wellness, Inc.

THOMSON
WADSWORTH

Australia • Brazil • Canada • Mexico • Singapore
Spain • United Kingdom • United States

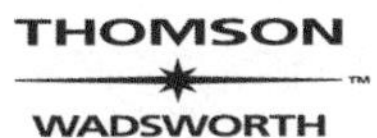

Principles and Labs for Physical Fitness, **Sixth Edition**

Werner W.K. Hoeger and Sharon A. Hoeger

Executive Editor: *Peter Adams*
Development Editor: *Nedah Rose*
Assistant Editor: *Kate Franco*
Editorial Assistant: *Jean Blomo*
Technology Project Manager: *Ericka Yeoman-Saler*
Marketing Manager: *Jennifer Somerville*
Marketing Assistant: *Catie Ronquillo*
Marketing Communications Manager: *Jessica Perry*
Project Manager, Editorial Production: *Sandra Craig*
Creative Director: *Rob Hugel*
Art Director: *John Walker*
Print Buyer: *Doreen Suruki*
Permissions Editor: *Bob Kauser*
Production/Composition: *Graphic World Inc.*
Text and Cover Designer: *Ellen Pettengell*
Photo Researcher: *Terri Wright*
Copy Editor: *Carol Lombardi*
Illustrator: *Graphic World Inc.*
Cover Image: © *Hughes Martin/Corbis*
Printer: *Courier Corporation/Kendallville*

Printed in the United States of America
1 2 3 4 5 6 7 11 10 09 08 07

Library of Congress Control Number: 2006940839

ISBN-10: 0-495-11193-7
ISBN-13: 978-0-495-11193-1

Thomson Higher Education
10 Davis Drive
Belmont, CA 94002-3098
USA

For more information about our products, contact us at:

Thomson Learning Academic Resource Center
1-800-423-0563

For permission to use material from this text or product, submit a request online at **http://www.thomsonrights.com.**

Any additonal questions about permissions can be submitted by e-mail to **thomsonrights@thomson.com.**

Brief Contents

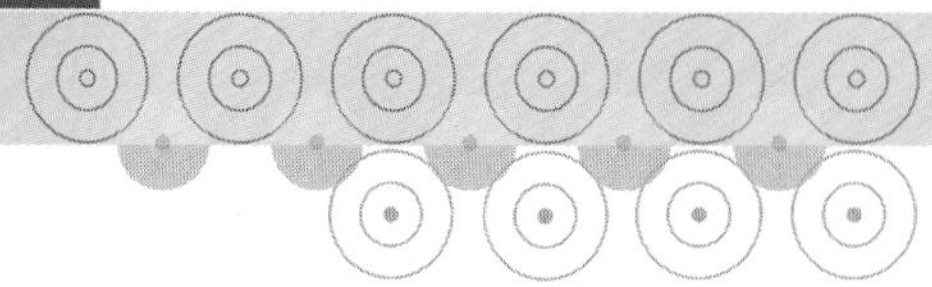

Contents

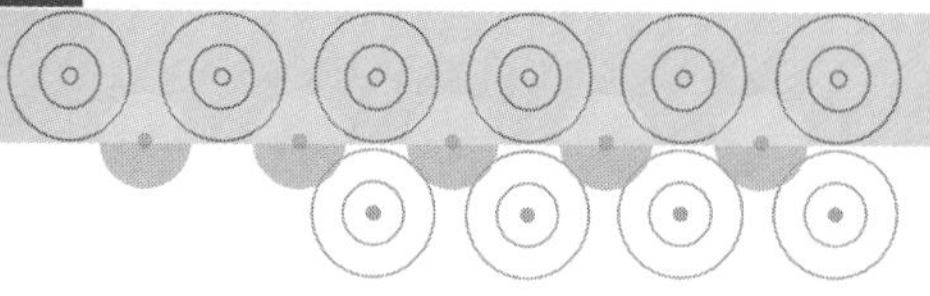

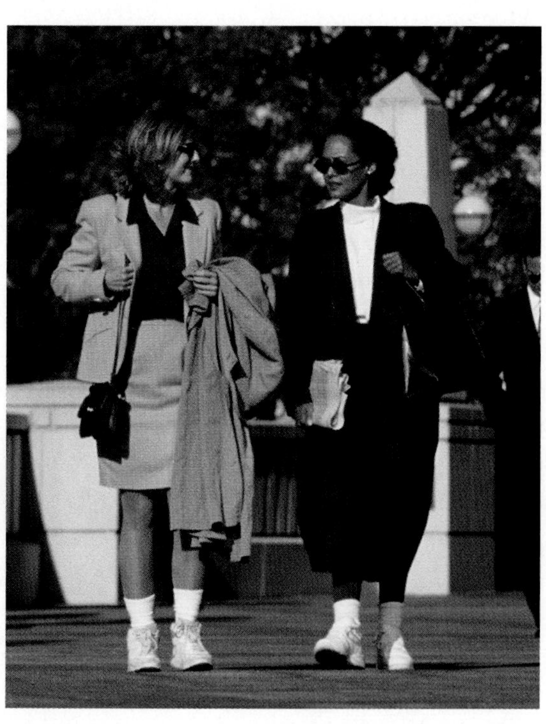

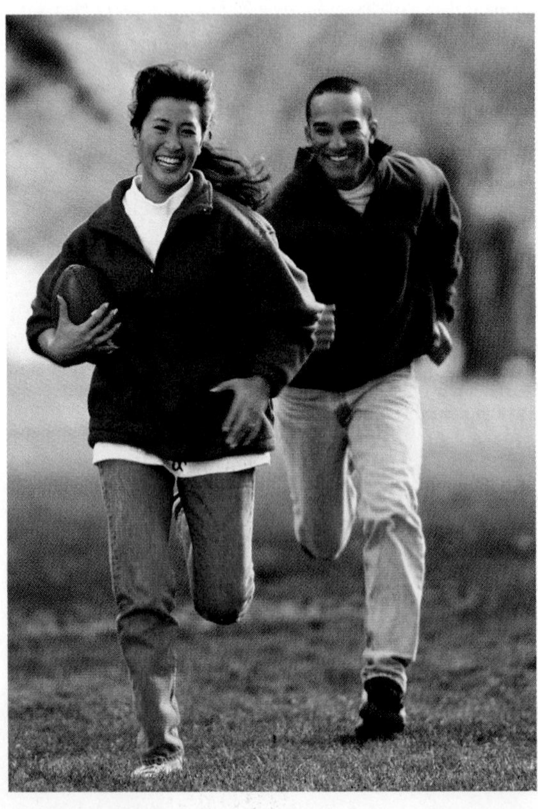

CHAPTER 7
Muscular Strength and Endurance 207

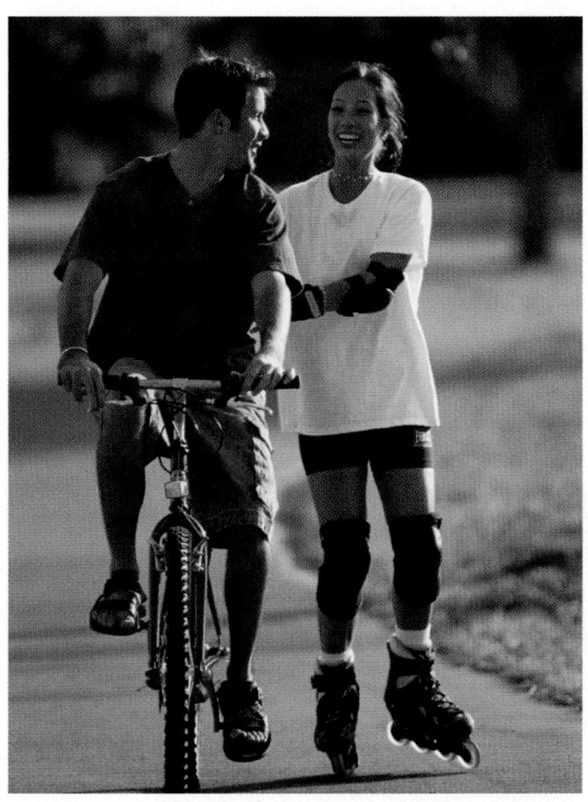

CHAPTER 8
Muscular Flexibility 257

CHAPTER 9
Skill Fitness and Fitness Programming 289

CHAPTER 10
Stress Management 325

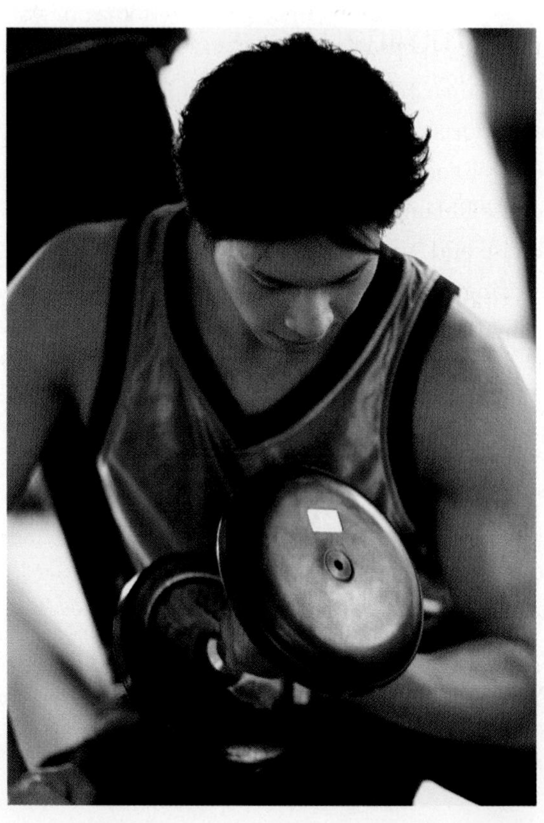

CHAPTER 11
A Healthy Lifestyle 361

Preface

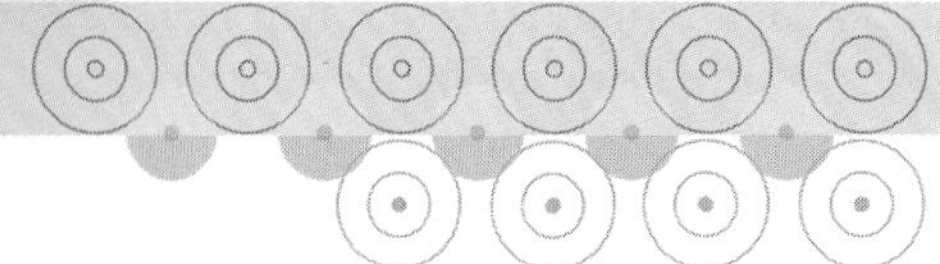

Most people go to college to learn how to make a living. Making a good living, however, won't help unless people live an active lifestyle that will allow them to enjoy what they have.

This text will teach you how to improve your personal fitness, health, and wellness—from becoming more physically active to losing weight, to gaining strength, and to dropping bad habits and adopting new, healthier ones. We believe that you control many of the factors that determine your health, and we've written this book to show you how to take command of your own fitness and wellness and live a longer, healthier life.

The Unwelcome Truth

The American way of life does not provide the human body with sufficient physical activity to maintain adequate health. Many present lifestyle patterns are such a serious threat to our health that they actually increase the deterioration rate of the human body and often lead to premature illness and mortality.

Research indicates that people who lead an active lifestyle live longer and enjoy a better quality of life. The U.S. Surgeon General has determined that lack of physical activity is detrimental to good health. As a result, the importance of sound fitness programs has assumed an entirely new dimension. The office of the Surgeon General identified physical fitness as a top health priority by stating that "The nation's top health goals as we begin the new millennium are: exercise, increased consumption of fruits and vegetables, smoking cessation, and the practice of safe sex." All four of these fundamental healthy lifestyle factors are thoroughly addressed in this book.

Because of the impressive scientific evidence supporting the benefits of physical activity, most people in this country are aware that physical fitness promotes a healthier, happier, and more productive life. Nevertheless, the vast majority do not enjoy a better quality of life because they either are led astray by a multi-billion dollar "quick fix" industry or they simply do not know how to implement a sound physical activity program that will yield positive results. Only in a fitness course will people learn sound principles to create a healthy lifestyle, including exercise prescriptions, that, if implemented, will teach them how to truly live life to its fullest potential.

Principles and Labs for Physical Fitness, sixth edition, contains 11 chapters and 33 laboratories (labs) that serve as a guide to implement a comprehensive lifetime fitness program. Students are encouraged to adhere to a well-balanced diet and a healthy lifestyle to help them achieve wellness. To promote this, the book includes information on motivation and behavioral modification techniques that help the reader eliminate negative behaviors and implement a healthier way of life.

The emphasis throughout the book is on teaching students how to take control of their own fitness and lifestyle habits so they can stay healthy and achieve the highest potential for well-being.

New in the Sixth Edition

This sixth edition of *Principles and Labs for Physical Fitness* has been revised and updated to conform to advances and recommendations since the publication of the fifth edition. New contents are based on information reported in literature and at professional health, physical education, exercise science, and sports medicine meetings. (The "running figure" icon next to captions, headings, and text indicates the presence of data from the American College of Sports Medicine [ACSM].)

Significant changes in this new edition include additional Behavior Modification Planning (BMP) boxes in several chapters—each with a "Try It" activity to further personalize the lesson—a new "Assess Your Behavior" questionnaire at the end of each chapter to help students reflect upon the chapter's contents, four new labs (1A, 2A, 3B, and 9B), several new graphs, and extensive new photography throughout the textbook. Individual chapter revisions include the following:

- New contents in Chapter 1 include information on the prevalence of physical activity in the United States, ways to monitor daily physical activity, use of pedometers, benefits of physical activity based on diverse public health recommendations (30, 60, or 60 to 90 minutes per day), and physiological fitness and its components (according to *ACSM's Guidelines for Exercise Testing and Prescription,* 2006). A new "Daily Physical Activity Log" lab also was added.

• Information on behavior modification theories, including learning theories, problem solving, social cognitive theory, and relapse prevention, has been added to Chapter 2. A new section on "Living in a Toxic Health and Fitness Environment" and a new lab to help students understand environmental influences on physical activity and nutrition further enhance an already-excellent chapter on behavior modification.

• The Nutrition for Wellness chapter has been revised to include information on the new MyPyramid guidelines. Trans fat intake guidelines and new sections on the benefits of vitamin D and probiotics are included. The information on fiber, nutrient supplementation, and antioxidants also was updated. New Behavior Modification Planning boxes for healthy eating and selecting nutritious foods are provided.

• Chapter 4, Body Composition, incorporates extensive changes, including standard error of estimates for the various body composition assessment techniques. The role of body mass index (BMI) as the most widely used technique to determine overweight and obesity in the general population is discussed in greater detail. Further, the chapter emphasizes the importance of BMI in combination with waist circumference (WC) to help identify individuals with high abdominal visceral fat and increased risk for disease. The chapter labs were revised to conform to updated standards for BMI, WC, and an assessment of recommended body weight based on BMI.

• The Weight Management chapter includes updated information on the health consequences of being overweight or obese, the role of the glycemic index of foods in weight management, activity guidelines for weight gain prevention and weight loss maintenance, and new estimated energy requirement equations (EER) to determine daily caloric intake by the Dietary Reference Intake committee of the Institute of Medicine of the National Academy of Sciences.

• Chapter 6, Cardiorespiratory Endurance, has been revised to conform to the current *ACSM's Guidelines for Exercise Testing and Prescription* (2006). In addition, the importance of increasing daily physical activity as a means to enhance health and quality of life is emphasized, accompanied by new Behavior Modification Planning boxes to increase daily activity and tips for inactive individuals to get started with exercise.

• The muscular strength prescription guidelines in Chapter 7 have been updated according to the 2006 *ACSM's Guidelines for Exercise Testing and Prescription.* A discussion of the benefits of core strength training with exercise balls and a series of stability ball exercises have been added to the chapter, along with dietary guidelines for strength development.

• In Chapter 8, Muscular Flexibility, the benefits of good posture were updated and the flexibility programming guidelines were revised according to the 2006 *ACSM's Guidelines for Exercise Testing and Prescription.*

• In Chapter 9, Skill Fitness and Fitness Programming, a new table on the contribution of selected activities to skill-related fitness has been added. Updates are also provided for several of the questions related to specific exercise considerations, as well as to the section "Preparing for Sports Participation." A new lab for students to demonstrate their competence in writing their personal comprehensive fitness program has been included in the chapter.

• Chapter 10, Stress Management, now includes information on the power of the mind over the body, how emotions affect health and wellness, the explanatory style and resultant health outcomes, the effects of self-esteem on health, and a description of the fighting spirit.

• All statistics on the incidence and prevalence of cardiovascular disease, cancer, addictive behavior, and sexually transmitted infections have been updated in Chapter 11. Included also are the *2006 Diet and Lifestyle Recommendations* by the American Heart Association to decrease cardiovascular disease risk, information on trans fat and updates on dietary and lifestyle guidelines to prevent and manage heart disease and prevent cancer, information on the role of physical activity in cancer prevention; and additional information on smokeless tobacco based on the 2006 U. S. Surgeon General's report on *The Health Consequences of Involuntary Exposure to Tobacco Smoke.* New Behavior Modification Planning boxes also were added to the chapter.

Ancillaries

ThomsonNOW™ Class-tested and student-praised, ThomsonNOW offers a variety of features that support course objectives and interactive learning, including pre- and post-tests and additional activities designed to get students involved in their learning progress and to be better prepared for class participation, quizzes, and tests.

Instructor's Manual with Test Bank These two essential ancillaries are bound together for convenience. The Instructor's Manual with Test Bank helps instructors plan and coordinate lectures by providing for each chapter a detailed outline, a lab list, and ideas for incorporating the material into classroom activities and discussions. A full test bank containing approximately 50 questions per chapter also is included.

PowerLecture for the Principles and Labs Series This teaching tool contains lecture presentations that feature more than 100 PowerPoint slides, including a text outline, art, and resources such as the Instructor's Manual with Test Bank, all on one convenient CD-ROM. PowerLecture also includes:

- **JoinIn® on TurningPoint™** Enhance your students' interaction with you, your lecture, and each other using JoinIn® content for Response Systems tailored to this text. Thomson's exclusive agreement to offer TurningPoint® software lets you pose book-specific questions and display students' answers seamlessly within the PowerPoint slides of your own lecture, in conjunction with the "clicker" hardware of your choice.

- **ExamView® Computerized Testing** Create, deliver, and customize tests and study guides (both print and online) in minutes with this easy-to-use assessment and tutorial system. ExamView offers a Quick Test Wizard that guides you step by step through the process of creating tests, while allowing you to see the test you are creating on the screen exactly as it will print or display online. You can build tests of up to 250 questions and, using ExamView's word processing capabilities, you can enter an unlimited number of questions and can edit existing questions.

Transparencies Approximately 100 color transparency acetates of charts, tables, and illustrations from the text can be used to enhance lectures.

Personal Daily Log This log contains an exercise pyramid, ethnic food pyramid, time-management strategies, and goal-setting worksheets. It also includes cardiorespiratory endurance and strength training forms and much more.

Behavior Change Workbook This workbook includes a brief discussion of current theories about making positive lifestyle changes, plus exercises to help students make changes in everyday life.

Diet Analysis+ 8.0 Diet Analysis+, the market-leading diet assessment program used by colleges and universities, allows students to create personal profiles and determine the nutritional value of the diet. The program calculates nutrition intakes, goal percentages, and actual percentages of nutrients, vitamins, and minerals, customized to the student's profile. Students can use this tool to gain an understanding of the way nutrition relates to personal health goals. The software is available online or on a Windows/Mac® CD-ROM.

Testwell This online assessment tool allows students to complete a 100-question wellness inventory related to the dimensions of wellness. Students can evaluate their nutrition, emotional health, spirituality, sexuality, physical health, self-care, safety, environmental health, occupational health, and intellectual health.

Careers in Health, Physical Education, and Sport This essential manual for majors who are interested in pursuing a position in their chosen field guides them through the complicated process of picking the type of career they want to pursue. The manual also provides suggestions on how to prepare for the working world and offers information about different career paths, education requirements, and reasonable salary expectations. The supplement also describes the differences in credentials found in the field and testing requirements for certain professions.

InfoTrac® College Edition This extensive online library gives professors and students access to the latest news and research articles online—updated daily and spanning 20 years. Conveniently accessible from a personal computer or the library, InfoTrac College Edition opens the door to the full extent of articles from hundreds of scholarly and popular journals and publications.

Wadsworth Video Library for Fitness, Wellness, and Personal Health This comprehensive library of videos includes such topics as weight control and fitness, AIDS, sexual communication, peer pressure, compulsive and addictive behaviors, and the relationship between alcohol and violence. Available to qualified adopters. Please consult your local sales representative for details.

Trigger Video Series Exclusive to Thomson Wadsworth, these videos are designed to promote classroom discussion on a variety of important topics related to physical fitness and stress. Each 60-minute video contains five 8–10 minute clips, followed by questions for discussion and material appropriate to the chapters in Hoeger and Hoeger's text. Available to qualified adopters. Please consult your local sales representative for details.

Health and Wellness Resource Center at http://www.gale.com/HealthRC/index.htm Gale's Health and Wellness Resource Center is a new, comprehensive Website that provides easy-to-find answers to health questions.

Walk4life® Elite Model Pedometer This pedometer tracks steps, elapsed time, distance, and calories burned. Whether used as a class activity or simply to encourage students to track their steps and walk toward better fitness, this is a valuable item for everyone.

Website (http://thomsonedu.com/health) When you adopt *Principles and Labs for Physical Fitness*, sixth edition, you and your students will have access to a rich array of teaching and learning resources that you won't find anywhere else. Resources include self-quizzes, Web links, suggested online readings, and more.

Acknowledgments

The authors wish to extend special gratitude to the following people, who provided feedback and reviewed this and the previous edition of *Principles and Labs for Physical Fitness:*

Lewis Bowling, *North Carolina Central University*
Mary Conway, *Sierra College*
Jesse DeMello, *Louisiana State University, Shreveport*
Britney Finley, *University of Arkansas, Little Rock*
Steve Gaskill, *University of Montana*
Tabitha Halfmann, *Southwest Texas State University*
Rebecca Hess, *California University of Pennsylvania*
John R. Hjelm, *North Park University*
Lawrence C. Rohner, *New Mexico State University*
Barbara Rostick, *Pennsylvania State University*
Judy Sloan, *Southern Adventist University*
Susan M. Todd, *Langara College*

We express gratitude to Amber Lee Fawson for her research and writing contributions to the new section on "Living in a Toxic Health and Fitness Environment" in Chapter 2. We thank John Kelly, Jonathan Hoeger, Christine Popadics, Kristin Aldrich, Alia Loan, Josh Bean, Cherie Hoeger, Michelle Hoeger, Christopher Hoeger, Daniel Fawson, and Neely Falgout for their time and assistance with new photography in this edition.

Brief Author Biographies

Werner W.K. Hoeger is the most successful fitness and wellness college textbook author. Dr. Hoeger is a full-time professor and director of the Human Performance Laboratory at Boise State University. He completed his undergraduate and master's degrees in physical education at the age of 20 and received his doctorate degree with an emphasis in exercise physiology at the age of 24. Dr. Werner Hoeger is a fellow of the American College of Sports Medicine. He was recognized as the Outstanding Alumnus from the College of Health and Human Performance at Brigham Young University in 2002 and was the first recipient of the Presidential Award for Research and Scholarship in the College of Education at Boise State University in 2004.

Dr. Hoeger uses his knowledge and personal experiences to write engaging, informative books that thoroughly address today's fitness and wellness issues in a format accessible to students. He has written several textbooks for Thomson Wadsworth, including *Lifetime Physical Fitness and Wellness,* ninth edition; *Fitness and Wellness,* seventh edition; *Principles and Labs for Physical Fitness,* sixth edition; *Wellness: Guidelines for a Healthy Lifestyle,* fourth edition; and *Water Aerobics for Fitness and Wellness,* third edition (with Terry-Ann Spitzer Gibson).

He was the first author to write a college fitness textbook that incorporated the "wellness" concept. In 1986, with the release of the first edition of *Lifetime Physical Fitness and Wellness,* he introduced the principle that to truly improve fitness, health, and quality of life and achieve wellness, a person needed to go beyond the basic health-related components of physical fitness. His work was so well received that almost every fitness author immediately followed his lead in their own publications.

As an innovator in the field, Dr. Hoeger has developed many fitness and wellness assessment tools, including fitness tests such as the modified sit-and-reach, total body rotation, shoulder rotation, muscular endurance, muscular strength and endurance, and soda pop coordination tests. Proving that he "practices what he preaches," at 48, he was the oldest male competitor in the 2002 Winter Olympics in Salt Lake City, Utah. He raced in the sport of luge along with his then-17-year-old son Christopher. It was the first time in Winter Olympics history that father and son competed in the same event. In 2006, at the age of 52, he was the oldest competitor at the Winter Olympics in Turin, Italy.

Sharon A. Hoeger is vice-president of Fitness & Wellness, Inc., of Boise, Idaho. Sharon received her degree in computer science from Brigham Young University. She is the developer of innovative fitness and wellness software and is a co-author of five of the seven fitness and wellness titles. Husband and wife have been jogging and strength training together for more than 30 years. They are the proud parents of five children, all of whom are involved in sports and lifetime fitness activities. Their motto: "Families that exercise together, stay together."

Why Physical Fitness?

CHAPTER 1

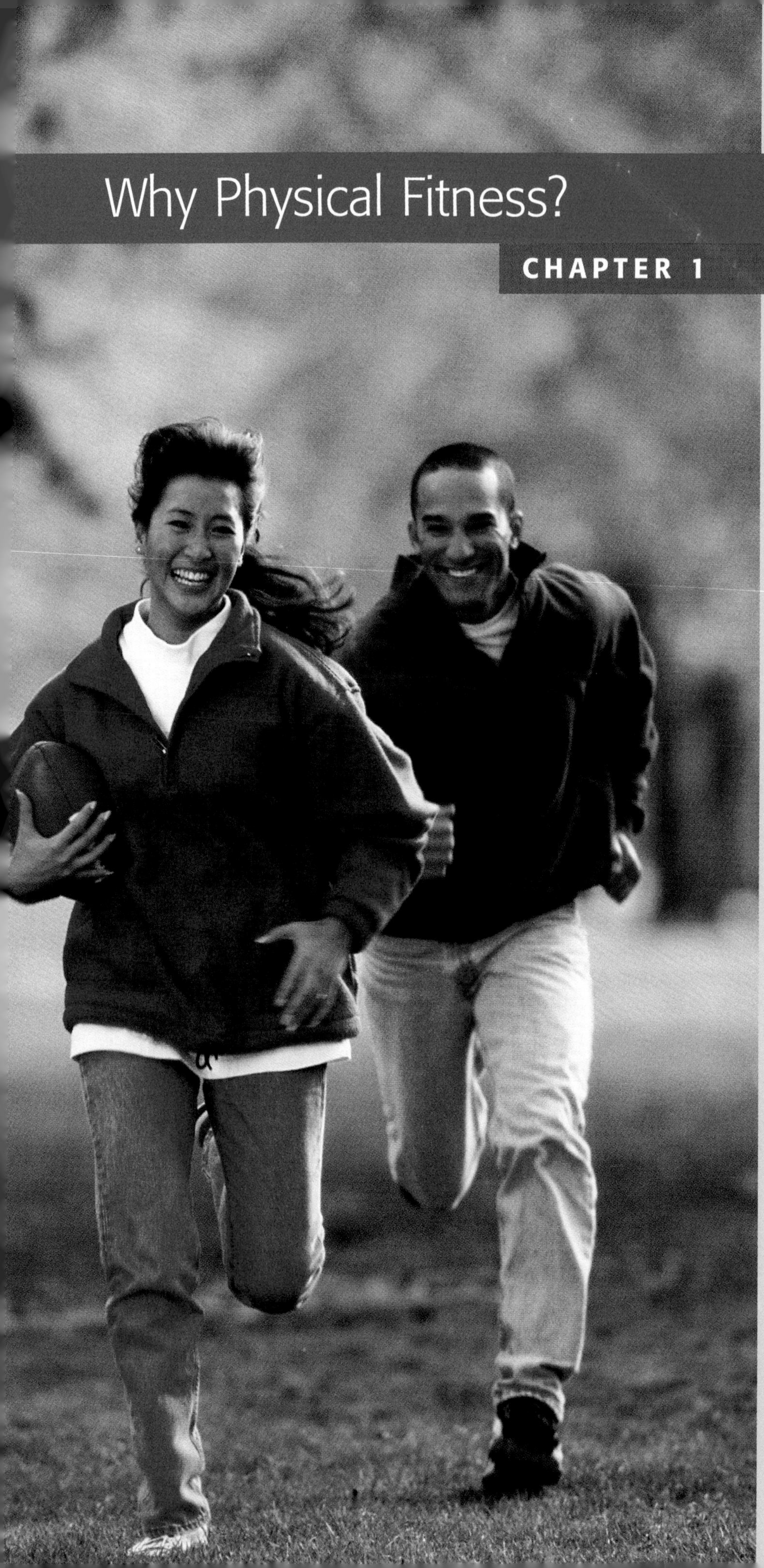

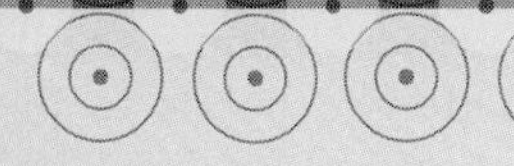

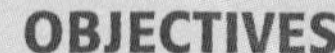

OBJECTIVES

- Identify the major health problems in the United States.
- Describe the difference between physical activity and exercise.
- Explain the relationships between an active lifestyle and health and longevity.
- Define physical fitness and list the components of health-related and skill-related fitness.
- Differentiate health fitness standards from physical fitness standards.
- Point out the benefits and the significance of participating in a lifetime exercise program.
- List national health objectives for the year 2010.
- Identify risk factors that may interfere with safe exercise participation.

Thomson NOW! The ThomsonNOW logo indicates an opportunity for online self-assessment and self-study, which:

- Allows you to create a personalized behavior change plan.
- Assesses your knowledge of important concepts and provides a personalized study plan.
- Helps to test your knowledge of material and prepare for exams.

Visit ThomsonNOW at www.thomsonedu.com/login to access these resources.

Widespread interest in **health** and preventive medicine over the last three decades has led to an increase in the number of people participating in organized fitness and wellness programs. Initially a fitness fad in the early 1970s, physical activity and wellness programs became a trend that now is very much part of the North American way of life. The growing number of participants is attributed primarily to scientific evidence linking regular physical activity and positive lifestyle habits to better health, longevity, quality of life, and total well-being.

Research findings in the last few years have shown that physical inactivity and a negative lifestyle seriously threaten health and hasten the deterioration rate of the human body. Physically active people live longer than their inactive counterparts, even if activity begins later in life. Estimates indicate that more than 112,000 deaths in the United States yearly are attributed to poor diet and physical inactivity.[1] Similar trends are found in most industrialized nations throughout the world.

The human organism needs movement and activity to grow, develop, and maintain health. Advances in modern technology, however, have almost completely eliminated the necessity for physical exertion in daily life. Physical activity is no longer a natural part of our existence. We live in an automated society, where most of the activities that used to require strenuous exertion can be accomplished by machines with the simple pull of a handle or push of a button. This epidemic of physical inactivity is the second greatest threat to U.S. public health and has been termed **"Sedentary Death Syndrome"** or **SeDS**[2] (the number-one threat is tobacco use—the largest cause of preventable deaths).

At the beginning of the 20th century, **life expectancy** for a child born in the United States was only 47 years. The most common health problems in the Western world were infectious diseases, such as tuberculosis, diphtheria, influenza, kidney disease, polio, and other diseases of infancy. Progress in the medical field largely eliminated these diseases. Then, as more North American people started to enjoy the "good life" (sedentary living, alcohol, fatty foods, excessive sweets, tobacco, drugs), we saw a parallel increase in the incidence of **chronic diseases** such as hypertension, coronary heart disease, atherosclerosis, strokes, diabetes, cancer, emphysema, and cirrhosis of the liver (see Figure 1.1).

As the incidence of chronic diseases climbed, we recognized that prevention is the best medicine. Consequently, a fitness and wellness movement developed gradually in the 1980s. People began to realize that good health is mostly self-controlled and that the leading causes of premature death and illness in North America could be prevented by adhering to positive lifestyle habits. We all desire to live a long life, and a healthy lifestyle program focuses on enhancing the overall quality of life for as long as we live.

FIGURE 1.1 Causes of deaths in United States for selected years.

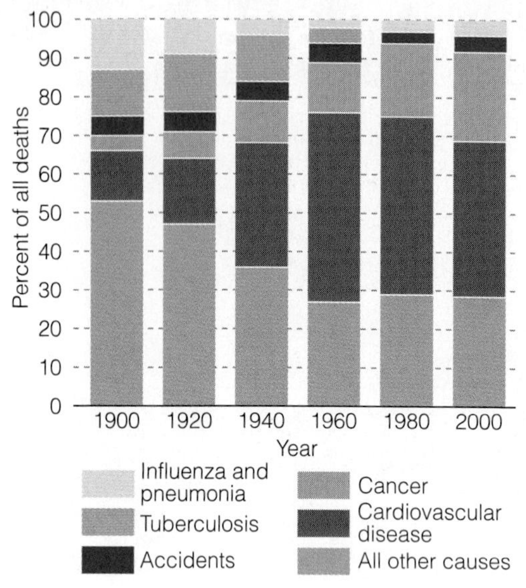

Source: National Center for Health Statistics, Division of Vital Statistics.

Life Expectancy Versus Healthy Life Expectancy

Based on 2006 government data, the average life expectancy in the United States is now 78.1 for men and 82.6 for women. The World Health Organization (WHO), however, has calculated **healthy life expectancy (HLE)** estimates for 191 nations. HLE is obtained by subtracting the years of ill health from total life expectancy. The United States ranked 24th in this report with an HLE of 70 years, and Japan was first with an HLE of 74.5 years (see Figure 1.2). This finding was a major surprise, given the status of the United States as a developed country with one of the best medical care systems in the world. The rating indicates that Americans spend more time disabled and die earlier than people in most other advanced countries. The WHO points to several factors that may account for this unexpected finding:

1. The extremely poor health of some groups, such as Native Americans, rural African Americans, and the inner-city poor. Their health status is more characteristic of poor developing nations than a rich industrialized country.
2. The HIV epidemic, which causes more deaths and disabilities in the United States than in other developed nations.
3. The high incidence of tobacco use.
4. The high incidence of coronary heart disease.
5. Fairly high levels of violence, notably homicides, compared with other developed countries.

FIGURE 1.2 Healthy life expectancy for selected countries.

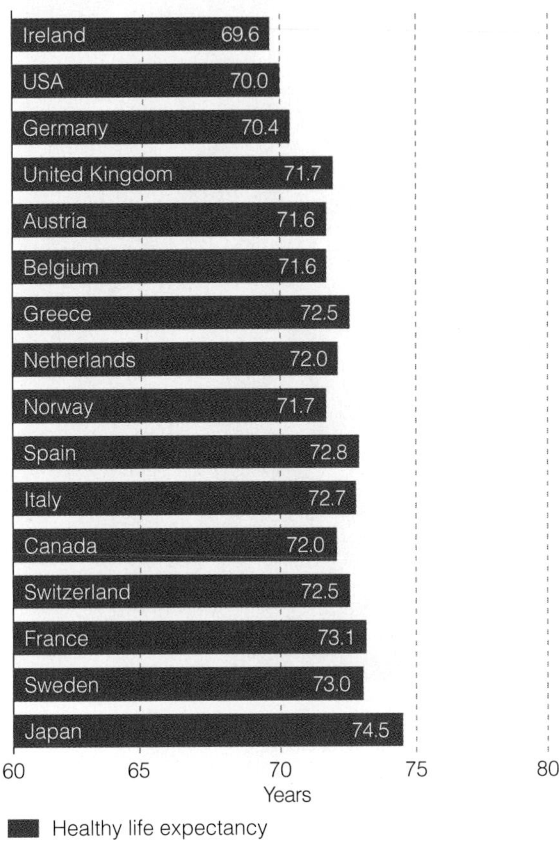

Source: World Health Organization, http://www.who.int/inf-pr-2000/en/pr2000-life.html. Retrieved June 4, 2000.

FIGURE 1.3 Factors that affect health and well-being.

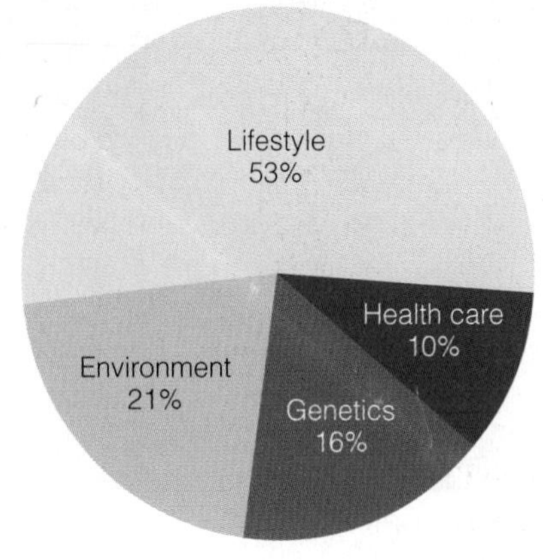

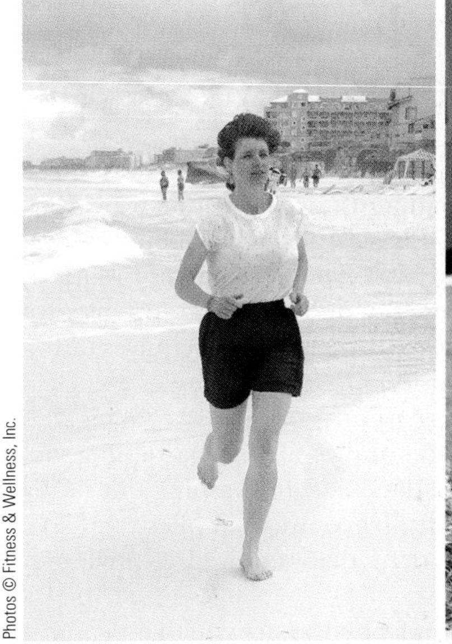
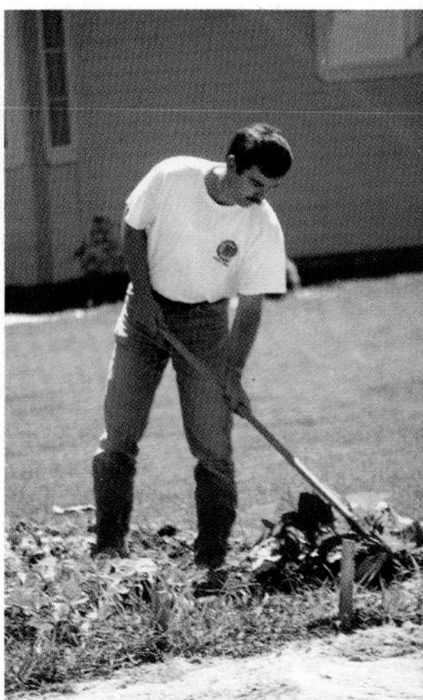

Photos © Fitness & Wellness, Inc.

Exercise and an active lifestyle increase health, fitness, and longevity.

Lifestyle as a Health Problem

As the incidence of chronic diseases rose, it became obvious that prevention was—and remains—the best medicine. According to Dr. David Satcher, former U.S. Surgeon General, more than 50 percent of the people who die in this country each year die because of what they do.

According to estimates, more than half of disease is lifestyle-related, a fifth is attributed to the environment, and a tenth is influenced by the health care the individual receives. Only 16 percent is related to genetic factors (see Figure 1.3).[3] Thus, the individual controls as much as 84 percent of his or her vulnerability to disease—and, therefore, quality of life. The data also indicate that 83 percent of deaths before age 65 are preventable. In essence, most people in the United States are threatened by the very lives they lead today.

Because of the unhealthy lifestyles that many young adults lead, their bodies may be middle-aged or older! Healthy choices made today influence health for decades. Many physical education programs do not emphasize the skills necessary for youth to maintain a high level of fitness and health throughout life. The intent of this book is to provide those skills and to help prepare you for a lifetime of physical fitness and wellness. A healthy lifestyle is self-controlled, and you can learn how to be responsible for your own health and fitness.

Health A state of complete well-being, and not just the absence of disease or infirmity.

Sedentary Death Syndrome (SeDS) Cause of deaths that are attributed to a lack of regular physical activity.

Life expectancy Number of years a person is expected to live based on the person's birth year.

Chronic diseases Illnesses that develop as a result of an unhealthy lifestyle and last a long time.

Healthy life expectancy (HLE) Number of years a person is expected to live in good health. This number is obtained by subtracting ill-health years from the overall life expectancy.

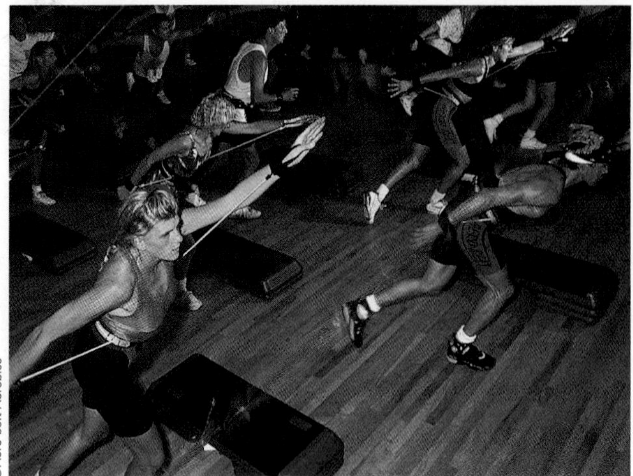
©Aero-belt Aerobics

Combined upper/lower body exercises increase the energy demands of the activity.

Physical Activity and Exercise Defined

Abundant scientific research over the last three decades has established a distinction between physical activity and exercise. **Physical activity** is bodily movement that is produced by skeletal muscles and requires the expenditure of energy and produces progressive health benefits. Physical activity typically requires only a low-to-moderate intensity of effort. Examples of physical activity are walking to and from work, taking the stairs instead of elevators and escalators, gardening, doing household chores, dancing, and washing the car by hand. Physical inactivity, by contrast, implies a level of activity that is lower than that required to maintain good health.

Exercise is a type of physical activity that requires planned, structured, and repetitive bodily movement to improve or maintain one or more components of physical fitness. Examples of exercise are walking, running, cycling, aerobics, swimming, and strength training. Exercise is usually viewed as an activity that requires a high-intensity effort.

Surgeon General's Report on Physical Activity and Health

According to a 1996 landmark report by the U.S. Surgeon General, poor health as a result of lack of physical activity is a serious public health problem that we must meet head-on at once.[4] The report stated that physical inactivity is more prevalent in

1. Women than men,
2. African Americans and Hispanic Americans than whites,
3. Older than younger adults,
4. Less affluent than more affluent people, and
5. Less educated than more educated adults.

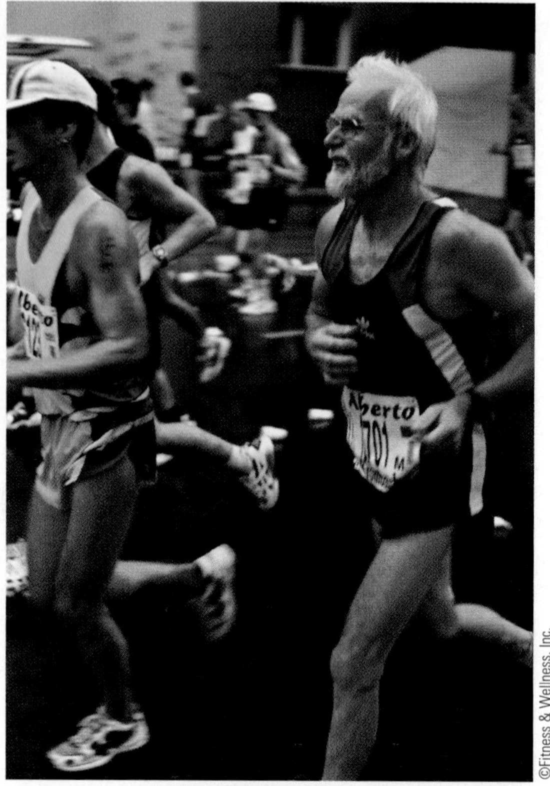

©Fitness & Wellness, Inc.

Regular participation in a lifetime physical activity program increases quality of life at all ages.

Furthermore, the number of people who are not physically active is more than twice the number of people who have hypertension, have high cholesterol, or smoke cigarettes. This report became a nationwide call to action.

The report states that regular **moderate physical activity** can prevent premature death, unnecessary illness, and disability. It could provide substantial benefits in health and well-being for the vast majority of people who are not physically active. Individuals who are already moderately active can achieve even greater health benefits by increasing their amount of physical activity.

Among the benefits of regular physical activity and exercise listed in the report and subsequent studies are significantly reduced risks for developing or dying from heart disease, stroke, type 2 diabetes, colon and breast cancers, high blood pressure, and osteoporotic fractures.[5] Regular physical activity also is important for the health of muscles, bones, and joints, and it seems to reduce symptoms of depression and anxiety, improve mood, and enhance one's ability to perform daily tasks throughout life. It also can help control health-care costs and maintain a high quality of life into old age.

Moderate physical activity has been defined as any activity that requires an energy expenditure of 150 calo-

TABLE 1.1 Daily Physical Activity Recommendations

Total Time	Outcome
30 minutes	Health benefits
60 minutes	Weight gain prevention
60–90 minutes	Weight regain prevention

ries per day, or 1,000 calories per week. The general health recommendation is that people strive to accumulate at least 30 minutes of physical activity per day most days of the week (see Table 1.1). Although 30 minutes of continuous activity is preferred, on days when time is limited, three activity sessions of at least 10 minutes each provide about half the aerobic benefits. Examples of moderate physical activity are walking, cycling, playing basketball or volleyball, swimming, doing water aerobics, dancing fast, pushing a stroller, raking leaves, shoveling snow, washing or waxing a car, washing windows or floors, and even gardening.

Because of the ever-growing epidemic of obesity in the United States, a 2002 guideline by American and Canadian scientists from the Institute of Medicine of the National Academy of Sciences increased the recommendation to 60 minutes of moderate-intensity physical activity every day.[6] This recommendation was based on evidence indicating that people who maintain healthy weight typically accumulate one hour of daily physical activity.

Critical Thinking

Do you consciously incorporate physical activity into your daily lifestyle? Can you provide examples? Do you believe you get sufficient daily physical activity to maintain good health?

Subsequently, the 2005 Dietary Guidelines for Americans released by the U.S. Department of Health and Human Services and Department of Agriculture noted that up to 60 minutes of moderate- to vigorous-intensity physical activity per day may be necessary to prevent weight gain, and between 60 and 90 minutes of moderate-intensity physical activity daily is recommended to sustain weight loss for previously overweight people.[7] Although health benefits are derived with 30 minutes per day, people with a tendency to gain weight need to be physically active daily for an hour to an hour and a half to prevent weight gain. And 60 to 90 minutes of activity per day provides additional health benefits, including a lower risk for cardiovascular disease and diabetes.

Monitoring Daily Physical Activity

According to the Centers for Disease Control and Prevention, the majority of U.S. adults are not sufficiently physically active to promote good health. The data indicate that only 46 percent of adults meet the minimal recommendation of 30 minutes of moderate physical activity at least 5 days per week, 25 percent report no leisure physical activity at all, and 16 percent are completely inactive (engaging in less than 10 minutes per week of moderate or vigorous-intensity physical activity). The prevalence of physical activity by state in the United States is displayed in Figure 1.4.

Other than carefully monitoring actual time engaged in activity, an excellent tool to monitor daily physical activity is through the use of **pedometers.** A pedometer is a small mechanical device that senses vertical body motion and counts footsteps. Wearing a pedometer throughout the day allows you to determine the total steps you take in a day. Some pedometers also record distance, calories burned, speeds, and actual time of activity each day. A pedometer is a great motivational tool to help increase, maintain, and monitor daily physical activity that involves lower body motion (walking, jogging, running). The use of pedometers most likely will increase in the next few years to help promote and quantify daily physical activity.

Before purchasing a pedometer, be sure to verify its accuracy. Many of the free and low-cost pedometers provided by corporations for promotion and advertisement purposes are inaccurate, so their use is discouraged. Pedometers also tend to lose accuracy at very slow walking speed (slower than 30 minutes per mile) because the vertical movement of the hip is too small to trigger the spring-mounted lever arm inside the pedometer to properly record the steps taken.

You can obtain a good pedometer for about $25, and ratings are available online. The most accurate pedometer brands are Walk4Life, Yamax, Kenz, and New Lifestyles. To test the accuracy of a pedometer, follow these steps: clip the pedometer on the waist directly above the kneecap, reset the pedometer to zero, carefully close the pedometer, walk exactly 50 steps at your normal pace, carefully open the pedometer, and look at the num-

Physical activity Bodily movement produced by skeletal muscles; requires expenditure of energy and produces progressive health benefits.

Exercise A type of physical activity that requires planned, structured, and repetitive bodily movement with the intent of improving or maintaining one or more components of physical fitness.

Moderate physical activity Activity that uses 150 calories of energy per day, or 1,000 calories per week.

Pedometer An electronic device that senses body motion and counts footsteps. Some pedometers also record distance, calories burned, speeds, "aerobic steps," and time spent being physically active.

FIGURE 1.4 Prevalence of recommended physical activity in the United States, 2003.

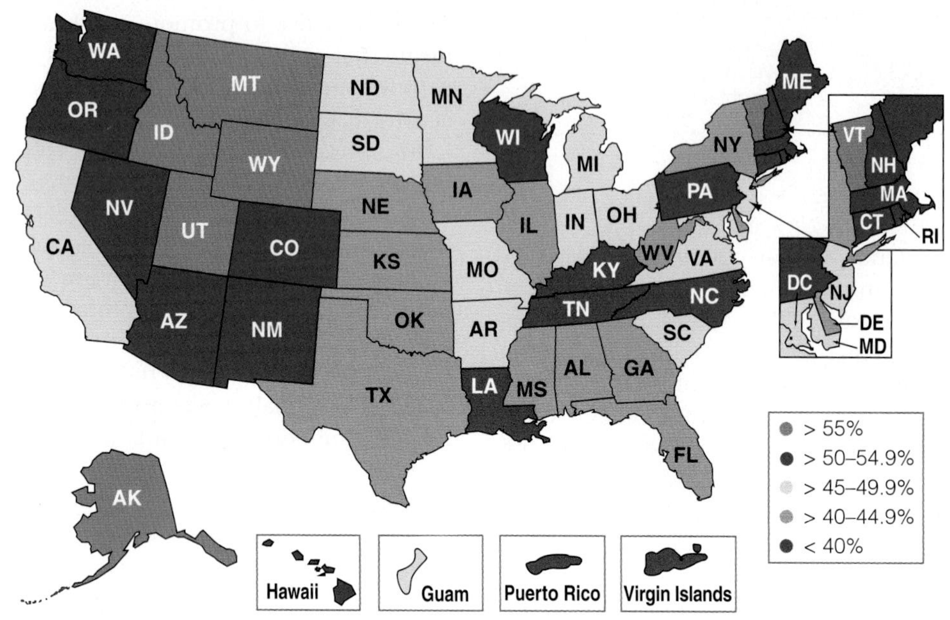

Note: Recommended physical activity is moderate-intensity physical activity at least 5 days a week for 30 minutes a day, or vigorous-intensity physical activity 3 days a week for 20 minutes a day.
Source: Centers for Disease Control and Prevention, Atlanta, 2005.

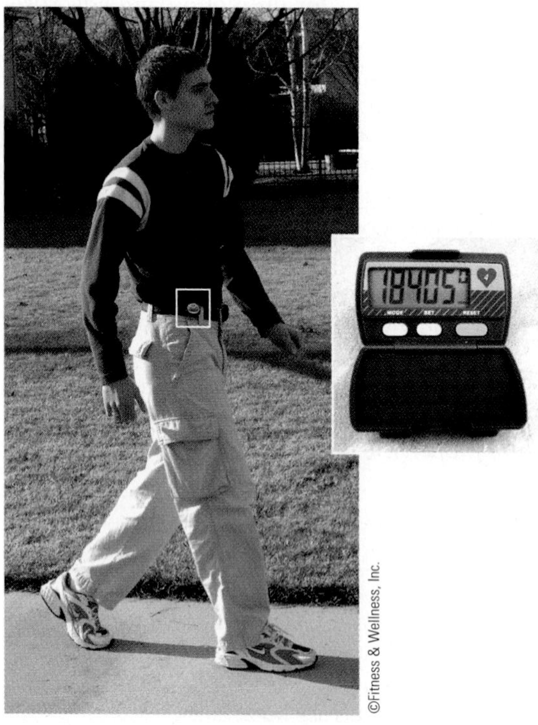

©Fitness & Wellness, Inc.

Pedometers are used to monitor daily physical activity by determining the total number of steps taken each day.

ber of steps recorded. A reading within 10 percent of the actual steps taken (45 to 55 steps) is acceptable.

The typical male American takes about 6,000 steps per day, in comparison to women, who take about 5,300 steps. A general recommendation for adults is 10,000 steps per day, and Table 1.2 provides specific activity categories based on the number of daily steps taken.

All daily steps count, but some of your steps should come in bouts of at least 10 minutes, so as to meet the national physical activity recommendation of accumulating 30 minutes of moderate-intensity physical activity in at least three 10-minute sessions most days of the week. A 10-minute brisk walk (a distance of about 1,300 yards at a 15-minute per mile pace) is approximately 1,300 steps. A 15-minute mile walk (1,760 yards) is about 1,900 steps. Thus, new pedometer brands have an "aerobic steps" function that records steps taken in excess of 60 steps per minute over a 10-minute period of time.

The first practical application that you can undertake in this course is to determine your current level of daily activity. The log provided in Lab 1A will help you do this. Keep a 4-day log of all physical activities that you do daily. On this log, record the time of day, type and duration of the exercise/activity, and if possible, steps taken while engaged in the activity. The results will indicate how active you are and serve as a basis to monitor changes in the next few months and years.

TABLE 1.2 Adult Activity Levels Based on Total Number of Steps Taken per Day

Steps per Day	Category
<5,000	Sedentary Lifestyle
5,000–7,499	Low Active
7,500–9,999	Somewhat Active
10,000–12,499	Active
≥12,500	Highly Active

Source: C. Tudor-Locke and D. R. Basset, "How many steps/day are enough? Preliminary pedometer indices for public health," *Sports Medicine* 34 (2004): 1–8.

Fitness and Longevity

During the second half of the 20th century, scientists began to realize the importance of good fitness and improved lifestyle in the fight against chronic diseases, particularly those of the cardiovascular system. Because of more participation in wellness programs, cardiovascular mortality rates dropped. The decline began in about 1963, and between 1960 and 2000 the incidence of cardiovascular disease dropped by 26 percent, according to national vital statistics from the Centers for Disease Control and Prevention. This decrease is credited to higher levels of wellness and better health care in the United States. More than half of the decline is attributed specifically to improved diet and reduction in smoking.

Furthermore, several studies showed an inverse relationship between physical activity and premature mortality rates. The first major study in this area, conducted among 16,936 Harvard alumni, linked physical activity habits and mortality rates.[8] The results showed that as the amount of weekly physical activity increased, the risk of cardiovascular deaths decreased. The largest decrease in cardiovascular deaths was observed among alumni who used more than 2,000 calories per week through physical activity. Figure 1.5 graphically illustrates the study results.

A landmark study subsequently conducted at the Aerobics Research Institute in Dallas upheld the findings of the Harvard alumni study.[9] Based on data from 13,344 people followed over an average of 8 years, the study revealed a graded and consistent inverse relationship between physical activity levels and mortality, regardless of age and other **risk factors.** As illustrated in Figure 1.6, the higher the level of physical activity, the longer the lifespan. The death rate during the 8-year study from all causes for the least-fit men was 3.4 times higher than that of the most-fit men. For the least-fit women, the death rate was 4.6 times higher than that of the most-fit women.

This study also reported a greatly reduced rate of premature death, even at moderate fitness levels that most adults can achieve easily. Greater protection is attained by combining higher fitness levels with reduction in other risk factors such as hypertension, serum cholesterol, cigarette smoking, and excessive body fat.

FIGURE 1.5 Death rates by physical activity index.

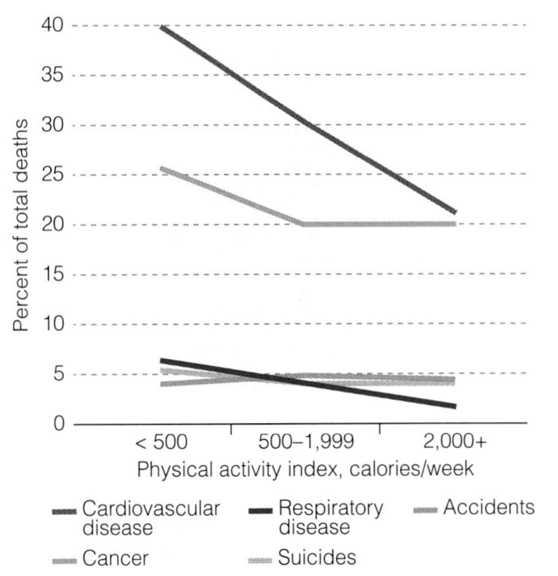

Note: The graph represents cause-specific death rates per 10,000 person-years of observation among 16,936 Harvard alumni, 1962–1978, by physical activity index; adjusted for differences in age, cigarette smoking, and hypertension.
Source: R. S. Paffenbarger, R. T. Hyde, A. L. Wing, and C. H. Steinmetz, "A Natural History of Athleticism and Cardiovascular Health," *Journal of the American Medical Association* 252 (1984): 491–495. Used by permission.

A follow-up 5-year research study on fitness and mortality found a substantial (44 percent) reduction in mortality risk when people abandoned a **sedentary** lifestyle and became moderately fit.[10] The lowest death rate was found in people who were fit at the start of the study and remained fit; and the highest death rate was found in men who were unfit at the beginning of the study and remained unfit (see Figure 1.7).

In another major research study, a healthy lifestyle was shown to contribute to some of the lowest cancer mortality rates ever reported in the literature.[11] The investigators in this study looked at three general health habits among the participants: regular physical activity, sufficient sleep, and lifetime abstinence from smoking. In addition, study participants abstained from alcohol, drugs, and all forms of tobacco.

Compared with the general white population, this group of over 10,000 people had much lower cancer, cardiovascular disease, and overall death rates (see Figure 1.8). Men in the study had one-third the death rate

Risk factors Lifestyle and genetic variables that may lead to disease.

Sedentary Description of a person who is relatively inactive and whose lifestyle is characterized by a lot of sitting.

FIGURE 1.6 Death rates by physical fitness groups.

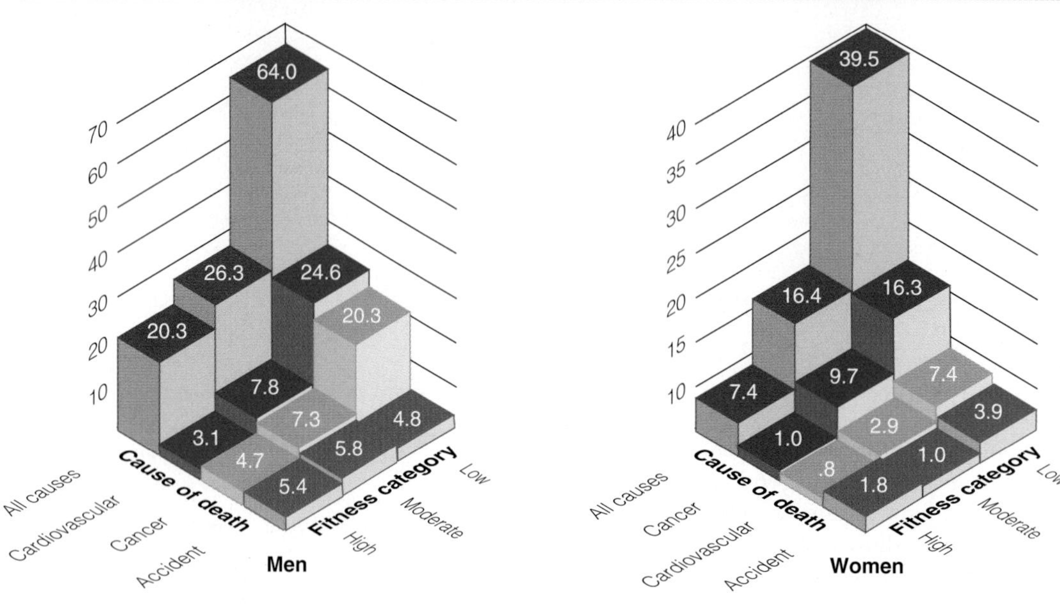

Numbers on top of the bars are all-cause death rates per 10,000 person-years of follow-up for each cell; 1 person-year indicates one person who was followed up one year later.

Source: Based on data from S. N. Blair, H. W. Kohl III, R. S. Paffenbarger, Jr., D. G. Clark, K. H. Cooper and L. W. Gibbons, "Physical Fitness and All-Cause Mortality: A Prospective Study of Healthy Men and Women," *Journal of the American Medical Association* 262 (1989): 2395–2401.

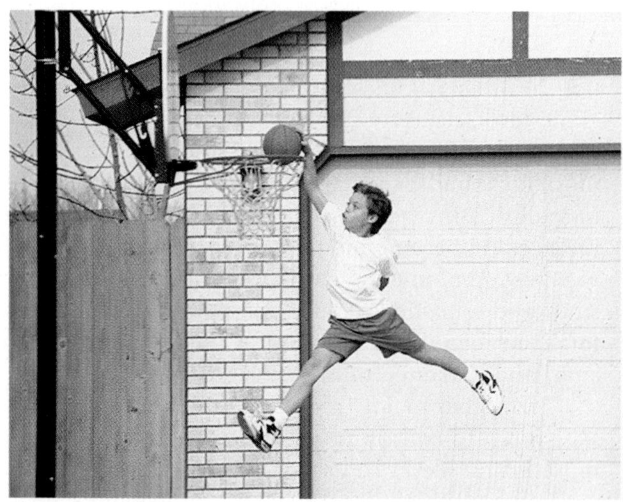

Individuals who initiate physical activity and exercise habits at a young age are more likely to participate throughout life.

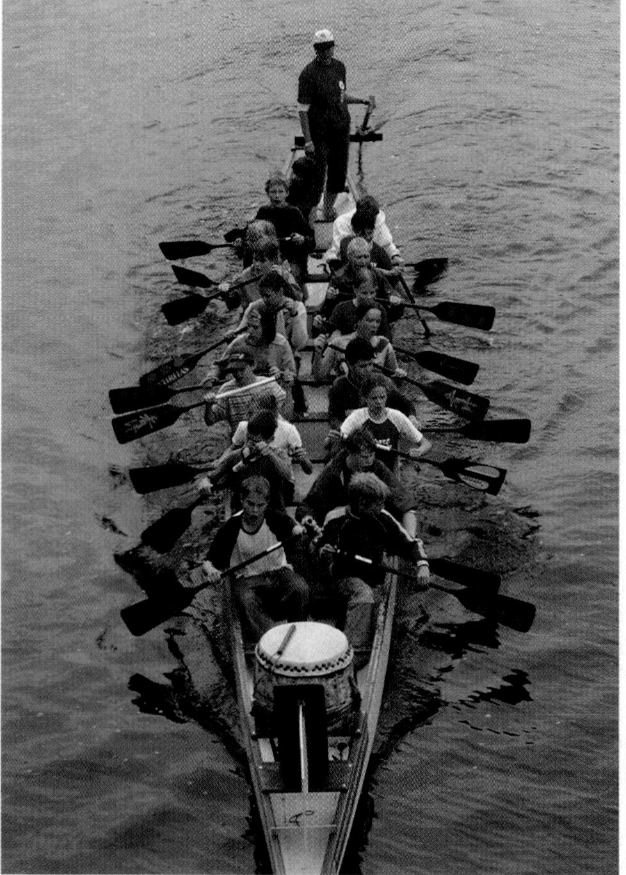

FIGURE 1.7 Effects of fitness changes on mortality rates.

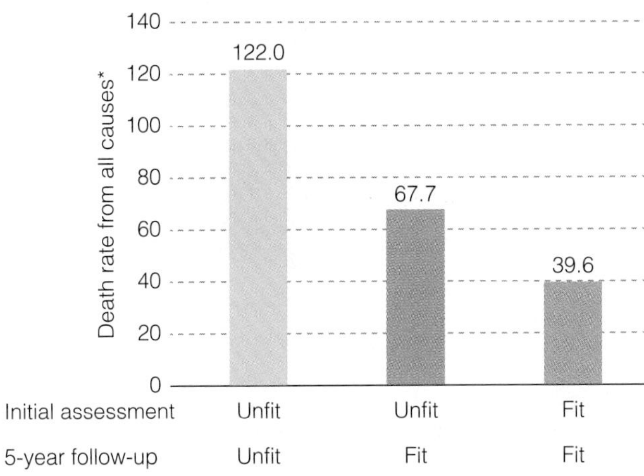

*Death rates per 10,000 man-years observation. Based on data from "Changes in Physical Fitness and All-Cause Mortality: A Prospective Study of Healthy Men," *Journal of the American Medical Association* 273 (1995): 1193–1198.
Source: S. N. Blair, H. W. Kohl III, C. E. Barlow, R. S. Paffenbarger, Jr., L. W. Gibbons, and C. A. Macera, "Changes in Physical Fitness and All-Cause Mortality: A Prospective Study of Healthy and Unhealthy Men," *Journal of the American Medical Association* 273 (1995): 1193–1198.

FIGURE 1.8 Effects of a healthy lifestyle on all causes, cancer, and cardiovascular death rates in white men and women.

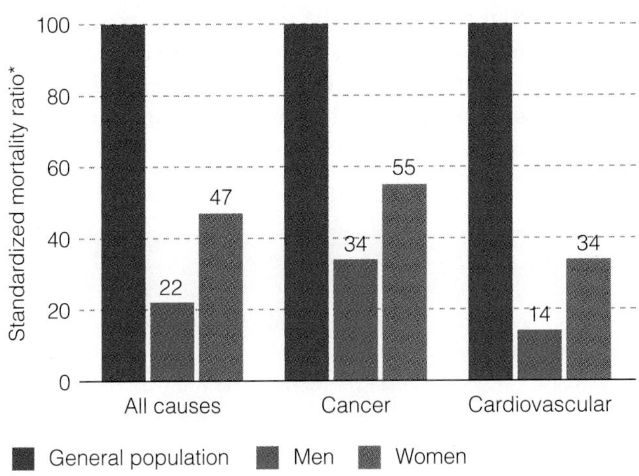

*Standardized Mortality Ration (SMR) relative to those in the general population (SMR = 100)
Source: J. E. Enstrom, "Health Practices and Cancer Mortality Among Active California Mormons," *Journal of the National Cancer Institute* 81 (1989): 1807–1814.

from cancer, one-seventh the death rate from cardiovascular disease, and one-fifth the rate of overall mortality. Women had about half the rate of cancer and overall mortality and one-third the death rate from cardiovascular disease. Life expectancies for 25-year-olds who adhered to the three health habits were 85 and 86 years, respectively, compared with 74 and 80 for the average U.S. white man and woman (see Figure 1.9). The additional 6 to 11 "golden years" are precious—and more enjoyable—for those who maintain a lifetime wellness program.

FIGURE 1.9 Life expectancy for 25-year-olds who adhere to a lifetime healthy lifestyle program as compared to the average U.S. white population.

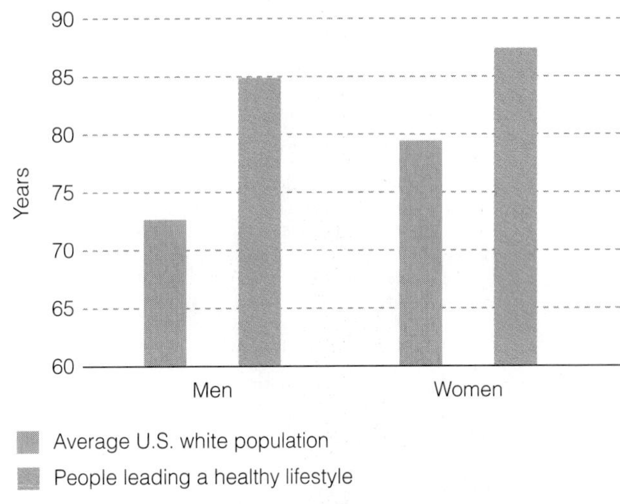

Source: J. E. Enstrom, "Health Practices and Cancer Mortality Among Active California Mormons," *Journal of the National Cancer Institute* 81 (1989): 1807–1814.

The results of these studies clearly indicate that fitness improves wellness, quality of life, and longevity. Moderate-intensity exercise does provide substantial health benefits. Research data also show a dose-response relationship between physical activity and health. That is, greater health and fitness benefits occur at higher duration and/or intensity of physical activity. Thus, **vigorous activity** and longer duration are preferable to the extent of one's capabilities because it is most clearly associated with better health and longer life.

Much scientific research has been conducted since the above-mentioned landmark studies. Almost universally, the results confirm the benefits of physical activity and exercise to health, longevity, and quality of life. The benefits are so impressive that researchers and sports medicine leaders state that if the benefits of exercise could be packaged in a pill, it would be the most widely prescribed medication throughout the world today.

Vigorous activity Any exercise that requires a MET level equal to or greater than 6 METs (21 ml/kg/min); 1 MET is the energy expenditure at rest, 3.5 ml/kg/min, whereas METs are defined as multiples of this resting metabolic rate (examples of activities that require a 6-MET level include aerobics, walking uphill at 3.5 mph, cycling at 10 to 12 mph, playing doubles in tennis, and vigorous strength training).

FIGURE 1.10 Health-related components of physical fitness.

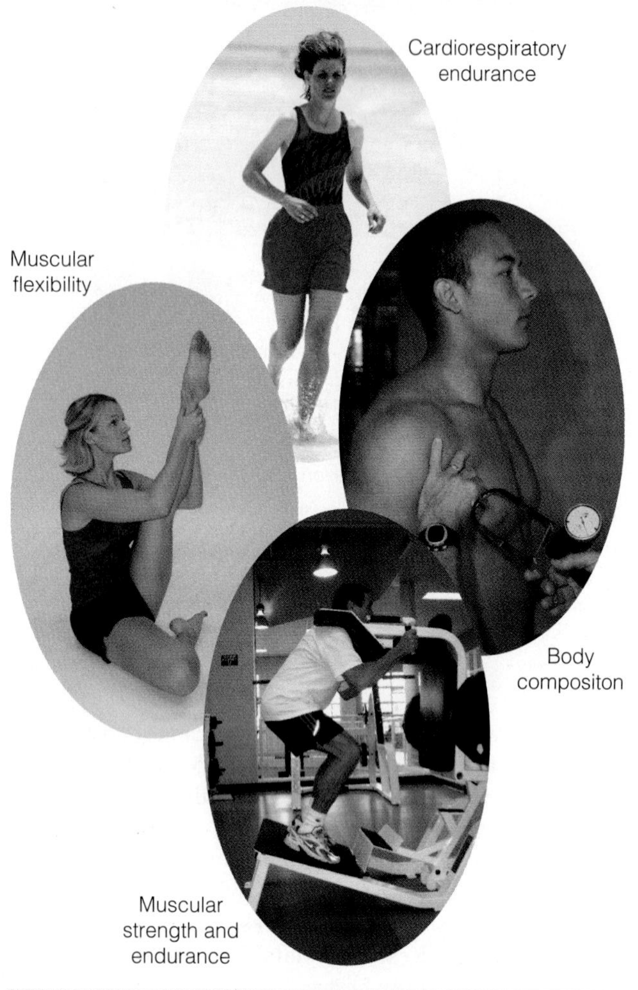

FIGURE 1.11 Motor skill-related components of physical fitness.

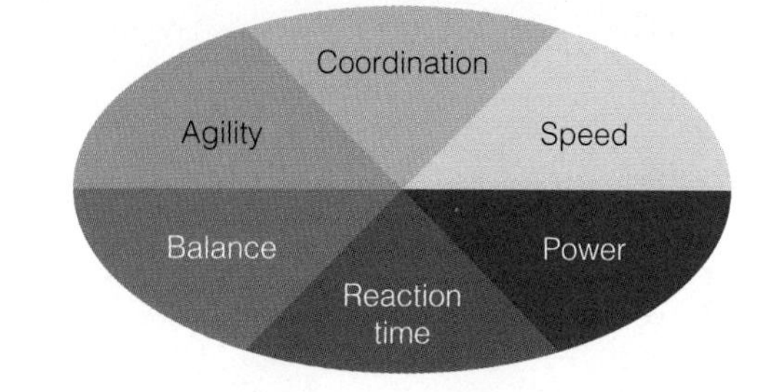

FIGURE 1.12 Components of physiologic fitness.

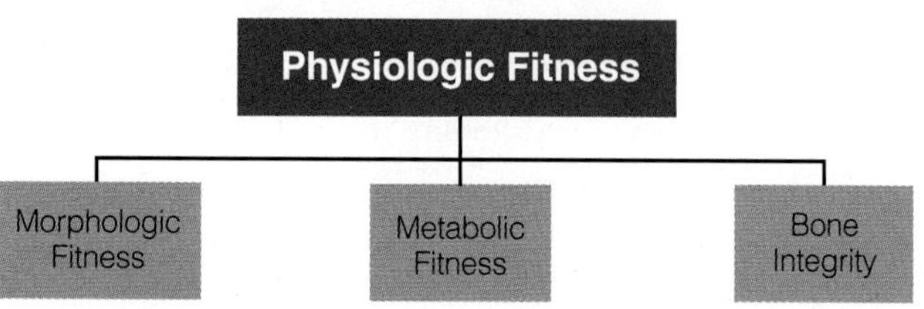

Types of Physical Fitness 

As the fitness concept grew at the end of the last century, it became clear that several specific components contribute to an individual's overall level of fitness. **Physical fitness** is classified into health-related, skill-related, and physiological fitness.

1. **Health-related fitness** is related to the ability to perform activities of daily living without undue fatigue and is conducive to a low risk of premature **hypokinetic diseases.**[12] The health-related fitness components are cardiorespiratory (aerobic) endurance, muscular strength and endurance, muscular flexibility, and body composition (Figure 1.10).
2. **Skill-related fitness** components consist of agility, balance, coordination, reaction time, speed, and power (Figure 1.11). These components are related primarily to successful sports and motor skill performance and may not be as crucial to better health.
3. **Physiologic fitness** is a term used primarily in the field of medicine in reference to biological systems that are affected by physical activity and the role the latter plays in preventing disease. The components of physiologic fitness are **metabolic fitness, morphological fitness,** and **bone integrity** (Figure 1.12).[13]

Critical Thinking

What role do the four health-related components of physical fitness play in your life? Can you rank them in order of importance to you and explain the rationale you used?

Fitness Standards: Health Versus Physical Fitness

A meaningful debate regarding age- and gender-related fitness standards has resulted in the two standards: health fitness (also referred to as criterion-referenced) and physical fitness. Following are definitions of both. The assessment of health-related fitness is presented in Chapters 4, 6, 7, and 8; where appropriate, physical fitness standards are included for comparison.

Health Fitness Standards

The **health fitness standards** proposed here are based on data linking minimum fitness values to disease pre-

FIGURE 1.13 Health and fitness benefits based on lifestyle and a physical activity program.

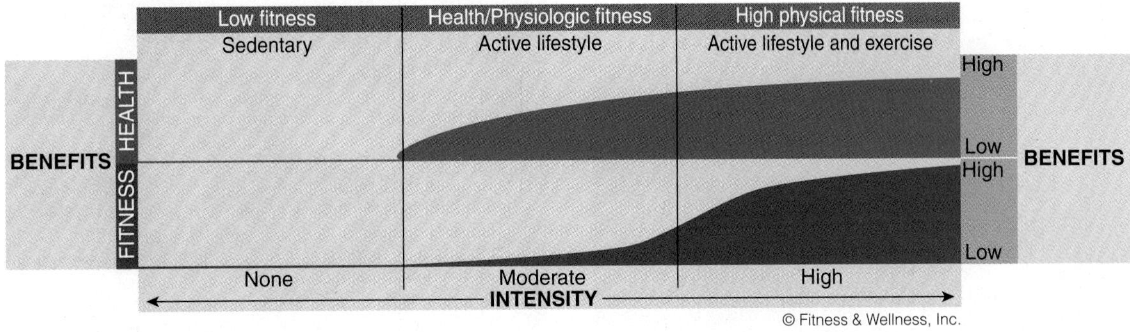

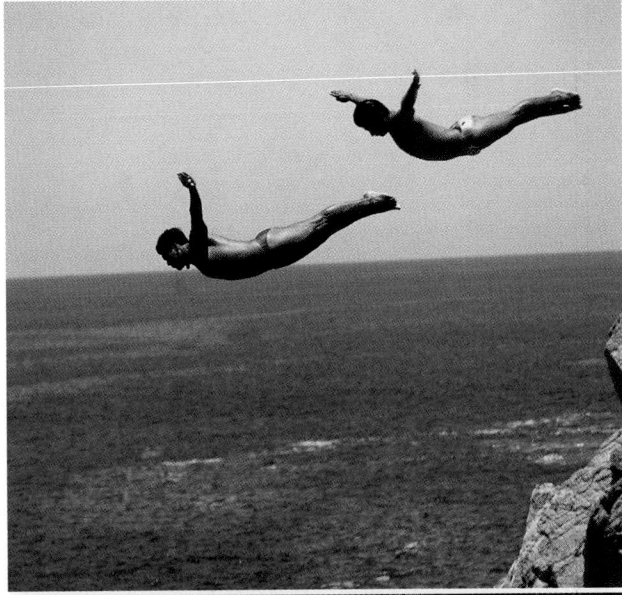

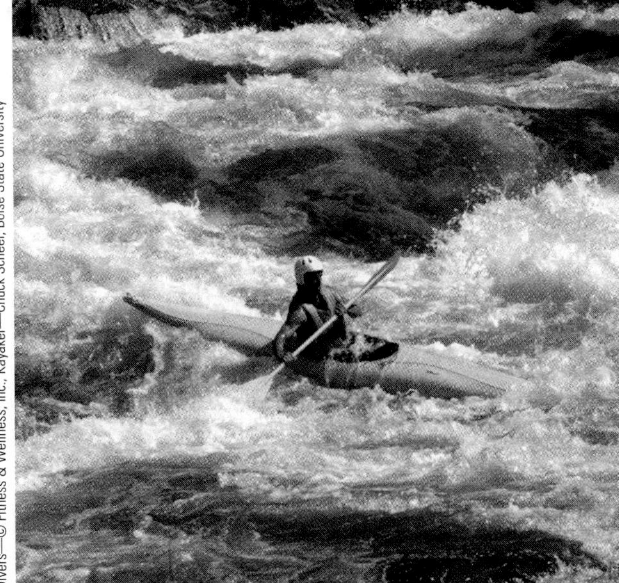

Divers—© Fitness & Wellness, Inc.; Kayaker—Chuck Scheer, Boise State University

Good health- and skill-related fitness are required to participate in highly skilled activities.

vention and health. Attaining the health fitness standard requires only moderate physical activity. For example, a 2-mile walk in less than 30 minutes, five to six times per week, seems to be sufficient to achieve the health fitness standard for cardiorespiratory endurance.

As illustrated in Figure 1.13, significant health benefits can be reaped with such a program, although fitness (expressed in terms of oxygen uptake or VO_{2max}—explained on page 12 and in Chapter 6) improvements are not as notable. Nevertheless, health improvements are quite striking, and only slightly greater benefits are obtained with a more intense exercise program. These benefits include reduction in blood lipids, lower blood

Physical fitness The ability to meet the ordinary as well as the unusual demands of daily life safely and effectively without being overly fatigued and still have energy left for leisure and recreational activities.

Health-related fitness Fitness programs that are prescribed to improve the overall health of the individual.

Hypokinetic diseases "Hypo" denotes "lack of"; therefore, illnesses related to lack of physical activity.

Skill-related fitness Fitness components important for success in skillful activities and athletic events; encompasses agility, balance, coordination, power, reaction time, and speed.

Physiologic fitness A term used primarily in the field of medicine to mean biological systems affected by physical activity and the role of activity in preventing disease.

Metabolic fitness A component of physiologic fitness that denotes reduction in the risk for diabetes and cardiovascular disease through a moderate-intensity exercise program in spite of little or no improvement in cardiorespiratory fitness.

Morphological fitness A component of physiological fitness used in reference to body composition factors such as percent body fat, body fat distribution, and body circumference.

Bone integrity A component of physiological fitness used to determine risk for osteoporosis based on bone mineral density.

Health fitness standards The lowest fitness requirements for maintaining good health, decreasing the risk for chronic diseases, and lowering the incidence of muscular-skeletal injuries.

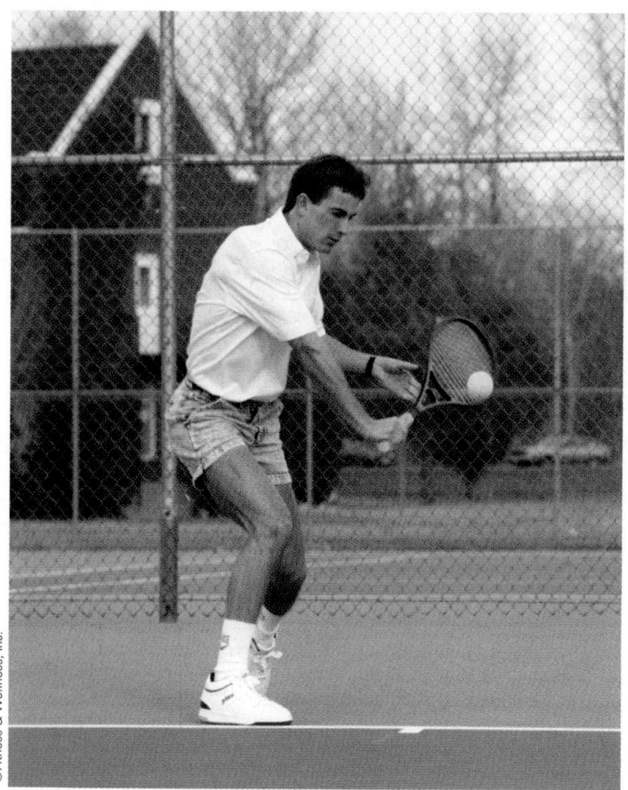

The health fitness standard can be achieved with moderate-intensity activities.

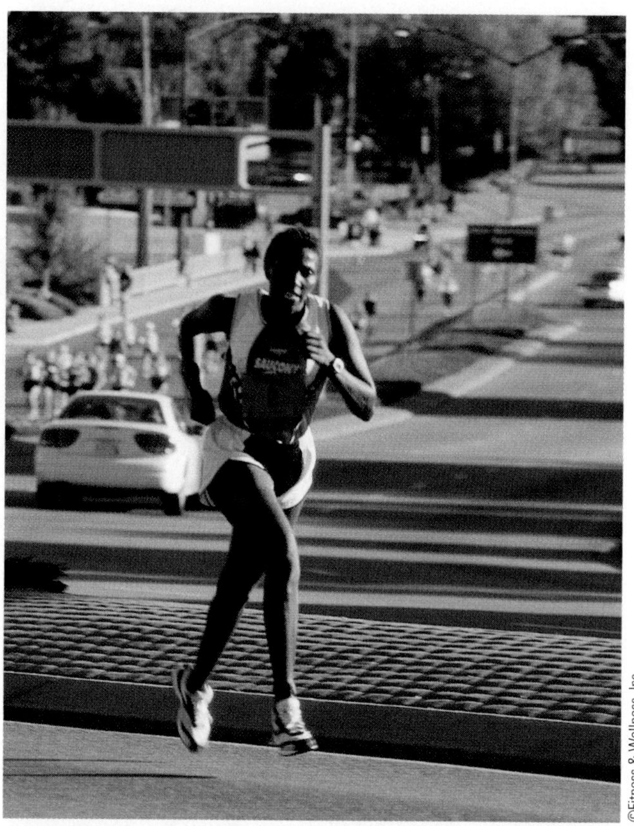

Maximal oxygen uptake, a measure of aerobic fitness, is best increased through high-intensity physical activity.

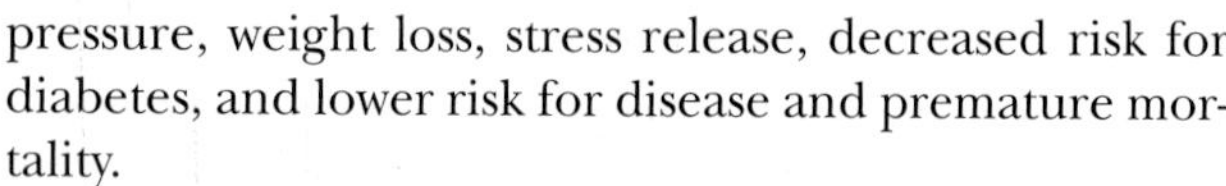

pressure, weight loss, stress release, decreased risk for diabetes, and lower risk for disease and premature mortality.

More specifically, improvements in the **metabolic profile** (measured by insulin sensitivity, glucose tolerance, and improved cholesterol levels) can be notable despite little or no weight loss or improvement in aerobic capacity. Physiological and metabolic fitness can be attained through an active lifestyle and moderate-intensity physical activity.

An assessment of health-related fitness uses **cardiorespiratory endurance,** measured in terms of the maximal amount of oxygen the body is able to utilize per minute of physical activity (maximal oxygen uptake, or VO_{2max})—essentially, a measure of how efficiently your heart, lungs, and muscles can operate during aerobic exercise (see Chapter 6). VO_{2max} is commonly expressed in milliliters (ml) of oxygen (volume of oxygen) per kilogram (kg) of body weight per minute (ml/kg/min). Individual values can range from about 10 ml/kg/min in cardiac patients to over 80 ml/kg/min in world-class runners, cyclists, and cross-country skiers.

Research data from the study presented in Figure 1.6 reported that achieving VO_{2max} values of 35 and 32.5 ml/kg/min for men and women, respectively, may be sufficient to lower the risk for all-cause mortality significantly. Although greater improvements in fitness yield a slightly lower risk for premature death, the largest drop is seen between the least-fit and the moderately fit. Therefore, the 35 and 32.5 ml/kg/min values could be selected as the health fitness standards.

Physical Fitness Standards

Physical fitness standards are set higher than the health fitness standards and require a more intense exercise program. Physically fit people of all ages have the freedom to enjoy most of life's daily and recreational activities to their fullest potential. Current health fitness standards may not be enough to achieve these objectives.

Sound physical fitness gives the individual a degree of independence throughout life that many people in the United States no longer enjoy. Most adults should be able to carry out activities similar to those they conducted in their youth, though not with the same intensity. These standards do not require being a championship athlete, but activities such as changing a tire, chopping wood, climbing several flights of stairs, playing basketball, mountain biking, playing soccer with children or grandchildren, walking several miles around a lake, and hiking through a national park do require more than the current "average fitness" level in the United States.

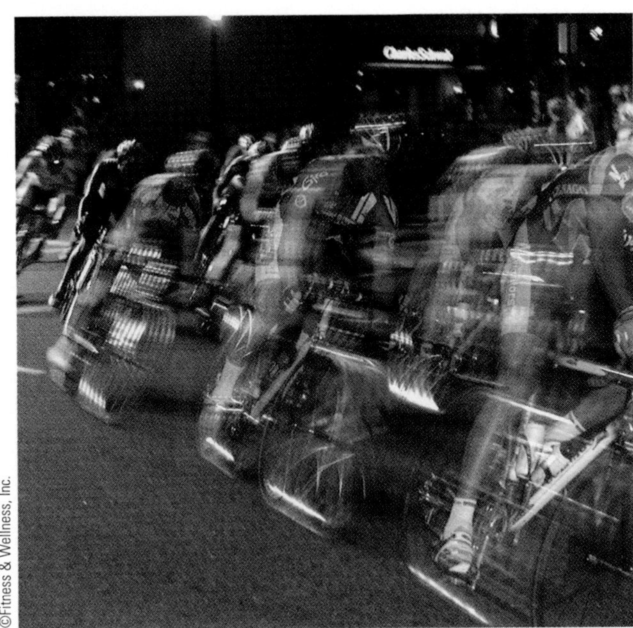

Vigorous exercise is required to achieve the high physical fitness standard.

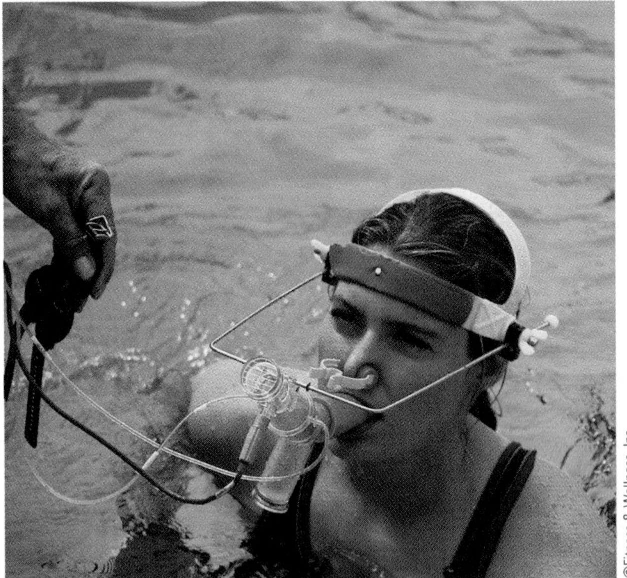

An oxygen uptake test is used to assess cardiorespiratory fitness by measuring the amount of oxygen used per minute of physical activity.

Which Program Is Best?

Your own personal objectives will determine the fitness program you decide to use. If the main objective of your fitness program is to lower the risk for disease, attaining the health fitness standards may be enough to ensure better health. If, however, you want to participate in vigorous fitness activities, achieving a high physical fitness standard is recommended. This book gives both health fitness and physical fitness standards for each fitness test so you can personalize your approach.

Benefits of Fitness

An inspiring story illustrating what fitness can do for a person's health and well-being is that of George Snell from Sandy, Utah. At age 45, Snell weighed approximately 400 pounds, his blood pressure was 220/180, he was blind because of undiagnosed diabetes, and his blood glucose level was 487.

Snell had determined to do something about his physical and medical condition, so he started a walking/jogging program. After about 8 months of conditioning, Snell had lost almost 200 pounds, his eyesight had returned, his glucose level was down to 67, and he was taken off medication. Just 2 months later—less than 10 months after beginning his personal exercise program—he completed his first marathon, a running course of 26.2 miles!

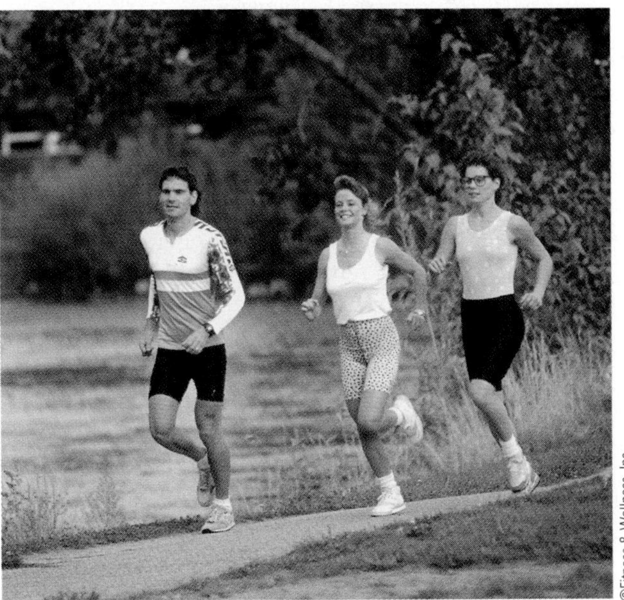

Good fitness enhances confidence and self-esteem.

Metabolic profile A measurement of plasma insulin, glucose, lipid, and lipoprotein levels to assess risk for diabetes and cardiovascular disease.

Cardiorespiratory endurance The ability of the lungs, heart, and blood vessels to deliver adequate amounts of oxygen to the cells to meet the demands of prolonged physical activity.

Physical fitness standards A fitness level that allows a person to sustain moderate-to-vigorous physical activity without undue fatigue and the ability to closely maintain this level throughout life.

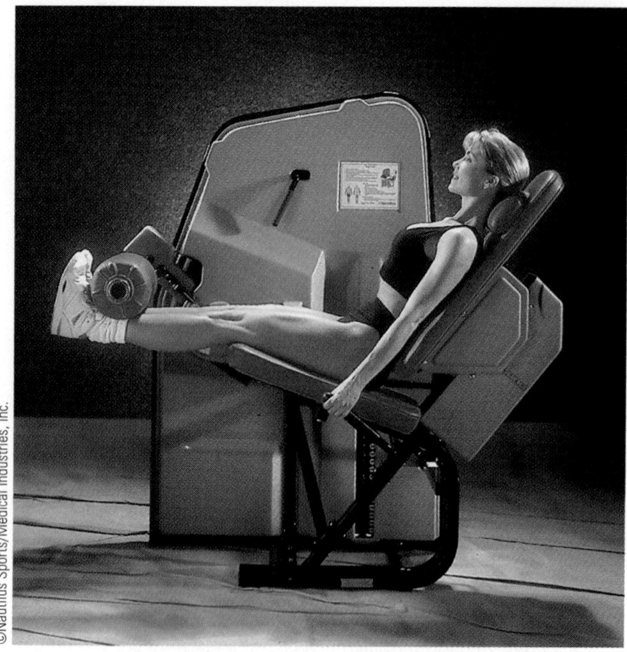

Good muscular strength is a key component of health-related fitness.

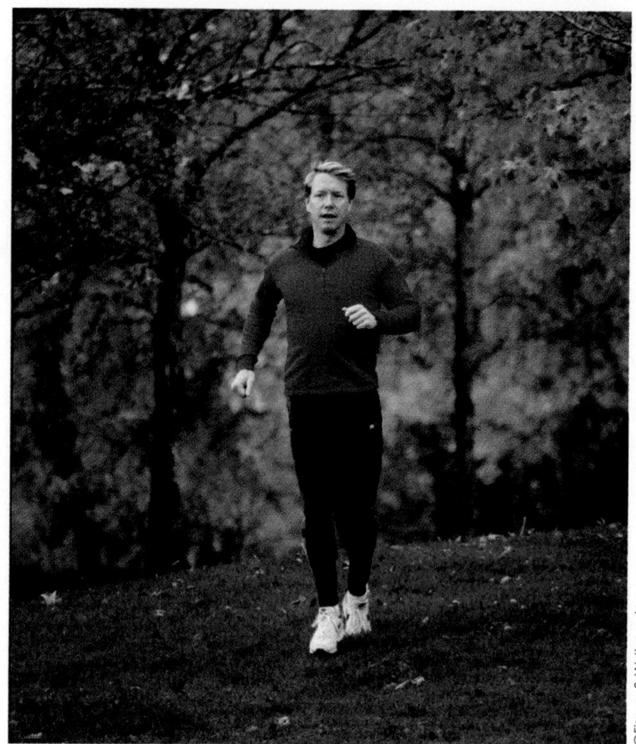

Health-care costs for physically active people are lower than for inactive individuals.

Health Benefits

Most people exercise because it improves their personal appearance and makes them feel good about themselves. Although many benefits accrue from participating in a regular fitness and wellness program and active people generally live longer, the greatest benefit of all is that physically fit individuals enjoy a better quality of life. These people live life to its fullest, with fewer health problems than inactive individuals (who also may indulge in other negative lifestyle behaviors). Although compiling an all-inclusive list of the benefits reaped from participating in a fitness and wellness program is difficult, the following list summarizes many of them. A fitness and wellness program

- Improves and strengthens the cardiorespiratory system.
- Maintains better muscle tone, muscular strength, and endurance.
- Improves muscular flexibility.
- Enhances athletic performance.
- Helps maintain recommended body weight.
- Helps preserve lean body tissue.
- Increases resting metabolic rate.
- Improves the body's ability to use fat during physical activity.
- Improves posture and physical appearance.
- Improves functioning of the immune system.
- Lowers the risk for chronic diseases and illness (such as cardiovascular diseases and cancer).
- Decreases the mortality rate from chronic diseases.
- Thins the blood so it doesn't clot as readily (thereby decreasing the risk for coronary heart disease and strokes).
- Helps the body manage cholesterol levels more effectively.
- Prevents or delays the development of high blood pressure and lowers blood pressure in people with hypertension.
- Helps prevent and control diabetes.
- Helps achieve peak bone mass in young adults and maintain bone mass later in life, thereby decreasing the risk for osteoporosis.
- Helps people sleep better.
- Helps prevent chronic back pain.
- Relieves tension and helps cope with life stresses.
- Raises levels of energy and job productivity.
- Extends longevity and slows down the aging process.
- Promotes psychological well-being and better morale, self-image, and self-esteem.
- Reduces feelings of depression and anxiety.
- Encourages positive lifestyle changes (improving nutrition, quitting smoking, controlling alcohol and drug use).
- Speeds recovery time following physical exertion.
- Speeds recovery following injury or disease.
- Regulates and improves overall body functions.
- Improves physical stamina and counteracts chronic fatigue.

FIGURE 1.14 U.S. health-care cost increments since 1950.

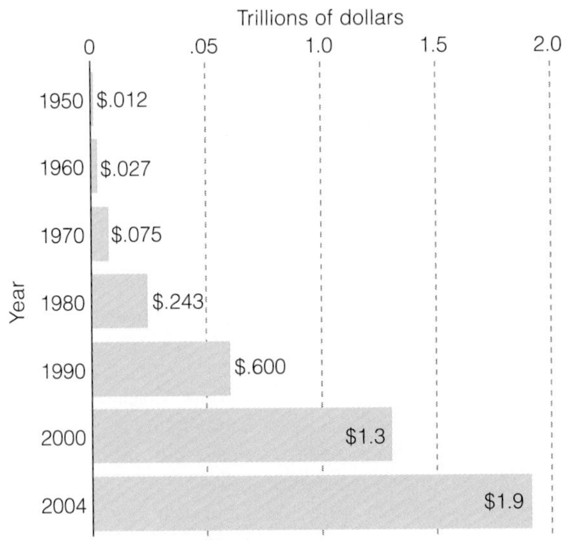

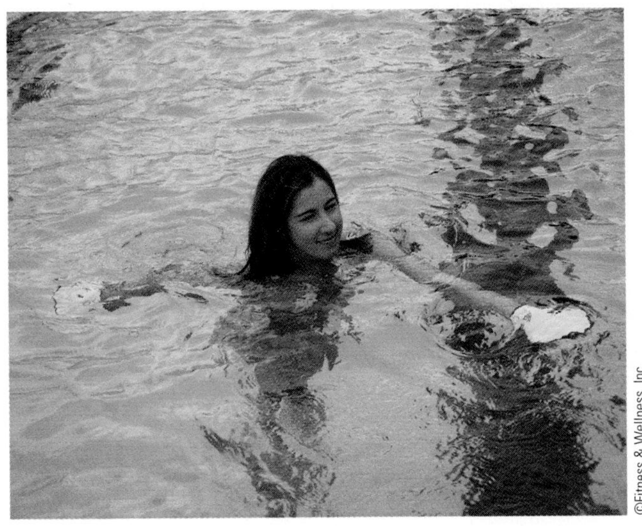

Good fitness improves overall body functions.

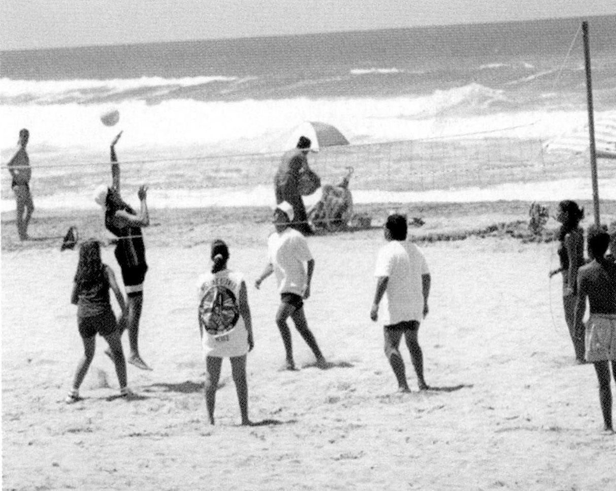

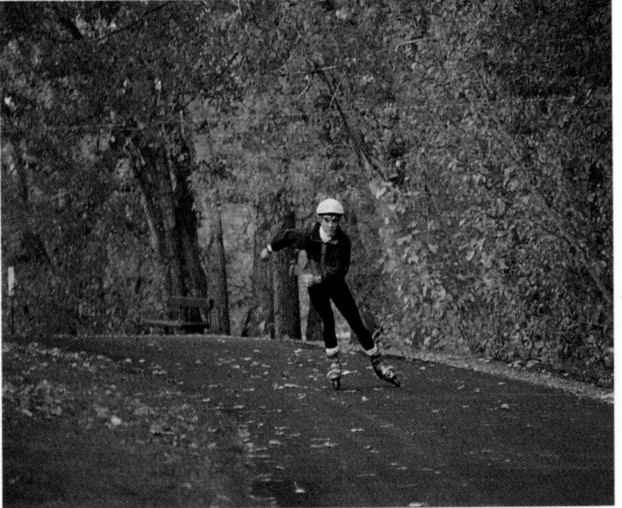

Many people refrain from physical activity because they lack the necessary skills to enjoy and reap the benefits of regular participation.

- Helps to maintain independent living, especially in older adults.
- Enhances quality of life; people feel better and live a healthier and happier life.

Economic Benefits

Sedentary living can have a strong impact on a nation's economy. As the need for physical exertion in Western countries decreased steadily during the last century, health-care expenditures increased dramatically. Health-care costs in the United States rose from $12 billion in 1950 to $1.9 trillion in 2004 (Figure 1.14), or about 13 percent of the gross national product (GNP). In 1980, health-care costs represented 8.8 percent of the GNP, and they are projected to reach about 16 percent by the year 2010.

In terms of yearly health-care costs per person, the United States spends more per person than any other industrialized nation. In 2004, U.S. health-care costs per capita were about $6,280 and are expected to reach almost $9,000 in 2010. Yet, overall, the U.S. health-care system ranks only 37th in the world.

One of the reasons for the low overall ranking is the overemphasis on state-of-the-art cures instead of prevention programs. The United States is the best place in the world to treat people once they are sick, but the system does a poor job of keeping people healthy in the first place. Ninety-five percent of our health-care dollars are spent on treatment strategies, and less than five percent is spent on prevention. In addition, the United States fails to provide good health care for all: More than 44 million residents do not have health insurance.

Behavior Modification Planning

HEALTHY LIFESTYLE HABITS

Research indicates that adhering to the following 12 lifestyle habits will significantly improve health and extend life.

1. *Participate in a lifetime physical activity program.* Exercise regularly at least 3 times per week and try to accumulate a minimum of 60 minutes of moderate-intensity physical activity each day of your life. The 60 minutes should include 20 to 30 minutes of aerobic exercise at least 3 times per week, along with strengthening and stretching exercises 2 to 3 times per week.
2. *Do not smoke cigarettes.* Cigarette smoking is the largest preventable cause of illness and premature death in the United States. If we include all related deaths, smoking is responsible for more than 440,000 unnecessary deaths each year.
3. *Eat right.* Eat a good breakfast and two additional well-balanced meals every day. Avoid eating too many calories, processed foods, and foods with a lot of sugar, fat, and salt. Increase your daily consumption of fruits, vegetables, and whole-grain products.
4. *Avoid snacking.* Some researchers recommend refraining from frequent between-meal snacks. Every time a person eats, insulin is released to remove sugar from the blood. Such frequent spikes in insulin may contribute to the development of heart disease. Less frequent increases of insulin are more conducive to good health.
5. *Maintain recommended body weight through adequate nutrition and exercise.* This is important in preventing chronic diseases and in developing a higher level of fitness.
6. *Get enough rest.* Sleep 7 to 8 hours each night.
7. *Lower your stress levels.* Reduce your vulnerability to stress and practice stress management techniques as needed.
8. *Be wary of alcohol.* Drink alcohol moderately or not at all. Alcohol abuse leads to mental, emotional, physical, and social problems.
9. *Surround yourself with healthy friendships.* Unhealthy friendships contribute to destructive behaviors and low self-esteem. Associating with people who strive to maintain good fitness and health reinforces a positive outlook in life and encourages positive behaviors. Constructive social interactions enhance well-being. Researchers have also found that mortality rates are much higher among people who are socially isolated. People who aren't socially integrated are more likely to "give up when seriously ill"—which accelerates dying.
10. *Be informed about the environment.* Seek clean air, clean water, and a clean environment. Be aware of pollutants and occupational hazards: asbestos fibers, nickel dust, chromate, uranium dust, and so on. Take precautions when using pesticides and insecticides.
11. *Increase education.* Data indicate that people who are more educated live longer. The theory is that as education increases, so do the number of connections between nerve cells. The increased number of connections in turn helps the individual make better survival (healthy lifestyle) choices.
12. *Take personal safety measures.* Although not all accidents are preventable, many are. Taking simple precautionary measures—such as using seat belts and keeping electrical appliances away from water—lessens the risk for avoidable accidents.

Try It

Look at the list above and indicate which habits are already a part of your lifestyle. What changes could you make to incorporate some additional healthy habits into your daily life?

Unhealthy behaviors are contributing to the staggering U.S. health-care costs. Risk factors for disease such as obesity and smoking carry a heavy price tag. An estimated 1 percent of the people account for 30 percent of health-care costs.[14] Half of the people use up about 97 percent of health-care dollars. Furthermore, the average health-care cost per person in the United States is almost twice as high as that in most other industrialized nations.

Scientific evidence now links participation in fitness and wellness programs to better health and also to lower medical costs and higher job productivity. As a result of the staggering rise in medical costs, many organizations offer health-promotion programs because keeping employees healthy costs less than treating them once they are sick.

Another reason some organizations are offering health promotion programs to their employees—overlooked by many because it does not seem to affect the bottom line directly—is simply top management's concern for the employees' well-being. Whether the program lowers medical costs is not the main issue; more important is that wellness helps individuals feel better about themselves and improve their quality of life.

A Healthy Lifestyle Challenge for the 21st Century

Because every person should strive for a better and healthier life, our biggest challenge as we begin the new century is to teach people how to take control of their personal health habits and adhere to a positive lifestyle. A wealth of information on the benefits of fitness and wellness programs indicates that improving the quality and possible length of our lives is a matter of personal choice.

Even though people in the United States believe a positive lifestyle has a great impact on health and

FIGURE 1.15 National Health Objectives 2010: Healthy People in Healthy Communities.

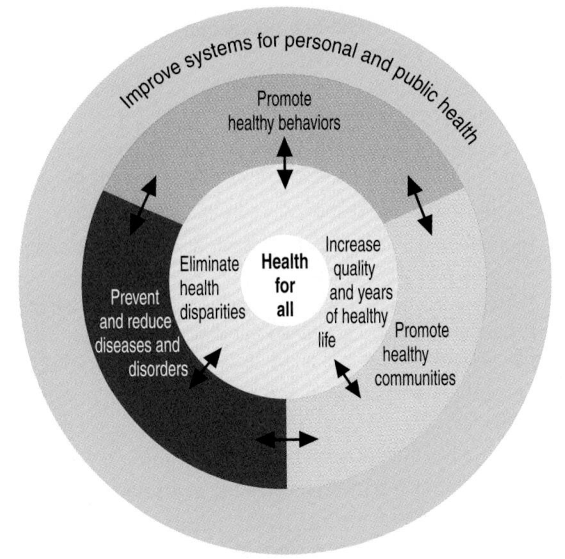

longevity, most do not reap the benefits because they don't know how to implement a safe and effective fitness and wellness program. Others are exercising incorrectly and, therefore, are not reaping the full benefits of their program. How, then, can we meet the health challenges of the 21st century? That is the focus of this book—to provide the necessary tools that will enable you to write, implement, and regularly update your personal lifetime fitness and wellness program.

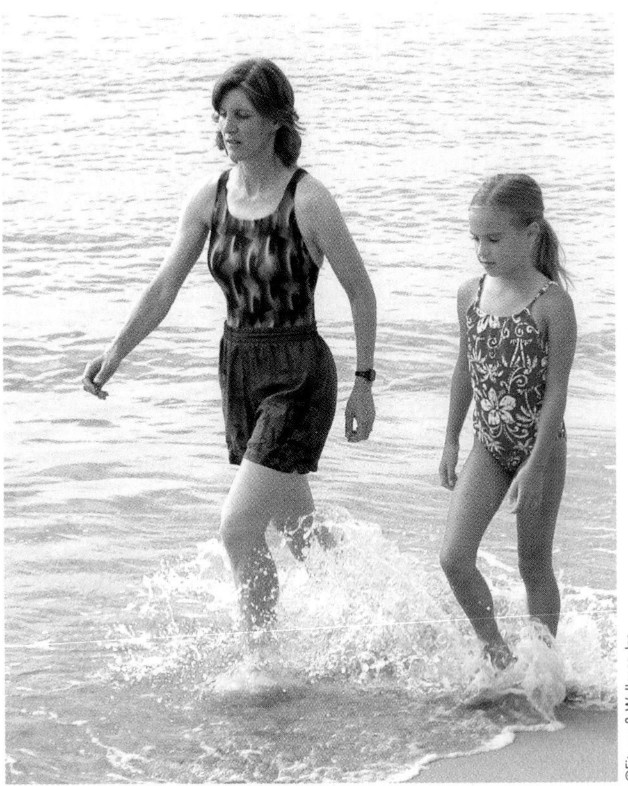

No current drug or medication provides as many health benefits as a regular physical activity program.

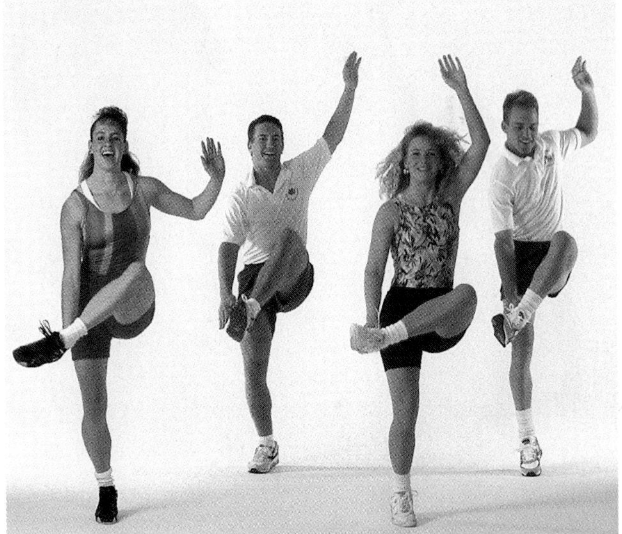

Exercising with others enhances adherence to fitness programs.

National Health Objectives for the Year 2010

Every 10 years, the U.S. Department of Health and Human Services releases a list of objectives for preventing disease and promoting health. Since its initiation in 1980, this 10-year plan has helped instill a new sense of purpose and focus for public health and preventive medicine. These national health objectives are intended to be realistic goals to improve the health of all Americans. Two unique goals of the 2010 objectives emphasize increased quality and years of healthy life and seek to eliminate health disparities among all groups of people (see Figure 1.15). The objectives address three important points:[15]

1. **Personal responsibility for health behavior.** Individuals need to become ever more health-conscious. Responsible and informed behaviors are key to good health.
2. **Health benefits for all people and all communities.** Lower socioeconomic conditions and poor health often are interrelated. Extending the benefits of good health to all people is crucial to the health of the nation.
3. **Health promotion and disease prevention.** A shift from treatment to preventive techniques will drastically cut health-care costs and help all Americans achieve a better quality of life.

Development of these health objectives usually involves more than 10,000 people representing 300 national organizations, including the Institute of Medicine of the National Academy of Sciences, all state health departments, and the federal Office of Disease Prevention

FIGURE 1.16 Selected health objectives for the year 2010.

1. Increase quality and years of healthy life.
2. Eliminate health disparities.
3. Improve the health, fitness, and quality of life of all Americans through the adoption and maintenance of regular, daily physical activity.
4. Promote health and reduce chronic disease risk, disease progression, debilitation, and premature death associated with dietary factors and nutritional status among all people in the United States.
5. Reduce disease, disability, and death related to tobacco use and exposure to secondhand smoke.
6. Increase the quality, availability, and effectiveness of educational and community-based programs designed to prevent disease and improve the health and quality of life of the American people.
7. Promote health for all people through a healthy environment.
8. Reduce the incidence and severity of injuries from unintentional causes, as well as violence and abuse.
9. Promote worker health and safety through prevention.
10. Improve access to comprehensive, high quality health care.
11. Ensure that every pregnancy in the United States is intended.
12. Improve maternal and pregnancy outcomes and reduce rates of disability in infants.
13. Improve the quality of health-related decisions through effective communication.
14. Decrease the incidence of functional limitations due to arthritis, osteoporosis, and chronic back conditions.
15. Decrease cancer incidence, morbidity, and mortality.
16. Promote health and prevent secondary conditions among persons with disabilities.
17. Enhance the cardiovascular health and quality of life of all Americans through prevention and control of risk factors and promotion of healthy lifestyle behaviors.
18. Prevent HIV transmission and associated morbidity and mortality.
19. Improve the mental health of all Americans.
20. Raise the public's awareness of the signs and symptoms of lung disease.
21. Increase awareness of healthy sexual relationships and prevent all forms of sexually transmitted diseases.
22. Reduce the incidence of substance abuse by all people, especially children.

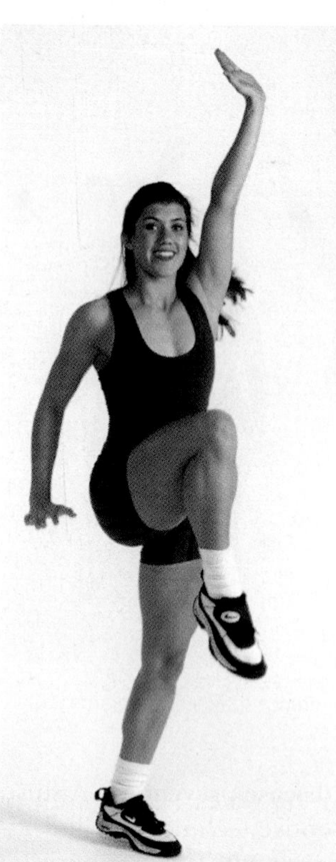

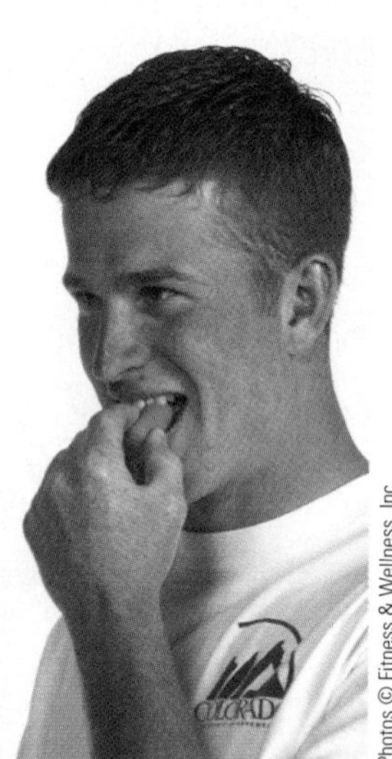

Photos © Fitness & Wellness, Inc.

Responsible and informed behaviors are the key to good health.

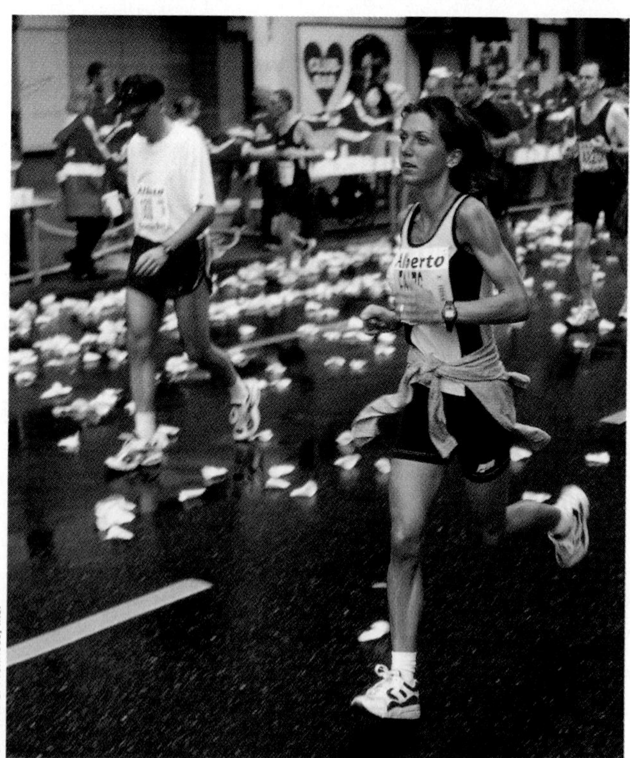

©Fitness & Wellness, Inc.

Proper conditioning is required prior to participating in high-intensity activities.

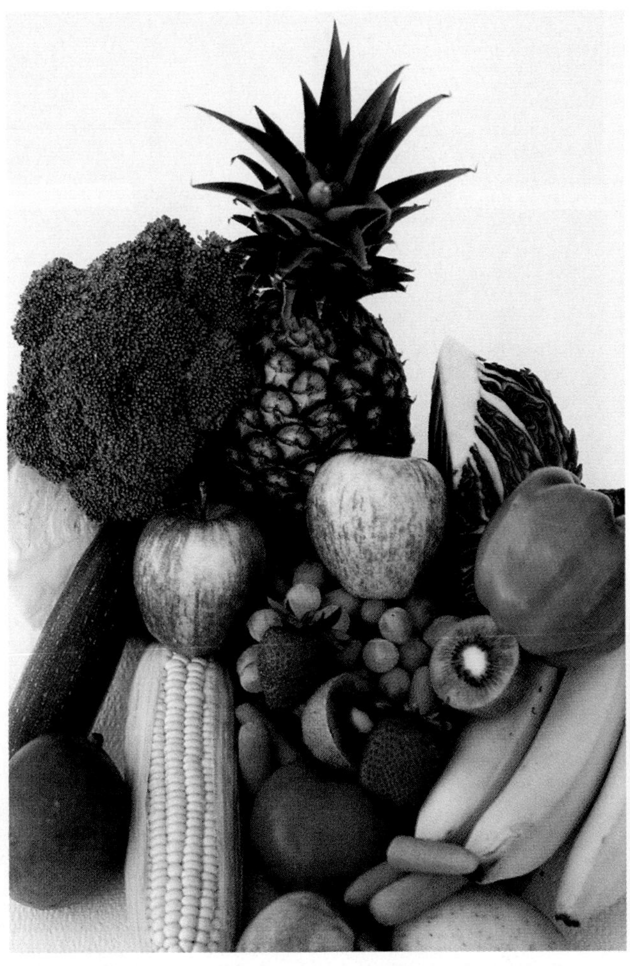

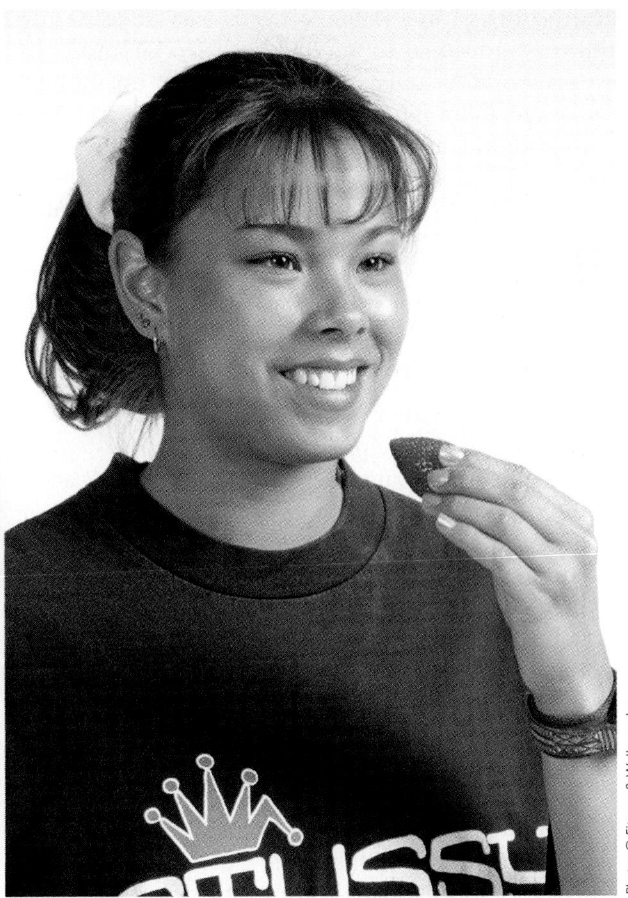

Photos © Fitness & Wellness, Inc.

Good nutrition is essential to achieve good health and fitness.

and Health Promotion. A summary of key 2010 objectives is provided in Figure 1.16. Living the fitness and wellness principles provided in this book will enhance the quality of your life and also will allow you to be an active participant in achieving the Healthy People 2010 Objectives.

Guidelines for a Healthy Lifestyle: Using This Book

Most people go to college to learn how to make a living, but a fitness and wellness course will teach you how to *live*—how to truly live life to its fullest potential. Some people think that success is measured by how much money they make. Making a good living will not help you unless you live a wellness lifestyle that will allow you to enjoy what you earn.

Although everyone would like to enjoy good health and wellness, most people don't know how to reach this objective. Lifestyle is the most important factor affecting personal well-being. Granted, some people live long because of genetic factors, but quality of life during middle age and the "golden years" is more often related to wise choices initiated during youth and continued throughout life.

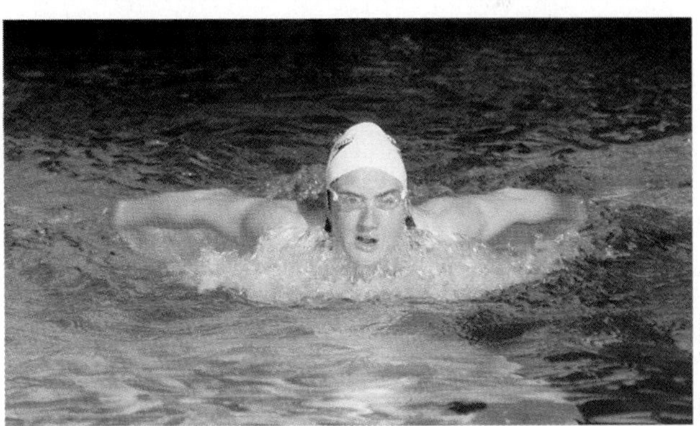

©Fitness & Wellness, Inc.

A very high level of physical fitness is necessary to participate in competitive sports.

In a few short years, lack of wellness can lead to a loss of vitality and gusto for life, as well as premature **morbidity** and mortality. The time to start is now.

Morbidity A condition related to, or caused by, illness or disease.

An Individualized Approach

Because fitness and wellness needs vary significantly from one individual to another, all exercise and wellness prescriptions must be personalized to obtain best results. The following chapters and their respective laboratory experiences set forth the guidelines to help you develop a personal lifetime program that will improve your fitness and promote your own preventive health care and personal wellness.

The laboratory experiences have been prepared on tear-out sheets so they can be turned in to class instructors. As you study this book and complete the respective worksheets, you will learn to

- determine whether medical clearance is needed for your safe participation in exercise.
- implement motivational and behavior modification techniques to help you adhere to a lifetime fitness and wellness program.
- conduct nutritional analyses and follow the recommendations for adequate nutrition.
- write sound diet and weight-control programs.
- assess your health-related components of fitness (cardiorespiratory endurance, muscular strength and endurance, muscular flexibility, and body composition).
- write exercise prescriptions for cardiorespiratory endurance, muscular strength and endurance, and muscular flexibility.
- assess your skill-related components of fitness (agility, balance, coordination, power, reaction time, and speed).
- understand the relationship between fitness and aging.
- determine your levels of tension and stress, lessen your vulnerability to stress, and implement a stress management program if necessary.
- learn healthy lifestyle guidelines to decrease your risk for chronic diseases—including cardiovascular disease, cancer, sexually transmitted infections—and for chemical dependency.
- write objectives to improve your fitness and wellness and chart a wellness program for the future.
- differentiate myths and facts about exercise and health-related concepts.

Critical Thinking

What are your feelings about lifestyle habits that enhance health and longevity? How important are they to you? What obstacles keep you from adhering to such habits or incorporating new ones into your life?

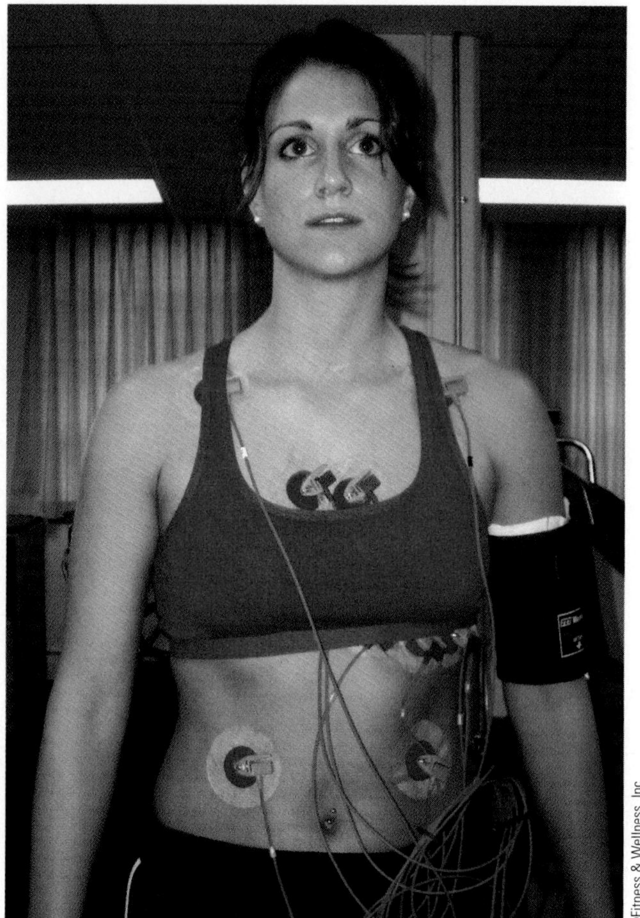

An exercise tolerance test (stress ECG test) with electrocardiographic monitoring may be required of some individuals prior to initiating an exercise program.

Exercise Safety

Even though testing and participation in exercise are relatively safe for most apparently healthy individuals under age 45, the reaction of the cardiovascular system to higher levels of physical activity cannot be totally predicted.[16] Consequently, a small but real risk exists for exercise-induced abnormalities in people with a history of cardiovascular problems and those who are at higher risk for disease. These factors include abnormal blood pressure, irregular heart rhythm, fainting, and, in rare instances, a heart attack or cardiac arrest.

Before you engage in an exercise program or participate in any exercise testing, you should fill out the questionnaire in Lab 1B. If your answer to any of the questions is yes, you should see a physician before participating in a fitness program. Exercise testing and participation are not wise under some of the conditions listed in Lab 1B and may require a medical evaluation, including a stress electrocardiogram (ECG) test. If you

TABLE 1.3 Resting Heart Rate Ratings

Heart Rate (beats/minute)	Rating
≤59	Excellent
60–69	Good
70–79	Average
80–89	Fair
≥90	Poor

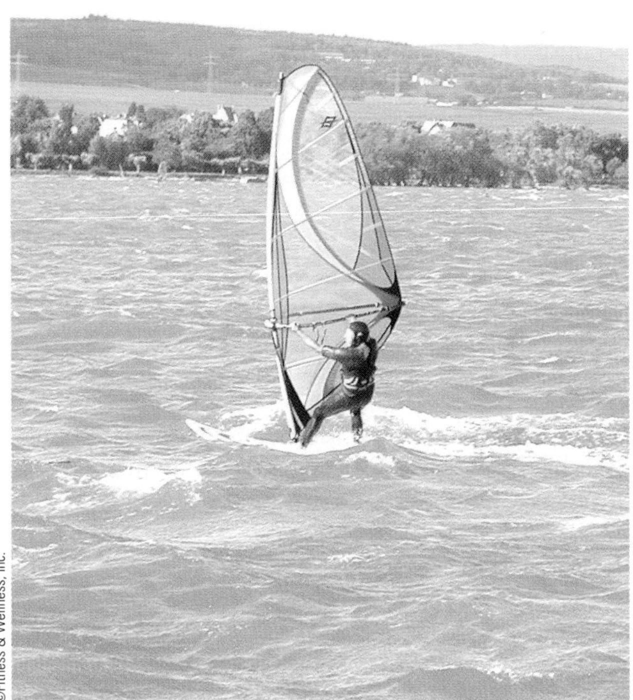

Good fitness and a healthy lifestyle allow people the freedom to perform most of life's leisure and recreational activities without limitations.

have any questions regarding your current health status, consult your doctor before initiating, continuing, or increasing your level of physical activity.

Resting Heart Rate and Blood Pressure Assessment

In Lab 1C you have the opportunity to assess your heart rate and blood pressure. Heart rate can be obtained by counting your pulse either on the wrist over the radial artery or over the carotid artery in the neck (see Chapter 6, page 179).

You may count your pulse for 30 seconds and multiply by 2 or take it for a full minute. The heart rate usually is at its lowest point (resting heart rate) late in the evening after you have been sitting quietly for about half an hour watching a relaxing TV show or reading in bed, or early in the morning just before you get out of bed.

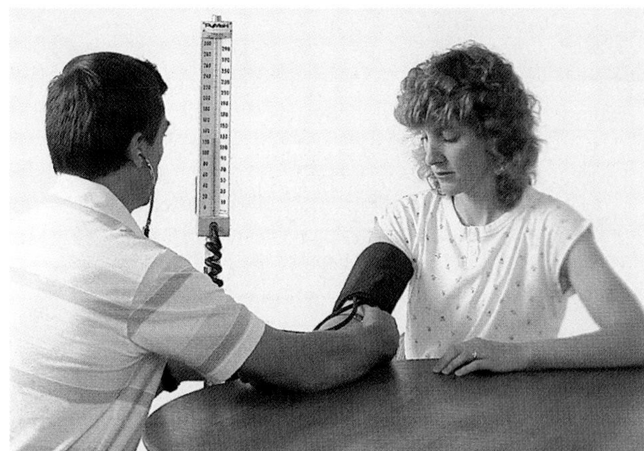

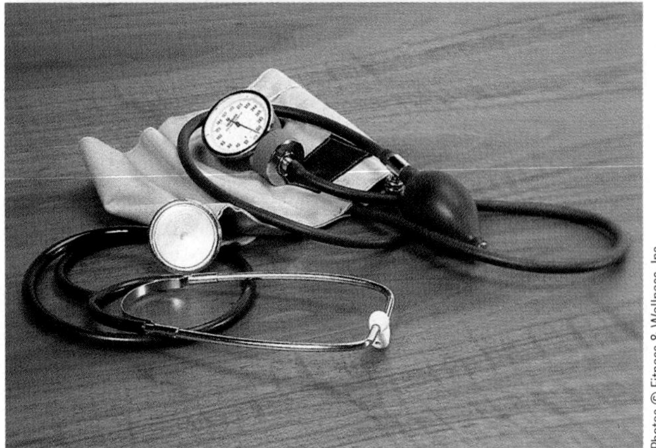

Blood pressure can be measured with a stethoscope and a mercury gravity manometer or an aneroid blood pressure gauge.

Unless you have a pathological condition, a lower resting heart rate indicates a stronger heart. To adapt to cardiorespiratory or aerobic exercise, blood volume increases, the heart enlarges, and the muscle gets stronger. A stronger heart can pump more blood with fewer strokes.

Resting heart rate categories are given in Table 1.3. Although resting heart rate decreases with training, the extent of **bradycardia** depends not only on the amount of training but also on genetic factors. Although most highly trained athletes have a resting heart rate around 40 beats per minute, occasionally, one of these athletes has a resting heart rate in the 60s or 70s even during peak training months of the season. For most individuals, however, the resting heart rate decreases as the level of cardiorespiratory endurance increases.

Blood pressure is assessed using a **sphygmomanometer** and a stethoscope. Use a cuff of the appro-

Bradycardia Slower heart rate than normal.

Sphygmomanometer Inflatable bladder contained within a cuff and a mercury gravity manometer (or aneroid manometer) from which the pressure is read.

TABLE 1.4 Blood Pressure Guidelines (expressed in mm Hg)

Rating	Systolic	Diastolic
Normal	≤120	≤80
Prehypertension	120–139	80–89
Hypertension	≥140	≥90

Source: National Heart, Lung and Blood Institute.

priate size to get accurate readings. Size is determined by the width of the inflatable bladder, which should be about 80 percent of the circumference of the midpoint of the arm.

Blood pressure usually is measured while the person is in the sitting position, with the forearm and the manometer at the same level as the heart. At first, the pressure is recorded from each arm, and after that from the arm with the highest reading.

The cuff should be applied approximately an inch above the antecubital space (natural crease of the elbow), with the center of the bladder directly over the medial (inner) surface of the arm. The stethoscope head should be applied firmly, but with little pressure, over the brachial artery in the antecubital space. The arm should be flexed slightly and placed on a flat surface.

To determine how high the cuff should be inflated, the person recording the blood pressure monitors the subject's radial pulse with one hand and, with the other hand, inflates the manometer's bladder to about 30 to 40 mm Hg above the point at which the feeling of the pulse in the wrist disappears. Next, the pressure is released, followed by a wait of about one minute, then the bladder is inflated to the predetermined level to take the blood pressure reading. The cuff should not be overinflated, as this may cause blood vessel spasm, resulting in higher blood pressure readings. The pressure should be released at a rate of 2 to 4 mm Hg per second.

As the pressure is released, **systolic blood pressure** is recorded as the point where the sound of the pulse becomes audible. The **diastolic blood pressure** is the point where the sound disappears. The recordings should be expressed as systolic over diastolic pressure—for example, 124/80.

If you take more than one reading, be sure the bladder is completely deflated between readings and allow at least a full minute before making the next recording. The person measuring the pressure also should note whether the pressure was recorded from the left or the right arm. Resting blood pressure ratings are given in Table 1.4.

In some cases the pulse sounds become less intense (point of muffling sounds) but still can be heard at a lower pressure (50 or 40 mm Hg) or even all the way down to zero. In this situation the diastolic pressure is recorded at the point of a clear, definite change in the loudness of the sound (also referred to as fourth phase), and at complete disappearance of the sound (fifth phase) (for example, 120/78/60 or 120/82/0).

To establish the real values for resting blood pressure, have several readings taken by different people or at different times of the day. A single reading may not be an accurate value because of the various factors that can affect blood pressure.

Systolic blood pressure Pressure exerted by blood against walls of arteries during forceful contraction (systole) of the heart.

Diastolic blood pressure Pressure exerted by the blood against the walls of the arteries during the relaxation phase (diastole) of the heart.

Assess Your Behavior

Thomson NOW! *Log on to www.thomsonedu.com/login and take a wellness inventory to assess the behaviors that might most benefit from healthy change.*

1. Are you aware of your family health history and lifestyle factors that may negatively impact your health?
2. Do you accumulate at least 30 minutes of moderate-intensity physical activity on most days of the week?
3. Are you accumulating at least 10,000 steps on most days of the week?

Assess Your Knowledge

Thomson NOW! *Log on to www.thomsonedu.com/login to assess your understanding of this chapter's topics by taking the Student Practice Test and exploring the modules recommended in your Personalized Study Plan.*

1. Bodily movement produced by skeletal muscles is called
   a. physical activity.
   b. kinesiology.
   c. exercise.
   d. aerobic exercise.
   e. muscle strength.

2. Most people in the United States
   a. get adequate physical activity on a regular basis.
   b. meet health-related fitness standards.
   c. regularly participate in skill-related activities.
   d. Choices a, b, and c are correct.
   e. do not get sufficient physical activity to maintain good health.

3. Which of the following statements is correct?
   a. The United States has one of the best medical care systems in the world.
   b. Americans die earlier than people in most other developed nations.
   c. The United States does not rank among the top 10 nations in the world in terms of healthy life expectancy.
   d. Americans spend more time disabled than people in most other advanced countries.
   e. All statements are correct.

4. Physical inactivity in the United States is more prevalent in
   a. men than women.
   b. whites than African Americans and Hispanic Americans.
   c. less-educated than more-educated adults.
   d. younger than older adults.
   e. All statements are correct.

5. Research on the effects of fitness on mortality indicates that the largest drop in premature mortality is seen between
   a. the average and excellent fitness groups.
   b. the low and moderately fit groups.
   c. the high and excellent fitness groups.
   d. the moderately fit and good fitness groups.
   e. The drop is similar between all fitness groups.

6. Which of the following is *not* a component of health-related fitness?
   a. cardiorespiratory endurance
   b. body composition
   c. agility
   d. muscular strength and endurance
   e. muscular flexibility

7. Metabolic fitness can be achieved
   a. with an active lifestyle and moderate physical activity.
   b. through a high-intensity speed-training program.
   c. through an increased basal metabolic rate.
   d. with anaerobic training.
   e. through an increase in lean body mass.

8. Achieving health fitness standards
   a. leads to improvements in the metabolic profile.
   b. decreases the risk for chronic diseases.
   c. can be accomplished through a moderate fitness training program.
   d. can be done without achieving a high fitness standard.
   e. All choices are correct.

9. During the last decade, health-care costs in the United States
   a. have decreased.
   b. have stayed about the same.
   c. have continued to increase.
   d. have increased in some years and decreased in others.
   e. are unknown.

10. What is the greatest benefit of being physically fit?
   a. absence of disease
   b. a higher quality of life
   c. improved sports performance
   d. better personal appearance
   e. maintenance of ideal body weight

Correct answers can be found at the back of the book.

III. Effects of Aerobic Activity on Resting Heart Rate

Using your actual resting heart rate (RHR) from Part I of this lab, compute the total number of times your heart beats each day and each year:

A. Beats per day = ______ (RHR bpm) × 60 (min per hour) × 24 (hours per day) = ______ beats per day

B. Beats per year = ______ (heart rate in beats per day, use item A) × 365 = ______ beats per year

If your RHR dropped 20 bpm through an aerobic exercise program, determine the number of beats that your heart would save each year at that lower RHR:

C. Beats per day = ______ (your current RHR − 20) × 60 × 24 = ______ beats per day

D. Beats per year = ______ (heart rate in beats per day, use item C) × 365 = ______ beats per year

E. Number of beats saved per year (B − D) = ______ − ______ = ______ beats saved per year

Assuming that you will reach the average U.S. life expectancy of 80 years for women or 73 for men, determine the additional number of "heart rate life years" available to you if your RHR were 20 bpm lower:

F. Years of life ahead = ______ (use 80 for women and 73 for men) − ______ (current age) = ______ years

G. Number of beats saved = ______ (use item E) × ______ (use item F) = ______ beats saved

H. Number of heart rate life years based on the lower RHR = ______ (use item G) ÷ ______ (use item D) = ______ years

IV. Mean Blood Pressure Computation

During a normal resting contraction/relaxation cycle of the heart, the heart spends more time in the relaxation (diastolic) phase than in the contraction (systolic) phase. Accordingly, mean blood pressure (MBP) cannot be computed by taking an average of the systolic (SBP) and diastolic (DBP) blood pressures. The following equations are, therefore, used to determine MBP:

MBP = DBP + ⅓ PP   Where PP = pulse pressure or the difference between the systolic and diastolic pressures.

A. Compute your MBP using your own blood pressure results:

PP = ______ (systolic) − ______ (diastolic) = ______ mm Hg

MBP = ______ (DBP) + $\frac{\text{\_\_\_\_\_\_ (PP)}}{3}$ = ______ mm Hg

B. Determine the MBP for a person with a BP of 130/80 and a second person with a BP of 120/90.

Which subject has the lower MBP? ______

V. What I Learned

Draw conclusions based on your observed resting and activity heart rates and blood pressures. Discuss the importance of a lower resting heart rate to your health and comment on the effects of a higher systolic versus diastolic blood pressure on the mean arterial blood pressure.

Behavior Modification

CHAPTER 2

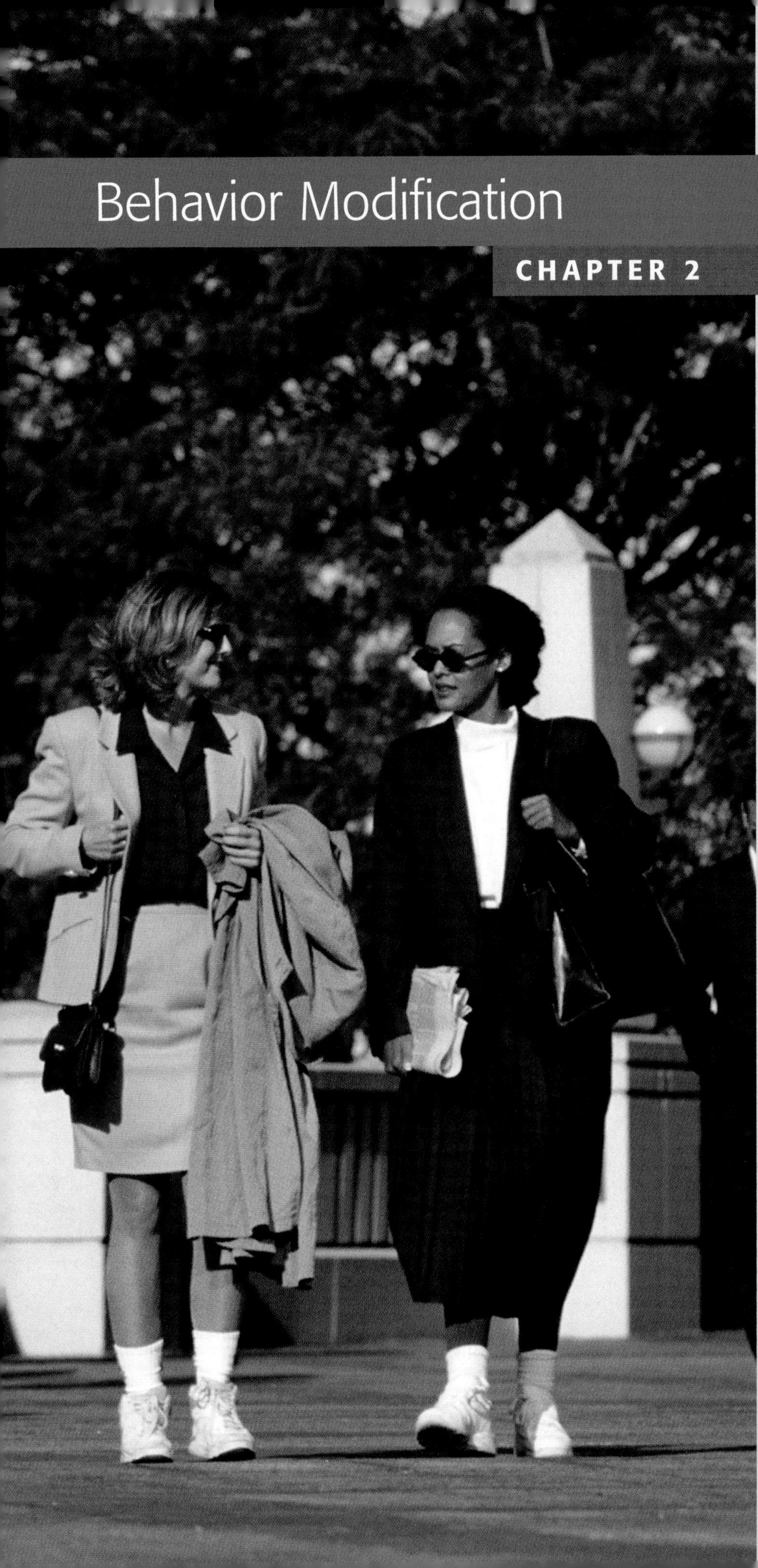

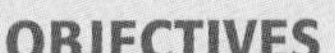

OBJECTIVES

- Learn the effects of environment on human behavior.
- Understand obstacles that hinder the ability to change behavior.
- Explain the concepts of motivation and locus of control.
- Identify the stages of change.
- Describe the processes of change.
- Explain techniques that will facilitate the process of change.
- Describe the role of SMART goal setting in the process of change.
- Be able to write specific objectives for behavioral change.

Thomson™ NOW! Go to www.thomsonedu.com/login to:

- Prepare for a healthy change in lifestyle.
- Check how well you understand the chapter's concepts.

The importance of regular physical activity and living a healthy lifestyle to maintain health and achieve wellness is well documented. Nearly all Americans accept that exercise is beneficial to health and see a need to incorporate it into their lives. Seventy percent of new and returning exercisers, however, are at risk for early dropout.[1] As the scientific evidence continues to mount each day, most people still are not adhering to a healthy lifestyle program.

Let's look at an all-too-common occurrence on college campuses. Most students understand that they should be exercising, and they contemplate enrolling in a fitness course. The motivating factor might be improved physical appearance, health benefits, or simply fulfillment of a college requirement. They sign up for the course, participate for a few months, finish the course—and stop exercising! They offer a wide array of excuses: too busy, no one to exercise with, already have the grade, inconvenient open-gym hours, job conflicts, and so on. A few months later they realize once again that exercise is vital, and they repeat the cycle (see Figure 2.1).

FIGURE 2.1 Exercise/exercise dropout cycle.

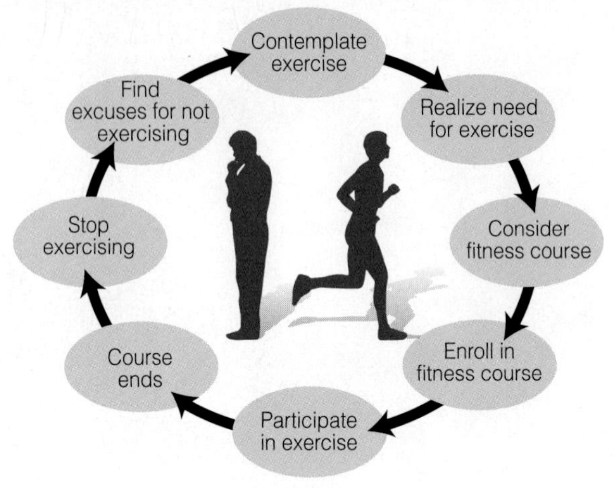

The information in this book will be of little value to you if you are unable to abandon your negative habits and adopt and maintain healthy behaviors. Before looking at any physical fitness and wellness guidelines, you will need to take a critical look at your behaviors and lifestyle—and most likely make some permanent changes to promote your overall health and wellness.

Living in a Toxic Health and Fitness Environment

Most of the behaviors we adopt are a product of our environment—the forces of social influences we encounter and the thought processes we go through. This environment includes family, friends, peers, homes, schools, workplaces, television, radio, and movies, as well as our communities, country, and culture in general.

Unfortunately, when it comes to fitness and wellness, we live in a "toxic" environment. Becoming aware of how the environment affects us is vital if we wish to achieve and maintain wellness. Yet, we are so habituated to the environment that we miss the subtle ways it influences our behaviors, personal lifestyle, and health each day.

From a young age, we observe, we learn, we emulate, and without realizing it, we incorporate into our own lifestyle the behaviors of people around us. We are transported by parents, relatives, and friends who drive us nearly any place we need to go. We watch them drive short distances to run errands. We see them take escalators and elevators and ride moving sidewalks at malls and airports. We notice that the adults around us use remote controls, pagers, and cell phones. We observe them stop at fast-food restaurants and pick up supersized, calorie-dense, high-fat meals. They watch television and surf the 'Net for hours at a time. Some smoke, some drink heavily, and some have hard-drug addictions. Others engage in risky behaviors by not wearing seat belts, by drinking and driving, and by having unprotected sex. All of these unhealthy habits can be passed along, unquestioned, to the next generation.

Environmental Influences on Physical Activity

Among the leading underlying causes of death in the United States are physical inactivity and poor diet. This is partially because most activities of daily living, which a few decades ago required movement or physical activity, now require almost no effort and negatively impact health, fitness, and body weight. Small movements that have been streamlined out of daily life quickly add up, especially when we consider these over 7 days a week and 52 weeks a year.

We can examine the decrease in the required daily energy (caloric) expenditure as a result of modern-day conveniences that lull us into physical inactivity. For example, short automobile trips that replace walking or riding a bike decrease energy expenditure by 50 to 300 calories per day; automatic car window and door openers represent about 1 calorie at each use; automatic garage door openers, 5 calories; drive-through windows at banks, fast-food restaurants, dry cleaners, and pharmacies add up to about 5 to 10 calories each time; elevators and escalators, 3 to 10 calories per trip; food processors, 5 to 10 calories; riding lawnmowers, about 100 calories; automatic car washes, 100 calories; hours of computer use to e-mail, surf the 'Net, and conduct

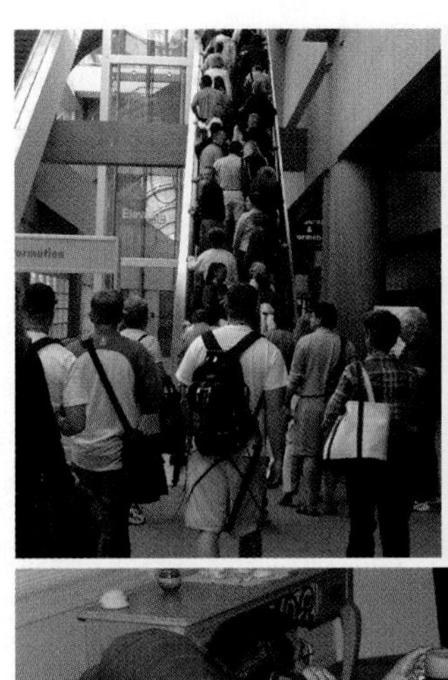
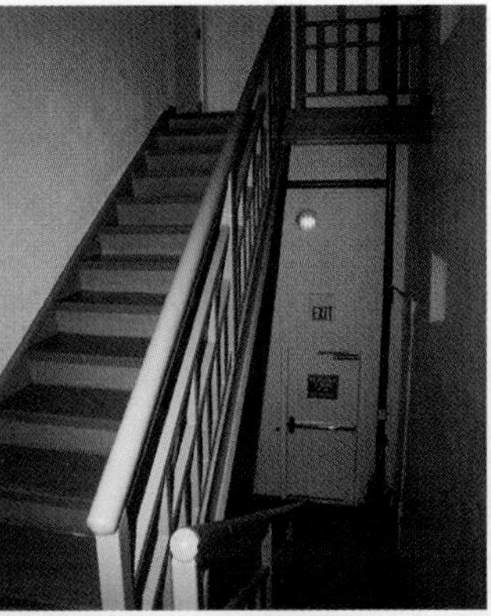
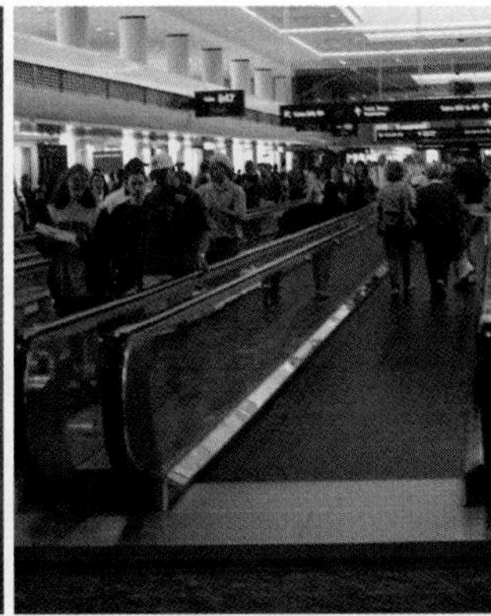
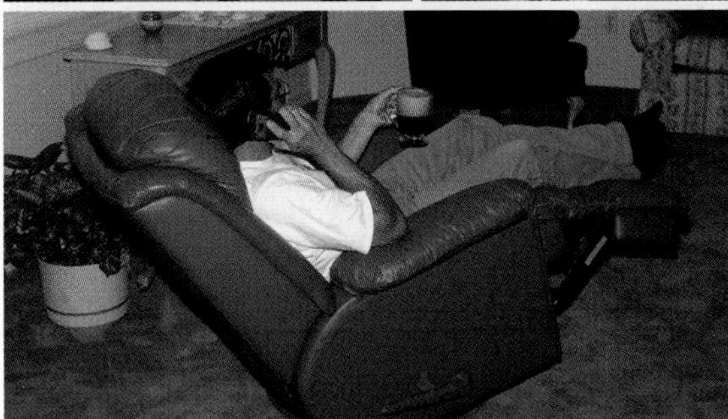
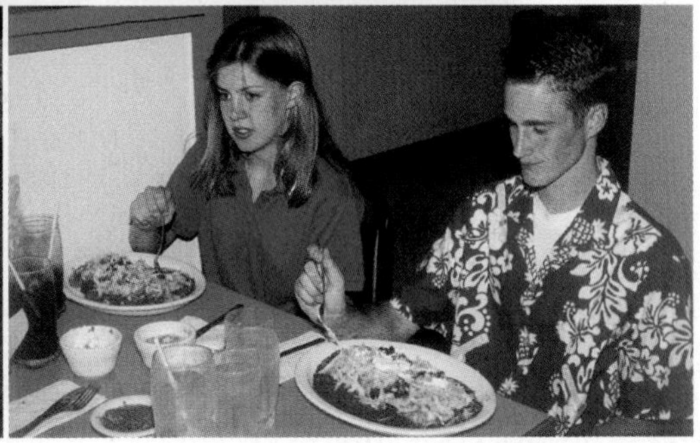

Our environment is not conducive to a healthy, physically active lifestyle.

Internet transactions represent another 50 to 300 calories; and excessive television viewing can add up to 200 or more calories. Little wonder that we have such a difficult time maintaining a healthy body weight.

Health experts recommend that, to be considered active, a person accumulate the equivalent of 5 to 6 miles of walking per day. This level of activity equates to about 10,000 to 12,000 daily steps. If you have never clipped on a pedometer, try to do so. When you look at the total number of steps it displays at the end of the day, you may be shocked by how few steps you took.

With the advent of now-ubiquitous cell phones, people are moving even less. Family members call each other on the phone even within the walls of their own home. Some people don't get out of the car anymore to ring a doorbell. Instead, they wait in front and send a text message to have the person come out.

Even modern-day architecture reinforces unhealthy behaviors. Elevators and escalators are often of the finest workmanship and located conveniently. Many of our newest, showiest shopping centers and convention centers don't provide accessible stairwells, so people are all but forced to ride escalators. If they want to walk up the escalator, they can't because the people in front of them obstruct the way. Entrances to buildings provide electric sensors and automatic door openers. Without a second thought, people walk through automatic doors instead of taking the time to push a door open.

At work, most people have jobs that require them to sit most of the day. We don't even get up and walk a short distance to talk to co-workers. Instead, we use intercoms and telephones.

Leisure time is no better. When people arrive home after work, they surf the 'Net, play computer games, or watch television for hours at a time. The first thing people consider when setting up a family room is where to put the television. This little (or big-screen) box has truly lulled us into inactivity. Excessive TV viewing is directly linked to obesity, and the amount of time people choose to spend watching television and movies made for TV is climbing. The average household watches close to 8 hours of programming each day—up one hour from 1982 and two from 1970.[2]

Television viewing is more than just a sedentary activity. Think about people's habits before they sit down to watch a favorite show. They turn on the television, then stop by the kitchen for a box of crackers and processed cheese. They return to watch the show, start snacking, and are bombarded with commercials about soft drinks, beer, and unhealthy foods. Viewers are enticed to purchase and eat unhealthy calorie-dense foods in an unnecessary and mindless "snacking setting." Television viewing even has been shown to reduce the number of fruits and vegetables some people consume, most likely because people are eating the unhealthy foods advertised on television.[3]

Our communities aren't much help either. Walking, jogging, and bicycle trails are too sparse in most cities, further discouraging physical activity. Places for safe exercise are hard to find in many metropolitan areas, motivating many people to remain indoors during

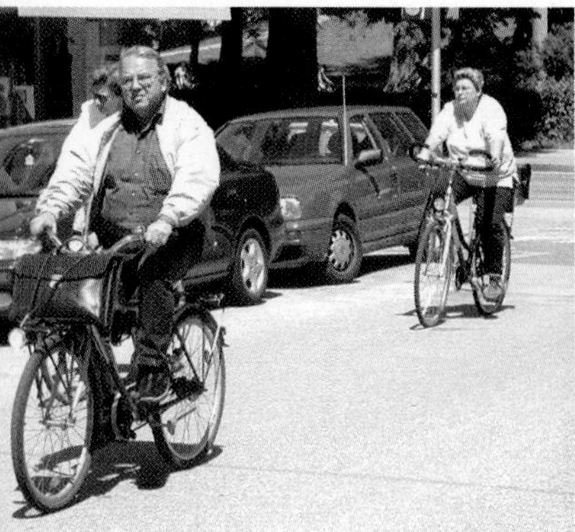
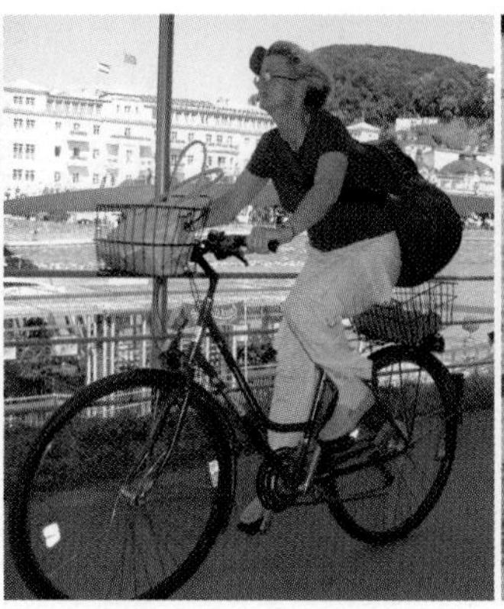
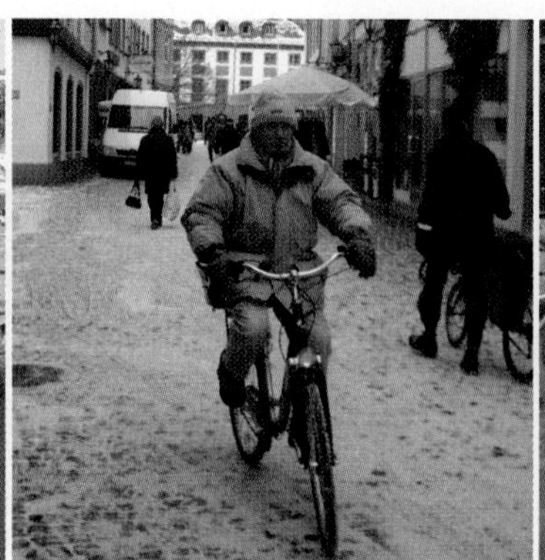
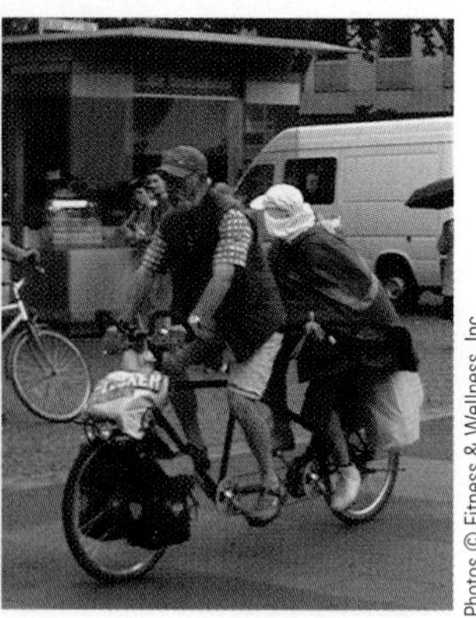

Photos © Fitness & Wellness, Inc.

Walking and cycling are priority activities in many European communities.

leisure hours for fear of endangering their personal safety and well-being.

In addition to sitting most of the day at work and at home, we also sit in our cars. We are transported or drive everywhere we have to go. Safety concerns also keep people in cars instead of on sidewalks and in parks. And communities are designed around the automobile. City streets make driving convenient and walking or cycling difficult, impossible, or dangerous. Streets typically are rated by traffic engineers according to their "level of service"—that is, based on how well they facilitate motorized traffic. A wide, straight street with few barriers to slow motorized traffic gets a high score. According to these guidelines, pedestrians are "obstructions." Only recently have a few local governments and communities started to devise standards to determine how useful streets are for pedestrians and bicyclists.

For each car in the United States, there are seven parking spaces.[4] Drivers can almost always find a parking spot, but walkers often run out of sidewalks and crosswalks in modern streets. Sidewalks have not been a priority in city, suburban, or commercial development. Whereas British street design manuals recommend sidewalks on both sides of the street, American manuals recommend sidewalks on one side of the street only.

One measure that encourages activity is the use of "traffic-calming" strategies: intentionally slowing traffic to make the pedestrian's role easier. These strategies were developed and are widely used in Europe. Examples include narrower streets, rougher pavement (cobblestone), pedestrian islands, and raised crosswalks.

Many European communities place a high priority on walking and cycling. Walking or biking makes up 40 to 54 percent of all daily trips taken by people in Austria, the Netherlands, Denmark, Italy, and Sweden. In the United States, walking and biking account for 10 percent of daily trips, whereas the automobile accounts for 84 percent of trips.[5]

Granted, many people drive because the distances to cover are far. We live in bedroom communities and commute to work. When people live near frequently visited destinations, they are more likely to walk or bike for transportation. Neighborhoods that mix commercial and residential use of land encourage walking over driving because of the short distances between home, shopping, and work.[6]

Children also walk or cycle to school today less frequently than in the past. The reasons? Distance, traffic, weather, perceived crime, and school policy. Distance is a significant barrier because the trend during the last few decades has been to build larger schools on the outskirts of communities instead of small schools within neighborhoods.

Environmental Influence on Diet and Nutrition

The present obesity epidemic in the United States and other developed countries has been getting worse every year. We are becoming a nation of overweight and obese people. You may ask why. Let's examine the evidence.

According to the USDA's Center for Nutrition Policy and Promotion, the amount of daily food supply available in the United States is about 3,900 calories per person, before wastage. This figure represents a 700-calorie rise over the early 1980s,[7] which means that we have taken the amount of food available to us and tossed in a Cinnabon for every person in the country.

The overabundance of food increases pressure on food suppliers to advertise and try to convince consumers to buy their products. The food industry spends more than $33 billion each year on advertising and promotion, and most of this money goes toward highly processed foods. The few ads and campaigns promoting healthy foods and healthful eating simply cannot compete. Most of us would be hard-pressed to recall a jingle for brown rice or kale. The money spent advertising a single food product across the United States is often 10 to 50 times more than the money the federal government spends promoting MyPyramid or encouraging us to eat fruits and vegetables.[8]

Coupled with our sedentary lifestyle, many activities of daily living in today's culture are associated with eating. We seem to be eating all the time. We eat during coffee breaks, when we socialize, when we play, when we watch sports, at the movies, during television viewing, and when the clock tells us it's time for a meal. Our lives seem to be centered on food, a nonstop string of occasions to eat and overeat. And much of the overeating is done without a second thought. For instance, when people rent a video, they usually end up in line with the video and also with popcorn, candy, and soft drinks. Do we really have to eat while watching a movie?

As a nation, we now eat out more often than in the past, portion sizes are larger, and we have an endless variety of foods to choose from. We also snack more than ever before. Unhealthy food is relatively inexpensive and is sold in places where it was not available in the past.

Increasingly, people have decided that they no longer require special occasions to eat out. Mother's Day, a birthday, or someone's graduation are no longer reasons to eat at a restaurant. Eating out is part of today's lifestyle. In the late 1970s, food eaten away from home represented about 18 percent of our energy intake. In the mid-1990s, this figure rose to 32 percent. Almost half of the money Americans spend on food today is on meals away from home.[9]

Eating out would not be such a problem if portion sizes were reasonable or if restaurant food were similar to food prepared at home. Compared to home meals, restaurant and fast-food meals are higher in fat and calories and lower in essential nutrients and fiber.

Food portions in restaurants have increased substantially in size. Patrons consume huge amounts of food, almost as if this were the last meal they will ever have. They drink entire pitchers of soda pop or beer instead of the traditional 8-ounce-cup size. Some restaurant menus may include selections that are called healthy choices, but these items may not provide nutritional information, including calories. In all likelihood, the menu has many other choices that look delicious but provide larger serving sizes with more fat and calories and fewer fruits and vegetables. Making a healthy selection is difficult, because people tend to choose food for its taste, convenience, and cost instead of nutrition.

Restaurant food is often less healthy than we think. Trained dieticians were asked to estimate nutrition information for five restaurant meals. The results showed that these dieticians underestimated the number of calories and fat by 37 and 49 percent, respectively.[10] Results such as these do not offer much hope for the average consumer who tries to make healthy choices when eating out.

We can also notice that most restaurants are pleasurable places to be: colorful, well lit, and thoughtfully decorated. These intentional features are designed to enhance comfort, appetite, and length of stay, with the intent to entice more eating. Employees are formally trained in techniques that urge patrons to eat more and spend more. Servers are prepared to approach the table and suggest specific drinks, with at least one from the bar. When the drink is served, they recommend selected appetizers. Drink refills are often free while dining out. Following dinner, the server offers desserts and coffee. A person could literally get a full day's worth of calories in one meal without ever ordering an entree.

Fast-food restaurants do not lag far behind. Menu items frequently are introduced at one size and, over time, popular items are increased two to five times their introductory size.[11] Large portion sizes are a major problem because people tend to eat what has been served. A study by the American Institute for Cancer Research found that with bigger portion sizes, 67 percent of Americans ate the larger amount of food they were served.[12] The tendency of most patrons is to "clean the plate."

Individuals seem to have the same disregard for hunger cues when snacking. Participants in one study were randomly given an afternoon snack of potato chips in different bag sizes. The participants received bags from 1 to 20 ounces for 5 days. The results showed that the larger the bag, the more the person ate. Men ate 37 percent more chips from the largest than the smallest bag. Women ate 18 percent more. Of significant interest, the size of the snack did not change the amount of food the person ate during the next meal.[13] Another study found no major difference in reported hunger or fullness after participants ate different sizes of sandwiches that were served to them, even though they ate more when they were given larger sandwiches.[14]

Other researchers set out to see if the size of the package—not just the amount of food—affects how much people eat. Study participants received two different sized packages with the same number of spaghetti strands. The larger package was twice the size of the smaller package. When participants were asked to take out enough spaghetti to prepare a meal for two adults, they took out an average of 234 strands from the small package versus 302 strands from the larger package.[15] In our own kitchens, and in restaurants, we seem to have taken away from our internal cues the decision of how much to eat. Instead we have turned that choice over to businesses that profit from our overindulgence.

Also working against our hunger cues is our sense of thrift. Many of us consider cost ahead of nutrition when we choose foods. Restaurants and groceries often appeal to this sense of thrift by using "value marketing," meaning they offer us a larger portion for only a small price increase. Customers think they are getting a bargain, and the food providers turn a better profit because the cost of additional food is small compared to the cost of marketing, production, and labor.

The National Alliance for Nutrition has further shown that a little more money buys a lot more calories. Ice cream upsizing from a kid's scoop to a double scoop, for example, adds an extra 390 calories for only an extra $1.62. A medium-size movie theater popcorn (unbuttered) provides 500 additional calories over a small-size popcorn for just an extra 71 cents. Equally, king-size candy bars provide about 230 additional calories for just another 33 cents over the standard size.[16] We often eat more simply because we get more for our money without taking into consideration the detrimental consequences to our health and waistline.

Another example of financial but not nutritional sense is free soft-drink refills. When people choose a high-calorie drink over diet soda or water, the person does not compensate by eating less food later that day.[17] Liquid calories seem to be difficult for people to account for. A 20-ounce bottle of regular soda contains the equivalent of one-third cup of sugar. One extra can of soda (160 calories) per day represents an extra 16.5 pounds of fat per year (160 calories × 365 days ÷ 3,500 calories). Even people who regularly drink diet sodas tend to gain weight. In their minds, they may rationalize that a calorie-free drink allows them to consume more food.

A larger variety of food also entice overeating. Think about your own experiences at parties that have a buffet of snacks. Do you eat more when everyone brings something to contribute to the snack table? When unhealthy choices outnumber healthy choices, people are less likely to follow their natural cues to choose healthy food.[18]

The previously mentioned environmental factors influence our thought process and hinder our ability to determine what constitutes an appropriate meal based on actual needs. The result: On average, American women consume 335 more daily calories than they did 20 years ago, and men an additional 170 calories.[19]

Now you can analyze and identify the environmental influences on your behaviors. Lab 2A provides you with the opportunity to determine whether you control your environment or the environment controls you.

Living in the 21st century, we have all the modern-day conveniences that lull us into overconsumption and sedentary living. By living in America, we adopt behaviors that put our health at risk. And though we understand that lifestyle choices affect our health and well-being, we still have an extremely difficult time making changes.

Let's look at weight gain. Most people do not start life with a weight problem. By age 20, a man may weigh 160 pounds. A few years later, the weight starts to climb and may reach 170 pounds. He now adapts and accepts 170 pounds as his weight. He may go on a diet but not make the necessary lifestyle changes. Gradually his weight climbs to 180, 190, 200 pounds. Although he may not like it and would like to weigh less, once again he adapts and accepts 200 pounds as his stable weight.

The time comes, usually around middle age, when most people want to make changes in their lives but find this difficult to accomplish, illustrating the adage that "old habits die hard." Acquiring positive behaviors that will lead to better health and well-being is a long-term process and requires continual effort. Understanding why so many people are unsuccessful at changing their behaviors and are unable to live a healthy lifestyle may increase your readiness and motivation for change. Next we will examine barriers to change, what motivates people to change, behavior change theories, the transtheoretical or stages-of-change model, the process of change, techniques for change, and actions required to make permanent changes in behavior.

Barriers to Change

In spite of the best intentions, people make unhealthy choices daily. The most common reasons are:

1. **Procrastination**. People seem to think that tomorrow, next week, or after the holiday is the best time to start change.

   Tip to initiate change. Ask yourself: Why wait until tomorrow when you can start changing today? Lack of motivation is a key factor in procrastination (motivation is discussed on pages 40–41).
2. **Preconditioned cultural beliefs**. If we accept the idea that we are a product of our environment, our cultural beliefs and our physical surroundings pose significant barriers to change. In Salzburg, Austria, people of both genders and all ages use bicycles as a primary mode of transportation. In the United States, few people other than children ride bicycles.

   Tip to initiate change. Find a like-minded partner. In the pre-Columbian era, people thought the world was flat. Few dared to sail long distances for fear that they would fall off the edge. If your health and fitness are at stake, preconditioned cultural beliefs shouldn't keep you from making changes. Finding people who are willing to "sail" with you will help overcome this barrier.
3. **Gratification**. People prefer instant gratification to long-term benefits. Therefore, they will overeat (instant pleasure) instead of using self-restraint to eat moderately to prevent weight gain (long-term satisfaction). We like tanning (instant gratification) and avoid paying much attention to skin cancer (long-term consequence).

   Tip to initiate change. Think ahead and ask yourself: How did I feel the last time I engaged in this behavior? How did it affect me? Did I really feel good about myself or about the results? In retrospect, was it worth it?
4. **Risk complacency**. Consequences of unhealthy behaviors often don't manifest themselves until years

later. People tell themselves, "If I get heart disease, I'll deal with it then. For now, let me eat, drink, and be merry."

Tip to initiate change. Ask yourself: How long do I want to live? How do I want to live the rest of my life and what type of health do I want to have? What do I want to be able to do when I am 60, 70, or 80 years old?

5. **Complexity**. People think the world is too complicated, with too much to think about. If you are living the typical lifestyle, you may feel overwhelmed by everything that seems to be required to lead a healthy lifestyle, for example:
   - getting exercise
   - decreasing intake of saturated and trans fats
   - eating high-fiber meals and cutting total calories
   - controlling use of substances
   - managing stress
   - wearing seat belts
   - practicing safe sex
   - getting annual physicals, including blood tests, Pap smears, and so on
   - fostering spiritual, social, and emotional wellness

   Tip to initiate change. Take it one step at a time. Work on only one or two behaviors at a time so the task won't seem insurmountable.
6. **Indifference and helplessness**. A defeatist thought process often takes over, and we may believe that the way we live won't really affect our health, that we have no control over our health, or that our destiny is all in our genes (also see discussion of locus of control, pages 40–41).

   Tip to initiate change. As much as 84 percent of the leading causes of death in the United States are preventable. Realize that only you can take control of your personal health and lifestyle habits and affect the quality of your life. Implementing many of the behavioral modification strategies and programs outlined in this book will get you started on a wellness way of life.
7. **Rationalization**. Even though people are not practicing healthy behaviors, they often tell themselves that they do get sufficient exercise, that their diet is fine, that they have good, solid relationships, or that they don't smoke/drink/get high enough to affect their health.

   Tip to initiate change. Learn to recognize when you're glossing over or minimizing a problem. You'll need to face the fact that you have a problem before you can commit to change. Your health and your life are at stake. Monitoring lifestyle habits through daily logs and then analyzing the results can help you change self-defeating behaviors.
8. **Illusions of invincibility**. At times people believe that unhealthy behaviors will not harm them.

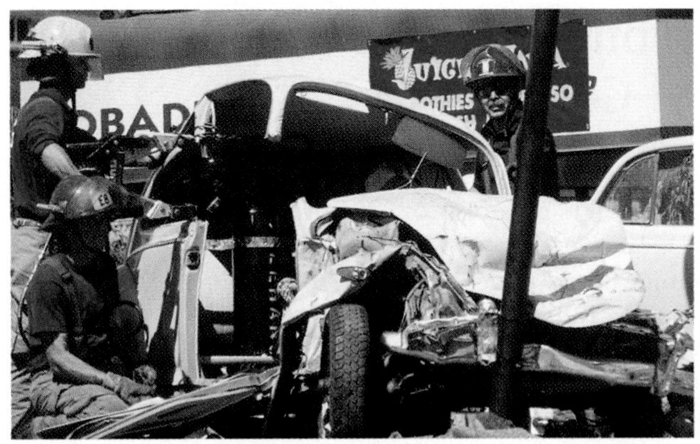

Feelings of invincibility are a strong barrier to change that can bring about life-threatening consequences.

Young adults often have the attitude that "I can smoke now, and in a few years I'll quit before it causes any damage." Unfortunately, nicotine is one of the most addictive drugs known to us, so quitting smoking is not an easy task. Health problems may arise before you quit, and the risk of lung cancer lingers for years after you quit. Another example is drinking and driving. The feeling of "I'm in control" or "I can handle it" while under the influence of alcohol is a deadly combination.

Others perceive low risk when engaging in negative behaviors with people they like (for example, sex with someone you've recently met and feel attracted to) but perceive themselves at risk just by being in the same classroom with an HIV-infected person.

Tip to initiate change. No one is immune to sickness, disease, and tragedy. The younger you are when you implement a healthy lifestyle, the better are your odds to attain a long and healthy life. Thus, initiating change right now will help you enjoy the best possible quality of life for as long as you live.

Critical Thinking

What barriers to exercise do you encounter most frequently? How about barriers that keep you from managing your daily caloric intake?

When health and appearance begin to deteriorate—usually around middle age—people seek out health-care professionals in search of a "magic pill" to reverse and cure the many ills they accumulated during years of abuse and overindulgence. The sooner we implement a healthy lifestyle program, the greater will be the health benefits and quality of life that lie ahead.

Motivation and Locus of Control

The explanation given for why some people succeed and others do not is often **motivation.** Although motivation comes from within, external factors trigger the inner desire to accomplish a given task. These external factors, then, control behavior.

When studying motivation, understanding **locus of control** is helpful. People who believe they have control over events in their lives are said to have an internal locus of control. People with an external locus of control believe that what happens to them is a result of chance or the environment and is unrelated to their behavior. People with an internal locus of control generally are healthier and have an easier time initiating and adhering to a wellness program than those who perceive that they have no control and think of themselves as powerless and vulnerable. The latter people also are at greater risk for illness. When illness does strike a person, establishing a sense of control is vital to recovery.

Few people have either a completely external or a completely internal locus of control. They fall somewhere along a continuum. The more external one's locus of control is, the greater is the challenge to change and adhere to exercise and other healthy lifestyle behaviors. Fortunately, people can develop a more internal locus of control. Understanding that most events in life are not determined genetically or environmentally helps people pursue goals and gain control over their lives. Three impediments, however, can keep people from taking action: lack of competence, confidence, and motivation.[20]

1. *Problems of competence.* Lacking the skills to get a given task done leads to reduced competence. If your friends play basketball regularly but you don't know how to play, you might be inclined not to participate. The solution to this problem of competence is to master the skills you require to participate. Most people are not born with all-inclusive natural abilities, including playing sports.

   Another alternative is to select an activity in which you are skilled. It may not be basketball, but it well could be aerobics. Don't be afraid to try new activities. Similarly, if your body weight is a problem, you could learn to cook healthy, low-calorie meals. Try different recipes until you find foods that you like.
2. *Problems of confidence.* Problems with confidence arise when you have the skill but don't believe you can get it done. Fear and feelings of inadequacy often interfere with ability to perform the task. You shouldn't talk yourself out of something until you have given it a fair try. If you have the skills, the sky is the limit. Initially, try to visualize yourself doing the task and getting it done. Repeat this several times, then actually try it. You will surprise yourself.

   Sometimes, lack of confidence arises when the task seems insurmountable. In these situations, dividing a goal into smaller, more realistic objectives helps to accomplish the task. You might know how to swim but may need to train for several weeks to swim a continuous mile. Set up your training program so you swim a little farther each day until you are able to swim the entire mile. If you don't meet your objective on a given day, try it again, reevaluate, cut back a little, and, most important, don't give up.
3. *Problems of motivation.* With problems of motivation, both the competence and the confidence are there but individuals are unwilling to change because the reasons to change are not important to them. For example, people begin contemplating a smoking-cessation program only when the reasons for quitting outweigh the reasons for smoking. The primary causes of unwillingness to change are lack of knowledge and lack of goals. Knowledge often determines goals, and goals determine motivation. How badly you want something dictates how hard you'll work at it.

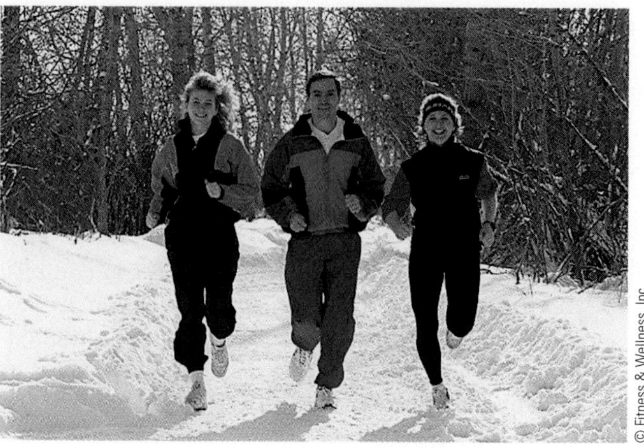

The higher quality of life experienced by people who are physically fit is hard to explain to someone who has never achieved good fitness.

Many people are unaware of the magnitude of benefits of a wellness program. When it comes to a healthy lifestyle, however, you may not get a second chance. A stroke, a heart attack, or cancer can have irreparable or fatal consequences. Greater understanding of what leads to disease may be all you need to initiate change.

Also, feeling physically fit is difficult to explain unless you have experienced it yourself. Feelings of fitness, self-esteem, confidence, health, and better quality of life cannot be conveyed to someone who is constrained by sedentary living. In a way, wellness is like reaching the top of a mountain. The quiet, the clean air, the lush vegetation, the flowing water in the river, the wildlife, and the majestic valley below are difficult to explain to someone who has spent a lifetime within city limits.

Changing Behavior

The very first step in addressing behavioral change is to recognize that you indeed have a problem. The five general categories of behaviors addressed in the process of willful change are:

1. Stopping a negative behavior
2. Preventing relapse of a negative behavior
3. Developing a positive behavior
4. Strengthening a positive behavior
5. Maintaining a positive behavior

Most people do not change all at once. Thus, psychotherapy has been used successfully to help people change their behavior. But most people do not seek professional help. They usually attempt to change by themselves with limited or no knowledge of how to achieve change. In essence, the process of change moves along a continuum from not willing to change, recognizing the need for change, and taking action and implementing change.

The simplest model of change is the two-stage model of unhealthy behavior and healthy behavior. This model states that either you do it or you don't. Most people who use this model attempt self-change but end up asking themselves why they're unsuccessful. They just can't do it (exercise, perhaps, or quit smoking). Their intent to change may be good, but to accomplish it, they need knowledge about how to achieve change.

Behavior Change Theories

For most people, changing chronic/unhealthy behaviors to stable, healthy behaviors is challenging. The "do it or don't do it" approach seldom works when attempting to implement lifestyle changes. Thus, several theories or models have been developed over the years. Among the most accepted models are **learning theories, problem solving model, social cognitive theory, relapse prevention model,** and the **transtheoretical model.**

Learning Theories

Learning theories maintain that most behaviors are learned and maintained under complex schedules of reinforcement and anticipated outcomes. The process involved in learning a new behavior requires modifying many small behaviors that shape the new pattern behavior. For example, a previously inactive individual who wishes to accumulate 10,000 steps per day may have to gradually increase the number of steps daily, park farther away from the office and stores, decrease television and Internet use, take stairs instead of elevators and escalators, and avoid the car and telephone when running errands that are only short distances away. The outcomes are better health, body weight management, and feelings of well-being.

Problem Solving Model

The problem solving model proposes that many behaviors are the result of making decisions as we seek to change the problem behavior. The process of change requires conscious attention, setting goals, and designing a specific plan of action. For instance, to quit smoking cigarettes, one has to understand the reasons for smoking, know under what conditions each cigarette is smoked, decide that one will quit, select a date to do so, and then draw up a plan of action to reach the goal (a complete smoking cessation program is outlined in Chapter 13).

Social Cognitive Theory

In the social cognitive approach, behavior change is influenced by the environment, self-efficacy, and characteristics of the behavior itself. You can encourage **self-efficacy** (believing that you can do the task) by educating yourself about the behavior, developing the skills to master the behavior, performing smaller mastery experiences successfully, and receiving verbal reinforcement and modeling (observing others perform the behavior). If you desire to lose weight, for example, you need to learn the principles of proper weight man-

---

Motivation The desire and will to do something.

Locus of control A concept examining the extent to which a person believes he or she can influence the external environment.

Learning theories Behavioral modification perspective stating that most behaviors are learned and maintained under complex schedules of reinforcement and anticipated outcomes.

Problem solving model Behavioral modification model proposing that many behaviors are the result of making decisions as the individual seeks to solve the problem behavior.

Social cognitive theory Behavioral modification model holding that behavior change is influenced by the environment, self-efficacy, and characteristics of the behavior itself.

Relapse prevention model Behavioral modification model based on the principle that high-risk situations can be anticipated through the development of strategies to prevent lapses and relapses.

Transtheoretical model Behavioral modification model proposing that change is accomplished through a series of progressive stages in keeping with a person's readiness to change.

Self-efficacy A belief in one's own ability to perform a given task.

FIGURE 2.2 Stages of change model.

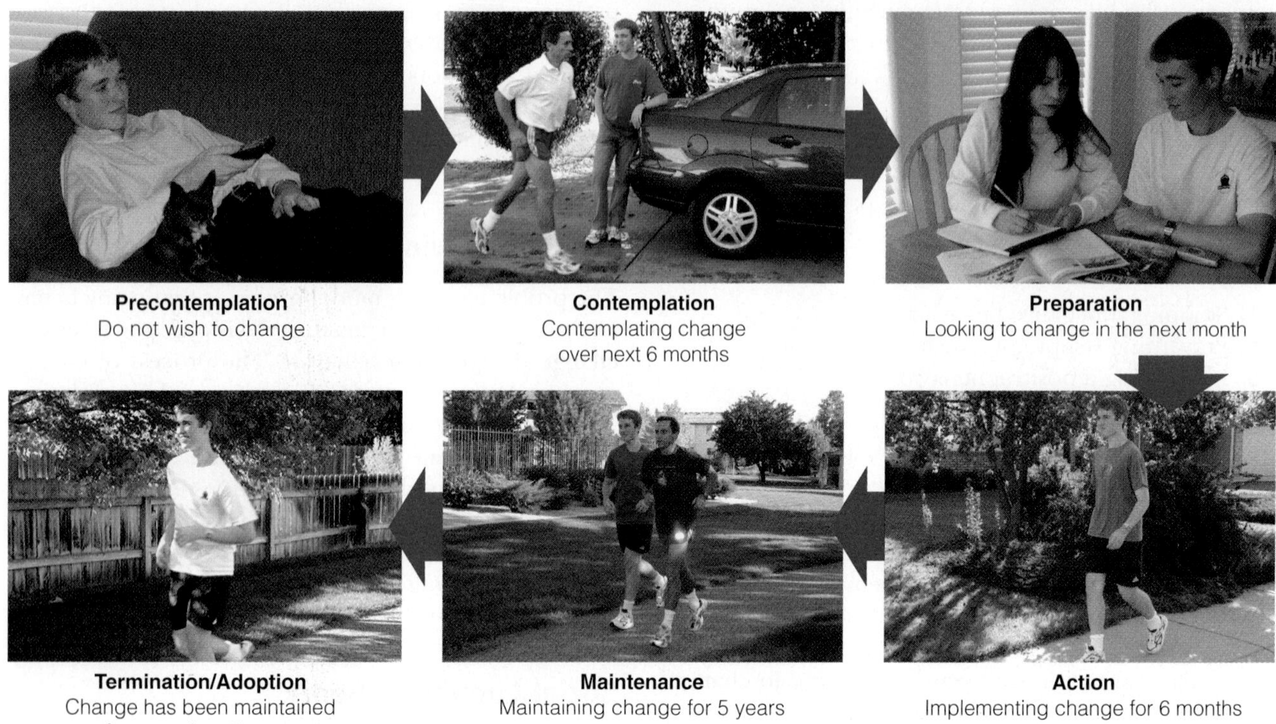

agement, eat less, shop and cook wisely, be more active, set small weight loss goals of 1 to 2 pounds per week, praise yourself for your accomplishments, and visualize losing the weight as others you admire have done.

Relapse Prevention Model

In relapse prevention, people are taught to anticipate high-risk situations and develop action plans to prevent **lapses** and **relapses.** Examples of factors that disrupt behavior change include negative physiological or psychological states (stress, illness), social pressure, lack of support, limited coping skills, change in work conditions, and lack of motivation. For example, if the weather turns bad for your evening walk, you can choose to walk around the indoor track (or at the mall), do water aerobics, swim, or play racquetball.

Transtheoretical Model

The transtheoretical model, developed by psychologists James Prochaska, John Norcross, and Carlo DiClemente, is based on the theory that change is a gradual process that involves several stages.[21] The model is used most frequently to change health-related behaviors such as physical inactivity, smoking, poor nutrition, weight problems, stress, and alcohol abuse.

An individual goes through five stages in the process of willful change. The stages describe underlying processes that people go through to change problem behaviors and replace them with healthy behaviors. A sixth stage (termination/adoption) was subsequently added to this model. The six stages of change are precontemplation, contemplation, preparation, action, maintenance, and termination/adoption (see Figure 2.2).

After years of study, researchers indicate that applying specific behavioral-change processes during each stage of the model increases the success rate for change (the specific processes for each stage are shown in Table 2.1, page 45). Understanding each stage of this model will help you determine where you are in relation to your personal healthy-lifestyle behaviors. It also will help you identify processes to make successful changes. The discussion in the remainder of the chapter focuses on the transtheoretical model, with the other models integrated as applicable with each stage of change.

1. **Precontemplation**
   Individuals in the **precontemplation stage** are not considering change or do not want to change a given behavior. They typically deny having a problem and have no intention of changing in the immediate future. These people are usually unaware

or underaware of the problem. Other people around them, including family, friends, healthcare practitioners, and co-workers, however, identify the problem clearly. Precontemplators do not care about the problem behavior and may even avoid information and materials that address the issue. They tend to avoid free screenings and workshops that might help identify and change the problem, even if they receive financial compensation for attending. Often they actively resist change and seem resigned to accepting the unhealthy behavior as their "fate."

Precontemplators are the most difficult people to inspire toward behavioral change. Many think that change isn't even a possibility. At this stage, knowledge is power. Educating them about the problem behavior is critical to help them start contemplating the process of change. The challenge is to find ways to help them realize that they are ultimately responsible for the consequences of their behavior. Typically, they initiate change only when people they respect or job requirements pressure them to do so.

2. **Contemplation**
   In the **contemplation stage,** individuals acknowledge that they have a problem and begin to think seriously about overcoming it. Although they are not quite ready for change, they are weighing the pros and cons of changing. Even though they may remain in this stage for years, in their minds they are planning to take some action within the next 6 months. Education and peer support remain valuable during this stage.
3. **Preparation**
   In the **preparation stage,** individuals are seriously considering change and planning to change a behavior within the next month. They are taking initial steps for change and may even try the new behavior for a short while, such as stopping smoking for a day or exercising a few times during the month. During this stage, people define a general goal for behavioral change (for example, to quit smoking by the last day of the month) and write specific objectives (or strategies) to accomplish this goal. The discussion on "Goal Setting" later in this chapter will help you write SMART goals and specific objectives to reach your goal. Continued peer and environmental support is helpful during the preparation stage.

   A key concept to keep in mind during the preparation stage is that in addition to being prepared to address the behavioral change or goal you are attempting to reach, you must prepare to address the specific objectives (supportive behaviors) required to reach that goal (see Figure 2.3). For example, you may be willing to give weight loss a try, but are you prepared to start eating less, eat out less often, eat less calorie-dense foods, shop and cook wisely, exercise more, watch television less, and become much more active? Achieving goals generally requires changing these supportive behaviors, and you must be prepared to do so.

FIGURE 2.3 Goal setting and supportive behaviors.

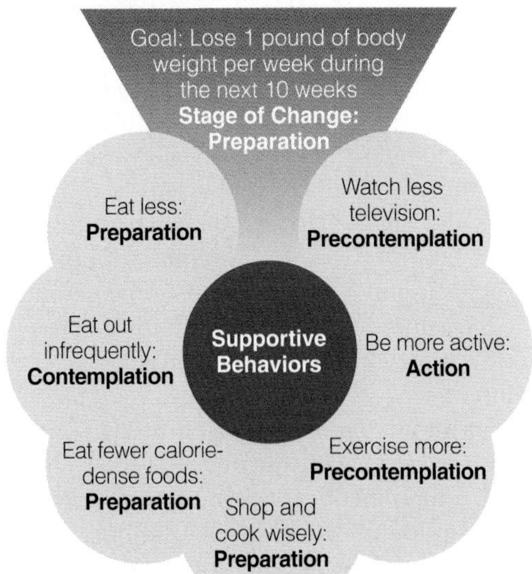

NOTE: This Figure 2.3 may not lead to goal achievement. All supportive behaviors should be in the preparation stage to enhance success in the action stage.

4. **Action**
   The **action stage** requires the greatest commitment of time and energy. Here, the individual is actively doing things to change or modify the problem behavior or to adopt a new, healthy behavior. The action stage requires that the person follow the specific guidelines set forth for that be-

Lapse (v.) To slip or fall back temporarily into unhealthy behavior(s); (n.) short-term failure to maintain healthy behaviors.

Relapse (v.) To slip or fall back into unhealthy behavior(s) over a longer time; (n.) longer-term failure to maintain healthy behaviors.

Precontemplation stage Stage of change in the transtheoretical model in which an individual is unwilling to change behavior.

Contemplation stage Stage of change in the transtheoretical model in which the individual is considering changing behavior within the next 6 months.

Preparation stage Stage of change in the transtheoretical model in which the individual is getting ready to make a change within the next month.

Action stage Stage of change in the transtheoretical model in which the individual is actively changing a negative behavior or adopting a new, healthy behavior.

havior. For example, a person has actually stopped smoking completely, is exercising aerobically three times per week according to exercise prescription guidelines, or is maintaining a healthy diet.

Relapse is common during this stage, and the individual may regress to a previous stage. If unsuccessful, a person should reevaluate his or her readiness to change supportive behaviors as required to reach the overall goal. Problem solving that includes identifying barriers to change and specific strategies (objectives) to overcome supportive behaviors is useful during relapse. Once people are able to maintain the action stage for 6 consecutive months, they move into the maintenance stage.

5. **Maintenance**
During the **maintenance stage,** the person continues the new behavior for up to 5 years. This stage requires the person to continue to adhere to the specific guidelines that govern the behavior (such as complete smoking cessation, exercising aerobically three times per week, or practicing proper stress management techniques). At this time, the person works to reinforce the gains made through the various stages of change and strives to prevent lapses and relapse.
6. **Termination/Adoption**
Once a person has maintained a behavior more than 5 years, he or she is said to be in the **termination** or **adoption** stage and exits from the cycle of change without fear of relapse. In the case of negative behaviors that are terminated, the stage of change is referred to as *termination.* If a positive behavior has been adopted successfully for more than 5 years, this stage is designated as *adoption.* Some researchers have also labeled this stage the "transformed" stage of change because the word literally means "to have changed."[22]

Many experts believe that, once an individual enters the termination/adoption stage, former addictions, problems, or lack of compliance with healthy behaviors no longer presents an obstacle in the quest for wellness. The change has become part of one's lifestyle. This phase is the ultimate goal for all people searching for a healthier lifestyle.

For addictive behaviors such as alcoholism and hard drug use, however, some health-care practitioners believe that the individual never enters the termination stage. Chemical dependency is so strong that most former alcoholics and hard-drug users must make a lifetime effort to prevent relapse. Similarly, some behavioral scientists suggest that the adoption stage might not be applicable to health behaviors such as exercise and weight control, because the likelihood of relapse is always high.

Use the guidelines provided in Lab 2B to determine where you stand in respect to behaviors you want to change or new ones you wish to adopt. As you follow the guidelines, you will realize that you might be at different stages for different behaviors. For instance, you might be in the preparation stage for aerobic exercise and smoking cessation, in the action stage for strength training, but only in the contemplation stage for a healthy diet. Realizing where you are with respect to different behaviors will help you design a better action plan for a healthy lifestyle.

FIGURE 2.4 Model of progression and relapse.

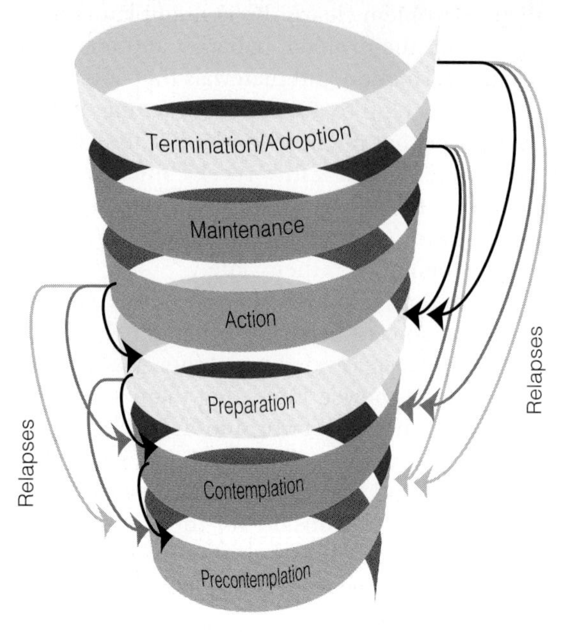

Relapse

After the precontemplation stage, relapse may occur at any level of the model. Even individuals in the maintenance and termination/adoption stages may regress to any of the first three stages of the model (see Figure 2.4). Relapse, however, does not mean failure. Failure comes only to those who give up and don't use prior experiences as a building block for future success. The chances of moving back up to a higher stage of the model are far better for someone who has previously made it into one of those stages.

The Process of Change

Using the same plan for everyone who wishes to change a behavior will not work. With exercise, for instance, we provide different prescriptions to people of varying fitness levels (see Chapter 6). The same prescription would not provide optimal results for a person who has been inactive for 20 years, compared with one who already walks regularly three times each week. This principle also holds true for individuals who are attempting to change their behaviors.

TABLE 2.1 Applicable Processes of Change During Each Stage of Change

Precontemplation	Contemplation	Preparation	Action	Maintenance	Termination/Adoption
Consciousness-raising	Consciousness-raising	Consciousness-raising			
Social liberation	Social liberation	Social liberation	Social liberation		
	Self-analysis	Self-analysis			
	Emotional arousal	Emotional arousal			
	Positive outlook	Positive outlook	Positive outlook		
		Commitment	Commitment	Commitment	Commitment
		Behavior analysis	Behavior analysis		
		Goal setting	Goal setting	Goal setting	
		Self-reevaluation	Self-reevaluation	Self-reevaluation	
			Countering	Countering	
			Monitoring	Monitoring	Monitoring
			Environment control	Environment control	Environment control
			Helping relationships	Helping relationships	Helping relationships
			Rewards	Rewards	Rewards

Source: Adapted from J. O. Prochaska, J. C. Norcross, and C. C. DiClemente, *Changing for Good* (New York: William Morrow, 1994); and W. W. K. Hoeger and S. A. Hoeger, *Fitness & Wellness* (Belmont, CA: Wadsworth/Thomson Learning, 2007).

Timing is also important in the process of willful change. People respond more effectively to selected **processes of change** in keeping with the stage of change they have reached at any given time.[23] Thus, applying appropriate processes at each stage of change enhances the likelihood of changing behavior permanently. The following description of 14 of the most common processes of change will help you develop a personal plan for change. The respective stages of change where each process works best are summarized in Table 2.1.

Consciousness-Raising

The first step in a **behavior modification** program is consciousness-raising. This step involves obtaining information about the problem so you can make a better decision about the problem behavior. For example, the problem could be physical inactivity. Learning about the benefits of exercise or the difference in benefits between physical activity and exercise (see Chapter 1) can help you decide the type of fitness program (health or high fitness) that you want to pursue. Possibly, you don't even know that a certain behavior is a problem, such as being unaware of saturated and total fat content in many fast-food items. Consciousness-raising may continue from the precontemplation stage through the preparation stage.

Social Liberation

Social liberation stresses external alternatives that make you aware of problem behaviors and begin to contemplate change. Examples of social liberation include pedestrian-only traffic areas, non-smoking areas, health-oriented cafeterias and restaurants, advocacy groups, civic organizations, policy interventions, and self-help groups. Social liberation often provides opportunities to get involved, stir up emotions, and enhance self-esteem—helping you gain confidence in your ability to change.

Self-Analysis

The next process in modifying behavior is developing a decisive desire to do so, called self-analysis. If you have no interest in changing a behavior, you won't do it. You will remain a precontemplator or a contemplator. A person who has no intention of quitting smoking will not quit, regardless of what anyone may say or how strong the evidence in favor of quitting may be. In your self-analysis, you may want to prepare a list of reasons for continuing or discontinuing the behavior. When the reasons for changing outweigh the reasons for not changing, you are ready for the next stage—either the contemplation stage or the preparation stage.

Emotional Arousal

In emotional arousal, a person experiences and expresses feelings about the problem and its solutions. Also referred to as "dramatic release," this process often involves deep emotional experiences. Watching a loved

Maintenance stage Stage of change in the transtheoretical model in which the individual maintains behavioral change for up to 5 years.

Termination/adoption stage Stage of change in the transtheoretical model in which the individual has eliminated an undesirable behavior or maintained a positive behavior for more than 5 years.

Processes of change Actions that help you achieve change in behavior.

Behavior modification The process of permanently changing negative behaviors to positive behaviors that will lead to better health and well-being.

one die from lung cancer caused by cigarette smoking may be all that is needed to make a person quit smoking. As in other examples, emotional arousal might be prompted by a dramatization of the consequences of drug use and abuse, a film about a person undergoing open-heart surgery, or a book illustrating damage to body systems as a result of unhealthy behaviors.

Positive Outlook

Having a positive outlook means taking an optimistic approach from the beginning and believing in yourself. Following the guidelines in this chapter will help you design a plan so you can work toward change and remain enthused about your progress. Also, you may become motivated by looking at the outcome—how much healthier you will be, how much better you will look, or how far you will be able to jog.

Commitment

Upon making a decision to change, you accept the responsibility to change and believe in your ability to do so. During the commitment process, you engage in preparation and may draw up a specific plan of action. Write down your goals and, preferably, share them with others. In essence, you are signing a behavioral contract for change. You will be more likely to adhere to your program if others know you are committed to change.

Behavior Modification Planning

STEPS FOR SUCCESSFUL BEHAVIOR MODIFICATION

1. Acknowledge that you have a problem.
2. Describe the behavior to change (increase physical activity, stop overeating, quit smoking).
3. List advantages and disadvantages of changing the specified behavior.
4. Decide positively that you will change.
5. Identify your stage of change.
6. Set a realistic goal (SMART goal), completion date, and sign a behavioral contract.
7. Define your behavioral change plan: List processes of change, techniques of change, and objectives that will help you reach your goal.
8. Implement the behavior change plan.
9. Monitor your progress toward the desired goal.
10. Periodically evaluate and reassess your goal.
11. Reward yourself when you achieve your goal.
12. Maintain the successful change for good.

Try It

In your Online Journal or class notebook, record your answers to the following questions:

Have you consciously attempted to incorporate a healthy behavior into or eliminate a negative behavior from your lifestyle? If so, what steps did you follow, and what helped you achieve your goal?

Behavior Analysis

How you determine the frequency, circumstances, and consequences of the behavior to be altered or implemented is known as behavior analysis. If the desired outcome is to consume less trans and saturated fats, you first must find out what foods in your diet are high in these fats, when you eat them, and when you don't eat them—all part of the preparation stage. Knowing when you don't eat them points to circumstances under which you exert control over your diet and will help as you set goals.

Goals

Goals motivate change in behavior. The stronger the goal or desire, the more motivated you'll be either to change unwanted behaviors or to implement new, healthy behaviors. The discussion on goal setting (pages 49–50) will help you write goals and prepare an action plan to achieve those goals. This will aid with behavior modification.

Self-Reevaluation

During the process of self-evaluation, individuals analyze their feelings about a problem behavior. The pros and cons or advantages and disadvantages of a certain behavior can be reevaluated at this time. For example, you may decide that strength training will help you get stronger and tone up, but implementing this change will require you to stop watching an hour of TV three times per week. If you presently have a weight problem and are unable to lift certain objects around the house, you may feel good about weight loss and enhanced physical capacity as a result of a strength-training program. You also might visualize what it would be like if you were successful at changing.

Countering

The process whereby you substitute healthy behaviors for a problem behavior, known as countering, is critical in changing behaviors as part of the action and maintenance stages. You need to replace unhealthy behaviors with new, healthy ones. You can use exercise to combat sedentary living, smoking, stress, or overeating. Or you may use exercise, diet, yard work, volunteer work, or reading to prevent overeating and achieve recommended body weight.

Monitoring

During the action and maintenance stages, continuous behavior monitoring increases awareness of the desired outcome. Sometimes this process of monitoring is suffi-

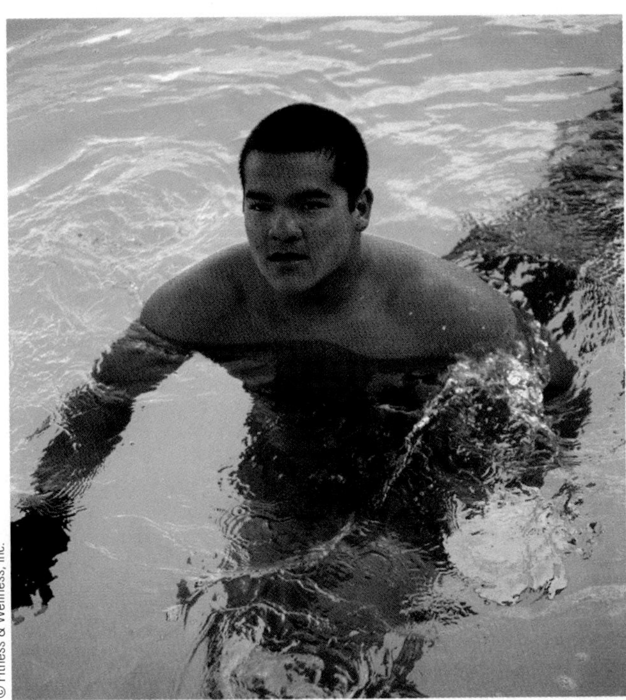

Countering: Substituting healthy behaviors for problem behaviors facilitates change.

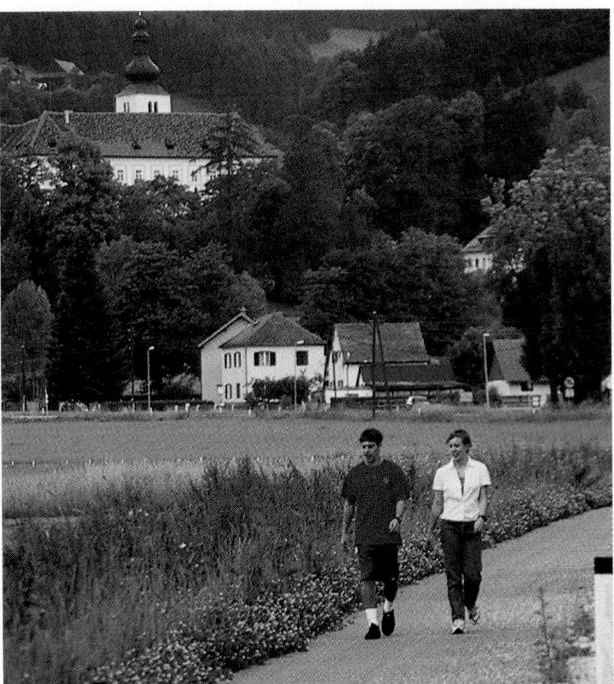

Rewarding oneself when a goal is achieved, such as scheduling a weekend getaway, is a powerful tool during the process of change.

cient in itself to cause change. For example, keeping track of daily food intake reveals sources of excessive fat in the diet. This can help you gradually cut down or completely eliminate high-fat foods. If the goal is to increase daily intake of fruit and vegetables, keeping track of the number of servings consumed each day raises awareness and may help increase intake.

Environment Control

In environment control, the person restructures the physical surroundings to avoid problem behaviors and decrease temptations. If you don't buy alcohol, you can't drink any. If you shop on a full stomach, you can reduce impulse-buying of junk food.

Similarly, you can create an environment in which exceptions become the norm, and then the norm can flourish. Instead of bringing home cookies for snacks, bring fruit. Place notes to yourself on the refrigerator and pantry to avoid unnecessary snacking. Put baby carrots or sugarless gum where you used to put cigarettes. Post notes around the house to remind you of your exercise time. Leave exercise shoes and clothing by the door so they are visible as you walk into your home. Put an electric timer on the TV so it will shut off automatically at 7:00 PM. All of these tactics will be helpful throughout the action, maintenance, and termination/adoption stages.

Helping Relationships

Surrounding yourself with people who will work toward a common goal with you or those who care about you and will encourage you along the way—helping relationships—will be supportive during the action, maintenance, and termination/adoption stages.

Attempting to quit smoking, for instance, is easier when a person is around others who are trying to quit as well. The person also could get help from friends who have quit smoking already. Losing weight is difficult if meal planning and cooking are shared with roommates who enjoy foods that are high in fat and sugar. This situation can be even worse if a roommate also has a weight problem but does not desire to lose weight.

Although peer support is a strong incentive for behavioral change, the individual should avoid people who will not be supportive. Friends who have no desire to quit smoking or to lose weight, or whatever behavior a person is trying to change, may tempt one to smoke or overeat and encourage relapse into unwanted behaviors.

People who have achieved the same goal already may not be supportive either. For instance, someone may say, "I can do six consecutive miles." Your response should be, "I'm proud that I can jog three consecutive miles."

Rewards

People tend to repeat behaviors that are rewarded and disregard those that are not rewarded or are punished. Rewarding oneself or being rewarded by others is a powerful tool during the process of change in all stages. If you have successfully cut down your caloric intake during the week, reward yourself by going to a movie or buying a new pair of shoes. Do not reinforce yourself

TABLE 2.2 Sample Techniques for Use with Processes of Change

Process	Techniques
Consciousness-Raising	Become aware that there is a problem, read educational materials about the problem behavior or about people who have overcome this same problem, find out about the benefits of changing the behavior, watch an instructional program on television, visit a therapist, talk and listen to others, ask questions, take a class.
Social Liberation	Seek out advocacy groups (Overeaters Anonymous, Alcoholics Anonymous), join a health club, buy a bike, join a neighborhood walking group, work in non-smoking areas.
Self-Analysis	Become aware that there is a problem, question yourself on the problem behavior, express your feelings about it, analyze your values, list advantages and disadvantages of continuing (smoking) or not implementing a behavior (exercise), take a fitness test, do a nutrient analysis.
Emotional Arousal	Practice mental imagery of yourself going through the process of change, visualize yourself overcoming the problem behavior, do some role-playing in overcoming the behavior or practicing a new one, watch dramatizations (a movie) of the consequences or benefits of your actions, visit an auto salvage yard or a drug rehabilitation center.
Positive Outlook	Believe in yourself, know that you are capable, know that you are special, draw from previous personal successes.
Commitment	Just do it, set New Year's resolutions, sign a behavioral contract, set start and completion dates, tell others about your goals, work on your action plan.
Behavior Analysis	Prepare logs of circumstances that trigger or prevent a given behavior and look for patterns that prompt the behavior or cause you to relapse.
Goal Setting	Write goals and objectives; design a specific action plan.
Self-Reevaluation	Determine accomplishments and evaluate progress, rewrite goals and objectives, list pros and cons, weigh sacrifices (can't eat out with others) versus benefits (weight loss), visualize continued change, think before you act, learn from mistakes, and prepare new action plans accordingly.
Countering	Seek out alternatives: Stay busy, walk (don't drive), read a book (instead of snacking), attend alcohol-free socials, carry your own groceries, mow your yard, dance (don't eat), go to a movie (instead of smoking), practice stress management.
Monitoring	Use exercise logs (days exercised, sets and resistance used in strength training), keep journals, conduct nutrient analyses, count grams of fat, count number of consecutive days without smoking, list days and type of relaxation technique(s) used.
Environment Control	Rearrange your home (no TVs, ashtrays, large-sized cups), get rid of unhealthy items (cigarettes, junk food, alcohol), then avoid unhealthy places (bars, happy hour), avoid relationships that encourage problem behaviors, use reminders to control problem behaviors or encourage positive ones (post notes indicating "don't snack after dinner" or "lift weights at 8:00 PM"). Frequent healthy environments (a clean park, a health club, restaurants with low-fat/low-calorie/nutrient-dense menus, friends with goals similar to yours).
Helping Relationships	Associate with people who have and want to overcome the same problem, form or join self-help groups, join community programs specifically designed to deal with your problem.
Rewards	Go to a movie, buy a new outfit or shoes, buy a new bike, go on a weekend get-away, reassess your fitness level, use positive self-talk ("good job," "that felt good," "I did it," "I knew I'd make it," "I'm good at this").

with destructive behaviors such as eating a high-fat/calorie-dense dinner. If you fail to change a desired behavior (or to implement a new one), you may want to put off buying those new shoes you had planned for that week. When a positive behavior becomes habitual, give yourself an even better reward. Treat yourself to a weekend away from home or buy a new bicycle.

Critical Thinking

Your friend John is a 20-year-old student who is not physically active. Exercise has never been a part of his life, and it has not been a priority in his family. He has decided to start a jogging and strength-training course in 2 weeks. Can you identify his current stage of change and list processes and techniques of change that will help him maintain a regular exercise behavior?

Techniques of Change

Not to be confused with the *processes* of change, you can apply any number of **techniques of change** within each process to help you through that specific process (see Table 2.2). For example, following dinner, people with a weight problem often can't resist continuous snacking during the rest of the evening until it is time to retire for the night. In the process of countering, for example, you can use various techniques to avoid unnecessary snacking. Examples include going for a walk, flossing and brushing your teeth immediately after dinner, going for a drive, playing the piano, going to a show, or going to bed earlier.

As you develop a behavior modification plan, you need to identify specific techniques that may work for you within each process of change. A list of techniques

FIGURE 2.5 Stage of change identification.

Please indicate which response most accurately describes your current ______ behavior (in the blank space identify the behavior: smoking, physical activity, stress, nutrition, weight control). Next, select the statement below (select only one) that best represents your current behavior pattern. To select the most appropriate statement, fill in the blank for one of the first three statements if your current behavior is a problem behavior. (For example, you may say, "I currently smoke and I do *not* intend to change in the foreseeable future," or "I currently *do not exercise* but I am contemplating changing in the next 6 months.") If you have already started to make changes, fill in the blank in one of the last three statements. (In this case, you may say: "I currently *eat a low-fat diet* but I have only done so within the last 6 months," or "I currently *practice adequate stress management techniques* and I have done so for over 6 months.") As you can see, you may use this form to identify your stage of change for any type of health-related behavior.

1. I currently ______, and I do not intend to change in the foreseeable future.
2. I currently ______, but I am contemplating changing in the next 6 months.
3. I currently ______, regularly, but I intend to change in the next month.
4. I currently ______, but I have done so only within the last 6 months.
5. I currently ______, and I have done so for more than 6 months.
6. I currently ______, and I have done so for more than 5 years.

for each process is provided in Table 2.2. This is only a sample list; dozens of other techniques could be used as well. For example, a discussion of behavior modification and adhering to a weight management program starts on page 153, getting started and adhering to a lifetime exercise program is presented on pages 191–193, stress management techniques are provided in Chapter 10, and tips to help stop smoking on pages 440–445. Some of these techniques also can be used with more than one process. Visualization, for example, is helpful in emotional arousal and self-reevaluation.

Now that you are familiar with the stages of change in the process of behavior modification, use Figure 2.5 and Lab 2B to identify two problem behaviors in your life. In this lab activity, you will be asked to determine your stage of change for two behaviors according to six standard statements. Based on your selection, determine the stage of change classification according to the ratings provided in Table 2.3. Next, develop a behavior modification plan according to the processes and techniques for change that you have learned in this chapter. (Similar exercises to identify stages-of-change for other fitness and wellness behaviors are provided in activities for subsequent chapters.)

Goal Setting and Evaluation

To initiate change, **goals** are essential, as goals motivate behavioral change. Whatever you decide to accomplish, setting goals will provide the road map to help make your dreams a reality. Setting goals, however, is not as simple as it looks. Setting goals is more than just deciding what you want to do. A vague statement such as "I will lose weight" is not sufficient to help you achieve this goal.

TABLE 2.3 Stage of Change Classification

Selected Statements (see Figure 2.5 and Lab 2B)	Classification
1	Precontemplation
2	Contemplation
3	Preparation
4	Action
5	Maintenance
6	Termination/Adoption

SMART Goals

Only a well-conceived action plan will help you attain goals. Determining what you want to accomplish is the starting point, but to reach your goal you need to write **SMART goals.** The SMART acronym is used in reference to goals that are **S**pecific, **M**easurable, **A**cceptable, **R**ealistic, and **T**ime-specific. In Lab 2C, you have an opportunity to set SMART goals for two behaviors that you wish to change or adopt.

1. Specific. When writing goals, state exactly and in a positive manner what you would like to accomplish. For example, if you are overweight at 150 pounds and at 27 percent body fat, to simply state "I will lose weight," is not a specific goal. Instead, rewrite your goal to state "I

Techniques of change Methods or procedures used during each process of change.

Goals The ultimate aims toward which effort is directed.

SMART An acronym used in reference to Specific, Measurable, Attainable, Realistic, and Time-specific goals.

will reduce my body fat to 20 percent body fat (137 pounds) in 12 weeks."

Write down your goals. An unwritten goal is simply a wish. A written goal, in essence, becomes a contract with yourself. Show this goal to a friend or an instructor, and have him or her witness the contract you made with yourself by signing alongside your signature.

Once you have identified and written down a specific goal, write the specific **objectives** that will help you reach that goal. These objectives are necessary steps required to reach your goal. For example, a goal might be to achieve recommended body weight. Several specific objectives could be to

a. lose an average of 1 pound (or 1 fat percentage point) per week,
b. monitor body weight before breakfast every morning,
c. assess body composition at 3-week intervals,
d. limit fat intake to less than 25 percent of total daily caloric intake,
e. eliminate all pastries from the diet during this time, and
f. walk/jog in the proper target zone for 60 minutes, six times per week.

2. Measurable. Whenever possible, goals and objectives should be measurable. For example, "I will lose weight" is not measurable, but "to reduce body fat to 20 percent" is measurable. Also note that all of the sample-specific objectives (a) through (f) in Item 1 above are measurable. For instance, you can figure out easily whether you are losing a pound or a percentage point per week; you can conduct a nutrient analysis to assess your average fat intake; or you can monitor your weekly exercise sessions to make sure you are meeting this specific objective.

3. Acceptable. Goals that you set for yourself are more motivational than goals that someone else sets for you. These goals will motivate and challenge you and should be consistent with your other goals. As you set an acceptable goal, ask yourself: Do I have the time, commitment, and necessary skills to accomplish this goal? If not, you need to restate your goal so it is acceptable to you.

When successful completion of a goal involves others, such as an athletic team or an organization, an acceptable goal must be compatible with those of the other people involved. If a team's practice schedule is set Monday through Friday from 4:00 to 6:00 PM, it is unacceptable for you to train only three times per week or at a different time of the day.

Acceptable goals also embrace positive thoughts. Visualize and believe in your success. As difficult as some tasks may seem, where there's a will, there's a way. A plan of action, prepared according to the guidelines in this chapter, will help you achieve your goals.

4. Realistic. Goals should be within reach. On the one hand, if you currently weigh 190 pounds and your target weight is 140 pounds, setting a goal to lose 50 pounds in a month would be unsound, if not impossible. Such a goal does not allow you to implement adequate behavior modification techniques or ensure weight maintenance at the target weight. Unattainable goals only set you up for failure, discouragement, and loss of interest.

On the other hand, do not write goals that are too easy to achieve and do not challenge you. If a goal is too easy, you may lose interest and stop working toward it.

You can write both short-term and long-term goals. If the long-term goal is to attain recommended body weight and you are 53 pounds overweight, you might set a short-term goal of losing 10 pounds and write specific objectives to accomplish this goal. Then the immediate task will not seem as overwhelming and will be easier.

At times, problems arise even with realistic goals. Try to anticipate potential difficulties as much as possible, and plan for ways to deal with them. If your goal is to jog for 30 minutes on 6 consecutive days, what are the alternatives if the weather turns bad? Possible solutions are to jog in the rain, find an indoor track, jog at a different time of day when the weather is better, or participate in a different aerobic activity such as stationary cycling, swimming, or step aerobics.

Monitoring your progress as you move toward a goal also reinforces behavior. Keeping an exercise log or doing a body composition assessment periodically enables you to determine your progress at any given time.

5. Time-specific. A goal always should have a specific date set for completion. The above example to reach 20 percent body fat in 12 weeks is time-specific. The chosen date should be realistic but not too distant in the future. Allow yourself enough time to achieve the goal, but not too much time, as this could affect your performance. With a deadline, a task is much easier to work toward.

Goal Evaluation

In addition to the SMART guidelines provided above, you should conduct periodic evaluations of your goals. Reevaluations are vital to success. You may find that after you have fully committed and put all your effort into a goal, that goal may be unreachable. If so, reassess the goal.

Recognize that you will face obstacles and you will not always meet your goals. Use your setbacks and learn from them. Rewrite your goal and create a plan that will help you get around self-defeating behaviors in the future. Once you achieve a goal, set a new one to improve upon or maintain what you have achieved. Goals keep you motivated.

Assess Your Behavior

Thomson NOW! *Log on to www.thomsonedu.com/login to create a behavior change contract.*

1. What are your feelings about the science of behavior modification and how its principles may help you on your journey to health and wellness?
2. Do you have behaviors you'd like to change? Are you in the precontemplation or contemplation stage of change for healthy lifestyle factors (for example, regular exercise, healthy eating, not smoking, stress management, prevention of sexually transmitted infections)? If you are, are you willing to learn what is required to change or eliminate unhealthy behaviors and adopt healthy lifestyle behaviors?
3. Are you now in the action phase (or above) for exercise and healthy eating? If not, examine and list the barriers that keep you from moving to the action stage.

Assess Your Knowledge

Thomson NOW! *Log on to www.thomsonedu.com/login to assess your understanding of this chapter's topics by taking the Student Practice Test and exploring the modules recommended in your Personalized Study Plan.*

1. Most of the behaviors that people adopt in life are
   a. a product of their environment.
   b. learned early in childhood.
   c. learned from parents.
   d. genetically determined.
   e. the result of peer pressure.
2. Instant gratification is
   a. a barrier to change.
   b. a factor that motivates change.
   c. one of the six stages of change.
   d. the end result of successful change.
   e. a technique in the process of change.
3. The desire and will to do something is referred to as
   a. invincibility.
   b. confidence.
   c. competence.
   d. external locus of control.
   e. motivation.
4. People who believe they have control over events in their lives
   a. tend to rationalize their negative actions.
   b. exhibit problems of competence.
   c. often feel helpless over illness and disease.
   d. have an internal locus of control.
   e. often engage in risky lifestyle behaviors.
5. A person who is unwilling to change a negative behavior because the reasons for change are not important enough is said to have problems of
   a. competence.
   b. conduct.
   c. motivation.
   d. confidence.
   e. risk complacency.
6. Which of the following is a stage of change in the transtheoretical model?
   a. recognition
   b. motivation
   c. relapse
   d. preparation
   e. goal setting
7. A precontemplator is a person who
   a. has no desire to change a behavior.
   b. is looking to make a change in the next 6 months.
   c. is preparing for change in the next 30 days.
   d. willingly adopts healthy behaviors.
   e. is talking to a therapist to overcome a problem behavior.
8. An individual who is trying to stop smoking and has not smoked for 3 months is in the
   a. maintenance stage.
   b. action stage.
   c. termination stage.
   d. adoption stage.
   e. evaluation stage.
9. The process of change in which an individual obtains information to make a better decision about a problem behavior is known as
   a. behavior analysis.
   b. self-reevaluation.
   c. commitment.
   d. positive outlook.
   e. consciousness-raising.

10. A goal is effective when it is
a. specific.
b. measurable.
c. realistic.
d. time-specific.
e. all of the above.

Correct answers can be found at the back of the book.

Media Menu

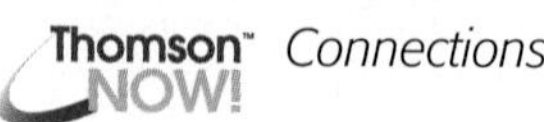

Connections

- Prepare for a healthy change in lifestyle.
- Check how well you understand the chapter's concepts.

Internet Connections

Transtheoretical Model

The model is described by its originators, James O. Prochaska, Ph.D., and Carlo C. DiClemente, Ph.D. This site, from the University of South Florida Community and Family Health, traces the historical development of the transtheoretical model and features several useful print references.
http://www.hsc.usf.edu/~kmbrown/Stages_of_Change_Overview.htm

Transtheoretical Model–
Cancer Prevention Research Center

This site also describes the transtheoretical model, including descriptions of effective interventions to promote change in health behavior, focusing on the individual's decision-making strategies.
http://www.uri.edu/research/cprc/TTM/detailedoverview.htm

Behavior Change Theories

This comprehensive site, by the Department of Health Promotion at California Polytechnic University at Pomona, describes all of the theories of behavioral change, including Learning Theories, Transtheoretical Model, Health Belief Model, Relapse Prevention Model, Reasoned Action and Planned Behavior, Social Learning/Social Cognitive Theory, and Social Support.
http://www.csupomona.edu/~jvgrizzell/

How to Fit Exercise into Your Daily Routine

Sponsored by the Centers for Disease Control and Prevention, this site describes how you can incorporate simple exercises into your daily schedule—whether you're at home, at work, or spending time away with the family. Make time to exercise!
http://www.cdc.gov/nccdphp/dnpa/physical/life/tips.htm

Notes

1. J. Annesi, "Using Emotions to Empower Members for Long-Term Exercise Success," *Fitness Management* 17 (2001): 54–58.
2. Television Bureau of Advertising Web site, "Time Spent Viewing per TV Home: per Day Annual Averages," http://www.tvb.org/nav/build_frameset.asp?url=/rcentral/index.asp (accessed March 26, 2005).
3. R. Boynton-Jarret, T. N. Thomas, K. E. Peterson, J. Wiecha, A. M. Sobol, and S. L. Gortmaker, "Impact of Television Viewing Patterns on Fruit and Vegetable Consumption among Adolescents," *Pediatrics* 113 (2003): 1321–1326.
4. League of California Cities Planners Institute, Pasadena Conference Center (April 13–15, 2005).
5. J. Pucher and C. Lefevre, *The Urban Transport Crisis in Europe and North America* (London: Macmillan Press Ltd., 1996).
6. B. E. Saelens, J. F. Sallis, and L. D. Frank, "Environmental Correlates of Walking and Cycling: Findings from the Transportation, Urban Design, and Planning Literatures," *Annals of Behavioral Medicine* 25 (2003): 80–91.
7. S. Gerrior, L. Bente, and H. Hiza, "Nutrient Content of the U.S. Food Supply, 1909–2000," *Home Economics Research Report No. 56* (U.S. Department of Agriculture, Center for Nutrition Policy and Promotion, 2004): 74, http://www.usda.gov/cnpp/nutrient_content.html (accessed April 18, 2005).
8. Marion Nestle, *Food Politics* (Berkeley: University of California Press, 2002), 1, 8, 22.
9. "Food Prepared Away from Home Is Increasing and Found to Be Less Nutritious," *Nutrition Research Newsletter* 21, no. 8 (August 2002): 10(2); A. Clauson, "Shares of Food Spending for Eating Reaches 47 Percent," *Food Review* 22 (1999): 20–22.
10. "A Diner's Guide to Health and Nutrition Claims on Restaurant Menus" (New York: Center for Science in the Public Interest, 1997), http://www.cspinet.org/reports/dinersgu.html (accessed March 25, 2005).
11. Lisa R. Young and Marion Nestle, "Expanding Portion Sizes in the U.S. Marketplace: Implications for Nutrition Counseling," *Journal of the American Dietetic Association* 103, no. 2 (February 2003): 231.
12. American Institute for Cancer Research, "As Restaurant Portions Grow, Vast Majority of Americans Still Belong to 'Clean Plate Club,' New Survey

Finds" (Washington, DC: AICR News Release, January 15, 2001).

13. T. V. E. Kral, L. S. Roe, J. S. Meengs, and D. E. Wall, "Increasing the Portion Size of a Packaged Snack Increases Energy Intake," *Appetite* 39 (2002): 86.
14. J. A. Ello-Martin, L. S. Roe, J. S. Meengs, D. E. Wall, and B. J. Rolls, "Increasing the Portion Size of a Unit Food Increases Energy Intake" *Appetite* 39 (2002): 74.
15. B. Wansink, "Can Package Size Accelerate Usage Volume?" *Journal of Marketing* 60 (1996): 1–14.
16. National Alliance for Nutrition and Activity (NANA), "From Wallet to Waistline: The Hidden Costs of Super Sizing" (Washington, DC: NANA, 2002), http://www.preventioninstitute.org/portionsizerept.html.
17. S. H. A. Holt, N. Sandona, and J. C. Brand-Miller, "The Effects of Sugar-Free vs. Sugar-Rich Beverages on Feelings of Fullness and Subsequent Food Intake," *International Journal of Food Sciences and Nutrition* 51, no. 1 (January 2000): 59.
18. M. G. Tordoff, "Obesity by Choice: The Powerful Influence of Nutrient Availability on Nutrient Intake," *American Journal of Physiology: Regulatory, Integrative and Comparative Physiology* 282 (2001): 1536–1539.
19. "Wellness Facts," *University of California at Berkeley Wellness Letter* (Palm Coast, FL: The Editors, May 2004).
20. G. S. Howard, D. W. Nance, and P. Myers, *Adaptive Counseling and Therapy* (San Francisco: Jossey-Bass, 1987).
21. J. O. Prochaska, J. C. Norcross, and C. C. DiClemente, *Changing for Good* (New York: William Morrow, 1994).
22. B. J. Cardinal, "Extended Stage Model of Physical Activity Behavior," *Journal of Human Movement Studies* 37 (1999): 37–54.
23. See note 21; also B. H. Marcus et al., "Evaluation of Motivationally Tailored vs. Standard Self-help Physical Activity Interventions at the Workplace," *American Journal of Health Promotion* 12 (1998): 246–253.

Suggested Readings

Blair, S. N., et al. *Active Living Every Day.* Champaign, IL: Human Kinetics, 2001.

Bouchard, C., et al. *Physical Activity, Fitness, and Health.* Champaign, IL: Human Kinetics, 1994.

Brehm, B. *Successful Fitness Motivation Strategies.* Champaign, IL: Human Kinetics, 2004.

Burgand, M., and K. Gallagher. "Self-Monitoring: Influencing Effective Behavior Change in Your Clients." *ACSM's Health & Fitness Journal* 10, no. 1 (2006): 14–19.

Dishman, R. *Advances in Exercise Adherence.* Champaign, IL: Human Kinetics, 1994.

Marcus, B., and L. Forsyth. *Motivating People To Be Physically Active.* Champaign, IL: Human Kinetics, 2003.

Prochaska, J. O., J. C. Norcross, and C. C. DiClemente. *Changing for Good.* New York: William Morrow, 1994.

Samuelson, M. "Stages of Change: From Theory to Practice." *The Art of Health Promotion* 2 (1998): 1–7.

Lab 2A Controlling Your Physical Activity and Nutrition

Name: | **Date:** | **Gender/Age:**

Instructor: | **Course:** | **Section:**

Objective

To aid in the identification of environemntal factors that have an effect on your physical activity and nutrition habits.

Instructions

Select the appropriate answer to each question and obtain a final score according to the guidelines provided at the end of each section.

I. Physical Activity

Note: Based on the definitions of *physical activity* and *exercise* (see page 5), as you take this questionnaire, keep in mind that you can be physically active without exercising but you cannot exercise without being physically active.

	Nearly always	Often	Seldom	Never
1. Do you identify daily time slots to be *physically active*?	4	3	2	1
2. Do you seek additional opportunities to be active each day (walk, cycle, park farther away, do yard work/gardening)?	4	3	2	1
3. Do you avoid labor-saving devices/activities (escalators, elevators, self-propelled lawn mowers, snow blowers, drive-through windows)?	4	3	2	1
4. Does physical activity improve your health and well-being?	4	3	2	1
5. Does physical activity increase your energy level?	4	3	2	1
6. Do you seek professional and/or medical (if necessary) advice prior to starting an exercise program or when increasing the intensity, duration, and frequency of exercise?	4	3	2	1
7. Do you identify time slots to *exercise* most days of the week?	4	3	2	1
8. Do you schedule exercise during times of the day when you feel most energetic?	4	3	2	1
9. Do you have an alternative plan to be active or exercise during adverse weather conditions (walk at the mall, swim at the health club, climb stairs, skip rope, dance)?	4	3	2	1
10. Do you cross-train (participate in a variety of activities)?	4	3	2	1
11. Do you surround yourself with people who support your physical activity/exercise goals?	4	3	2	1
12. Do you let family and friends know of your physical activity/exercise interests?	4	3	2	1
13. Do you invite family and friends to exercise with you?	4	3	2	1
14. Do you seek new friendships with people who are physically active?	4	3	2	1
15. Do you select friendships with people whose fitness and skill levels are similar to yours?	4	3	2	1
16. Do you plan social activities that involve physical activity?	4	3	2	1
17. Do you plan activity/exercise when you are away from home (during business and vacation trips)?	4	3	2	1
18. When you have a desire to do so, do you take classes to learn new activity/sport skills?	4	3	2	1
19. Do you limit daily television viewing and Internet and computer game time?	4	3	2	1
20. Do you spend leisure hours being physically active?	4	3	2	1

Physical Activity Score: __________

Total number of daily steps: [ ]

II. Nutrition	Nearly always	Often	Seldom	Never
1. Do you prepare a shopping list prior to going to the store?	4	3	2	1
2. Do you select food items primarily from the perimeter of the store (site of most fresh/unprocessed foods)?	4	3	2	1
3. Do you limit the unhealthy snacks you bring into the home and the workplace?	4	3	2	1
4. Do you plan your meals and is your pantry well stocked so you can easily prepare a meal without a quick trip to the store?	4	3	2	1
5. Do you help cook your meals?	4	3	2	1
6. Do you pay attention to how hungry you are before and during a meal?	4	3	2	1
7. When reaching for food, do you remind yourself that you have a choice about what and how much you eat?	4	3	2	1
8. Do you eat your meals at home?	4	3	2	1
9. Do you eat your meals at the table only?	4	3	2	1
10. Do you include whole-grain products in your diet each day (whole-grain bread/cereal/crackers/rice/pasta)?	4	3	2	1
11. Do you make a deliberate effort to include a variety of fruits and vegetables in your diet each day?	4	3	2	1
12. Do you limit your daily saturated fat and trans fat intake (red meat, whole milk, cheese, butter, hard margarines, luncheon meats, baked goods)?	4	3	2	1
13. Do you avoid unnecessary/unhealthy snacking (at work or play, during TV viewing, at the movies or socials)?	4	3	2	1
14. Do you plan caloric allowances prior to attending social gatherings that include food and eating?	4	3	2	1
15. Do you limit alcohol consumption to two drinks a day if you are a man or one drink a day if you are a woman?	4	3	2	1
16. Are you aware of strategies to decrease caloric intake when dining out (resist the server's offerings for drinks and appetizers, select a low-calorie/nutrient-dense item, drink water, resist cleaning your plate, ask for a doggie bag, share meals, request whole-wheat substitutes, get dressings on the side, avoid cream sauces, skip desserts)?	4	3	2	1
17. Do you avoid ordering larger meal sizes because you get more food for your money?	4	3	2	1
18. Do you avoid buying food when you hadn't planned to do so (gas stations, convenience stores, video rental stores)?	4	3	2	1
19. Do you fill your time with activities that will keep you away from places where you typically consume food (kitchen, coffee room, dining room)?	4	3	2	1
20. Do you know what situations trigger your desire for unnecessary snacking and overeating (vending machines, TV viewing, food ads, cookbooks, fast-food restaurants, buffet restaurants)?	4	3	2	1

Nutrition Score: __________

Environmental Control Ratings

≥71	You have good control over your environment
51–70	There is room for improvement
31–50	Your environmental control is poor
≤30	You are controlled by your environment

Lab 2B Behavior Modification Plan

Name: ____ **Date:** ____ **Grade:** ____

Instructor: ____ **Course:** ____ **Section:** ____

Necessary Lab Equipment

None.

Objective

To help you identify the stage of change for two problem behaviors and the processes and techniques for change.

Instructions

Chapter 2 must be read prior to this lab.

I. Stages of Change Instructions

Please indicate which response most accurately describes your current ____ behavior (in the blank space identify the behavior: smoking, physical activity, stress, nutrition, weight control). Next, select the statement below (select only one) that best represents your current behavior pattern. To select the most appropriate statement, fill in the blank for one of the first three statements if your current behavior is a problem behavior. For example, you may say:

"I currently smoke, and I do not intend to change in the foreseeable future" or

"I currently do not exercise, but I am contemplating changing in the next 6 months."

If you have already started to make changes, fill in the blank in one of the last three statements. In this case you may say:

"I currently eat a low-fat diet, but I have only done so within the last 6 months" or

"I currently practice adequate stress management techniques, and I have done so for over 6 months."

You may use this form to identify your stage of change for any health-related behavior. After identifying two problem behaviors, look up your stage of change for each one using Table 2.3 (on page 49).

Behavior #1. Fill in only one blank.

☐ 1. I currently ____, and do not intend to change in the foreseeable future.

☐ 2. I currently ____, but I am contemplating changing in the next 6 months.

☐ 3. I currently ____ regularly, but I intend to change in the next month.

☐ 4. I currently ____, but I have only done so within the last 6 months.

☐ 5. I currently ____, and I have done so for over 6 months.

☐ 6. I currently ____, and I have done so for over 5 years.

Stage of change: ____ (see Table 2.3 on page 49).

Behavior #2. Fill in only one blank.

☐ 1. I currently ____, and do not intend to change in the foreseeable future.

☐ 2. I currently ____, but I am contemplating changing in the next 6 months.

☐ 3. I currently ____ regularly, but I intend to change in the next month.

☐ 4. I currently ____, but I have only done so within the last 6 months.

☐ 5. I currently ____, and I have done so for over 6 months.

☐ 6. I currently ____, and I have done so for over 5 years.

Stage of change: ____ (see Table 2.3 on page 49).

II. Processes of Change

According to your stage of change for the two behaviors identified above, list the processes of change that apply to each behavior (see Table 2.1 on page 45).

Behavior #1:

Behavior #2:

III. Techniques for Change

List a minimum of three techniques that you will use with each process of change (see Table 2.2 on page 48).

Behavior #1: 1.

2.

3.

Behavior #2: 1.

2.

3.

Will you continue to use techniques as a process of behavior modification in the future? Briefly, discuss the techniques that were most beneficial to you.

Today's date: Completion Date: Signature:

Lab 2C Setting SMART Goals

Name: ______ Date: ______ Grade: ______

Instructor: ______ Course: ______ Section: ______

Objective

To learn to write SMART goals.

Instructions

In Lab 2B you identified two behaviors that you wish to change. Using SMART goal guidelines, write goals and objectives that will provide a road map for behavioral change. In the spaces provided in this lab, indicate how your stated goals meet each one of the SMART goal guidelines.

I. SMART Goals

Goal 1:

Indicate what makes your goal specific.

How is your goal measurable?

Why is this an acceptable goal?

State why you consider this goal realistic.

How is this goal time-specific?

II. Specific Objectives

Write a minimum of five specific objectives that will help you reach your two SMART goals.

Goal 1:

Objectives:

1.

2.

3.

4.

5.

Goal 2:

Objectives:

1.

2.

3.

4.

5.

Nutrition for Wellness

CHAPTER 3

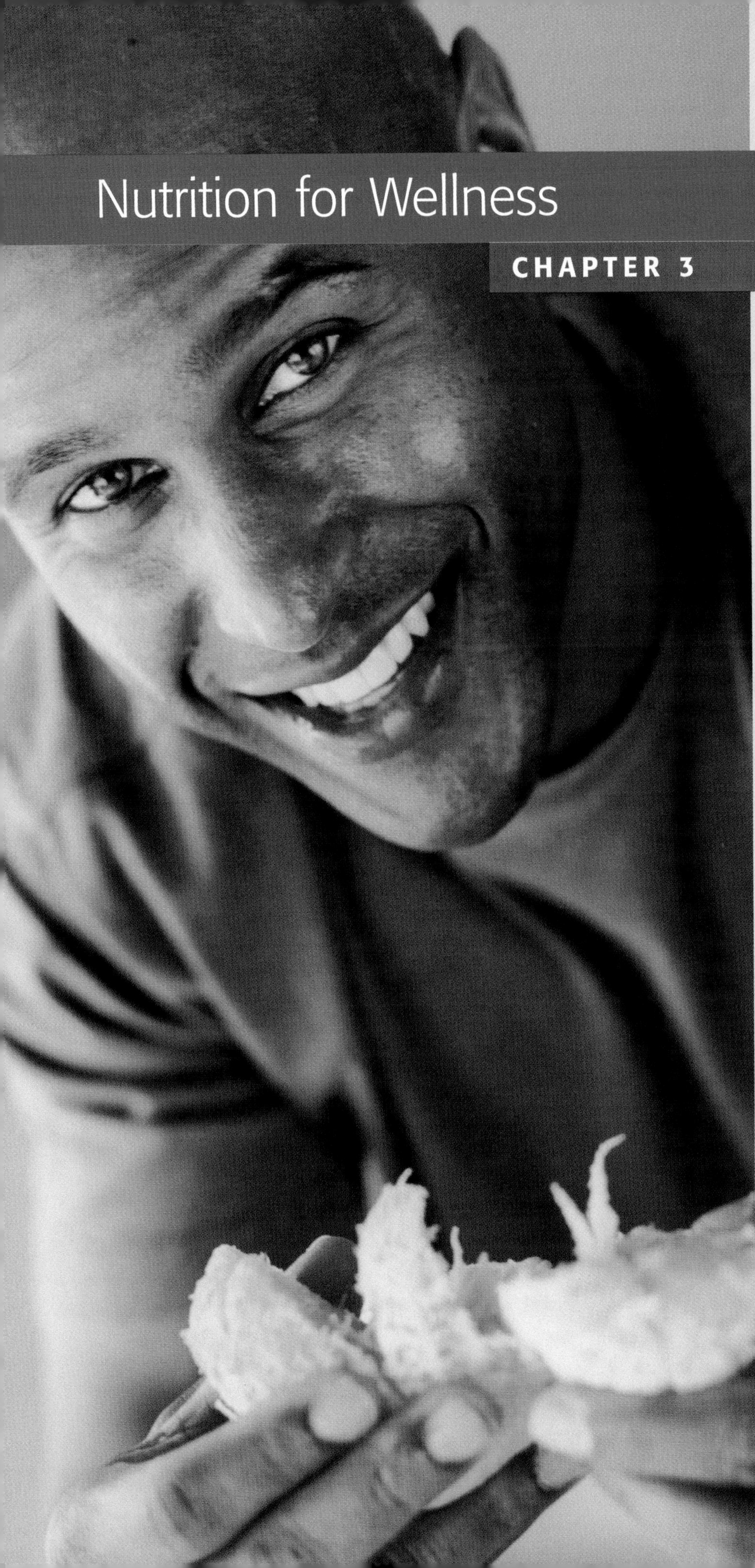

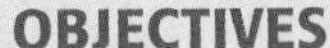

OBJECTIVES

- Define *nutrition* and describe its relationship to health and well-being.
- Learn to use the USDA MyPyramid guidelines for healthier eating.
- Describe the functions of the nutrients—carbohydrates, fiber, fats, proteins, vitamins, minerals, and water—in the human body.
- Define the various energy production mechanisms of the human body.
- Be able to conduct a comprehensive nutrient analysis and implement changes to meet the Dietary Reference Intakes (DRIs).
- Identify myths and fallacies regarding nutrition.
- Become aware of guidelines for nutrient supplementation.
- Learn the 2005 Dietary Guidelines for Americans.

Thomson NOW! Go to www.thomsonedu.com/login to:

- Assess your eating habits.
- Check how well you understand the chapter's concepts.

Good **nutrition** is essential to overall health and wellness. Proper nutrition means that a person's diet supplies all the essential nutrients for healthy body functioning, including normal tissue growth, repair, and maintenance. The diet should also provide enough **substrates** to produce the energy necessary for work, physical activity, and relaxation.

Nutrients should be obtained from a wide variety of sources. Figure 3.1 shows MyPyramid nutrition guidelines and recommended daily food amounts according to various caloric requirements. To lower the risk for chronic disease, an effective wellness program must incorporate healthy eating guidelines. These guidelines will be discussed throughout this chapter and in later chapters.

Too much or too little of any nutrient can precipitate serious health problems. The typical U.S. diet is too high in calories, sugar, saturated fat, trans fat, and sodium, and not high enough in whole grains, fruits, and vegetables—factors that undermine good health. On a given day, nearly half of the people in the United States eat no fruit and almost a fourth eat no vegetables.

Food availability is not a problem. The problem is overconsumption of the wrong foods. Diseases of dietary excess and imbalance are among the leading causes of death in many developed countries throughout the world, including the United States.

Diet and nutrition often play a crucial role in the development and progression of chronic diseases. A diet high in saturated fat and cholesterol increases the risk for diseases of the cardiovascular system, including atherosclerosis, coronary heart disease, and strokes. In sodium-sensitive individuals, high salt intake has been linked to high blood pressure. Up to 50 percent of all cancers may be diet-related. Obesity, diabetes, and osteoporosis also have been associated with faulty nutrition.

Nutrients

The essential nutrients the human body requires are carbohydrates, fat, protein, vitamins, minerals, and water. The first three are called "fuel nutrients" because they are the only substances the body uses to supply the energy (commonly measured in calories) needed for work and normal body functions. The three others—vitamins, minerals, and water—are regulatory nutrients. They have no caloric value, but are still necessary for a person to function normally and maintain good health. Many nutritionists add to this list a seventh nutrient: fiber. This nutrient is vital for good health. Recommended amounts seem to provide protection against several diseases, including cardiovascular disease and some cancers.

Carbohydrates, fats, proteins, and water are termed *macronutrients* because we need them in proportionately large amounts daily. Vitamins and minerals are required in only small amounts—grams, milligrams, and micrograms instead of, say, ounces—and nutritionists refer to them as *micronutrients.*

Depending on the amount of nutrients and calories they contain, foods can be classified by their **nutrient density.** Foods that contain few or a moderate number of calories but are packed with nutrients are said to have high nutrient density. Foods that have a lot of calories but few nutrients are of low nutrient density and are commonly called "junk food."

A **calorie** is the unit of measure indicating the energy value of food to the person who consumes it. It also is used to express the amount of energy a person expends in physical activity. Technically, a kilocalorie (kcal), or large calorie, is the amount of heat necessary to raise the temperature of 1 kilogram of water 1 degree Centigrade. For simplicity, people call it a calorie rather than a kcal. For example, if the caloric value of a food is 100 calories (that is, 100 kcal), the energy in this food would raise the temperature of 100 kilograms of water 1 degree Centigrade. Similarly, walking 1 mile would burn about 100 calories (again, 100 kcal).

Carbohydrates

Carbohydrates constitute the major source of calories the body uses to provide energy for work, maintain cells, and generate heat. They also help regulate fat and metabolize protein. Each gram of carbohydrates provides the human body with 4 calories. The major sources of carbohydrates are breads, cereals, fruits, vegetables, and milk and other dairy products. Carbohydrates are classified into simple carbohydrates and complex carbohydrates (Figure 3.2).

Simple Carbohydrates

Often called "sugars," **simple carbohydrates** have little nutritive value. Examples are candy, soda, and cakes. Simple carbohydrates are divided into monosaccha-

---

Nutrition Science that studies the relationship of foods to optimal health and performance.

Substrates Substances acted upon by an enzyme (examples: carbohydrates, fats).

Nutrients Substances found in food that provide energy, regulate metabolism, and help with growth and repair of body tissues.

Nutrient density A measure of the amount of nutrients and calories in various foods.

Calorie The amount of heat necessary to raise the temperature of 1 gram of water 1 degree Centigrade; used to measure the energy value of food and cost (energy expenditure) of physical activity.

Carbohydrates A classification of a dietary nutrient containing carbon, hydrogen, and oxygen; the major source of energy for the human body.

Simple carbohydrates Formed by simple or double sugar units with little nutritive value; divided into monosaccharides and disaccharides.

FIGURE 3.1 MyPyramid: Steps to a healthier you.

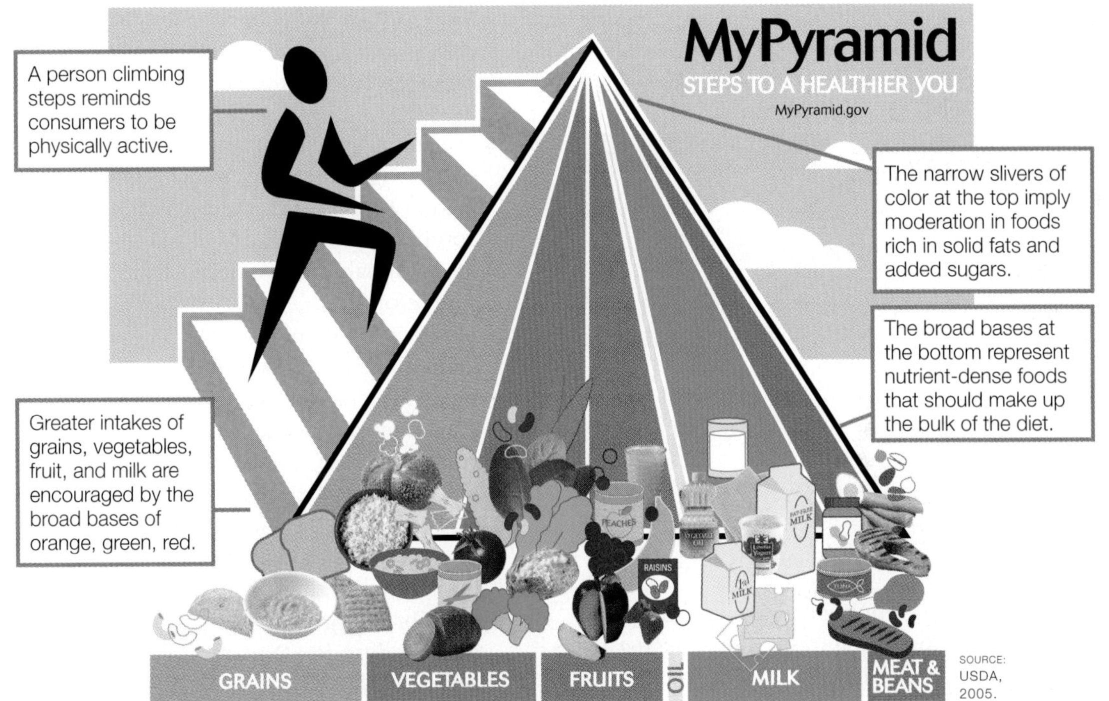

GRAINS	VEGETABLES	FRUITS	OILS	MILK	MEATS & BEANS
In general: 1 slice of bread, 1 cup of ready-to-eat cereal, ½ cup of cooked rice, cooked pasta, or cooked cereal can be considered as 1 oz equivalent of grains. Look for "whole" before the grain name on the list of ingredients and make at least half your grains whole.	In general: 1 cup of raw or cooked vegetables or vegetable juice, or 2 cups of raw leafy greens can be considered as 1 cup from the vegetable group. Try to eat more dark green and orange veggies, as well as dry beans and peas.	In general: 1 cup of fruit or 100% fruit juice, or ½ cup of dried fruit can be considered as 1 cup from the fruit group. Eat a variety of fruit, including fresh, frozen, canned, or dried fruit. Go easy on fruit juices.	Measured in teaspoons of either oils or solid fats. Most sources should come from fish, nuts, and vegetable oils. Limit solid fats such as butter, stick margarine, shortening, and lard.	In general: 1 cup of milk or yogurt, 1½ oz of natural cheese, or 2 oz of processed cheese can be considered as 1 cup from the milk group. Go low-fat or fat free. If you can't consume milk, choose lactose-free products or other calcium sources.	In general: 1 oz of meat, poultry, or fish, ¼ cup cooked dry beans, 1 egg, 1 tbsp of peanut butter, or ½ oz of nuts or seeds can be considered as 1 oz equivalent from the Meats & Beans group.

Recommended Daily Amounts from Each Food Group

FOOD GROUP	1600 cal	1800 cal	2000 cal	2200 cal	2400 cal	2600 cal	2800 cal	3000 cal
Fruits	1½ c	1½ c	2 c	2 c	2 c	2 c	2½ c	2½ c
Vegetables	2 c	2½ c	2½ c	3 c	3 c	3½ c	3½ c	4 c
Grains	5 oz	6 oz	6 oz	7 oz	8 oz	9 oz	10 oz	10 oz
Meat and legumes	5 oz	5 oz	5½ oz	6 oz	6½ oz	6½ oz	7 oz	7 oz
Milk	3 c	3 c	3 c	3 c	3 c	3 c	3 c	3 c
Oils	5 tsp	5 tsp	6 tsp	6 tsp	7 tsp	8 tsp	8 tsp	10 tsp
Discretionary calorie allowance*	132 cal	195 cal	267 cal	290 cal	362 cal	410 cal	426 cal	512 cal

*Discretionary calorie allowance: At each calorie level, people who consistently choose calorie-dense foods may be able to meet their nutrient needs without consuming their full allotment of calories. The difference between the calories needed to supply nutrients and those needed for energy is known as the *discretionary calorie allowance.*

Source: http://mypyramid.gov/. Additional information on MyPyramid can be obtained at this site, including an online individualized MyPyramid eating plan based on your age, gender, and activity level.

FIGURE 3.2 Major types of carbohydrates.

Simple carbohydrates

Monosaccharides	Disaccharides
Glucose	Sucrose (glucose+fructose)
Fructose	Lactose (glucose+galactose)
Galactose	Maltose (glucose+glucose)

Complex carbohydrates

Polysaccharides	Fiber
Starches	Cellulose
Dextrins	Hemicellulose
Glycogen	Pectins
	Gums
	Mucilages

rides and disaccharides. These carbohydrates—whose names end with "-ose"—often take the place of more nutritive foods in the diet.

Monosaccharides. The simplest sugars are **monosaccharides.** The three most common monosaccharides are glucose, fructose, and galactose.

1. *Glucose* is a natural sugar found in food and also is produced in the body from other simple and complex carbohydrates. It is used as a source of energy, or it may be stored in the muscles and liver in the form of glycogen (a long chain of glucose molecules hooked together). Excess glucose in the blood is converted to fat and stored in **adipose tissue.**
2. *Fructose,* or fruit sugar, occurs naturally in fruits and honey and is converted to glucose in the body.
3. *Galactose* is produced from milk sugar in the mammary glands of lactating animals and is converted to glucose in the body.

Disaccharides. The three major **disaccharides** are:

1. *Sucrose* or table sugar (glucose + fructose).
2. *Lactose* (glucose + galactose).
3. *Maltose* (glucose + glucose).

These disaccharides are broken down in the body, and the resulting simple sugars (monosaccharides) are used as indicated above.

Complex Carbohydrates

Complex carbohydrates also are called *polysaccharides.* Anywhere from about 10 to thousands of monosaccharide molecules can unite to form a single polysaccharide. Examples of complex carbohydrates are starches, dextrins, and glycogen.

1. *Starch,* the storage form of glucose in plants, is needed to promote their earliest growth. Starch is commonly found in grains, seeds, corn, nuts, roots, potatoes, and legumes. In a healthful diet, grains, the richest source of starch, should supply most of the energy. Once eaten, starch is converted to glucose for the body's own energy use.
2. *Dextrins* are formed from the breakdown of large starch molecules exposed to dry heat, such as in baking bread or producing cold cereals. These complex carbohydrates of plant origin provide many valuable nutrients and can be an excellent source of fiber.
3. *Glycogen* is the animal polysaccharide synthesized from glucose and is found only in tiny amounts in meats. In essence, we manufacture it; we don't consume it. **Glycogen** constitutes the body's reservoir of glucose. Thousands of glucose molecules are linked, to be stored as glycogen in the liver and muscle. When a surge of energy is needed, enzymes in the muscle and the liver break down glycogen and thereby make glucose readily available for energy transformation. (This process is discussed under "Nutrition for Athletes," starting on page 91.)

Fiber

Fiber is a form of complex carbohydrate. A high-fiber diet gives a person a feeling of fullness without adding too many calories to the diet. **Dietary fiber** is present mainly in plant leaves, skins, roots, and seeds. Processing and refining foods removes almost all of their natural fiber. In our diet, the main sources of fiber are whole-grain cereals and breads, fruits, vegetables, and legumes.

Fiber is important in the diet because it decreases the risk for cardiovascular disease and cancer. Increased fiber intake also may lower the risk for coronary heart disease, because saturated fats often take the place of fiber in the diet, increasing the absorption and formation of cholesterol. Other health disorders that have been tied to low intake of fiber are constipation, diverticulitis, hemorrhoids, gallbladder disease, and obesity.

The recommended fiber intake for adults 50 years and younger is 25 grams per day for women and 38 grams for men. As a result of decreased food consumption in people over 50 years of age, an intake of 21 and 30 grams of fiber per day, respectively, is recommended.[1] Most people in the United States eat only 15 grams of fiber per day, putting them at increased risk for disease.

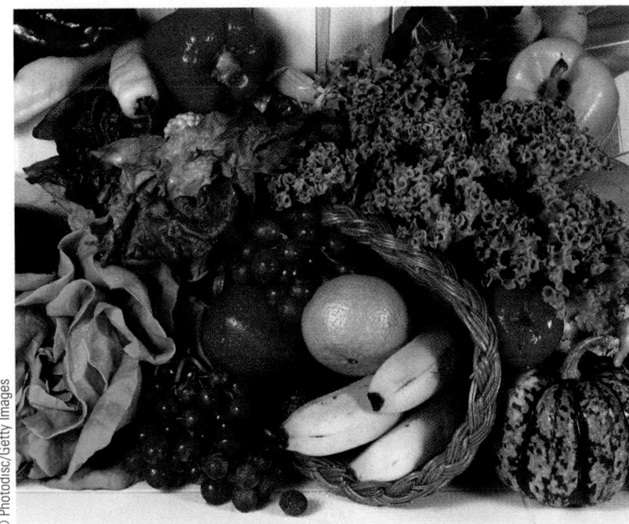

High-fiber foods are essential in a healthy diet.

A person can increase fiber intake by eating more fruits, vegetables, legumes, whole grains, and whole-grain cereals. Research provides evidence that increasing fiber intake to 30 grams per day leads to a significant reduction in heart attacks, cancer of the colon, breast cancer, diabetes, and diverticulitis. Table 3.1 provides the fiber content of selected foods. A practical guideline to obtain your fiber intake is to eat at least five daily servings of fruits and vegetables and three servings of whole-grain foods (whole-grain bread, cereal, and rice).

Fiber is typically classified according to its solubility in water.

1. *Soluble fiber* dissolves in water and forms a gel-like substance that encloses food particles. This property allows soluble fiber to bind and excrete fats from the body. This type of fiber has been shown to lower blood cholesterol and blood sugar levels. Soluble fiber is found primarily in oats, fruits, barley, legumes, and psyllium (an ancient Indian grain added to some breakfast cereals).
2. *Insoluble fiber* is not easily dissolved in water, and the body cannot digest it. This type of fiber is important because it binds water, causing a softer and bulkier stool that increases **peristalsis,** the involuntary muscle contractions of intestinal walls that force the stool through the intestines and enable quicker excretion of food residues. Speeding the passage of food residues through the intestines seems to lower the risk for colon cancer, mainly because it reduces the amount of time that cancer-causing agents are in contact with the intestinal wall. Insoluble fiber is also thought to bind with carcinogens (cancer-producing substances), and more water in the stool may dilute the cancer-causing agents, lessening their potency. Sources of insoluble fiber include wheat, cereals, vegetables, and skins of fruits.

TABLE 3.1 Dietary Fiber Content of Selected Foods

Food (gm)	Serving Size	Dietary Fiber
Almonds, shelled	¼ cup	3.9
Apple	1 medium	3.7
Banana	1 small	1.2
Beans (red kidney)	½ cup	8.2
Blackberries	½ cup	4.9
Beets, red, canned (cooked)	½ cup	1.4
Brazil nuts	1 oz	2.5
Broccoli (cooked)	½ cup	3.3
Brown rice (cooked)	½ cup	1.7
Carrots (cooked)	½ cup	3.3
Cauliflower (cooked)	½ cup	5.0
Cereal		
All Bran	1 oz	8.5
Cheerios	1 oz	1.1
Cornflakes	1 oz	0.5
Fruit and Fibre	1 oz	4.0
Fruit Wheats	1 oz	2.0
Just Right	1 oz	2.0
Wheaties	1 oz	2.0
Corn (cooked)	½ cup	2.2
Eggplant (cooked)	½ cup	3.0
Lettuce (chopped)	½ cup	0.5
Orange	1 medium	4.3
Parsnips (cooked)	½ cup	2.1
Pear	1 medium	4.5
Peas (cooked)	½ cup	4.4
Popcorn (plain)	1 cup	1.2
Potato (baked)	1 medium	4.9
Strawberries	½ cup	1.6
Summer squash (cooked)	½ cup	1.6
Watermelon	1 cup	0.1

The most common types of fiber are:

1. *Cellulose:* water-soluble fiber found in plant cell walls.
2. *Hemicellulose:* water-soluble fiber found in cereal fibers.

Monosaccharides The simplest carbohydrates (sugars), formed by five- or six-carbon skeletons. The three most common monosaccharides are glucose, fructose, and galactose.

Adipose tissue Fat cells in the body.

Disaccharides Simple carbohydrates formed by two monosaccharide units linked together, one of which is glucose. The major disaccharides are sucrose, lactose, and maltose.

Complex carbohydrates Carbohydrates formed by three or more simple sugar molecules linked together; also referred to as polysaccharides.

Glycogen Form in which glucose is stored in the body.

Dietary fiber A complex carbohydrate in plant foods that is not digested but is essential to digestion.

Peristalsis Involuntary muscle contractions of intestinal walls that facilitate excretion of wastes.

Behavior Modification Planning

TIPS TO INCREASE FIBER IN YOUR DIET

- Eat more vegetables, either raw or steamed
- Eat salads daily that include a wide variety of vegetables
- Eat more fruit, including the skin
- Choose whole-wheat and whole-grain products
- Choose breakfast cereals with more than 3 grams of fiber per serving
- Sprinkle a teaspoon or two of unprocessed bran or 100 percent bran cereal on your favorite breakfast cereal
- Add high-fiber cereals to casseroles and desserts
- Add beans to soups, salads, and stews
- Add vegetables to sandwiches: sprouts, green and red pepper strips, diced carrots, sliced cucumbers, red cabbage, onions
- Add vegetables to spaghetti: broccoli, cauliflower, sliced carrots, mushrooms
- Experiment with unfamiliar fruits and vegetables—collards, kale, broccoflower, asparagus, papaya, mango, kiwi, starfruit
- Blend fruit juice with small pieces of fruit and crushed ice
- When increasing fiber in your diet, drink plenty of fluids

Try It

Do you know your average daily fiber intake? If you do not know, keep a 3-day record of daily fiber intake. How do you fare against the recommended guidelines? If your intake is low, how can you change your diet to increase your daily fiber intake?

3. *Pectins:* water-insoluble fiber found in vegetables and fruits.
4. *Gums and mucilages:* water-insoluble fiber also found in small amounts in foods of plant origin.

Surprisingly, excessive fiber intake can be detrimental to health. It can produce loss of calcium, phosphorus, and iron, not to mention gastrointestinal discomfort. If your fiber intake is below the recommended amount, increase your intake gradually over several weeks to avoid gastrointestinal disturbances. While increasing your fiber intake, be sure to drink more water to avoid constipation and even dehydration.

Fats (Lipids)

The human body uses **fats** as a source of energy. Also called lipids, fats are the most concentrated energy source, with each gram of fat supplying 9 calories to the body (in contrast to 4 for carbohydrates). Fats are a part of the human cell structure. Deposits of fat cells are used as stored energy and as an insulator to preserve body heat. They absorb shock, supply essential fatty acids, and carry the fat-soluble vitamins A, D, E, and K. Fats can be classified into three main groups: simple, compound, and derived (see Figure 3.3). The most familiar sources of fat are whole milk and other dairy products, meats, and meat alternatives such as eggs and nuts.

FIGURE 3.3 Major types of fats (lipids).

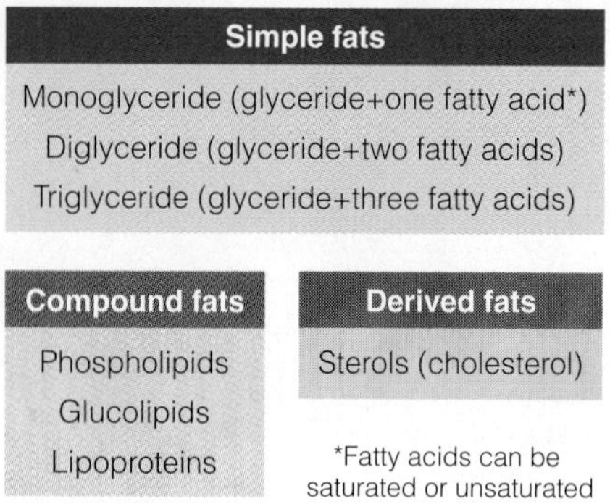

Simple fats
Monoglyceride (glyceride+one fatty acid*)
Diglyceride (glyceride+two fatty acids)
Triglyceride (glyceride+three fatty acids)

Compound fats	Derived fats
Phospholipids	Sterols (cholesterol)
Glucolipids	
Lipoproteins	

*Fatty acids can be saturated or unsaturated

Simple Fats

A simple fat consists of a glyceride molecule linked to one, two, or three units of fatty acids. Depending on the number of fatty acids attached, simple fats are divided into *monoglycerides* (one fatty acid), *diglycerides* (two fatty acids), and *triglycerides* (three fatty acids). More than 90 percent of the weight of fat in foods and more than 95 percent of the stored fat in the human body are in the form of triglycerides.

The length of the carbon atom chain and the amount of hydrogen saturation (that is, the number of hydrogen molecules attached to the carbon chain) in fatty acids vary. Based on the extent of saturation, fatty acids are said to be saturated or unsaturated. Unsaturated fatty acids are classified further into monounsaturated and polyunsaturated fatty acids. Saturated fatty acids are mainly of animal origin, and unsaturated fats are found mostly in plant products.

Saturated Fats. In saturated fatty acids (or "saturated fats"), the carbon atoms are fully saturated with hydrogen atoms; only single bonds link the carbon atoms on the chain (see Figure 3.4). Foods high in saturated fatty acids are meats, animal fat, lard, whole milk, cream, butter, cheese, ice cream, hydrogenated oils (hydrogenation makes oils saturated), coconut oil, and palm oils. Saturated fats typically do not melt at room temperature. Coconut and palm oils are exceptions. In general, saturated fats raise the blood cholesterol level. The data on coconut and palm oils are controversial, as

FIGURE 3.4 Chemical structure of saturated and unsaturated fats.

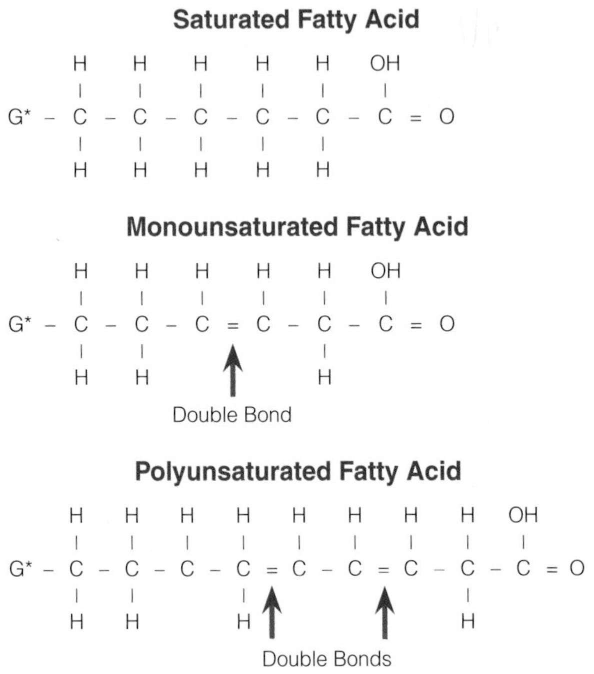

Saturated Fatty Acid

```
       H    H    H    H    H    OH
       |    |    |    |    |    |
G* -   C  - C  - C  - C  - C  - C = O
       |    |    |    |    |
       H    H    H    H    H
```

Monounsaturated Fatty Acid

```
       H    H    H    H    H    OH
       |    |    |    |    |    |
G* -   C  - C  - C  = C  - C  - C = O
       |    |              |
       H    H     ↑        H
              Double Bond
```

Polyunsaturated Fatty Acid

```
      H   H   H   H   H   H   H   H   OH
      |   |   |   |   |   |   |   |   |
G* -  C - C - C - C = C - C = C - C - C = O
      |   |       |               |
      H   H       H ↑       ↑     H
                   Double Bonds
```

*Glyceride component

some research indicates that these oils may be neutral in terms of their effects on cholesterol and actually may provide some health benefits.

Unsaturated Fats. In unsaturated fatty acids (or "unsaturated fats"), double bonds form between unsaturated carbons. These healthy fatty acids include monounsaturated and polyunsaturated fats, which are usually liquid at room temperature. Other shorter fatty acid chains also tend to be liquid at room temperature. Unsaturated fats help lower blood cholesterol. When unsaturated fats replace saturated fats in the diet, the former stimulate the liver to clear cholesterol from the blood.

In monounsaturated fatty acids (MUFA), only one double bond is found along the chain. Monounsaturated fatty acids are found in olive, canola, peanut, and sesame oils. They are also found in avocados, peanuts, and cashews.

Polyunsaturated fatty acids (PUFA) contain two or more double bonds between unsaturated carbon atoms along the chain. Corn, cottonseed, safflower, walnut, sunflower, and soybean oils are high in polyunsaturated fatty acids, also found in fish, almonds, and pecans.

Trans Fatty Acids. Hydrogen often is added to monounsaturated and polyunsaturated fats to increase shelf life and to solidify them so they are more spreadable. During this process, called "partial hydrogenation," the position of hydrogen atoms may be changed along the carbon chain, transforming the fat into a **trans fatty acid.** Margarine and spreads, shortening, some nut butters, crackers, cookies, dairy products, meats, processed foods, and fast foods often contain trans fatty acids.

Trans fatty acids are not essential and provide no known health benefit. In truth, health-conscious people minimize their intake of these types of fats because diets high in trans fatty acids increase rigidity of the coronary arteries, elevate cholesterol, and contribute to the formation of blood clots that may lead to heart attacks and strokes.

Trans fats are found in about 40 percent of supermarket foods, including almost all cookies, 80 percent of frozen breakfast foods, 75 percent of snacks and chips, most cake mixes, and almost 50 percent of all cereals. Doughnuts, french fries, stick margarine, vegetable shortening, and cookies and crackers are all high in trans fatty acid content.[2]

Paying attention to food labels is important, because the words "partially hydrogenated" and "trans fatty acids" indicate that the product carries a health risk just as high as that of saturated fat. Starting in 2006, the Food and Drug Administration requires that food labels list trans fatty acids so consumers can make healthier choices.

A type of polyunsaturated fatty acids that has gained attention in recent years are the **omega-3 fatty acids** (specifically alpha-linolenic acid), which are heart-healthy. Fish—especially fresh or frozen mackerel, herring, tuna, salmon, and lake trout—and flaxseed contain omega-3 fatty acids. Canned fish is not recommended, because the canning process destroys most of the omega-3 oil. These fatty acids are also found, but to a lesser extent, in flaxseeds, canola oil, walnuts, and wheat germ. Omega-3 fatty acids help to decrease the risk for blood clots, abnormal heart rhythms, high blood pressure, inflammation, heart attack, and stroke.

Potential contaminants in fish, in particular mercury, have created concerns among some people. Pregnant women and children should avoid mercury in fish. Farm-raised salmon also has slightly higher levels of polychlorinated biphenyls (PCBs), which the Environmental Protection Agency (EPA) lists as a "probable human carcinogen." The best recommendation is to balance the risks against the benefits. The American Heart

---

Fats A classification of nutrients containing carbon, hydrogen, some oxygen, and sometimes other chemical elements.

Trans fatty acid Solidified fat formed by adding hydrogen to monounsaturated and polyunsaturated fats to increase shelf life.

Omega-3 fatty acids Polyunsaturated fatty acids found primarily in cold-water seafood, flaxseed, and flaxseed oil; thought to lower blood cholesterol and triglycerides.

Association recommends consuming fish twice a week. At this point, the risk of adverse effects from eating fish is extremely low and primarily theoretical in nature.[3] If you are still concerned, use canned tuna and wild salmon, which are lower in contaminants.

One of the simplest ways to increase omega-3 fatty acids is to consume flaxseed, which is also high in fiber and plant chemicals known as *lignans*. The oil in flaxseed is high in alpha-linolenic acid and has been shown to reduce abnormal heart rhythms and prevent blood clots.[4] Studies are being conducted to investigate the potential cancer-fighting ability of lignans. In one report, the addition of a daily ounce (3 to 4 tablespoons) of ground flaxseeds to the diet seemed to lead to a decrease in the onset of tumors, preventing their formation, and even led to a shrinkage of tumors.[5]

Excessive flaxseed in the diet, however, is not recommended. High doses actually may be detrimental to health. Pregnant and lactating women, especially, should not consume large amounts of flaxseed.

Because flaxseeds have a hard outer shell, they should be ground to obtain the nutrients; whole seeds will pass through the body undigested. Flavor and nutrients are best preserved by grinding the seeds just before use. Pre-ground seeds should be kept sealed and refrigerated. Ground flaxseeds can be mixed with salad dressings, salads, wheat flour, pancakes, muffins, cereals, rice, cottage cheese, and yogurt. Flaxseed oil also may be used, but the oil has little or no fiber and lignans and must be kept refrigerated because it spoils quickly. The oil cannot be used for cooking either, because it scorches easily.

Other essential unsaturated fatty acids are the **omega-6 fatty acids** group, in particular linoleic acid. Our diets typically are high in omega-6-rich oils, found in corn, soybean, sunflower, cottonseed, and most oils in processed foods. Most of the polyunsaturated fatty acids consumed by Americans are omega-6 fatty acids. We usually consume 10 to 20 times more omega-6 than omega-3. Excessive omega-6 fatty acids amplify inflammatory processes that can damage organs in the body. To decrease your intake of linoleic acid, watch for corn, soybean, sunflower, and cottonseed oils in salad dressings, mayonnaise, and margarine.

The National Academy of Sciences has set recommended intakes for alpha-linolenic acid and linoleic acid. For alpha-linolenic acid, the recommendations are 1.6 and 1.1 grams per day for men and women, respectively. The standard for linoleic acid has been set at 17 grams per day for men and 12 grams for women.

Data suggest that the amount of fish oil obtained by eating one or two servings of fish weekly lessens the risk of mortality from coronary heart disease. But people who have diabetes or a history of hemorrhaging or strokes, who are on aspirin or blood-thinning therapy, or who are presurgical patients should not consume fish oil except under a physician's instruction.

Compound Fats

Compound fats are a combination of simple fats and other chemicals. Examples are:

1. *Phospholipids:* similar to triglycerides, except that choline (or another compound) and phosphoric acid take the place of one of the fatty acid units.
2. *Glucolipids:* a combination of carbohydrates, fatty acids, and nitrogen.
3. *Lipoproteins:* water-soluble aggregates of protein and triglycerides, phospholipids, or cholesterol.

Lipoproteins (a combination of lipids and proteins) are especially important because they transport fats in the blood. The major forms of lipoproteins are high-density (HDL), low-density (LDL), and very-low-density (VLDL) lipoproteins. Lipoproteins play a large role in developing or in preventing heart disease. High HDL ("good" cholesterol) levels have been associated with lower risk for coronary heart disease, whereas high LDL ("bad" cholesterol) levels have been linked to increased risk for this disease. HDL is more than 50 percent protein and contains little cholesterol. LDL is approximately 25 percent protein and nearly 50 percent cholesterol. VLDL contains about 50 percent triglycerides, only about 10 percent protein, and 20 percent cholesterol.

Derived Fats

Derived fats combine simple and compound fats. **Sterols** are an example. Although sterols contain no fatty acids, they are considered lipids because they do not dissolve in water. The sterol mentioned most often is cholesterol, which is found in many foods or can be manufactured in the body—primarily from saturated fats and trans fats.

Proteins

Proteins are the main substances the body uses to build and repair tissues such as muscles, blood, internal organs, skin, hair, nails, and bones. They form a part of hormone, antibody, and **enzyme** molecules. Enzymes play a key role in all of the body's processes. Because all enzymes are formed by proteins, this nutrient is necessary for normal functioning. Proteins also help maintain the normal balance of body fluids.

Proteins can be used as a source of energy, too, but only if sufficient carbohydrates are not available. Each gram of protein yields 4 calories of energy (the same as carbohydrates). The main sources of protein are meats and alternatives, milk, and other dairy products. Excess proteins may be converted to glucose or fat, or even excreted in the urine.

The human body uses 20 **amino acids** to form different types of protein. Amino acids contain nitrogen,

TABLE 3.2 Amino Acids

Essential Amino Acids*	Nonessential Amino Acids
Histidine	Alanine
Isoleucine	Arginine
Leucine	Asparagine
Lysine	Aspartic acid
Methionine	Cysteine
Phenylalanine	Glutamic acid
Threonine	Glutamine
Tryptophan	Glycine
Valine	Proline
	Serine
	Tyrosine

* Must be provided in the diet because the body cannot manufacture them.

carbon, hydrogen, and oxygen. Of the 20 amino acids, nine are called "essential amino acids" because the body cannot produce them. The other 11, termed "nonessential amino acids," can be manufactured in the body if food proteins in the diet provide enough nitrogen (see Table 3.2). For the body to function normally, all amino acids shown in the table must be present in the diet.

Proteins that contain all the essential amino acids, known as "complete" or "higher-quality" protein, are usually of animal origin. If one or more of the essential amino acids are missing, the proteins are termed "incomplete" or "lower-quality" protein. Individuals have to take in enough protein to ensure nitrogen for adequate production of amino acids and also to get enough high-quality protein to obtain the essential amino acids.

Protein deficiency is not a problem in the typical U.S. diet. Two glasses of skim milk combined with about 4 ounces of poultry or fish meet the daily protein requirement. But too much animal protein can cause health problems. Some people eat twice as much protein as they need. Protein foods from animal sources are often high in fat, saturated fat, and cholesterol, which can lead to cardiovascular disease and cancer. Too much animal protein also decreases the blood enzymes that prevent precancerous cells from developing into tumors.

As mentioned earlier, a well-balanced diet contains a variety of foods from all five basic food groups, including wise selection of foods from animal sources (see also "Balancing the Diet," page 72). Based on current nutrition data, meat (poultry and fish included) should be replaced by grains, legumes, vegetables, and fruits as main courses. Meats should be used more for flavoring than for volume. Daily consumption of beef, poultry, or fish should be limited to 3 ounces (about the size of a deck of cards) to 6 ounces.

Vitamins

Vitamins are necessary for normal bodily metabolism, growth, and development. Vitamins are classified into two types based on their solubility:

1. fat-soluble (A, D, E, and K)
2. water-soluble (B complex and C).

The body does not manufacture most vitamins, so they can be obtained only through a well-balanced diet. To decrease loss of vitamins during cooking, natural foods should be microwaved or steamed rather than boiled in water that is thrown out later.

A few exceptions, such as vitamins A, D, and K, are formed in the body. Vitamin A is produced from beta-carotene, found mainly in yellow foods such as carrots, pumpkin, and sweet potatoes. Vitamin D is created when ultraviolet light from the sun transforms 7-dehydrocholesterol, a compound in human skin. Vitamin K is created in the body by intestinal bacteria. The major functions of vitamins are outlined in Table 3.3.

Vitamins C, E, and beta-carotene also function as antioxidants, which are thought to play a key role in preventing chronic diseases. The specific functions of these antioxidant nutrients and of the mineral selenium (also an antioxidant) are discussed under "Antioxidants" (page 84).

Minerals

Approximately 25 **minerals** have important roles in body functioning. Minerals are inorganic substances contained in all cells, especially those in hard parts of the body (bones, nails, teeth). Minerals are crucial to maintaining water balance and the acid–base balance. They are essential components of respiratory pigments, enzymes, and enzyme systems, and they regulate mus-

Omega-6 fatty acids Polyunsaturated fatty acids found primarily in corn and sunflower oils and most oils in processed foods.

Lipoproteins Lipids covered by proteins, these transport fats in the blood. Types are LDL, HDL, and VLDL.

Sterols Derived fats, of which cholesterol is the best-known example.

Proteins A classification of nutrients consisting of complex organic compounds containing nitrogen and formed by combinations of amino acids; the main substances used in the body to build and repair tissues.

Enzymes Catalysts that facilitate chemical reactions in the body.

Amino acids Chemical compounds that contain nitrogen, carbon, hydrogen, and oxygen; the basic building blocks the body uses to build different types of protein.

Vitamins Organic nutrients essential for normal metabolism, growth, and development of the body.

Minerals Inorganic nutrients essential for normal body functions; found in the body and in food.

TABLE 3.3 Major Functions of Vitamins

Nutrient	Good Sources	Major Functions	Deficiency Symptoms
Vitamin A	Milk, cheese, eggs, liver, yellow and dark-green fruits and vegetables	Required for healthy bones, teeth, skin, gums, and hair; maintenance of inner mucous membranes, thus increasing resistance to infection; adequate vision in dim light.	Night blindness; decreased growth; decreased resistance to infection; rough, dry skin
Vitamin D	Fortified milk, cod liver oil, salmon, tuna, egg yolk	Necessary for bones and teeth; needed for calcium and phosphorus absorption.	Rickets (bone softening), fractures, muscle spasms
Vitamin E	Vegetable oils, yellow and green leafy vegetables, margarine, wheat germ, whole-grain breads and cereals	Related to oxidation and normal muscle and red blood cell chemistry.	Leg cramps, red blood cell breakdown
Vitamin K	Green leafy vegetables, cauliflower, cabbage, eggs, peas, potatoes	Essential for normal blood clotting.	Hemorrhaging
Vitamin B_1 (Thiamin)	Whole-grain or enriched bread, lean meats and poultry, fish, liver, pork, poultry, organ meats, legumes, nuts, dried yeast	Assists in proper use of carbohydrates, normal functioning of nervous system, maintenance of good appetite.	Loss of appetite, nausea, confusion, cardiac abnormalities, muscle spasms
Vitamin B_2 (Riboflavin)	Eggs, milk, leafy green vegetables, whole grains, lean meats, dried beans and peas	Contributes to energy release from carbohydrates, fats, and proteins; needed for normal growth and development, good vision, and healthy skin.	Cracking of the corners of the mouth, inflammation of the skin, impaired vision
Vitamin B_6 (Pyridoxine)	Vegetables, meats, whole-grain cereals, soybeans, peanuts, potatoes	Necessary for protein and fatty acids metabolism and for normal red blood cell formation.	Depression, irritability, muscle spasms, nausea
Vitamin B_{12}	Meat, poultry, fish, liver, organ meats, eggs, shellfish, milk, cheese	Required for normal growth, red blood cell formation, nervous system and digestive tract functioning.	Impaired balance, weakness, drop in red blood cell count
Niacin	Liver and organ meats, meat, fish, poultry, whole grains, enriched breads, nuts, green leafy vegetables, and dried beans and peas	Contributes to energy release from carbohydrates, fats, and proteins; normal growth and development; and formation of hormones and nerve-regulating substances.	Confusion, depression, weakness, weight loss
Biotin	Liver, kidney, eggs, yeast, legumes, milk, nuts, dark-green vegetables	Essential for carbohydrate metabolism and fatty acid synthesis.	Inflamed skin, muscle pain, depression, weight loss
Folic Acid	Leafy green vegetables, organ meats, whole grains and cereals, dried beans	Needed for cell growth and reproduction and for red blood cell formation.	Decreased resistance to infection
Pantothenic Acid	All natural foods, especially liver, kidney, eggs, nuts, yeast, milk, dried peas and beans, green leafy vegetables	Related to carbohydrate and fat metabolism.	Depression, low blood sugar, leg cramps, nausea, headaches
Vitamin C (Ascorbic acid)	Fruits, vegetables	Helps protect against infection; required for formation of collagenous tissue, normal blood vessels, teeth, and bones.	Slow-healing wounds, loose teeth, hemorrhaging, rough scaly skin, irritability

cular and nervous tissue impulses, blood clotting, and normal heart rhythm.

The four minerals mentioned most often are calcium, iron, sodium, and selenium. Calcium deficiency may result in osteoporosis, and low iron intake can induce iron-deficiency anemia (see pages 94–97). High sodium intake may contribute to high blood pressure. Selenium seems to be important in preventing certain types of cancer. Specific functions of some of the most important minerals are given in Table 3.4.

Water

The most important nutrient is **water,** as it is involved in almost every vital body process: in digesting and absorbing food, in producing energy, in the circulatory process, in regulating body heat, in removing waste products, in building and rebuilding cells, and in transporting other nutrients. In males, about 61 percent of total body weight is water. The proportion of body weight in women is 56 percent (see Figure 3.5). The difference is due primarily to the higher amount of muscle mass in men.

Almost all foods contain water, but it is found primarily in liquid foods, fruits, and vegetables. Although for decades the recommendation was to consume at least 8 cups of water per day, a panel of scientists of the Institute of Medicine of the National Academy of Sciences (NAS) indicated in 2004 that people are getting enough water from the liquids (milk, juices, sodas, coffee) and the moisture content of solid foods. Most Americans and Canadians remain well hydrated simply by using thirst as their guide. Caffeine-containing drinks also are acceptable as a water source because

TABLE 3.4 Major Functions of Minerals

Nutrient	Good Sources	Major Functions	Deficiency Symptoms
Calcium	Milk, yogurt, cheese, green leafy vegetables, dried beans, sardines, salmon	Required for strong teeth and bone formation; maintenance of good muscle tone, heartbeat, and nerve function.	Bone pain and fractures, periodontal disease, muscle cramps
Copper	Seafood, meats, beans, nuts, whole grains	Helps with iron absorption and hemoglobin formation; required to synthesize the enzyme cytochrome oxidase.	Anemia (although deficiency is rare in humans)
Iron	Organ meats, lean meats, seafood, eggs, dried peas and beans, nuts, whole and enriched grains, green leafy vegetables	Major component of hemoglobin; aids in energy utilization.	Nutritional anemia, overall weakness
Phosphorus	Meats, fish, milk, eggs, dried beans and peas, whole grains, processed foods	Required for bone and teeth formation and for energy release regulation.	Bone pain and fracture, weight loss, weakness
Zinc	Milk, meat, seafood, whole grains, nuts, eggs, dried beans	Essential component of hormones, insulin and enzymes; used in normal growth and development.	Loss of appetite, slow-healing wounds, skin problems
Magnesium	Green leafy vegetables, whole grains, nuts, soybeans, seafood, legumes	Needed for bone growth and maintenance, carbohydrate and protein utilization, nerve function, temperature regulation.	Irregular heartbeat, weakness, muscle spasms, sleeplessness
Sodium	Table salt, processed foods, meat	Needed for body fluid regulation, transmission of nerve impulses, heart action.	Rarely seen
Potassium	Legumes, whole grains, bananas, orange juice, dried fruits, potatoes	Required for heart action, bone formation and maintenance, regulation of energy release, acid-base regulation.	Irregular heartbeat, nausea, weakness
Selenium	Seafood, meat, whole grains	Component of enzymes; functions in close association with vitamin E.	Muscle pain, possible heart muscle deterioration, possible hair loss and nail loss

FIGURE 3.5 Approximate proportions of nutrients in the human body.

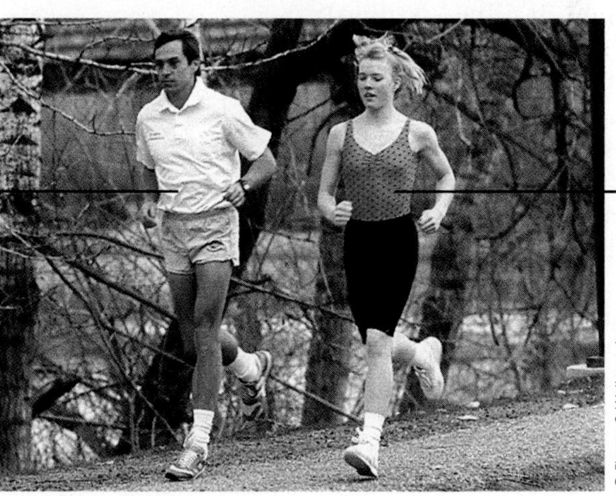

Higher percentage of fat tissue in women is normal and needed for reproduction

data indicate that people who regularly consume such beverages do not have more 24-hour urine output than those who don't.

An exception of not waiting for the thirst signal to replenish water loss is when an individual exercises in the heat or does so for an extended time (see Chapter 9, page 302). Water lost under these conditions must be replenished regularly. If you wait for the thirst signal, you may have lost too much water already. At 2 percent

Water The most important classification of essential body nutrients, involved in almost every vital body process.

TABLE 3.5 The American Diet: Current and Recommended Carbohydrate, Fat, and Protein Intake Expressed as a Percentage of Total Calories

	Current Percentage	Recommended Percentage*
Carbohydrates:	50%	45–65%
Simple	26%	Less than **25%**
Complex	24%	**20–40%**
Fat:	34%	**20–30%****
Monounsaturated:	11%	Up to **20%**
Polyunsaturated:	10%	Up to **10%**
Saturated:	13%	Less than **7%**
Protein:	16%	**10–35%**

* Source of recommended % is the 2002 recommended guidelines by the National Academy of Sciences.

** Up to 35% is allowed for individuals with metabolic syndrome who may need additional fat in the diet.

of body weight lost, a person is dehydrated. At 5 percent, one may become dizzy and disoriented, have trouble with cognitive skills and heart function, and even lose consciousness.

Balancing the Diet

One of the fundamental ways to enjoy good health and live life to its fullest is through a well-balanced diet. Several guidelines have been published to help you accomplish this. As illustrated in Table 3.5, the most recent recommended guidelines by the National Academy of Sciences (NAS) state that daily caloric intake should be distributed so that 45 to 65 percent of the total calories come from carbohydrates (mostly complex carbohydrates and less than 25 percent from sugar), 20 to 35 percent from fat, and 10 to 35 percent from protein.[6] The recommended ranges allow for flexibility in planning diets according to individual health and physical activity needs.

In addition to the macronutrients, the diet must include all of the essential vitamins, minerals, and water. The source of fat calories is also critical. The National Cholesterol Education Program recommends that, of total calories, saturated fat should constitute less than 7 percent, polyunsaturated up to 10 percent, and monounsaturated fat up to 20 percent. Rating a particular diet accurately is difficult without a complete nutrient analysis. You have an opportunity to perform this analysis in Labs 3A and 3B.

The NAS guidelines vary slightly from those previously issued by major national health organizations, which recommend 50 to 60 percent of total calories from carbohydrates, less than 30 percent from fat, and about 15 percent from protein. These percentages are within the ranges recommended by the NAS. The most drastic difference appears in the NAS allowed range of fat intake, up to 35 percent of total calories. This higher percentage, however, was included to accommodate individuals with metabolic syndrome (see Chapter 11, page 378) who have an abnormal insulin response to carbohydrates and may need additional fat in the diet. For all other individuals, daily fat intake should not exceed 30 percent of total caloric intake.

The NAS recommendations will be effective only if people consistently replace saturated and trans fatty acids with unsaturated fatty acids. The latter will require changes in the typical "unhealthy" American diet, which is generally high in red meats, whole dairy products, and fast foods—all of which are high in saturated and/or trans fatty acids.

Diets in most developed countries changed significantly after the turn of the 20th century. Today, people eat more calories and fat, fewer carbohydrates, and about the same amount of protein. People also weigh more than they did in 1900, an indication that we are eating more calories and are not as physically active as our forebears.

Nutrition Standards

Nutritionists use a variety of nutrient standards, the most widely known of which is the RDA, or Recommended Dietary Allowances. This, however, is not the only standard. Among others are the Dietary Reference Intakes and the Daily Values on food labels. Each standard has a different purpose and utilization in dietary planning and assessment.

Dietary Reference Intakes (DRI)

To help people meet dietary guidelines, the National Academy of Sciences developed a set of dietary nutrient intakes for healthy people in the United States and Canada, the **Dietary Reference Intakes (DRI).** The DRIs are based on a review of the most current research on nutrient needs of healthy people. The DRI reports are written by the Food and Nutrition Board of the Institute of Medicine in cooperation with scientists from Canada.

The DRIs encompass four types of reference values for planning and assessing diets and for establishing adequate amounts and maximum safe nutrient intakes in the diet: Estimated Average Requirement (EAR), Recommended Dietary Allowance (RDA), Adequate Intakes (AI), and Tolerable Upper Intake Levels (UL). The type of reference value used for a given nutrient and a specific age/gender group is determined according to available scientific information and the intended use of the dietary standard.

EAR. The **Estimated Average Requirement (EAR)** is the amount of a nutrient that is estimated to meet the nutrient requirement of half the healthy people in spe-

TABLE 3.6 Dietary Reference Intakes (DRIs): Recommended Dietary Allowances (RDA) and Adequate Intakes (AI) for Selected Nutrients

	Recommended Dietary Allowances (RDA)													Adequate Intakes (AI)					
	Thiamin (mg)	Riboflavin (mg)	Niacin (mg NE)	Vitamin B_6 (mg)	Folate (mcg DFE)	Vitamin B12 (mcg)	Phosphorus (mg)	Magnesium (mg)	Vitamin A (mcg)	Vitamin C (mg)	Vitamin E (mg)	Selenium (mcg)	Iron (mcg)	Calcium (mg)	Vitamin D (mcg)	Fluoride (mg)	Pantothenic acid (mg)	Biotin (mg)	Choline (mg)
Males																			
14–18	1.2	1.3	16	1.3	400	2.4	1,250	410	900	75	15	55	11	1,300	5	3	5.0	25	550
19–30	1.2	1.3	16	1.3	400	2.4	700	400	900	90	15	55	8	1,000	5	4	5.0	30	550
31–50	1.2	1.3	16	1.3	400	2.4	700	420	900	90	15	55	8	1,000	5	4	5.0	30	550
51–70	1.2	1.3	16	1.7	400	2.4	700	420	900	90	15	55	8	1,200	10	4	5.0	30	550
>70	1.2	1.3	16	1.7	400	2.4	700	420	900	90	15	55	8	1,200	15	4	5.0	30	550
Females																			
14–18	1.0	1.0	14	1.2	400	2.4	1,250	360	700	65	15	55	15	1,300	5	3	5.0	25	400
19–30	1.1	1.1	14	1.3	400	2.4	700	310	700	75	15	55	18	1,000	5	3	5.0	30	425
31–50	1.1	1.1	14	1.3	400	2.4	700	320	700	75	15	55	18	1,000	5	3	5.0	30	425
51–70	1.1	1.1	14	1.5	400	2.4	700	320	700	75	15	55	8	1,200	10	3	5.0	30	425
>70	1.1	1.1	14	1.5	400	2.4	700	320	700	75	15	55	8	1,200	15	3	5.0	30	425
Pregnant	1.4	1.4	18	1.9	600	2.6	*	+40	750	85	15	60	27	*	*	3	6.0	30	450
Lactating	1.5	1.6	17	2.0	500	2.8	*	*	1,300	120	19	70	10	*	*	3	7.0	35	550

* Values for these nutrients do not change with pregnancy or lactation. Use the value listed for women of comparable age.
Source: Adapted with permission from *Recommended Dietary Allowances,* 10th Edition, and the *Dietary Reference Intakes* series. Copyright © 1989 and 2002, respectively, by the National Academy of Sciences. Courtesy of the National Academies Press, Washington, DC.

cific age and gender groups. At this nutrient intake level, the nutritional requirements of 50 percent of the people are not met. For example, looking at 300 healthy women at age 26, the EAR would meet the nutritional requirement for only half of these women.

RDA. The **Recommended Dietary Allowance (RDA)** is the daily amount of a nutrient that is considered adequate to meet the known nutrient needs of nearly all healthy people in the United States. Because the committee must decide what level of intake to recommend for everybody, the RDA is set well above the EAR and covers about 98 percent of the population. Stated another way, the RDA recommendation for any nutrient is well above almost everyone's actual requirement. The RDA could be considered a goal for adequate intake. The process for determining the RDA depends on being able to set an EAR, because RDAs are determined statistically from the EAR values. If an EAR cannot be set, no RDA can be established.

AI. When data are insufficient or inadequate to set an EAR, an **Adequate Intake (AI)** value is determined instead of the RDA. The AI value is derived from approximations of observed nutrient intakes by a group or groups of healthy people. The AI value for children and adults is expected to meet or exceed the nutritional requirements of a corresponding healthy population.

Nutrients for which daily DRIs have been set are given in Table 3.6.

UL. The **Upper Intake Level (UL)** establishes the highest level of nutrient intake that seems to be safe for most healthy people, beyond which exists an increased

Dietary Reference Intakes (DRI) A general term that describes four types of nutrient standards that establish adequate amounts and maximum safe nutrient intakes in the diet: Estimated Average Requirements (EAR), Recommended Dietary Allowances (RDA), Adequate Intakes (AI), and Tolerable Upper Intake Levels (UL).

Estimated Average Requirement (EAR) The amount of a nutrient that meets the dietary needs of half the people.

Recommended Dietary Allowance (RDA) The daily amount of a nutrient (statistically determined from the EARs) that is considered adequate to meet the known nutrient needs of almost 98 percent of all healthy people in the United States.

Adequate Intake (AI) The recommended amount of a nutrient intake when sufficient evidence is not available to calculate the EAR and subsequent RDA.

Upper Intake Level (UL) The highest level of nutrient intake that seems safe for most healthy people, beyond which exists an increased risk of adverse effects.

TABLE 3.7 Tolerable Upper Intake Levels (UL) of Selected Nutrients for Adults (19–70 years)

Nutrient	UL per Day
Calcium	2.5 gr
Phosphorus	4.0 gr*
Magnesium	350 mg
Vitamin D	50 mcg
Fluoride	10 mg
Niacin	35 mg
Iron	45 mg
Vitamin B_6	100 mg
Folate	1,000 mcg
Choline	3.5 gr
Vitamin A	3,000 mcg
Vitamin C	2,000 mg
Vitamin E	1,000 mg
Selenium	400 mcg

* 3.5 gr per day for pregnant women.

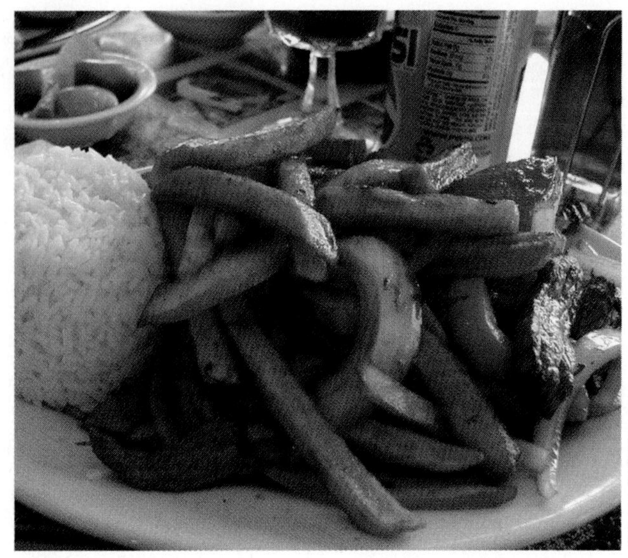

The typical American diet is too high in calories and saturated fat.

risk of adverse effects. As intakes increase above the UL, so does the risk of adverse effects. In general terms, the optimum nutrient range for healthy eating is between the RDA and the UL. The established ULs are presented in Table 3.7.

Daily Values

The **Daily Values (DVs)** are reference values for nutrients and food components for use on food labels. The DVs include fat, saturated fat, and carbohydrates (as a percent of total calories); cholesterol, sodium, and potassium (in milligrams); and fiber and protein (in grams). The DVs for total fat, saturated fat, and carbohydrate are expressed as percentages for a 2,000-calorie diet and therefore may require adjustments depending on an individual's daily **Estimated Energy Requirement (EER)** in calories. For example, on a 2,000-calorie diet (EER), the recommended carbohydrate intake is about 300 grams (about 60 percent of EER), and the recommendation for fat is 65 grams (about 30 percent of EER). The vitamin, mineral, and protein DVs were adapted from the RDAs. The DVs also are not as specific for age and gender groups as are the DRIs. Both the DRIs and the DVs apply only to healthy adults. They are not intended for people who are ill and may require additional nutrients. Figure 3.6 shows the food label with U.S. Recommended Daily Values.

Nutrient Analysis

The first step in evaluating your diet is to conduct a nutrient analysis. This can be quite educational, because most people do not realize how harmful and nonnutritious many common foods are. The top sources of calories in the American diet are soft drinks, sweet rolls, pastries, doughnuts, cakes, hamburgers, cheeseburgers, meatloaf, pizza, potato and corn chips, and buttered popcorn; all of which are low in essential nutrients and high in either fat and/or sugar and calories.

Most nutrient analyses cover calories, carbohydrates, fats, cholesterol, and sodium, as well as eight essential nutrients: protein, calcium, iron, vitamin A, thiamin, riboflavin, niacin, and vitamin C. If the diet has enough of these eight nutrients, the foods consumed in natural form to provide these nutrients typically contain all the other nutrients the human body needs.

To do your own nutrient analysis, keep a 3-day record of everything you eat using Figure 3A.1 in Lab 3A, (make additional copies of this form as needed). At the end of each day, look up the nutrient content for those foods in the list of Nutritive Values of Selected Foods (in Appendix A). Record this information on the form in Lab 3A. If you do not find a food in Appendix A, the information may be on the food container itself.

Critical Thinking

What do the nutrition standards mean to you? How much of a challenge would it be to apply those standards in your daily life?

Daily Values (DVs) Reference values for nutrients and food components used in food labels.

Estimated Energy Requirement (EER) The average dietary energy (caloric) intake that is predicted to maintain energy balance in a healthy adult of defined age, gender, weight, height, and level of physical activity, consistent with good health.

FIGURE 3.6 Food label with U.S. Recommended Daily Values.

1 Better by Design

How to recognize the new food labels

The new food labels feature a revamped nutrition panel titled "Nutrition Facts," with nutrient listings that reflect current health concerns. Now you'll be able to find information on fat, fiber, and other food components fundamental to lowering your risk of cancer and other chronic diseases. Listings for nutrients like thiamin and riboflavin will no longer be required, because Americans generally eat enough of them these days.

2 Size Up the Situation

All serving sizes are created equal

Now you can compare similar products and know that their serving sizes are basically identical. So when you realize how much fat is packed into that carton of double-dutch-chocolate-caramel-chew ice cream you're eyeing, you might opt for low-fat frozen yogurt instead. Serving sizes will also be standardized, so manufacturers can't make nutrition claims for unrealistically small portions. That means a chocolate cake, for example, must be divided into 8 servings sized to satisfy the average person—not 16 servings sized to satisfy the average munchkin.

3 Look Before You Leap

Use the Daily Values

You will find the Daily Values on the bottom half of the "Nutrition Facts" panel. Some represent maximum levels of nutrients that should be consumed each day for a healthful diet (as with fat) while others refer to minimum levels that can be exceeded (as with carbohydrates). They are based on both a 2,000 and 2,500 calorie diet. Your own needs may be more or less, but these figures give you a point from which to compare. For example, the sample label indicates that someone with a 2,000 calorie diet should eat no more than 65 grams of fat per day. This is based on a diet getting 30 percent of calories as fat. If you normally eat less calories, or want to eat less than 30 percent of calories as fat, your daily fat consumption will be lower.

4 Rate It Right

Scan the % Daily Values

The % Daily Values make judging the nutritional quality of a food a snap. For instance, you can look at the % Daily Value column and find that a food has 25 percent of the Daily Value for fiber. This means the product will give you a substantial portion of the recommended amount of fiber for the day. You can also use this column to compare nutrients in similar products. The % Daily Values are based on a 2,000 calorie diet.

5 Trust Adjectives

Descriptors have legal definitions

Terms like "low," "high," and "free" have long been used on food labels. What these words actually mean, however, could vary. Thanks to the new labeling laws, such descriptions must now meet legal definitions. For example, you may be shopping for foods high in vitamin A, which has been linked to lower risk of certain cancers. Under the new label laws, a food described as "high" in a particular nutrient must contain 20 percent or more of the Daily Value for that nutrient. So if the bottle of juice you're thinking of buying says "high in vitamin A," you can now feel confident that it really is a good source of the vitamin.

6 Read Health Claims with Confidence

The nutrient link to disease prevention

You can also expect to see food packages with health claims linking certain nutrients to reduced risk of cancer and other diseases. The federal government has approved three health claims dealing with cancer prevention: a low-fat diet may reduce your risk for cancer; high fiber foods may reduce your risk for cancer; and fruits and vegetables may reduce your risk for cancer. A food may not make such a health claim for one nutrient if it contains other nutrients that undermine its health benefits. A high fiber, but high fat, jelly doughnut cannot carry a health claim!

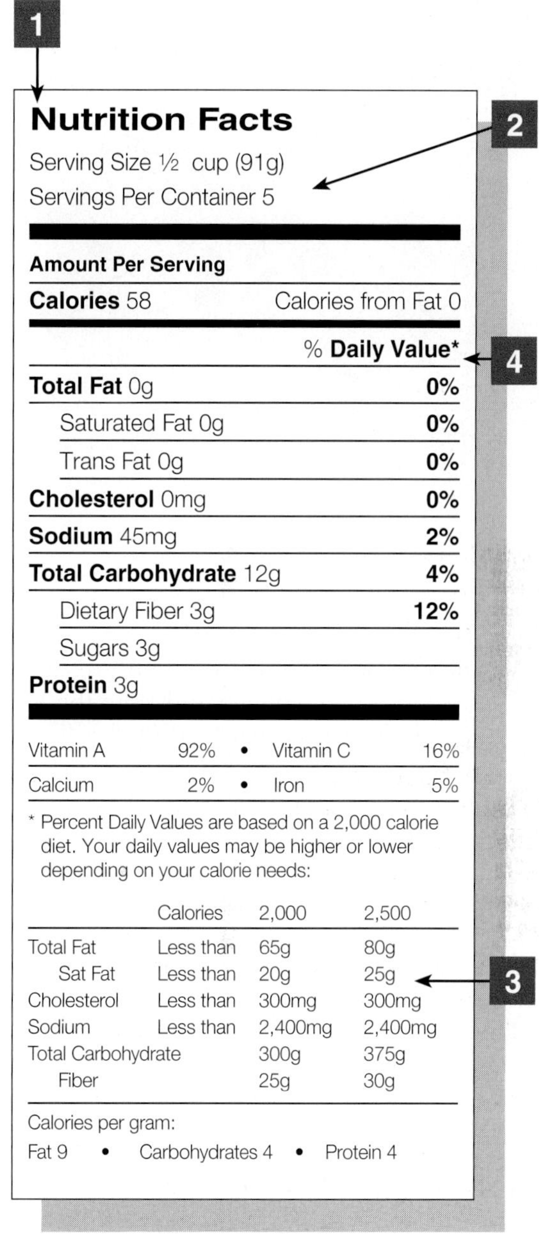

Nutrition Facts

Serving Size ½ cup (91g)
Servings Per Container 5

Amount Per Serving	
Calories 58	Calories from Fat 0
	% **Daily Value***
Total Fat 0g	**0%**
Saturated Fat 0g	**0%**
Trans Fat 0g	**0%**
Cholesterol 0mg	**0%**
Sodium 45mg	**2%**
Total Carbohydrate 12g	**4%**
Dietary Fiber 3g	**12%**
Sugars 3g	
Protein 3g	

Vitamin A	92%	•	Vitamin C	16%
Calcium	2%	•	Iron	5%

* Percent Daily Values are based on a 2,000 calorie diet. Your daily values may be higher or lower depending on your calorie needs:

	Calories	2,000	2,500
Total Fat	Less than	65g	80g
Sat Fat	Less than	20g	25g
Cholesterol	Less than	300mg	300mg
Sodium	Less than	2,400mg	2,400mg
Total Carbohydrate		300g	375g
Fiber		25g	30g

Calories per gram:
Fat 9 • Carbohydrates 4 • Protein 4

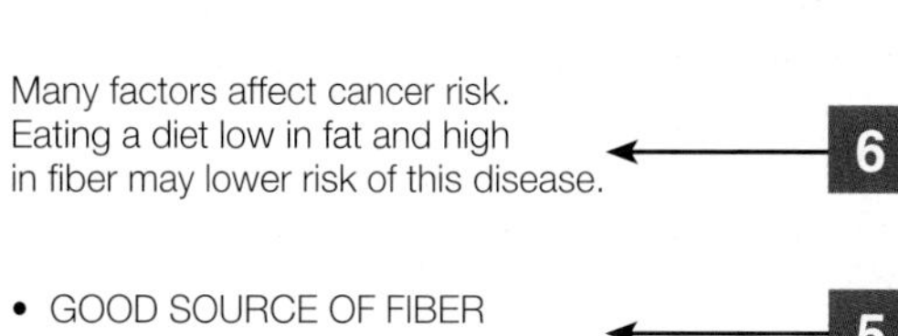

Reprinted with permission from the American Institute for Cancer Research

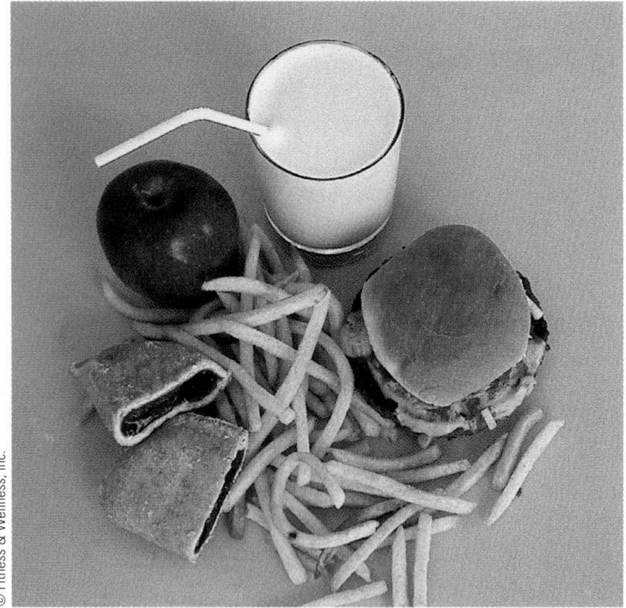

An apple a day will not keep the doctor away if most meals are high in fat content.

When you have recorded the nutritive values for each day, add up each column and write the totals at the bottom of the chart. After the third day, fill in your totals in Figure 3A.2 in Lab 3A and compute an average for the 3 days. To rate your diet, compare your figures with those in the Recommended Dietary Allowances (RDA) (Table 3.6). The results will give a good indication of areas of strength and deficiency in your current diet.

Some of the most revealing information learned in a nutrient analysis is the source of fat and saturated fat intake in the diet. The average daily fat consumption in the U.S. diet is about 34 percent of the total caloric intake, much of it from saturated and trans fatty acids, which increases the risk for chronic diseases such as cardiovascular disease, cancer, diabetes, and obesity. Although fat provides a smaller percentage of our total daily caloric intake as compared with two decades ago (37 percent), the decrease in percentage is simply because Americans now eat more calories than 20 years ago (335 additional daily calories for women and 170 for men).

As illustrated in Figure 3.7, 1 gram of carbohydrates or of protein supplies the body with 4 calories, and fat provides 9 calories per gram consumed (alcohol yields 7 calories per gram). Therefore, looking at only the total grams consumed for each type of food can be misleading.

For example, a person who eats 160 grams of carbohydrates, 100 grams of fat, and 70 grams of protein has a total intake of 330 grams of food. This indicates that 30 percent of the total grams of food is in the form of fat (100 grams of fat ÷ 30 grams of total food = .30; .30 × 100 = 30 percent)—and, in reality, almost half of that diet is in the form of fat calories.

FIGURE 3.7 Caloric value of food (fuel nutrients).

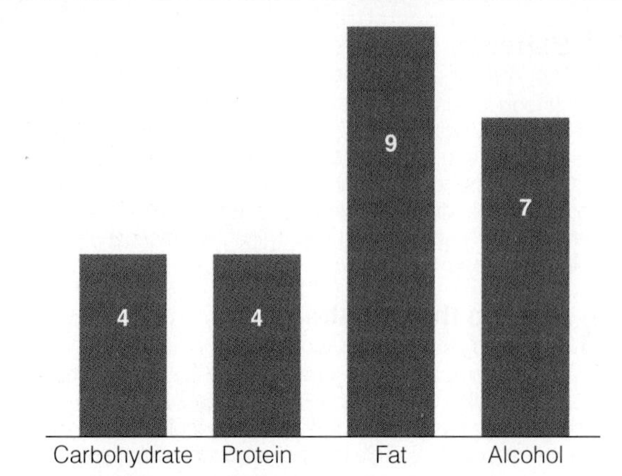

In the sample diet, 640 calories are derived from carbohydrates (160 grams × 4 calories per gram), 280 calories from protein (70 grams × 4 calories per gram), and 900 calories from fat (100 grams × 9 calories per gram), for a total of 1,820 calories. If 900 calories are derived from fat, almost half of the total caloric intake is in the form of fat (900 ÷ 1,820 × 100 = 49.5 percent).

Each gram of fat provides 9 calories—more than twice the calories of a gram of carbohydrates or protein. When figuring out the percent fat calories of individual foods, you may find Figure 3.8 a useful guideline. Multiply the Total Fat grams by 9 and divide by the total calories in that particular food (per serving). Then multiply that number by 100 to get the percentage. For example, the food label in Figure 3.8 (page 78) lists a total of 120 calories and 5 grams of fat, and the equation below it shows the fat content to be 38 percent of total calories. This simple guideline can help you decrease the fat in your diet.

The fat content of selected foods, given in grams and as a percent of total calories, is presented in Figure 3.9 (page 79). The percentage of fat is further subdivided into saturated, monounsaturated, polyunsaturated, and other fatty acids.

Achieving a Balanced Diet

Anyone who has completed a nutrient analysis and has given careful attention to Tables 3.3 (vitamins) and 3.4 (minerals) probably will realize that a well-balanced diet entails eating a variety of nutrient-dense foods and monitoring total daily caloric intake. The MyPyramid healthy eating guide in Figure 3.1 (page 63) contains five major food groups and oils. The food groups are grains, vegetables, fruits, milk, and meats and beans.

Behavior Modification Planning

CALORIC AND FAT CONTENT OF SELECTED FAST FOOD

	Calories	Total Fat (grams)	Saturated Fat (grams)	Percent Fat Calories
Burgers				
McDonald's Big Mac	590	34	11	52
McDonald's Big N' Tasty with Cheese	590	37	12	56
McDonald's Quarter Pounder with Cheese	530	30	13	51
Burger King Whopper	760	46	15	54
Burger King Bacon Double Cheeseburger	580	34	18	53
Burger King BK Smokehouse Cheddar Griller	720	48	19	60
Burger King Whopper with Cheese	850	53	22	56
Burger King Double Whopper	1,060	69	27	59
Burger King Double Whopper with Cheese	1,150	76	33	59
Sandwiches				
Arby's Regular Roast Beef	350	16	6	41
Arby's Super Roast Beef	470	23	7	44
Arby's Roast Chicken Club	520	28	7	48
Arby's Market Fresh Roast Beef & Swiss	810	42	13	47
McDonald's Crispy Chicken	430	21	8	43
McDonald's Filet-O-Fish	470	26	5	50
McDonald's Chicken McGrill	400	17	3	38
Wendy's Chicken Club	470	19	4	36
Wendy's Breast Fillet	430	16	3	34
Wendy's Grilled Chicken	300	7	2	21
Burger King Specialty Chicken	560	28	6	45
Subway Veggie Delight*	226	3	1	12
Subway Turkey Breast	281	5	2	16
Subway Sweet Onion Chicken Teriyaki	374	5	2	12
Subway Steak & Cheese	390	14	5	32
Subway Cold Cut Trio	440	21	7	43
Subway Tuna	450	22	6	44
Mexican				
Taco Bell Crunchy Taco	170	10	4	53
Taco Bell Taco Supreme	220	14	6	57
Taco Bell Soft Chicken Taco	190	7	3	33
Taco Bell Tostada	250	12	5	43
Taco Bell Bean Burrito	370	12	4	29
Taco Bell Fiesta Steak Burrito	370	12	4	29
Taco Bell Grilled Steak Soft Taco	290	17	4	53
Taco Bell Double Decker Taco	340	14	5	37
French Fries				
Wendy's, biggie (5½ oz)	440	19	7	39
McDonald's, large (6 oz)	540	26	9	43
Burger King, large (5½ oz)	500	25	13	45
Shakes				
Wendy's Frosty, medium (16 oz)	440	11	7	23
McDonald's McFlurry, small (12 oz)	610	22	14	32
Burger King, Old Fashioned Ice Cream Shake, medium (22 oz)	760	41	29	49
Hash Browns				
McDonald's Hash Browns (2 oz)	130	8	4	55
Burger King, Hash Browns, small (2½ oz)	230	15	9	59

Try It

Using the above information, record in your Online Journal or class notebook ways you can restructure fast-food consumption to decrease caloric value and fat and saturated fat content in your diet.

* 6-inch sandwich with no mayo

Source: Adapted from *Restaurant Confidential* by Michael F. Jacobson and Jayne Hurley (Workman, 2002), by permission of Center for Science in the Public Interest.

Whole grains, vegetables, fruits, and milk provide the nutritional base for a healthy diet. When increasing the intake of these food groups, it is important to decrease the intake of low-nutrient foods to effectively balance caloric intake with energy needs. Whole grains are a major source of fiber as well as other nutrients. Whole grains contain the entire grain kernel (the bran, germ, and endosperm). Examples include whole-wheat flour, whole cornmeal, oatmeal, cracked wheat (bulgur), and brown rice. Refined grains have been milled—a process that removes the bran and germ. The process also removes fiber, iron, and many B vitamins. Refined grains include white flour, white bread, white rice, and degermed cornmeal. Refined grains are often enriched to add back B vitamins and iron. Fiber, however, is not added back.

In addition to providing nutrients crucial to health, fruits and vegetables are the sole source of **phytonutrients** ("phyto" comes from the Greek word for plant). These compounds show promising results in the fight against cancer and heart disease. More than 4,000 phytonutrients have been identified. The main function of phytonutrients in plants is to protect them from sunlight. In humans, phytonutrients seem to have a powerful ability to block the formation of cancerous tumors. Their actions are so diverse that, at almost every stage of cancer, phytonutrients have the ability to block, disrupt, slow, or even reverse the process. In terms of heart

Phytonutrients Compounds thought to prevent and fight cancer; found in large quantities in fruits and vegetables.

FIGURE 3.8 Computation for fat content in food.

Nutrition Facts

Serving Size 1 cup (240 ml)
Servings Per Container 4

Amount Per Serving	
Calories 120	Calories from Fat 45
	% **Daily Value***
Total Fat 5g	**8%**
Saturated Fat 3g	**15%**
Cholesterol 20mg	**7%**
Sodium 120mg	**5%**
Total Carbohydrate 12g	**4%**
Dietary Fiber 0g	**0%**
Sugars 12g	
Protein 8g	

Vitamin A	10%	•	Vitamin C	4%
Calcium	30%	•	Iron	0%

* Percent Daily Values are based on a 2,000 calorie diet. Your daily values may be higher or lower depending on your calorie needs:

	Calories	2,000	2,500
Total Fat	Less than	65g	80g
Sat Fat	Less than	20g	25g
Cholesterol	Less than	300mg	300mg
Sodium	Less than	2,400mg	2,400mg
Total Carbohydrate		300g	375g
Fiber		25g	30g

Calories per gram:
Fat 9 • Carbohydrate 4 • Protein 4

Percent fat calories = (grams of fat × 9) ÷ calories per serving × 100

5 grams of fat × 9 calories per grams of fat = 45 calories from fat

45 calories from fat ÷ 120 calories per serving × 100 = 38% fat

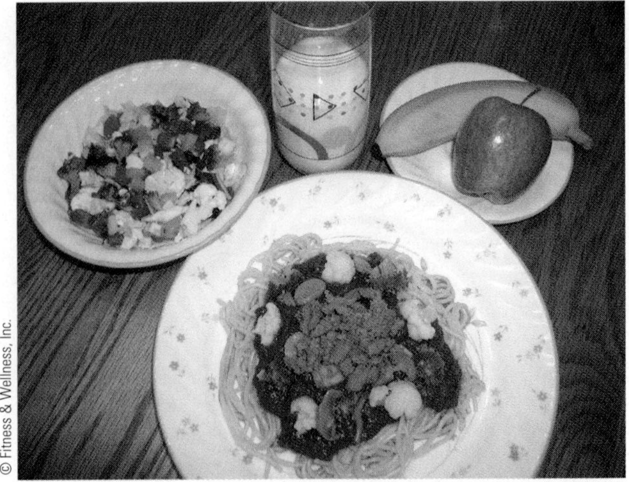

You can restructure your meals so rice, pasta, beans, breads, and vegetables are in the center of the plate; meats are on the side and added primarily for flavoring; fruits are used for desserts; and low- or non-fat milk products are used.

disease, they may reduce inflammation, inhibit blood clots, or prevent the oxidation of LDL cholesterol.

The consistent message is to eat a diet with ample fruits and vegetables. The daily recommended amount of fruits and vegetables has absolutely no substitute. Science has not yet found a way to allow people to eat a poor diet, pop a few pills, and derive the same benefits.

Milk and milk products (select low-fat or non-fat) can decrease the risk of low bone mass (osteoporosis) throughout life. Besides calcium, milk is a good source of potassium, vitamin D, and protein and may aid with managing body weight.

Foods in the meats and beans group consist of poultry, fish, eggs, nuts, legumes, and seeds. Nutrients in this group include protein, B vitamins, vitamin E, iron, zinc, and magnesium. Choose low-fat or lean meats and poultry and bake them, grill them, or broil them. Most Americans eat sufficient food in this group but need to choose leaner foods and a greater variety of fish, dry beans, nuts, and seeds. In terms of meat, poultry, and fish, the recommendation is to consume about 3 ounces and not to exceed 6 ounces daily. All visible fat and skin should be trimmed off meats and poultry before cooking.

Oils are fats that come from different plants and fish and are liquid at room temperature. Choose carefully and avoid oils that have trans fats (check the food label) or saturated fats. Solid fats at room temperature come from animal sources or can be made from vegetable oils through the process of hydrogenation.

As an aid to balancing your diet, the form in Lab 3B enables you to record your daily food intake. This record is much easier to keep than the complete dietary analysis in Lab 3A. Make one copy for each day you wish to record.

To start the activity, go to http://mypyramid.gov/ and establish your personal MyPyramid Plan based on your age, sex, and activity level. Record this information on the form provided in Figure 3B.1 in Lab 3B. Next, whenever you have something to eat, record the food and the amount eaten according to the MyPyramid standard amounts (oz, c, or tsp—see Figure 3.1). Do this immediately after each meal so you will be able to keep track of your actual food intake more easily. At the end of the day, evaluate your diet by checking whether you ate the minimum required amounts for each food

FIGURE 3.9 Fat content of selected foods.

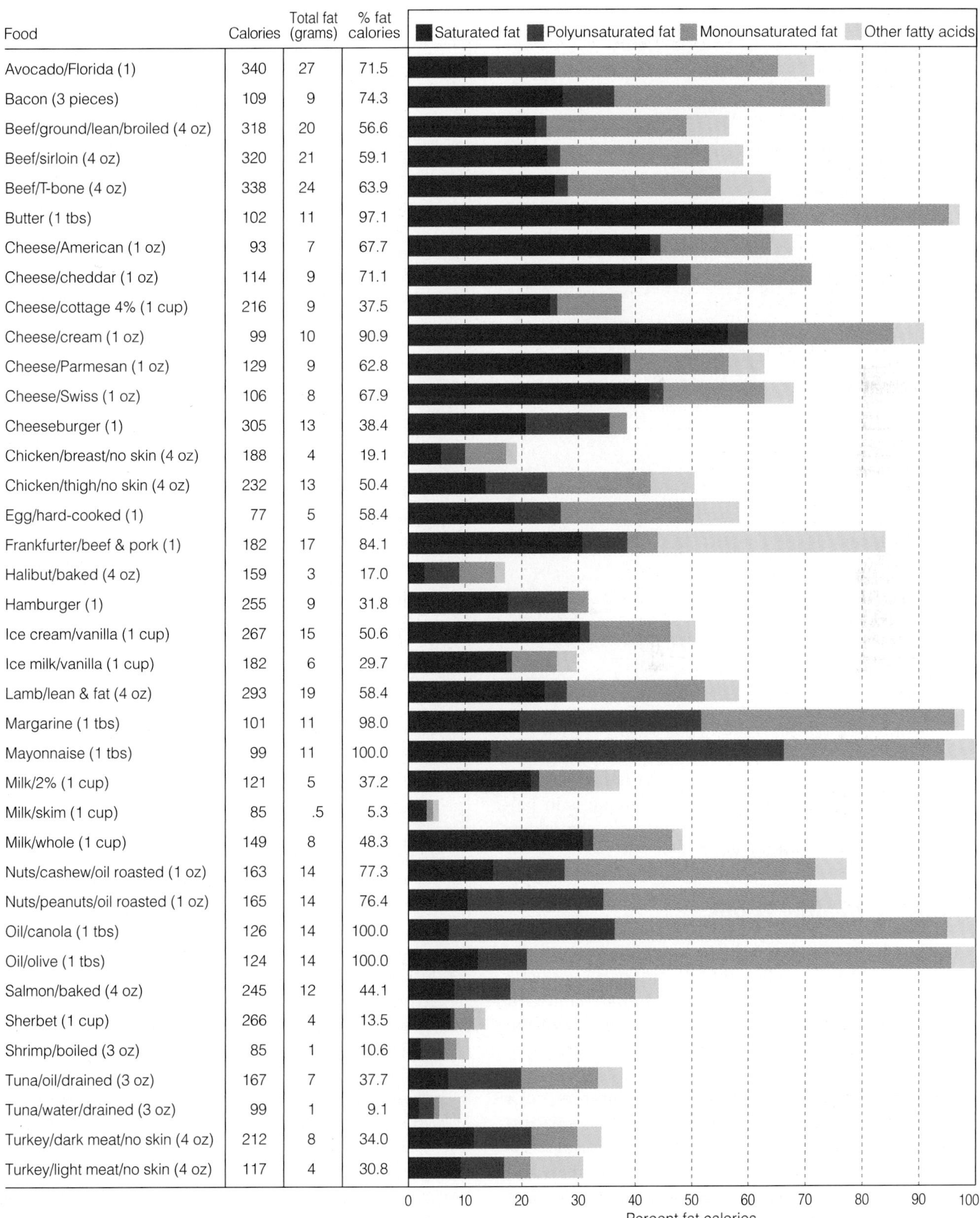

Food	Calories	Total fat (grams)	% fat calories
Avocado/Florida (1)	340	27	71.5
Bacon (3 pieces)	109	9	74.3
Beef/ground/lean/broiled (4 oz)	318	20	56.6
Beef/sirloin (4 oz)	320	21	59.1
Beef/T-bone (4 oz)	338	24	63.9
Butter (1 tbs)	102	11	97.1
Cheese/American (1 oz)	93	7	67.7
Cheese/cheddar (1 oz)	114	9	71.1
Cheese/cottage 4% (1 cup)	216	9	37.5
Cheese/cream (1 oz)	99	10	90.9
Cheese/Parmesan (1 oz)	129	9	62.8
Cheese/Swiss (1 oz)	106	8	67.9
Cheeseburger (1)	305	13	38.4
Chicken/breast/no skin (4 oz)	188	4	19.1
Chicken/thigh/no skin (4 oz)	232	13	50.4
Egg/hard-cooked (1)	77	5	58.4
Frankfurter/beef & pork (1)	182	17	84.1
Halibut/baked (4 oz)	159	3	17.0
Hamburger (1)	255	9	31.8
Ice cream/vanilla (1 cup)	267	15	50.6
Ice milk/vanilla (1 cup)	182	6	29.7
Lamb/lean & fat (4 oz)	293	19	58.4
Margarine (1 tbs)	101	11	98.0
Mayonnaise (1 tbs)	99	11	100.0
Milk/2% (1 cup)	121	5	37.2
Milk/skim (1 cup)	85	.5	5.3
Milk/whole (1 cup)	149	8	48.3
Nuts/cashew/oil roasted (1 oz)	163	14	77.3
Nuts/peanuts/oil roasted (1 oz)	165	14	76.4
Oil/canola (1 tbs)	126	14	100.0
Oil/olive (1 tbs)	124	14	100.0
Salmon/baked (4 oz)	245	12	44.1
Sherbet (1 cup)	266	4	13.5
Shrimp/boiled (3 oz)	85	1	10.6
Tuna/oil/drained (3 oz)	167	7	37.7
Tuna/water/drained (3 oz)	99	1	9.1
Turkey/dark meat/no skin (4 oz)	212	8	34.0
Turkey/light meat/no skin (4 oz)	117	4	30.8

Behavior Modification Planning

"SUPER" FOODS

The following "super" foods that fight disease and promote health should be included often in the diet.

- Avocados
- Bananas
- Beans
- Beets
- Blueberries
- Broccoli
- Butternut squash
- Carrots
- Grapes
- Kale
- Kiwifruit
- Flaxseeds
- Nuts (Brazil, walnuts)
- Salmon (wild)
- Soy
- Oats and oatmeal
- Olives and olive oil
- Onions
- Oranges
- Peppers
- Strawberries
- Spinach
- Tea (green, black, red)
- Tomatoes
- Yogurt

Try It

Using the above list, make a list of which super foods you can add to your diet and when you can eat them (snacks/meals). List meals that you can add these foods to.

group. If you meet the minimum required servings at the end of each day and your caloric intake is in balance with the recommended amount, you are taking good "Steps to a Healthier You."

Choosing Healthy Foods

Once you have completed the nutrient analysis and the healthy diet plan (Labs 3A and 3B), you may conduct a self-evaluation of your current nutritional habits. In Lab 3B, you can also assess your current stage of change regarding healthy nutrition and list strategies to help you improve your diet.

Initially, developing healthy eating habits requires a conscious effort to select nutritious foods (see adjacent box). You must learn the nutritive value of typical foods that you eat. You can do so by reading food labels and looking up the nutritive values using listings such as that provided in Appendix A or by using computer software available for such purposes. Healthy eating further requires proper meal planning and adequate coping strategies when confronted with situations that encourage unhealthy eating and overindulgence. Addi-

Behavior Modification Planning

SELECTING NUTRITIOUS FOODS

To select nutritious foods:

1. Given the choice between whole foods and refined, processed foods, choose the former (apples rather than apple pie, potatoes rather than potato chips). No nutrients have been refined out of the whole foods, and they contain less fat, salt, and sugar.
2. Choose the leaner cuts of meat. Select fish or poultry often, beef seldom. Ask for broiled, not fried, to control your fat intake.
3. Use both raw and cooked vegetables and fruits. Raw foods offer more fiber and vitamins, such as folate and thiamin, that are destroyed by cooking. Cooking foods frees other vitamins and minerals for absorption.
4. Include milk, milk products, or other calcium sources for the calcium you need. Use low-fat or non-fat items to reduce fat and calories.
5. Learn to use margarine, butter, and oils sparingly. A little gives flavor, a lot overloads you with fat and calories.
6. Vary your choices. Eat broccoli today, carrots tomorrow, and corn the next day. Eat Chinese today, Italian tomorrow, and broiled fish with brown rice and steamed vegetables the third day.
7. Load your plate with vegetables and unrefined starchy foods. A small portion of meat or cheese is all you need for protein.
8. When choosing breads and cereals, choose the whole-grain varieties.

To select nutritious fast foods:

9. Choose the broiled sandwich lettuce, tomatoes, and other goodies—and hold the mayo—rather than the fish or chicken patties coated with breadcrumbs and cooked in fat.
10. Select a salad—and use more plain vegetables than those mixed with oily or mayonnaise-based dressings.
11. Order chili with more beans than meat. Choose a soft bean burrito over tacos with fried shells.
12. Drink low-fat milk rather than a cola beverage.

When choosing from a vending machine:

13. Choose cracker sandwiches over chips and pork rinds (virtually pure fat). Choose peanuts, pretzels, and popcorn over cookies and candy.
14. Choose milk and juices over cola beverages.

Try It

Based on what you have learned, list strategies you can use to increase food variety, enhance the nutritive value of your diet, and decrease fat and caloric content in your meals.

Adapted from W. W. K. Hoeger, L. W. Turner, & B. Q. Hafen. *Wellness: Guidelines for a Healthy Lifestyle* (Wadsworth Thomson Learning, 2007).

tional information on these topics is provided in the weight management chapter (Chapter 5).

Vegetarianism

More than 12 million people in the United States follow vegetarian diets. **Vegetarians** rely primarily on foods from the bread, cereal, rice, pasta, and fruit and vegetable groups and avoid most foods from animal sources in the dairy and protein groups. The five basic types of vegetarians are as follows:

1. **Vegans** eat no animal products at all.
2. **Ovovegetarians** allow eggs in the diet.
3. **Lactovegetarians** allow foods from the milk group.
4. **Ovolactovegetarians** include egg and milk products in the diet.
5. **Semivegetarians** do not eat red meat, but do include fish and poultry in addition to milk products and eggs in their diet.

Vegetarian diets can be healthful and consistent with the Dietary Guidelines for Americans and can meet the DRIs for nutrients. Vegetarians who do not select their food combinations properly, however, can develop nutritional deficiencies of protein, vitamins, minerals, and even calories. Even greater attention should be paid when planning vegetarian diets for infants and children. Unless carefully planned, a strict plant-based diet will prevent proper growth and development.

Nutrient Concerns

In some vegetarian diets, protein deficiency can be a concern. Vegans in particular must be careful to eat foods that provide a balanced distribution of essential amino acids, such as grain products and legumes. Strict vegans also need a supplement of vitamin B_{12}. This vitamin is not found in plant foods; its only source is animal foods. Deficiency of this vitamin can lead to anemia and nerve damage.

The key to a healthful vegetarian diet is to eat foods that possess complementary proteins because most plant-based products lack one or more essential amino acids in adequate amounts. For example, both grains and legumes are good protein sources, but neither provides all the essential amino acids. Grains and cereals are low in the amino acid lysine, and legumes lack methionine. Foods from these two groups—such as combinations of tortillas and beans, rice and beans, rice and soybeans, or wheat bread and peanuts—complement each other and provide all required protein nutrients. These complementary proteins may be consumed over the course of one day, but it is best if they are consumed during the same meal.

Other nutrients likely to be deficient in vegetarian diets—and ways to compensate—are as follows:

- Vitamin D can be obtained from moderate exposure to the sun or by taking a supplement.

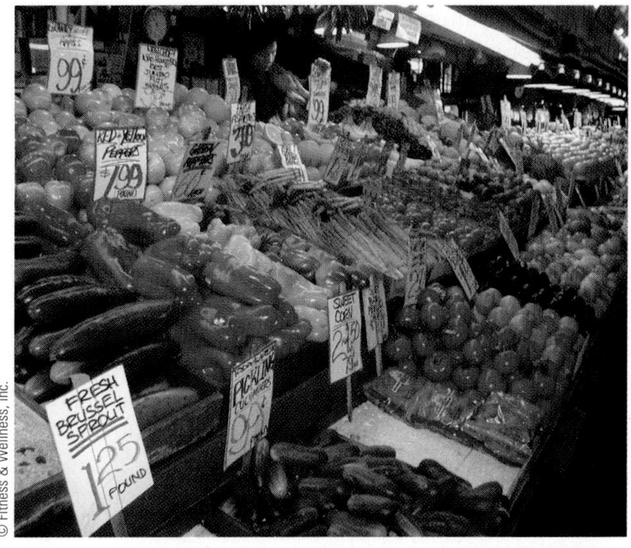

Most fruits and vegetables contain large amounts of cancer-preventing phytonutrients.

- Riboflavin can be found in green leafy vegetables, whole grains, and legumes.
- Calcium can be obtained from fortified soybean milk or fortified orange juice, calcium-rich tofu, and selected cereals. A calcium supplement is also an option.
- Iron can be found in whole grains, dried fruits and nuts, and legumes. To enhance iron absorption, a good source of vitamin C should be consumed with these foods (calcium and iron are the most difficult nutrients to consume in sufficient amounts in a strict vegan diet).
- Zinc can be obtained from whole grains, wheat germ, beans, nuts, and seeds.

MyPyramid also can be used as a guide for vegetarians. The key is food variety. Most vegetarians today eat dairy products and eggs. They can replace meat with legumes, nuts, seeds, eggs, and meat substitutes (tofu, tempeh, soy milk, and commercial meat replacers such as veggie burgers and soy hot dogs). For additional MyPyramid healthy eating tips for vegetarians and how to get enough of the previously mentioned nutrients, go to http://mypyramid.gov/. Those who are interested in vegetarian diets are encouraged to consult additional resources, because special vegetar-

---

Vegetarians Individuals whose diet is of vegetable or plant origin.

Vegans Vegetarians who eat no animal products at all.

Ovovegetarians Vegetarians who allow eggs in their diet.

Lactovegetarians Vegetarians who eat foods from the milk group.

Ovolactovegetarians Vegetarians who include eggs and milk products in their diet.

Semivegetarians Vegetarians who include milk products, eggs, and fish and poultry in the diet.

ian diet planning cannot be covered adequately in a few paragraphs.

Nuts

Consumption of nuts, commonly used in vegetarian diets, has received considerable attention in recent years. A few years ago, most people regarded nuts as especially high in fat and calories. Although they are 70 to 90 percent fat, most of this is unsaturated fat. And research indicates that people who eat nuts several times a week have a lower incidence of heart disease. Eating 2 to 3 ounces (about one-half cup) of almonds, walnuts, or macadamia nuts a day may decrease high blood cholesterol by about 10 percent. Nuts can even enhance the cholesterol-lowering effects of the Mediterranean diet.

Heart-health benefits are attributed not only to the unsaturated fats but also to other nutrients found in nuts, including vitamin E and folic acid. And nuts are also packed with additional B vitamins, calcium, copper, potassium, magnesium, fiber, and phytonutrients. Many of these nutrients are cancer- and cardio-protective, help lower homocysteine levels (page 374), and act as antioxidants, discussed in "Antioxidants" (page 84) and "Folate" (page 87).

Nuts do have a drawback: They are high in calories. A handful of nuts provides as many calories as a piece of cake, so nuts should be avoided as a snack. Excessive weight gain is a risk factor for cardiovascular disease. Nuts are recommended for use in place of high-protein foods such as meats, bacon, eggs, or as part of a meal in fruit or vegetable salads, homemade bread, pancakes, casseroles, yogurt, and oatmeal. Peanut butter is also healthier than cheese or some cold cuts in sandwiches.

Soy Products

The popularity of soy foods, including use in vegetarian diets, is attributed primarily to Asian research that points to less heart disease and fewer hormone-related cancers in people who regularly consume soy foods. The benefits of soy lie in its high protein content and plant chemicals, known as *isoflavones,* that act as antioxidants and may protect against estrogen-related cancers (breast, ovarian, and endometrial). The compound *genistein,* one of many phytonutrients in soy, may reduce the risk for breast cancer, and soy consumption also may lower the risk for prostate cancer. A benefit of eating soy foods is that they replace consumption of unhealthy animal products high in fat and saturated fat.

Probiotics

Yogurt is rated in the "super foods" category because, in addition to being a good source of calcium, riboflavin, and protein, it contains **probiotics.** These health-promoting microorganisms live in the intestines and help break down foods and prevent disease-causing organisms from settling in. Probiotics have been found to offer protection against gastrointestinal infections, boost immune activity, and even help fight certain types of cancer.

When selecting yogurt, look for products with L-acidophilus, Bifidus, and the prebiotic (substances on which probiotics feed) inulin. The latter, a soluble fiber, appears to enhance calcium absorption. Avoid yogurt with added fruit jam, sugar, and candy.

Diets from Other Cultures

Increasingly, Americans are eating foods reflecting the ethnic composition of people from other countries. Learning how to wisely select from the wide range of options is the task of those who seek a healthy diet.

Mediterranean Diet

The **Mediterranean diet** has received much attention because people in that region have notably lower rates of diet-linked diseases and a longer life expectancy. The diet features olive oil, grains (whole, not refined), legumes, vegetables, fruits, and, in moderation, fish, red wine, nuts, and dairy products. Although it is a semivegetarian diet, up to 40 percent of the total daily caloric intake may come from fat—mostly monounsaturated fat from olive oil. Moderate intake of red wine is included with meals. The dietary plan also encourages regular physical activity (see Figure 3.10).

More than a "diet," the Mediterranean diet is a dietary pattern that has existed for centuries. According to the largest and most comprehensive research on this dietary pattern, the health benefits and decreased mortality are not linked to any specific component of the diet (such as olive oil or red wine) but are achieved through the interaction of all the components of the pattern.[7] Those who adhered most closely to the dietary pattern had a lower incidence of heart disease (33 percent) and deaths from cancer (24 percent). Although most people in the United States focus on the olive oil component of the diet, olive oil is used mainly as a means to increase consumption of vegetables because vegetables sauteed in oil taste better than steamed vegetables.

Ethnic Diets

As people migrate, they take their dietary practices with them. Many ethnic diets are healthier than the typical American diet because they emphasize consumption of complex carbohydrates and limit fat intake. The predominant minority ethnic groups in America are African American, Hispanic American, and Asian American. Unfortunately, the generally healthier ethnic diets quickly become Americanized when these people enter the United States. Often, they cut back on vegetables and add meats and salt to the diet in conformity with the American consumer.

Ethnic dishes, nonetheless, can be prepared at home. They are easy to make and much healthier when using the typical (original) variety of vegetables, corn,

FIGURE 3.10 The Traditional Healthy Mediterranean Diet Pyramid.

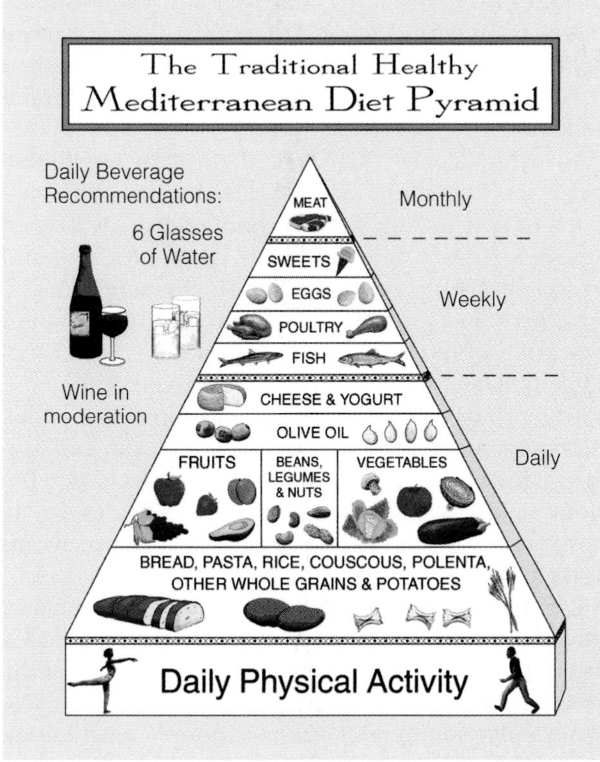

rice, spices, and condiments. Ethnic health recommendations also encourage daily physical activity and suggest no more than two alcoholic drinks per day. Three typical ethnic diets are as follows:

- The African-American diet (soul food) is based on the regional cuisine of the American South. Soul food includes yams, black-eyed peas, okra, and peanuts. The latter have been combined with American foods such as corn products and pork. Today, most people think of soul food as meat, fried chicken, sweet potatoes, and chitterling.
- Hispanic foods in the United States arrived with the conquistadores and evolved through combinations with other ethnic diets and local foods available in Latin America. For example, the Cuban cuisine combined Spanish, Chinese, and native foods; Puerto Rican cuisine developed from Spanish, African, and native products; Mexican diets evolved from Spanish and native food. Prominent in all of these diets were corn, beans, squash, chili peppers, avocados, papayas, and fish. The colonists later added rice and citrus foods. Today, the Hispanic diet incorporates a wide variety of foods, including red meat, but the staple still consists of rice, corn, and beans.
- Asian-American diets are characteristically rich in vegetables and use minimal meat and fat. The Okinawan diet in Japan, where some of the healthiest and oldest people in the world live, is high in fresh (versus pickled) vegetables, high in fiber, and low in fat and salt. The Chinese cuisine includes more than 200 vegetables, and fat-free sauces and seasoning are used to enhance flavor. The Chinese diet varies somewhat within regions of China. The lowest in fat is that of southern China, with most meals containing fish, seafood, and stir-fried vegetables. Chinese food in American restaurants contains a much higher percentage of fat and protein than the traditional Chinese cuisine.

Table 3.8 (page 84) provides a list of healthier foods to choose from when dining at selected ethnic restaurants.

All healthy diets have similar characteristics: They are high in fruits, vegetables, and grains and low in fat and saturated fat. Healthy diets also use low-fat or fat-free dairy products, and they emphasize portion control—essential in a healthy diet plan.

Many people now think that if a food item is labeled "low fat" or "fat free," they can consume it in large quantities. "Low fat" or "fat free" does not imply "calorie free." Many people who consume low-fat diets eat more (and thus increase their caloric intake), which in the long term leads to obesity and its associated health problems.

Nutrient Supplementation

Approximately half of all adults in the United States take daily nutrient **supplements.** Nutrient requirements for the body normally can be met by consuming as few as 1,200 calories per day, as long as the diet contains the recommended amounts of food from the different food groups. Still, many people consider it necessary to take vitamin supplements.

It's true that our bodies cannot retain water-soluble vitamins as long as fat-soluble vitamins. The body excretes excessive intakes readily, although the body can retain small amounts for weeks or months in various or-

---

Probiotics Healthy bacteria (abundant in yogurt) that help break down foods and prevent disease-causing organisms from settling in the intestines.

Mediterranean diet Typical diet of people around the Mediterranean region, focusing on olive oil, red wine, grains, legumes, vegetables, and fruits, with limited amounts of meat, fish, milk, and cheese.

Supplements Tablets, pills, capsules, liquids, or powders that contain vitamins, minerals, antioxidants, amino acids, herbs, or fiber that individuals take to increase their intake of these nutrients.

TABLE 3.8 Ethnic Eating Guide

	Choose Often	Choose Less Often
Chinese	Beef with broccoli Chinese greens Steamed rice, brown or white Steamed beef with pea pods Stir-fry dishes Teriyaki beef or chicken Wonton soup	Crispy duck Egg rolls Fried rice Kung pao chicken (fried) Peking duck Pork spareribs
Japanese	Chiri nabe (fish stew) Grilled scallops Sushi, sashimi (raw fish) Teriyaki Yakitori (grilled chicken)	Tempura (fried chicken, shrimp, or vegetables) Tonkatsu (fried pork)
Italian	Cioppino (seafood stew) Minestrone (vegetarian soup) Pasta with marinara sauce Pasta primavera (pasta with vegetables) Steamed clams	Antipasto Cannelloni, ravioli Fettuccini alfredo Garlic bread White clam sauce
Mexican	Beans and rice Black bean/vegetable soup Burritos, bean Chili Enchiladas, bean Fajitas Gazpacho Taco salad Tamales Tortillas, steamed	Chili relleno Chimichangas Enchiladas, beef or cheese Flautas Guacamole Nachos Quesadillas Tostadas Sour cream (as topping)
Middle Eastern	Tandoori chicken Curry (yogurt-based) Rice pilaf Lentil soup Shish kebab	Falafel
French	Poached salmon Spinach salad Consommé Salad niçoise	Beef Wellington Escargot French onion soup Sauces in general
Soul Food	Baked chicken Baked fish Roasted pork (not smothered or "etouffe") Sauteed okra Baked sweet potato	Fried chicken Fried fish Smothered pork tenderloin Okra in gumbo Sweet potato casserole or pie
Greek	Gyros Pita Lentil soup	Baklava Moussaka

Source: Adapted from P. A. Floyd, S. E. Mimms, and C. Yelding-Howard. *Personal Health: Perspectives & Lifestyles* (Belmont, CA: Wadsworth/Thomson Learning, 1998).

gans and tissues. Fat-soluble vitamins, by contrast, are stored in fatty tissue. Therefore, daily intake of these vitamins is not as crucial. Too much vitamin A and vitamin D actually can be detrimental to health.

People should not take **megadoses** of vitamins and minerals. For some nutrients, a dose of five times the RDA taken over several months may create problems. For other nutrients, it may not pose a threat to human health. Vitamin and mineral doses should not exceed the ULs. For nutrients that do not have an established UL, one day's dose should be no more than three times the RDA.

Iron deficiency (determined through blood testing) is more common in women than men. Iron supplementation is frequently recommended for women who have a heavy menstrual flow. Some pregnant and lactating women also may require supplements. The average pregnant woman who eats an adequate amount of a variety of foods should take a low dose of iron supplement daily. Women who are pregnant with more than one baby may need additional supplements. Folate supplements also are encouraged prior to and during pregnancy to prevent certain birth defects (see the following discussions of antioxidants and folate). In the above instances, individuals should take supplements under a physician's supervision.

Adults over the age of 60 are encouraged to take a daily multivitamin. Aging may decrease the body's ability to absorb and utilize certain nutrients. Nutrient deficiencies in older adults include vitamins C, D, B_6, B_{12}, folate, and the minerals calcium, zinc, and magnesium.

Other people who may benefit from supplementation are those with nutrient deficiencies, alcoholics and street-drug users who do not have a balanced diet, smokers, vegans (strict vegetarians), individuals on low-calorie diets (fewer than 1,200 calories per day), and people with disease-related disorders or who are taking medications that interfere with proper nutrient absorption.

Although supplements may help a small group of individuals, most supplements do not provide benefits to healthy people who eat a balanced diet. Supplements do not seem to prevent chronic diseases or help people run faster, jump higher, relieve stress, improve sexual prowess, cure a common cold, or boost energy levels.

Antioxidants

Much research and discussion are taking place regarding the effectiveness of **antioxidants** in thwarting several chronic diseases. Although foods probably contain more than 4,000 antioxidants, the four more studied antioxidants are vitamins C, E, and beta-carotene (a precursor to vitamin A), and the mineral selenium (see Table 3.9).

Oxygen is used during metabolism to change carbohydrates and fats into energy. During this process, oxygen is transformed into stable forms of water and carbon dioxide. A small amount of oxygen, however, ends up in an unstable form, referred to as **oxygen free radicals.** A free radical molecule has a normal proton

TABLE 3.9 Antioxidant Nutrients, Sources, and Functions

Nutrient	Good Sources	Antioxidant Effect
Vitamin C	Citrus fruit, kiwi fruit, cantaloupe, strawberries, broccoli, green or red peppers, cauliflower, cabbage	Appears to deactivate oxygen free radicals.
Vitamin E	Vegetable oils, yellow and green leafy vegetables, margarine, wheat germ, oatmeal, almonds, whole-grain breads, cereals	Protects lipids from oxidation.
Beta-carotene	Carrots, squash, pumpkin, sweet potatoes, broccoli, green leafy vegetables	Soaks up oxygen free radicals.
Selenium	Seafood, Brazil nuts, meat, whole grains	Helps prevent damage to cell structures.

FIGURE 3.11 Antioxidant protection: blocking and absorbing oxygen free radicals to prevent chronic disease.

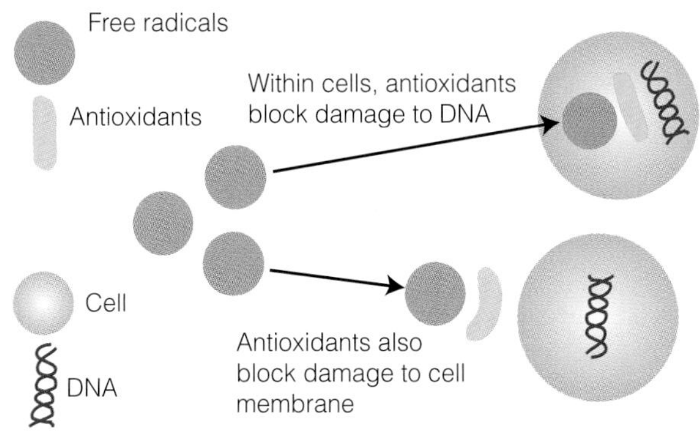

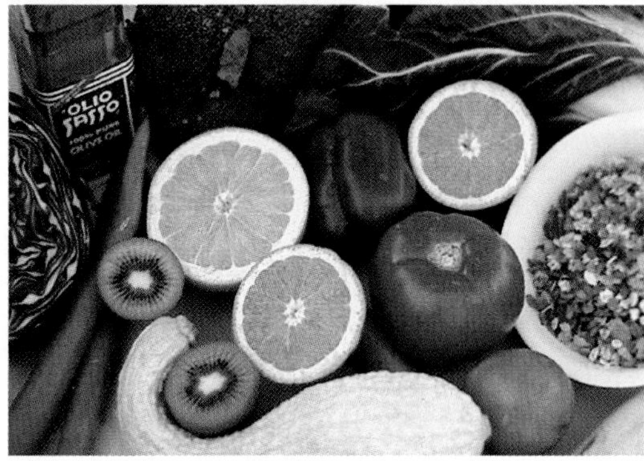

© Fitness & Wellness, Inc.

nucleus with a single unpaired electron. Having only one electron makes the free radical extremely reactive, and it looks constantly to pair its electron with one from another molecule. When a free radical steals a second electron from another molecule, that other molecule in turn becomes a free radical. This chain reaction goes on until two free radicals meet to form a stable molecule.

Free radicals attack and damage proteins and lipids—in particular, cell membranes and DNA. This damage is thought to contribute to the development of conditions such as cardiovascular disease, cancer, emphysema, cataracts, Parkinson's disease, and premature aging. Solar radiation, cigarette smoke, air pollution, radiation, some drugs, injury, infection, chemicals (such as pesticides), and other environmental factors also seem to encourage the formation of free radicals. Antioxidants are thought to offer protection by absorbing free radicals before they can cause damage and also by interrupting the sequence of reactions once damage has begun, thwarting certain chronic diseases (see Figure 3.11).

The body's own defense systems typically neutralize free radicals so they don't cause any damage. When free radicals are produced faster than the body can neutralize them, however, they can damage the cells.

Antioxidants are found abundantly in food, especially in fruits and vegetables. Unfortunately, most Americans do not eat the minimum recommended amounts of fruits and vegetables.

Antioxidants work best in the prevention and progression of disease but they cannot repair damage that has already occurred or cure people with disease. The benefits are obtained primarily from food sources themselves, and controversy surrounds the benefits of antioxidants taken in supplement form. Some researchers, however, believe that taking antioxidant supplements can further prevent free-radical damage.

Vitamin E

Vitamin E belongs to a group of eight compounds (four tocopherols and four tocotrienols) of which alpha-to-

---

Megadoses For most vitamins, 10 times the RDA or more; for vitamins A and D, 5 and 2 times the RDA, respectively.

Antioxidants Compounds such as vitamins C and E, beta-carotene, and selenium that prevent oxygen from combining with other substances in the body to form harmful compounds.

Oxygen free radicals Substances formed during metabolism that attack and damage proteins and lipids, in particular the cell membrane and DNA, leading to diseases such as heart disease, cancer, and emphysema.

TABLE 3.10 Antioxidant Content of Selected Foods

Beta-Carotene	IU
Apricot (1 medium)	675
Broccoli (½ cup, frozen)	1,740
Broccoli (½ cup, raw)	680
Cantaloupe (1 cup)	5,160
Carrot (1 medium, raw)	20,255
Green peas (½ cup, frozen)	535
Mango (1 medium)	8,060
Mustard greens (½ cup, frozen)	3,350
Papaya (1 medium)	6,120
Spinach (½ cup, frozen)	7,395
Sweet potato (1 medium, baked)	24,875
Tomato (1 medium)	1,395
Turnip greens (½ cup, boiled)	3,960

Vitamin E	IU	mg*
Almond oil (1 tbsp)		5.3
Almonds (1 oz)	10.1	
Canola oil (1 tbsp)		9.0
Cottonseed oil (1 tbsp)		5.2
Hazelnuts (1 oz)	4.4	
Kale (1 cup)	15.0	
Margarine (1 tbsp)		2.0
Peanuts (1 oz)	3.0	
Shrimp (3 oz, boiled)	3.1	
Sunflower seeds (1 oz, dry)	14.2	
Sunflower seed oil (1 tbsp)		6.9
Sweet potato (1 medium, baked)	7.2	
Wheat germ oil (1 tbsp)		20.0

Vitamin C	mg
Acerola (1 cup, raw)	1,640
Acerola juice (8 oz)	3,864
Cantaloupe (½ melon, medium)	90
Cranberry juice (8 oz)	90
Grapefruit (½, medium, white)	52
Grapefruit juice (8 oz)	92
Guava (1 medium)	165
Kiwi (1 medium)	75
Lemon juice (8 oz)	110
Orange (1 medium)	66
Orange juice (8 oz)	120
Papaya (1 medium)	85
Pepper (½ cup, red, chopped, raw)	95
Strawberries (1 cup, raw)	88

Selenium	mcg
Brazil nuts (1)	100
Bread, whole-wheat enriched (1 slice)	15
Beef (3 oz)	33
Cereals (3½ oz)	20
Chicken breast, roasted, no skin (3 oz)	24
Cod, baked (3 oz)	57
Egg, hard-boiled (1 large)	15
Fruits (3½ oz)	1
Noodles, enriched, boiled (1 cup)	50
Oatmeal, cooked (1 cup)	23
Red snapper (3 oz)	150
Rice, long grain, cooked (1 cup)	20
Salmon, baked (3 oz)	35
Spaghetti w/meat sauce (1 cup)	36
Tuna, canned, water, drained (3 oz)	68
Turkey breast, roasted, no skin (3 oz)	28
Walnuts, black, chopped (¼ cup)	5
Vegetables (3½ oz)	1

* Vitamin E values for oils are commonly expressed in milligrams (mg). One mg is almost equal to 1 IU (international unit).

copherol is the most active form. The recommended RDA for vitamin E is 15 mg or 22 **IU (international units).** Vitamin E is found primarily in oil-rich seeds and vegetable oils. As shown in Table 3.10, vitamin E is not found in large quantities in foods typically consumed in the diet.

Vitamin E supplements from natural sources contain d-alpha tocopherol, which is better absorbed by the body than dl-alpha tocopherol, a synthetic form composed of a variety of E compounds. Because vitamin E is fat-soluble, supplements should be taken with a meal that has some fat in it.

Based on early promising research, in 1994 the editorial board of the *University of California at Berkeley Wellness Letter* recommended 200 to 800 IU of vitamin E supplementation daily. Disappointing follow-up reviews of clinical trials in 2001, however, prompted the board to halve its daily recommendation. Based on new evidence and reviews of hundreds of previous studies, in 2005 the board withdrew the recommendation altogether.[8]

Although no evidence indicates that vitamin E supplementation below the upper limit of 1,000 mg per day is harmful, little or no clinical research supports any health benefits. Nuts, seeds, vegetable oils, whole grains, and leafy greens are good sources of vitamin E. Incorporate these foods regularly in the diet to obtain the RDA.

Vitamin C

Studies have shown that vitamin C may offer benefits against heart disease, cancer, and cataracts. Antioxidant recommendations for vitamin C over the years have ranged from 250 to 500 mg per day (the RDA is 75 to 90 mg). People who consume the recommended amounts of daily fruits and vegetables, nonetheless, need no supplementation because they obtain their daily vitamin C requirements through the diet alone. The daily UL for adults 19 to 70 years of age for vitamin C has been set at 2,000 mg.

Vitamin C is water-soluble, and the body eliminates it in about 12 hours. For best results, consume vitamin

C-rich foods twice a day. High intake of a vitamin C supplement, above 500 mg per day, is not recommended. The body absorbs very little vitamin C beyond the first 200 mg per serving or dose.

Beta-Carotene

Beta-carotene supplementation was encouraged in the early 1990s, but obtaining the daily recommended dose of beta-carotene (20,000 IU) from food sources rather than supplements is preferable. Clinical trials have found that beta-carotene supplements did not offer protection against heart disease or cancer and did not provide any other health benefits. Therefore, the recommendation is to "skip the pill and eat the carrot." One medium raw carrot contains about 20,000 IU of beta-carotene.

Selenium

Adequate intake of the mineral selenium is encouraged. Data indicate that individuals who take 200 micrograms (mcg) of selenium daily decreased their risk of prostate cancer by 63 percent, colorectal cancer by 58 percent, and lung cancer by 46 percent.[9] Selenium also may decrease the risk of cancers of the breast, liver, and digestive tract. According to Dr. Edward Giovannucci of the Harvard Medical School, the evidence for benefits of selenium in reducing the risk for prostate cancer is so strong that public health officials should recommend that people increase their selenium intake.

One Brazil nut (unshelled) that you crack yourself provides about 100 mcg of selenium. Shelled nuts found in supermarkets average only about 20 mcg each. Based on the current body of research, a dose of 100 to 200 mcg per day seems to provide the necessary amount of antioxidant for this nutrient. A person has no reason to take more than 200 mcg daily. In fact, the UL for selenium has been set at 400 mcg. Too much selenium can damage cells rather than protect them. If you choose to take supplements, take an organic form of selenium from yeast and not selenium selenite. The selenium content of various foods is provided in Table 3.10.

Selenium may interfere with the body's absorption of vitamin C. If taken in supplemental form, the two nutrients should be taken separately. Wait about an hour following vitamin C intake before taking selenium.

Multivitamins

Although much interest has been generated in the previously mentioned individual supplements, the American people still prefer multivitamins as supplements. A multivitamin complex that provides 100 percent of the DV for most nutrients can help fill in certain dietary deficiencies.[10] Some evidence suggests that regular intake decreases the risk for cardiovascular disease and colon cancer and improves immune function.

Multivitamins, however, are not magic pills. They may help, but they don't provide a license to eat carelessly. Multivitamins don't provide energy, fiber, or phytonutrients.

Vitamin D

Vitamin D is attracting a lot of attention because current research suggests that the vitamin possesses anticancer properties (especially against breast, colon, and prostate cancers and possibly lung and digestive cancers), decreases inflammation (fighting cardiovascular disease, periodontal disease, and arthritis), strengthens the immune system, controls blood pressure, helps maintain muscle strength, and may help deter diabetes and fight depression. Vitamin D is also necessary for calcium absorption, a nutrient critical for building and maintaining bones and teeth.

Most people are not getting enough vitamin D. The current recommended daily intake ranges between 200 to 600 IU (5 and 15 mcg) based on your age. Evidence suggests that we should get about 1,000 IU (25 mcg) per day.[11]

Good sources of vitamin D in the diet include salmon, mackerel, tuna, and sardines. Only fortified milk, orange juice, margarines, and cereals are also good sources. To obtain 1,000 IU per day from food sources alone, however, is difficult. The best source of vitamin D is sunshine. Ultraviolet rays lead to the production in the skin of an inactive form of vitamin D (D3). The inactive form is then transformed by the liver, and subsequently the kidneys, into the active form of vitamin D. Sun-generated vitamin D is also better than that obtained from foods or supplements.

Although excessive sun exposure can lead to skin damage, you should strive for daily "safe sun" exposure; that is, 5 to 10 minutes of unprotected sun exposure of the face, arms, and hands during peak daylight hours. Such exposure will generate between 1,000 and 2,000 IU of vitamin D. And even though the UL has been set at 2,000 IU, experts believe that this figure needs revision because there are no data implicating toxic effects up to 10,000 IU a day.[12] Generating too much vitamin D from the sun is impossible because the body only generates what it needs. People with limited sun exposure, and especially those in the northern United States and Canada during the winter months, should consider a daily multivitamin supplement that contains vitamin D3 (some multivitamins contain vitamin D2, which is a less potent form of the vitamin).

Folate

Although it is not an antioxidant, 400 mcg of **folate** (a B vitamin) is recommended for all premenopausal

---

International unit (IU) Measure of nutrients in foods.

Folate One of the B vitamins.

women. Folate helps prevent some birth defects and seems to offer protection against colon and cervical cancers. Women who might become pregnant should plan to take a folate supplement, because studies have shown that folate intake (400 mcg per day) during early pregnancy can prevent serious birth defects.

Some evidence also indicates that taking 400 mcg of folate along with vitamins B_6 and B_{12} prevents heart attacks by reducing homocysteine levels in the blood (see Chapter 11). High concentrations of homocysteine accelerate the process of plaque formation (atherosclerosis) in the arteries. Five servings of fruits and vegetables per day usually meet the needs for these nutrients. Almost 9 of 10 adults in the United States do not obtain the recommended 400 mcg of folate per day. Because of the vital role of folate in preventing heart disease, some experts recommend a daily supplement that includes 400 mcg of folate.

Side Effects

Toxic effects from antioxidant supplements are rare when they are taken under the ULs. If any of the following side effects arise while taking supplements, stop supplementation and check with a physician:

- Vitamin E: gastrointestinal disturbances, increase in blood lipids (determined through blood tests)
- Vitamin C: nausea, diarrhea, abdominal cramps, kidney stones, liver problems
- Selenium: nausea, vomiting, diarrhea, irritability, fatigue, flu-like symptoms, lesions of the skin and nervous tissue, loss of hair and nails, respiratory failure, liver damage

Substantial supplementation of vitamin E is not recommended for individuals on **anticoagulant** therapy, as vitamin E is an anticoagulant itself. Therefore, if you are on this type of therapy, check with your physician. Vitamin E also may be unsafe if taken with alcohol or by people who drink more than 4 ounces of pure alcohol per day (the equivalent of 8 beers). Pregnant women require a physician's approval prior to beta-carotene supplementation.

Benefits of Foods

Even though you may consider taking some supplements, fruits and vegetables are the richest sources of antioxidants and phytonutrients. Researchers at the U.S. Department of Agriculture compared the antioxidant effects of vitamins C and E with those of various common fruits and vegetables. The results indicated that three-fourths cup of cooked kale (which contains only 11 IU of vitamin E and 76 mg of vitamin C) neutralized as many free radicals as approximately 800 IU of vitamin E or 600 mg of vitamin C. Other excellent sources of antioxidants that these researchers found are blueberries, strawberries, spinach, Brussels sprouts, plums, broccoli, beets, oranges, and grapes. A list of top antioxidant foods is presented in Figure 3.12.

FIGURE 3.12 Top antioxidant foods.

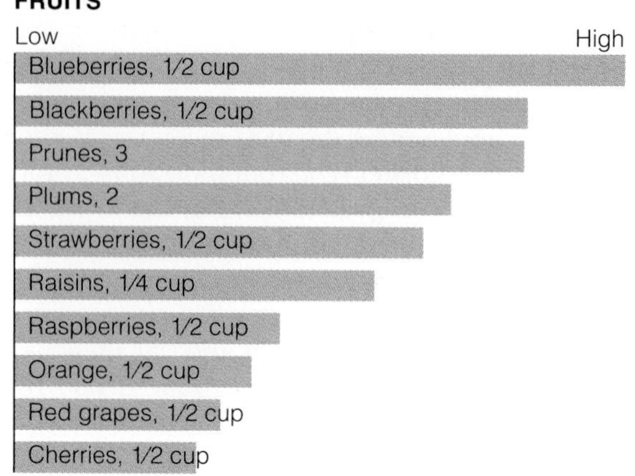

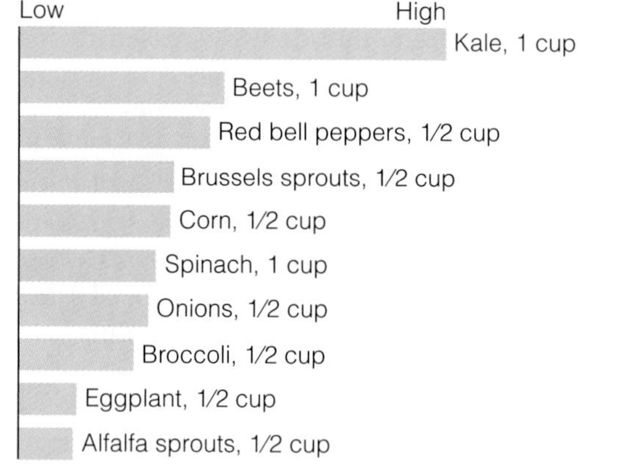

Source: Adapted from USDA, Agricultural Research Service, *Food & Nutrition Research Briefs,* April 1999 (downloaded from www.ars.usda.gov/is/np/fnrb).

Many people who eat unhealthy diets think they need supplementation to balance their diet. This is a fallacy about nutrition. The problem here is not necessarily a lack of vitamins and minerals but, rather, a diet too high in calories, saturated fat, and sodium. Vitamin, mineral, and fiber supplements do not supply all of the nutrients and other beneficial substances present in food and needed for good health.

Wholesome foods contain vitamins, minerals, carbohydrates, fiber, proteins, fats, phytonutrients, and other substances not yet discovered. Researchers do not know if the protective effects are caused by the antioxidants alone, or in combination with other nutrients (such as phytonutrients), or by some other nutrients in food that have not been investigated yet. Many nutrients work in **synergy,** enhancing chemical processes in the body.

Supplementation will not offset poor eating habits. Pills are no substitute for common sense. If you think your diet is not balanced, you first need to conduct a nutrient analysis (see Lab 3A, pages 103–105) to determine which nutrients you lack in sufficient amounts. Eat more of them, as well as foods that are high in antioxidants and phytonutrients. Following a nutrient assessment, a **registered dietitian** can help you decide what supplement(s), if any, might be necessary.

If you take supplements in pill form, look for products that meet the USP (U.S. Pharmacopoeia) disintegration standards on the bottle. The USP symbol suggests that the supplement should completely dissolve in 45 minutes or less. Supplements that do not dissolve, of course, cannot get into the bloodstream.

Critical Thinking

Do you take supplements? If so, for what purposes are you taking them—and do you think you could restructure your diet so you could do without them?

Functional Foods

Functional foods are foods or food ingredients that offer specific health benefits beyond those supplied by the traditional nutrients they contain. Many functional foods come in their natural form. A tomato, for example, is a functional food because it contains the phytonutrient lycopene, thought to reduce the risk for prostate cancer. Other examples of functional foods are kale, broccoli, blueberries, red grapes, and green tea.

The term "functional food," however, has been used primarily as a marketing tool by the food industry to attract consumers. Unlike **fortified foods,** which have been modified to help prevent nutrient deficiencies, the food industry creates functional foods by adding ingredients aimed at treating or preventing symptoms or disease. In functional foods, the added ingredient(s) is typically not found in the food item in its natural form but is added to allow manufacturers to make appealing health claims.

In most cases, only one extra ingredient is added (a vitamin, mineral, phytonutrient, or herb). An example is calcium added to orange juice to make the claim that this brand offers protection against osteoporosis. Food manufacturers now offer cholesterol-lowering margarines (enhanced with plant stanol), cancer-protective ketchup (fortified with lycopene), memory-boosting candy (with ginkgo added), calcium-fortified chips, and corn chips containing kava-kava (to enhance relaxation).

The use of some functional foods, however, may undermine good nutrition. Margarines still may contain saturated fats or partially hydrogenated oils. Regularly consuming ketchup on top of large orders of fries adds many calories and fat to the diet. Sweets are also high in calories and sugar. Chips are high in calories, salt, and fat. In all of these cases, the consumer would be better off taking the specific ingredient in a supplement form rather than consuming the functional food with its extra calories, sugar, salt, and/or fat.

Functional foods can provide added benefits if used in conjunction with a healthful diet. You may use nutrient-dense functional foods in your overall wellness plan as an adjunct to health-promoting strategies and treatments.

Genetically Modified Crops

A genetically modified organism (GMO) is one in which its DNA (or basic genetic material) is manipulated to obtain certain results. This is done by inserting genes with desirable traits from one plant, animal, or microorganism into another one to either introduce new traits or enhance existing traits.

Crops are genetically modified to make them better resist disease and extreme environmental conditions (such as heat and frost), require fewer fertilizers and pesticides, last longer, and improve their nutrient content and taste. GMO could help save billions of dollars by producing more crops and helping to feed the hungry in developing countries around the world.

Concern over the safety of **genetically modified foods (GM foods)** has led to heated public debates in Europe and, to a lesser extent, in the United States. The concern is that genetic modifications create "transgenic" organisms that have not previously existed and that have potentially unpredictable effects on the environment and on humans. Also, there is some concern that GM foods may cause illness or allergies in humans and that cross-pollination may de-

---

Anticoagulant Any substance that inhibits blood clotting.

Synergy A reaction in which the result is greater than the sum of its two parts.

Registered dietitian (RD) A person with a college degree in dietetics who meets all certification and continuing education requirements of the American Dietetic Association or Dietitians of Canada.

Functional foods Foods or food ingredients containing physiologically active substances that provide specific health benefits beyond those supplied by basic nutrition.

Fortified foods Foods that have been modified by the addition or increase of nutrients that either were not present or were present in insignificant amounts with the intent of preventing nutrient deficiencies.

Genetically modified foods (GM foods) Foods whose basic genetic material (DNA) is manipulated by inserting genes with desirable traits from one plant, animal, or microorganism into another one either to introduce new traits or to enhance existing ones.

FIGURE 3.15 2005 Dietary Guidelines for Americans.

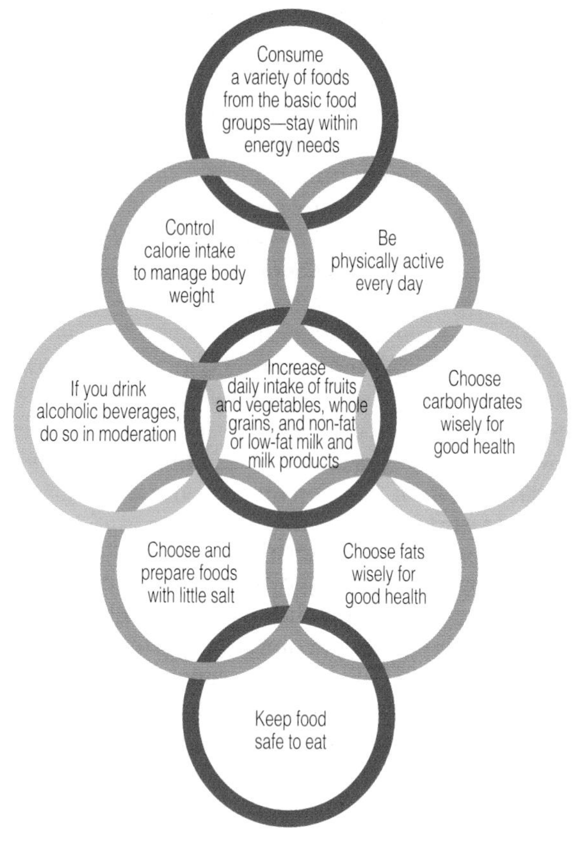

ents, intakes by Americans appear adequate. Still, efforts are warranted to promote increased dietary intakes of vitamin E, calcium, magnesium, potassium, and fiber by children and adults and to promote increased dietary intakes of vitamins A and C by adults. A basic premise of dietary guidance is to meet the recommended nutrient intakes while staying within energy needs.

- *Control calorie intake to manage body weight.* Calorie intake and physical activity go hand in hand in controlling a person's weight. To stem the obesity epidemic, most Americans need to consume fewer calories. In weight control, calories do count. Limiting portion sizes and monitoring weight regularly to adjust food intake as necessary are recommended.
- *Be physically active every day.* Making moderate physical activity a part of an adult's daily routine for at least 30 minutes per day promotes fitness and reduces the risk of acquiring chronic health conditions. Moderate physical activity for an hour each day can increase energy expenditure by about 150 to 200 calories, depending on body size. According to the committee, many adults need to participate in up to 60 minutes of moderate to vigorous physical activity on most days to prevent unhealthy weight gain; adults who previously have lost weight may need 60 and up to 90 minutes of moderate physical activity daily to avoid regaining weight. Compared with moderate physical activity, vigorous physical activity provides greater benefits for physical fitness and burns more calories per unit of time.
- *Increase daily intake of fruits and vegetables, whole grains, and non-fat or low-fat milk and milk products.* Fruits contain glucose, fructose, sucrose, and fiber, and most fruits are relatively low in calories. Also, fruits are important sources of at least eight additional nutrients, including vitamin C, folate, and potassium. Many vegetables provide only small amounts of sugars and/or starch, some are high in starch, and all provide fiber. Vegetables are important sources of 19 or more nutrients, including potassium, folate, and vitamins A and E.

  Moreover, increased consumption of fruits and vegetables may be a useful component of programs designed to achieve and sustain weight loss. Consuming a variety of fruits and vegetables daily is recommended (choose among citrus fruits, melons, and berries; other fruits; dark-green leafy vegetables; bright-orange vegetables; legumes; starchy vegetables; and other vegetables).

  Whole grains are high in starch, and they are important sources of 14 nutrients including fiber. Important sources of whole grains include whole wheat, oatmeal, popcorn, bulgur, and brown rice. The goal is to eat at least three 1-ounce equivalents per day of whole-grain foods, preferably in place of refined grains.

  Milk and milk products are important sources of at least 12 nutrients including calcium, magnesium, potassium, and vitamin D. Diets that provide three cups (or the equivalent) of non-fat or low-fat milk and/or milk products per day can improve bone mass and are not associated with weight gain.
- *Choose fats wisely for good health.* Keeping a low intake of saturated fat, trans fat, and cholesterol can reduce the risk of coronary heart disease. The lower the combined intake of saturated and trans fat and the lower the dietary cholesterol intake, the greater the cardiovascular benefit will be.

  The main way to keep saturated fat low is to limit one's intake of animal fats (such as those in cheese, milk, butter, ice cream, and other full-fat dairy products; fatty meat; bacon and sausage; and poultry skin and fat). The major way to limit trans fat intake is to limit the intake of foods made with partially hydrogenated vegetable oils. To limit dietary intake of cholesterol, a person has to limit the intake of eggs and organ meats especially, as well as limit the intake of meat, shellfish, poultry, and dairy products that contain fat.

2. Faulty nutrition o
velopment and p
a. cardiovascular
b. cancer
c. osteoporosis
d. diabetes
e. All are correc
3. According to MyI
tion is measured
a. servings.
b. ounces.
c. cups.
d. calories.
e. all of the abo
4. The recommen
adults 50 years a
a. 10 grams per
men.
b. 21 grams per
men.
c. 28 grams per
men.
d. 25 grams pe
men.
e. 45 grams pe
men.
5. Unhealthy fats i
a. unsaturated
b. monounsatu
c. polyunsatura
d. saturated fat
e. all of the ab
6. The daily recom
a. 45 to 65 per
b. 10 to 35 per
c. 20 to 35 per
d. 60 to 75 per
e. 35 to 50 per

Media Mer

Thomson NOW! Conne

- Analyze your ea
- Check how wel
cepts.

Internet Connection

American Dietetic Ass

This comprehensi
quently asked ques
to other reliable W
http://www.ea

A total fat intake of 20 to 35 percent of calories is recommended for all Americans age 18 years and older. Intakes of fat outside of this range are not recommended for most Americans because of the potential adverse effects on achieving recommended nutrient intakes and on risk factors for chronic diseases. The lower limit of fat intake is higher for children: 30 percent of calories from fat for children age 2 and 3 years, and 25 percent of calories from fat for those ages 4 to 18 years.

- *Choose carbohydrates wisely for good health.* When selecting foods from the fruit, vegetable, and grains groups, frequent fiber-rich choices are beneficial. This means, for example, choosing whole fruits rather than juices and whole grains rather than refined grains. Following the guidelines to increase the intake of fruits, vegetables, whole grains, and non-fat or low-fat milk and milk products is a healthful way to obtain the recommended amounts of carbohydrates. Compared with individuals who consume small amounts of foods and beverages that are high in added sugars, those who consume large amounts tend to consume more calories but smaller amounts of vitamins and minerals. A reduced intake of added sugars (especially sugar-sweetened beverages) may be helpful in achieving the recommended intakes of nutrients and in controlling weight.
- *Choose and prepare foods with little salt.* Reducing salt (sodium chloride) intake is one of several ways by which people can lower their blood pressure. Reducing blood pressure, ideally to the normal range, decreases the chance of developing a stroke, heart disease, heart failure, and kidney disease. The relationship between salt intake and blood pressure is direct and progressive without an apparent threshold. The goal is to consume less than 2,300 mg of sodium per day. On average, the higher a person's salt intake, the higher the blood pressure. Thus, reducing salt intake as much as possible is one way to lower blood pressure.
- *If you drink alcoholic beverages, do so in moderation.* Among middle-aged and older adults, the lowest all-cause mortality occurs at the level of one or two drinks per day. The mortality reduction likely stems from the protective effects of moderate alcohol consumption on coronary heart disease, primarily among males older than 45 years of age and women older than 55 years. Among younger people, alcohol consumption seems to provide little, if any, health benefit. Alcohol use among young adults is associated with increased risk of traumatic injury and death. Heavy drinking is hazardous, contributing to automobile injuries and deaths, assault, liver disease, and other health problems. Abstention is an important option.

  The goal for adults who choose to drink is to do so in moderation. "Moderation" is defined as consuming up to one drink per day for women and two drinks per day for men. One drink is defined as 12 ounces of regular beer, 5 ounces of wine (12 percent alcohol), or 1.5 ounces of 80-proof distilled spirits.

  Among those who should not consume alcoholic beverages are individuals who cannot restrict their drinking to moderate levels, children and adolescents, and individuals taking medications that can interact with alcohol or who have specific medical conditions. Alcoholic beverages should be avoided by women who may become pregnant or who are pregnant, by breastfeeding women, and by individuals who plan to drive or take part in other activities that require attention, skill, or coordination.
- *Keep food safe to eat.* According to the 2005 Dietary Guidelines report, foodborne diseases cause approximately 76 million illnesses, 325,000 hospitalizations, and 5,000 deaths in the United States each year. Three pathogens (salmonella, listeria, and toxoplasma) are responsible for more than 75 percent of these deaths. Actions by consumers can reduce the occurrence of foodborne illness substantially. The behaviors in the home that are most likely to prevent a problem with foodborne illnesses are

  Cleaning hands, contact surfaces, and fruits and vegetables (This does not apply to meat and poultry, which should not be washed.)
  Separating raw, cooked, and ready-to-eat foods while shopping, preparing, or storing
  Cooking foods to a safe temperature
  Chilling (refrigerating) perishable foods promptly
  Avoiding higher-risk foods (e.g., deli meats and frankfurters that have not been reheated to a safe temperature [may contain listeria]). This is especially important for high-risk groups (the very young, pregnant women, the elderly, and those who are immunocompromised).

Additional information on these guidelines is posted at www.health.gov/dietaryguidelines.

Proper Nutrition: A Lifetime Prescription for Healthy Living

The three factors that do the most for health, longevity, and quality of life are proper nutrition, a sound exercise program, and quitting (or never starting) smoking. Achieving and maintaining a balanced diet is not as difficult as most people think. If everyone were more educated about their own nutrition habits and the nutrition habits of their children, the current magnitude of nutrition-related health problems would be much

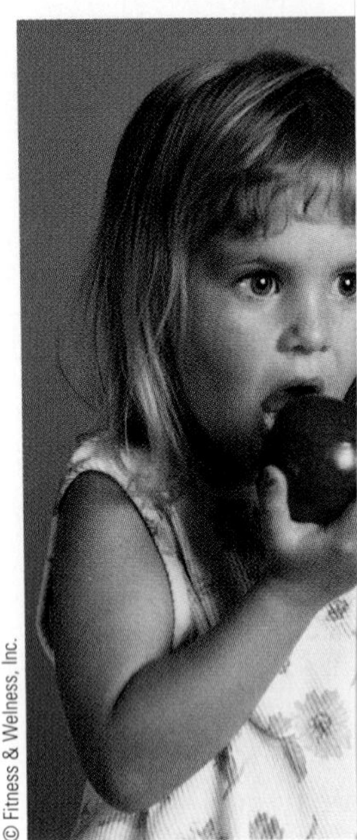
© Fitness & Welness, Inc.

smaller. Although trea
should place far grea
sity in youth and adul

Children tend to
parents adopt a healt
follow. The difficult p
themselves—to closel
learned from *their* par

Assess Your

Thomson NOW! Log on tc
and crea

1. Are whole grains
of your diet?
2. Are you meeting
mendations for d
(or substitutes) a
3. Will the inform
change in any ma

Assess Your

Thomson NOW! Log on t
this chap
modules

1. The science of nu
a. vitamins and
b. foods to optir
c. carbohydrate
opment and

Lab 3B MyPyramid Record Form

Body

Homework Assignment

Name: | Date: | Grade:

Instructor: | Course: | Section:

Assignment

This laboratory experience should be carried out as a homework assignment to be completed over the next 7 days.

Objective

To meet the minimum daily required amounts of the basic food groups and monitor total daily fat intake.

Lab Resources

"MyPyramid" at http://mypyramid.gov.

I. Instructions

Keep a 7-day record of your food consumption using the MyPyramid guidelines in Figure 3.1. Whenever you have something to eat, record the food item, the number of calories, the grams of fat (use the Nutritive Value of Selected Foods list given in Appendix A), and the amounts eaten based on the MyPyramid guidelines. If a particular food item is not listed in the Nutritive Value of Selected Foods list, the information can be obtained from the food container itself .

Record all information immediately after each meal, because it will be easier to keep track of foods and amounts eaten. If twice the amount of a particular serving is eaten, the calories, grams of fat, and amounts must be doubled as well.

At the end of the day, evaluate the diet by checking whether the minimum required amounts for each food group were met, and by total amount of calories and fat consumed. If you meet the required food group amounts and your daily caloric intake recommendation, you are well on your way to achieving a well-balanced diet. In addition, fat intake should not exceed 30 percent of the daily caloric consumption (may be up to 35 percent for individuals who suffer from metabolic syndrome—see Table 3.5, page 72). If you are on a diet, you may want to reduce fat intake to less than 20 percent of total daily calories (see Table 5.5, page 152).

II. Nutrition Stage of Change

Using Figure 2.5 (page 49) and Table 2.3 (page 49) identify your current stage of change for nutrition (healthy diet):

III. What I Learned and What I Can Do to Improve My Nutrition:

Based on the nutrient analysis conducted in Lab 3A and your daily diet analysis conducted in this lab, explain what these experiences have taught you and list specific changes and strategies that you can use to improve your present nutrition habits. Use an extra blank sheet of paper as needed.

I have learned the following about myself/my current diet: ____________________

____

____

Specific changes I plan to make: ____________________

____

____

Strategies I will use: ____________________

____

____

IV. Current number of daily steps: ☐ **Category** (Use Table 1.2, page 8): ____________________

To understand the concept of **body composition,** we must recognize that the human body consists of fat and non-fat components. The fat component is called fat mass or **percent body fat.** The non-fat component is termed **lean body mass.**

To determine **recommended body weight,** we need to find out what percent of total body weight is fat and what amount is lean tissue—in other words, assess body composition. Body composition should be assessed by a well-trained technician who understands the procedure being used.

Once the fat percentage is known, recommended body weight can be calculated from recommended body fat. Recommended body weight, also called "healthy weight," implies the absence of any medical condition that would improve with weight loss and a fat distribution pattern that is not associated with higher risk for illness.

Formerly, people relied on simple height/weight charts to determine their recommended body weight, but these tables can be highly inaccurate and fail to identify critical fat values associated with higher risk for disease.

Standard height/weight tables, first published in 1912, were based on average weights (including shoes and clothing) for men and women who obtained life insurance policies between 1888 and 1905—a notably unrepresentative population. The recommended body weight on these tables was obtained according to sex, height, and frame size. Because no scientific guidelines were given to determine frame size, most people chose their frame size based on the column in which the weight came closest to their own!

The best way to determine whether people are truly **overweight** or falsely at recommended body weight is through assessment of body composition. **Obesity** is an excess of body fat. If body weight is the only criterion, an individual might easily appear to be overweight according to height/weight charts, yet not have too much body fat. Typical examples are football players, body builders, weight lifters, and other athletes with large muscle size. Some athletes who appear to be 20 or 30 pounds overweight really have little body fat.

The inaccuracy of height/weight charts was illustrated clearly when a young man who weighed about 225 pounds applied to join a city police force but was turned down without having been granted an interview. The reason? He was "too fat," according to the height/weight charts. When this young man's body composition was assessed at a preventive medicine clinic, it was determined that only 5 percent of his total body weight was in the form of fat—considerably less than the recommended standard. In the words of the director of the clinic, "The only way this fellow could come down to the chart's target weight would have been through surgical removal of a large amount of his muscle tissue."

FIGURE 4.1 Typical body composition of an adult man and woman.

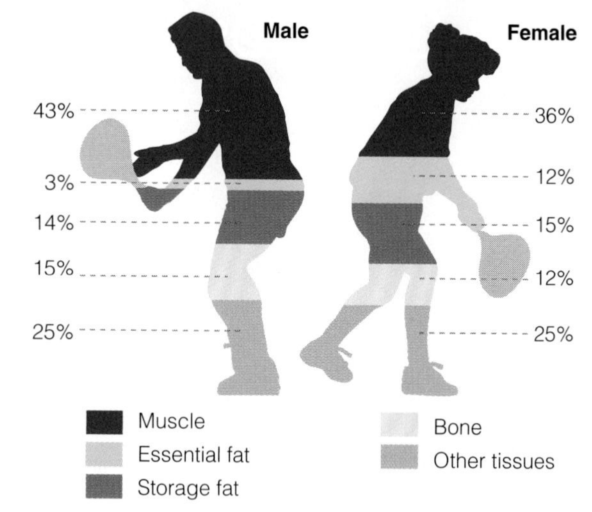

At the other end of the spectrum, some people who weigh very little (and may be viewed as skinny or underweight) actually can be classified as overweight because of their high body fat content. People who weigh as little as 120 pounds but are more than 30 percent fat (about one-third of their total body weight) are not rare. These cases are found more readily in the sedentary population and among people who are always dieting. Physical inactivity and a constant negative caloric balance both lead to a loss in lean body mass (see Chapter 5). These examples illustrate that body weight alone clearly does not tell the whole story.

Essential and Storage Fat

Total fat in the human body is classified into two types: **essential fat** and **storage fat.** Essential fat is needed for normal physiological function. Without it, human health and physical performance deteriorate. This type of fat is found within tissues such as muscles, nerve cells, bone marrow, intestines, heart, liver, and lungs. Essential fat constitutes about 3 percent of the total weight in men and 12 percent in women (see Figure 4.1). The percentage is higher in women because it includes sex-specific fat, such as that found in the breast tissue, the uterus, and other sex-related body parts.

Storage fat is the fat stored in adipose tissue, mostly just beneath the skin (subcutaneous fat) and around major organs in the body. This fat serves three basic functions:

1. as an insulator to retain body heat,
2. as energy substrate for metabolism, and
3. as padding against physical trauma to the body.

The amount of storage fat does not differ between men and women, except that men tend to store fat around the waist and women around the hips and thighs.

Critical Thinking

Mary is a cross-country runner whose coach has asked her to decrease her total body fat to 7 percent. Will Mary's performance increase at this lower percent body fat? How would you respond to this coach?

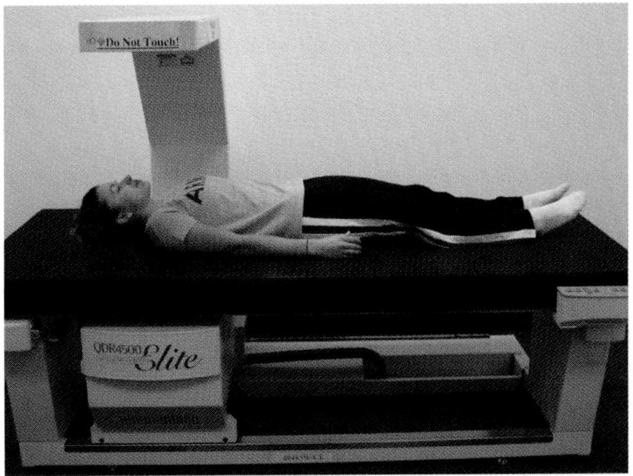

Dual energy X-ray absorptiometry (DEXA) technique to assess body composition and bone density.

Techniques to Assess Body Composition

Body composition can be estimated through the several procedures described in the following pages. Each procedure includes a standard error of estimate (SEE), a measure of the accuracy of the prediction made through the regression equation for that specific technique. For example, if the SEE for a given technique is ± 3.0 and the individual tests at a fat percentage of 18.0, the actual fat percentage may range from 15 to 21 percent.

Dual Energy X-Ray Absorptiometry

Dual energy X-ray absorptiometry (DEXA) is a method to assess body composition that is used most frequently in research and by medical facilities. A radiographic technique, DEXA uses very low-dose beams of X-ray energy (hundreds of times lower than a typical body X-ray) to measure total body fat mass, fat distribution pattern (see "Waist Circumference" on page 118), and bone density. Bone density is measured to assess the risk for osteoporosis. The procedure itself is simple and takes less than 15 minutes to administer. Many exercise scientists consider DEXA to be the standard technique to assess body composition. The SEE for this technique is ± 1.8 percent.

Because DEXA is not readily available to most fitness participants, other methods to estimate body composition are used. The most common of these are

1. hydrostatic or underwater weighing
2. air displacement
3. skinfold thickness
4. girth measurements
5. bioelectrical impedance

Because these procedures yield estimates of body fat, each technique may yield slightly different values. Therefore, when assessing changes in body composition, be sure to use the same technique for pre- and post-test comparisons.

The two most accurate techniques presently available in fitness laboratories are hydrostatic weighing and air displacement. Other techniques to assess body composition are available, but the equipment is costly and not easily accessible to the general population. In addition to percentages of lean tissue and body fat, some of these methods also provide information on total body water and bone mass. These techniques include magnetic resonance imaging (MRI), computed tomography (CT), and total body electrical conductivity (TOBEC). In terms of predicting percent body fat, these techniques do not seem to be more accurate than hydrostatic weighing or air displacement.

Body composition The fat and non-fat components of the human body; important in assessing recommended body weight.

Percent body fat Proportional amount of fat in the body based on the person's total weight; includes both essential fat and storage fat; also termed fat mass.

Lean body mass Body weight without body fat.

Recommended body weight Body weight at which there seems to be no harm to human health; healthy weight.

Overweight An excess amount of weight against a given standard, such as height or recommended percent body fat.

Obesity An excessive accumulation of body fat, usually at least 30 percent above recommended body weight.

Essential fat Minimal amount of body fat needed for normal physiological functions; constitutes about 3 percent of total weight in men and 12 percent in women.

Storage fat Body fat in excess of essential fat; stored in adipose tissue.

Dual energy X-ray absorptiometry (DEXA) Method to assess body composition that uses very low-dose beams of X-ray energy to measure total body fat mass, fat distribution pattern, and bone density.

FIGURE 4.2 Hydrostatic weighing procedure.

A small tank or pool, an autopsy scale, and a submersible chair are needed. The scale should measure up to about 10 kilograms (kg) and should be readable to the nearest .01 kilogram. The chair is suspended from the scale and submerged in a tank of water or pool measuring at least 5 × 5 × 5 feet. A swimming pool can be used in place of the tank.

The procedure for the technician is

1. Ask the person to be weighed to fast for approximately 6 to 8 hours and to have a bladder and bowel movement prior to underwater weighing.
2. Measure the individual's residual lung volume (RV, or amount of air left in the lungs following complete exhalation). If no equipment (spirometer) is available to measure the residual volume, estimate it using the following predicting equations* (to convert inches to centimeters, multiply inches by 2.54):

   Men: RV = [(0.027 × height in centimeters) + (0.017 × age)] − 3.447

   Women: RV = [(0.032 × height in centimeters) + (0.009 × age)] − 3.9

3. Have the person remove all jewelry prior to weighing. Weigh the person on land in a swimsuit and subtract the weight of the suit. Convert the weight from pounds to kilograms (divide pounds by 2.2046).
4. Record the water temperature in the tank in degrees Centigrade. Use that temperature to obtain the water density factor provided below, which is required in the formula to compute body density.

Temp (°C)	Water Density (gr/ml)	Temp (°C)	Water Density (gr/ml)
28	0.99626	35	0.99406
29	0.99595	36	0.99371
30	0.99567	37	0.99336
31	0.99537	38	0.99299
32	0.99505	39	0.99262
33	0.99473	40	0.99224
34	0.99440		

5. After the person is dressed in the swimsuit, have him or her enter the tank and completely wipe off all air clinging to the skin. Have the person sit in the chair with the water at chin level (raise or lower the chair as needed). Make sure the water and scale remain as still as possible during the entire procedure, because this allows for a more accurate reading. (During underwater weighing, you can decrease scale movement by holding and slowly releasing the neck of the scale until the subject is floating freely in the water.)

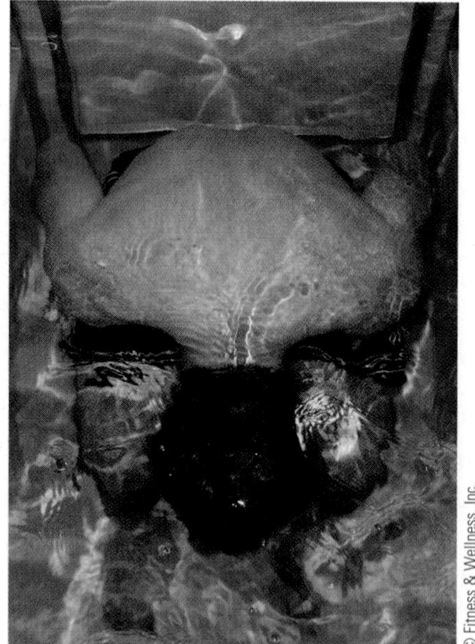

Hydrostatic or underwater weighing technique.

Hydrostatic Weighing

For decades, **hydrostatic weighing** has been the most common technique used in determining body composition in exercise physiology laboratories. In essence, a person's "regular" weight is compared with a weight taken underwater. Because fat is more buoyant than lean tissue, comparing the two weights can determine a person's percent of fat. Almost all other indirect techniques to assess body composition have been validated against hydrostatic weighing. The procedure requires a considerable amount of time, skill, space, and equipment and must be administered by a well-trained technician. The SEE for hydrostatic weighing is 2.5 percent.

This technique has several drawbacks. First, because each individual assessment can take as long as 30 minutes, hydrostatic weighing is not feasible when testing a lot of people. Furthermore, the person's residual lung volume (amount of air left in the lungs following complete forceful exhalation) should be measured before testing. If residual volume cannot be measured, as is the case in some laboratories and health/fitness centers, it is estimated using the predicting equations—which may decrease the accuracy of hydrostatic weighing. Also, the requirement of being completely under water makes hydrostatic weighing difficult to administer to **aquaphobic** people. For accurate results, the individual must be able to perform the test properly.

As described in Figure 4.2 and in Lab 4A, for each underwater weighing trial, the person has to (a) force out all of the air in the lungs, (b) lean forward and completely submerge underwater for about 5 to 10 seconds (long enough to get the underwater weight), and (c) remain as calm as possible (chair movement makes

6. Place a clip on the person's nose and have him or her forcefully exhale all of the air out of the lungs. The individual then totally submerges underwater. Make sure that all the air is exhaled from the lungs prior to submerging. Record the reading on the scale. Repeat this procedure 8 to 10 times, because practice and experience increase the accuracy of the underwater weight. Use the average of the three heaviest underwater weights as the gross underwater weight.

7. Because tare weight (the weight of the chair and chain or rope used to suspend the chair) accounts for part of the gross underwater weight, subtract this weight to obtain the person's net underwater weight. To determine tare weight, place a clothespin on the chain or rope at the water level when the person is submerged completely. After the person comes out of the water, lower the chair into the water to the pin level. Now record tare weight. Determine the net underwater weight by subtracting the tare weight from the gross underwater weight.

8. Compute body density and percent fat using the following equations:

$$\text{Body density} = \frac{BW}{\frac{BW - UW}{WD} - RV - .1}$$

$$\text{Percent fat}^{**} = \frac{495}{BD} - 450$$

Where:
BW = body weight in kg
UW = net underwater weight
WD = water density (determined by water temperature)
RV = residual volume
BD = body density

A sample computation for body fat assessment according to hydrostatic weighing is provided in Lab 4A.

*From H. L. Goldman and M. R. Becklake, "Respiratory Function Tests: Normal Values at Medium Altitudes and the Prediction of Nomal Results," in *American Review of Tuberculosis* 79 (1959): 457–467.
**From W. E. Siri, *Body Composition from Fluid Spaces and Density* (Berkeley: University of California, Donner Laboratory of Medical Physics, March 19, 1956).

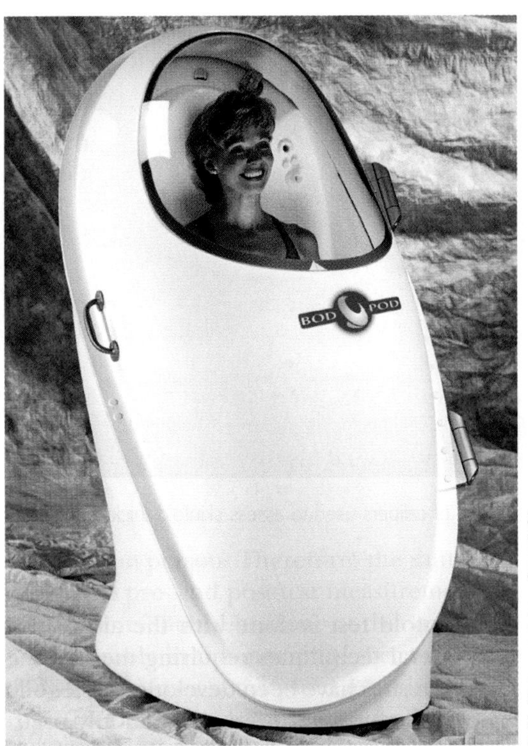

© Life Measurement, Inc.—Concord, CA

The Bod Pod, used to assess body composition.

reading the scale difficult). This procedure is repeated 8 to 10 times.

Forcing all of the air out of the lungs is not easy for everyone but is important to obtain an accurate reading. Leaving additional air (beyond residual volume) in the lungs makes a person more buoyant. Because fat is less dense than water, overweight individuals weigh less in water. Additional air in the lungs makes a person lighter in water, yielding a false, higher body fat percentage.

Air Displacement

Air displacement (also known as air displacement plethysmography) is a newer technique that holds considerable promise. With this method, an individual sits inside a small chamber, commercially known as the **Bod Pod.** Computerized pressure sensors determine the amount of air displaced by the person inside the chamber. Body volume is calculated by subtracting the air volume with the person inside the chamber from the volume of the empty chamber. The amount of air in the person's lungs also is taken into consideration when determining the actual body volume. Body density and percent body fat then are calculated from the obtained body volume.

Initial research has shown that this technique compares favorably with hydrostatic weighing, and it is less

Hydrostatic weighing Underwater technique to assess body composition; considered the most accurate of the body composition assessment techniques.

Aquaphobic Having a fear of water.

Air displacement Technique to assess body composition by calculating the body volume from the air replaced by an individual sitting inside a small chamber.

Bod Pod Commercial name of the equipment used to assess body composition through the air displacement technique.

FIGURE 4.5 Mortality risk versus Body Mass Index (BMI).

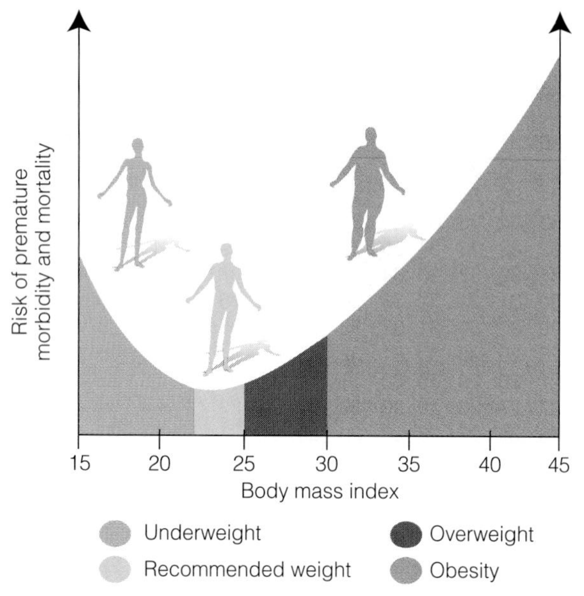

TABLE 4.5 Disease Risk According to Body Mass Index (BMI)

BMI	Disease Risk	Classification
<18.5	Increased	Underweight
18.5–21.99	Low	Acceptable
22.0–24.99	Very Low	Acceptable
25.0–29.99	Increased	Overweight
30.0–34.99	High	Obesity I
35.0–39.99	Very High	Obesity II
≥40.00	Extremely High	Obesity III

FIGURE 4.6 Overweight and obesity trends in the United States, 1960–2000.

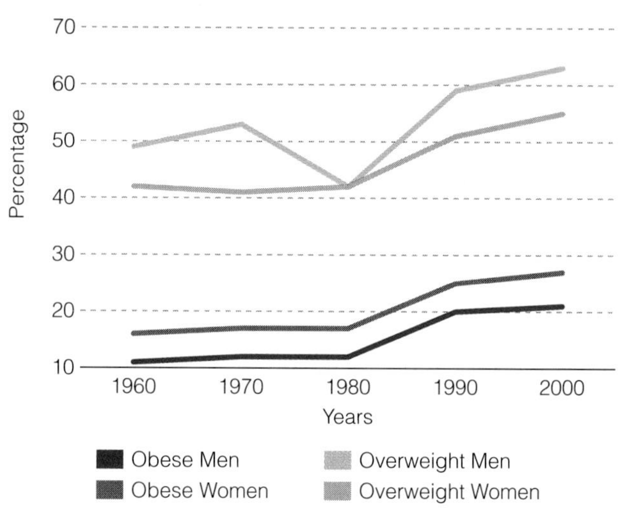

Adapted from the National Center for Health Statistics, Centers for Disease Control and Prevention, and the *Journal of the American Medical Association.*

as overweight if their indexes lie between 25 and 30. BMIs above 30 are defined as obese, and those below 18.5 as **underweight.** Scientific evidence has shown that the risk for premature illness and death is greater for those who are overweight, and the risk is also increased for individuals who are underweight[3] (see Figure 4.5).

Compared to individuals with a BMI between 22 and 25, people with a BMI between 25 and 30 (overweight) exhibit mortality rates up to 25 percent higher; rates for those with a BMI above 30 (obese) are 50 to 100 percent higher.[4] Table 4.5 provides disease risk categories when BMI is used as the sole criterion to identify people at risk. More than one-fifth of the U.S. adult population has a BMI of 30 or more. Overweight and obesity trends starting in 1960 according to BMI are given in Figure 4.6.

BMI is a useful tool to screen the general population, but its one weakness is that it fails to differentiate fat from lean body mass or note where most of the fat is located (waist circumference—see discussion that follows). Using BMI, athletes with a large amount of muscle mass (such as body builders and football players) can easily fall in the moderate- or even high-risk categories.

Waist Circumference

Scientific evidence suggests that the way people store fat affects their risk for disease. The total amount of body fat by itself is not the best predictor of increased risk for disease but, rather, the location of the fat. **Android obesity** is seen in individuals who tend to store fat in the trunk or abdominal area (which produces the "apple" shape). **Gynoid obesity** is seen in people who store fat primarily around the hips and thighs (which creates the "pear" shape).

Obese individuals with abdominal fat are clearly at higher risk for heart disease, hypertension, type 2 diabetes ("non-insulin-dependent" diabetes), and stroke than are obese individuals with similar amounts of body fat that is stored primarily in the hips and thighs.[5] Evidence also indicates that, among individuals with a lot of abdominal fat, those whose fat deposits are located around internal organs (intra-abdominal or abdominal visceral fat) have an even greater risk for disease than those with fat mainly just beneath the skin (subcutaneous fat).[6]

Complex scanning techniques to identify individuals at risk because of high intra-abdominal fatness are costly, so a simple **waist circumference (WC)** measure, designed by the National Heart, Lung, and Blood Institute, is used to assess this risk.[7] WC seems to predict abdominal visceral fat as accurately as the DEXA technique.[8] A waist circumference of more than 40 inches in men and 35 inches in women indicates a higher risk for cardiovascular disease, hypertension, and type 2 di-

TABLE 4.6 Disease Risk According to Waist Circumference (WC)

Men	Women	Disease Risk
<35.5	<32.5	Low
35.5–40.0	32.5–35.0	Moderate
>40.0	>35.0	High

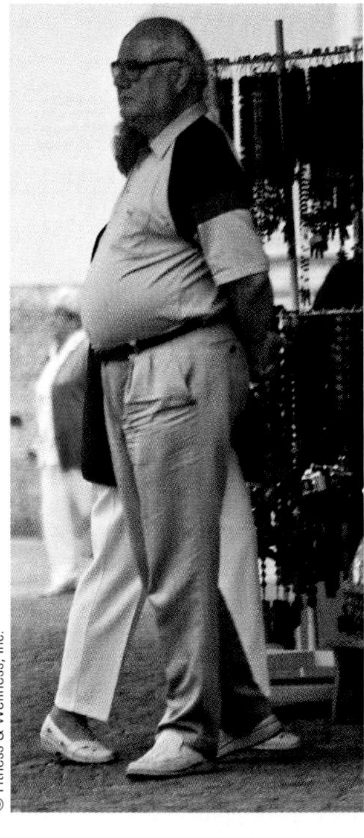

© Fitness & Wellness, Inc.

Individuals who accumulate body fat around the midsection are at greater risk for disease than those who accumulate body fat in other areas.

TABLE 4.7 Disease Risk According to Body Mass Index (BMI) and Waist Circumference (WC)

		Disease Risk Relative to Normal Weight and WC	
Classification	BMI (kg/m²)	Men ≤40″ (102 cm) Women ≤35″ (88 cm)	Men ≥40″ (102 cm) Women ≥35″ (88 cm)
Underweight	<18.5	Increased	Low
Normal	18.5–24.9	Very low	Increased
Overweight	25.0–29.9	Increased	High
Obesity Class I	30.0–34.9	High	Very high
Obesity Class II	35.0–39.9	Very high	Very high
Obesity Class III	≥40.0	Extremely high	Extremely high

Adapted from Expert Panel, *Executive Summary of the Clinical Guidelines on the Identification, Evaluation, and Treatment of Overweight and Obesity in Adults,* Archives of Internal Medicine 158 (1998): 1855–1867.

abetes (see Table 4.6). Weight loss is encouraged when individuals exceed these measurements.

A 2004 study concluded that WC is a better predictor than BMI of the risk for disease.[9] Thus, BMI in conjunction with WC provides the best combination to identify individuals at higher risk resulting from excessive body fat. Table 4.7 provides guidelines to identify people at risk according to BMI and WC.

A second procedure that was used for years to identify health risk based on the pattern of fat distribution is the waist-to-hip ratio (WHR) test. In recent years, however, several studies have found that WC is a better indicator than WHR of abdominal visceral obesity.[10] Thus, a combination of BMI and WC, rather than WHR, is now recommended by health-care professionals to assess potential risk for disease.

Determining Recommended Body Weight

If you are able to assess your percent body fat, you can determine your current body composition classification by consulting Table 4.8, which presents percentages of fat according to both the health fitness standard and the high physical fitness standard (see discussion in Chapter 1).

For example, the recommended health fitness fat percentage for a 20-year-old female is 28 percent or less. Although there are no clearly identified percent body fat levels at which the risk for disease definitely increases (as is the case with BMI), the health fitness standard in Table 4.8 is currently the best estimate of the point at which there seems to be no harm to health.

According to Table 4.8, the high physical fitness range for this same 20-year-old woman would be between 18 and 23 percent. The high physical fitness standard does not mean that you cannot be somewhat below this number. Many highly trained male athletes are as low as 3 percent, and some female distance runners have been measured at 6 percent body fat (which may not be healthy).

Scientists generally agree that the mortality rate is higher for obese people, and some evidence indicates that the same is true for underweight people. "Underweight" and "thin" do not necessarily mean the same thing. The body fat of a healthy thin person is near the high physical fitness standard, whereas an underweight person has extremely low body fat, even to the point of compromising the essential fat.

The 3 percent essential fat for men and 12 percent for women seem to be the lower limits for people to

Underweight Extremely low body weight.

Android obesity Obesity pattern seen in individuals who tend to store fat in the trunk or abdominal area.

Gynoid obesity Obesity pattern seen in people who store fat primarily around the hips and thighs.

Waist circumference (WC) A waist girth measurement to assess potential risk for disease based on intra-abdominal fat content.

TABLE 4.8 Body Composition Classification According to Percent Body Fat

MEN						
Age	Underweight	Excellent	Good	Moderate	Overweight	Significantly Overweight
≤19	<3	12.0	12.1–17.0	17.1–22.0	22.1–27.0	≥27.1
20–29	<3	13.0	13.1–18.0	18.1–23.0	23.1–28.0	≥28.1
30–39	<3	14.0	14.1–19.0	19.1–24.0	24.1–29.0	≥29.1
40–49	<3	15.0	15.1–20.0	20.1–25.0	25.1–30.0	≥30.1
≥50	<3	16.0	16.1–21.0	21.1–26.0	26.1–31.0	≥31.1
WOMEN						
Age	Underweight	Excellent	Good	Moderate	Overweight	Significantly Overweight
≤19	<12	17.0	17.1–22.0	22.1–27.0	27.1–32.0	≥32.1
20–29	<12	18.0	18.1–23.0	23.1–28.0	28.1–33.0	≥33.1
30–39	<12	19.0	19.1–24.0	24.1–29.0	29.1–34.0	≥34.1
40–49	<12	20.0	20.1–25.0	25.1–30.0	30.1–35.0	≥35.1
≥50	<12	21.0	21.1–26.0	26.1–31.0	31.1–36.0	≥36.1

☐ High physical fitness standard ☐ Health fitness standard

maintain good health. Below these percentages, normal physiological functions can be seriously impaired. Some experts point out that a little storage fat (in addition to the essential fat) is better than none at all. As a result, the health and high fitness standards for percent fat in Table 4.8 are set higher than the minimum essential fat requirements, at a point beneficial to optimal health and well-being. Finally, because lean tissue decreases with age, one extra percentage point is allowed for every additional decade of life.

Critical Thinking

Do you think you have a weight problem? Do your body composition results make you think differently about the way you perceive your current body weight and image?

Your recommended body weight is computed based on the selected health or high fitness fat percentage for your age and sex. Your decision to select a "desired" fat percentage should be based on your current percent body fat and your personal health/fitness objectives. Following are steps to compute your own recommended body weight:

1. Determine the pounds of body weight that are fat (FW) by multiplying your body weight (BW) by the current percent fat (%F) expressed in decimal form (FW = BW × %F).
2. Determine lean body mass (LBM) by subtracting the weight in fat from the total body weight (LBM = BW − FW). (Anything that is not fat must be part of the lean component.)
3. Select a desired body fat percentage (DFP) based on the health or high fitness standards given in Table 4.8.
4. Compute recommended body weight (RBW) according to the formula RBW = LBM ÷ (1.0 − DFP).

As an example of these computations, a 19-year-old female who weighs 160 pounds and is 30 percent fat would like to know what her recommended body weight would be at 22 percent:

Sex:	female
Age:	19
BW:	160 lbs
%F:	30% (.30 in decimal form)

1. FW = BW × %F
   FW = 160 × .30 = 48 lbs
2. LBM = BW − FW
   LBM = 160 − 48 = 112 lbs
3. DFP: 22% (.22 in decimal form)
4. RBW = LBM ÷ (1.0 − .DFP)
   RBW = 112 ÷ (1.0 − .22)
   RBW = 112 ÷ .78 = 143.6 lbs

In Lab 4A, you will have the opportunity to determine your own body composition and recommended body weight. A second column is provided in the activity for a follow-up assessment at a future date. The disease risk according to BMI and WC and recommended body weight according to BMI are determined in Lab 4B. You can also set goals to accomplish by the end of the term.

Behavior Modification Planning

TIPS FOR LIFETIME WEIGHT MANAGEMENT

Maintenance of recommended body composition is one of the most significant health issues of the 21st century. If you are committed to lifetime weight management, the following strategies will help:

- Accumulate 60 to 90 minutes of physical activity daily.
- Exercise at a brisk aerobic pace for a minimum of 20 minutes three times per week.
- Strength-train two to three times per week.
- Use common sense and moderation in your daily diet.
- Manage daily caloric intake by keeping in mind long-term benefits (recommended body weight) instead of instant gratification (overeating).
- "Junior-size" instead of "super-size."
- Regularly monitor body weight, body composition, body mass index, and waist circumference.
- Do not allow increases in body weight (percent fat) to accumulate; deal immediately with the problem through moderate reductions in caloric intake and maintenance of physical activity and exercise habits.

Try It

In your Online Journal or your class notebook, note which of these tips you are already using and which ones you can incorporate into your daily habits right away.

Other than hydrostatic weighing, skinfold thickness seems to be the most practical and valid technique to estimate body fat. If skinfold calipers are available, use this technique to assess your percent body fat. If none of these techniques is available to you, estimate your percent fat according to girth measurements (or another technique available to you) and use the resources at ThomsonNOW to obtain your body composition results. You also may wish to use several techniques and compare the results.

Critical Thinking

How do you feel about your current body weight, and what influence does society have on the way you perceive yourself in terms of your weight? Do your body composition results make you think differently about the way you see your current body weight and image?

FIGURE 4.7 Typical body composition changes for adults in the United States.

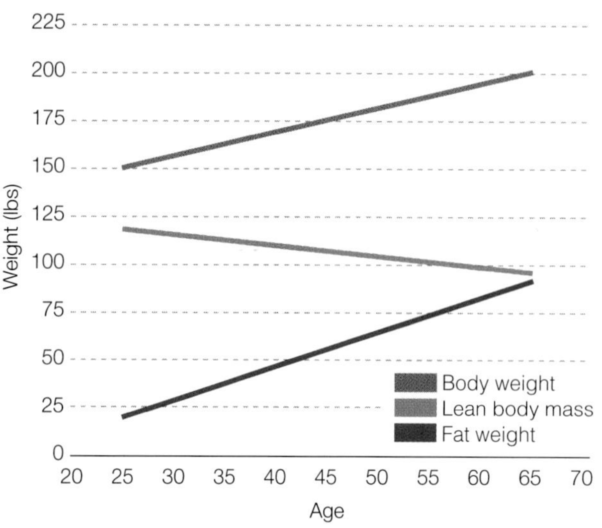

Importance of Regular Body Composition Assessment

Children in the United States do not start with a weight problem. Although a few struggle with weight throughout life, most are not overweight in the early years of life.

Trends indicate that, starting at age 25, the average person in the United States gains 1 to 2 pounds of weight per year. Thus, by age 65, the average American will have gained 40 to 80 pounds. Because of the typical reduction in physical activity in our society, however, the average person also loses $\frac{1}{2}$ pound of lean tissue each year. Therefore, this span of 40 years has produced an actual fat gain of 60 to 100 pounds accompanied by a 20-pound loss of lean body mass[11] (see Figure 4.7). These changes cannot be detected without assessing body composition periodically.

If you are on a diet/exercise program, you should repeat your percent body fat assessment and recommended weight computations about once a month. This is important because lean body mass is affected by weight-reduction programs and amount of physical activity. As lean body mass changes, so will your recommended body weight. To make valid comparisons, use the same technique for both pre- and post-program assessments. Knowing your percent body fat also is useful to identify fad diets that promote water loss and lean body mass, especially muscle mass (also see "Diet Crazes" in Chapter 5, page 133).

Changes in body composition resulting from a weight control/exercise program were illustrated in a co-ed aerobic dance course taught during a 6-week summer term. Students participated in a 60-minute aer-

FIGURE 4A.1 Sample computation for percent body fat according to hydrostatic weighing.

Name: Jane Doe Age: 20 Weight: 148.5 lbs

Height: 67 inches × 2.54 = 170.2 cm Water temperature: 33 °C Water density (WD): .99473 gr/ml

Residual volume (RV): 1.73 lt See Figure 4.2.

Body weight (BW) in kg = weight in pounds ÷ 2.2046

BW in kg = 148.5 ÷ 2.2046 = 67.36 kg

Gross underwater weights:

1.	6.15	kg	2.	6.12	kg	3.	6.24	kg	4.	6.26	kg	5.	6.21	kg
6.	6.26	kg	7.	6.29	kg	8.	6.28	kg	9.	6.24	kg	10.	6.27	kg

Average of three heaviest underwater weights (AUW): 6.28 kg

Tare weight (TW): 5.154 kg

Net underwater weight (UW) = AUW − TW

Net underwater weight (UW) = 6.28 − 5.154 = 1.126 kg

Body density (BD):

$$BD = \frac{BW}{\frac{BW - UW}{WD} - RV - .1} \qquad BD = \frac{67.36}{\frac{67.36 - 1.126}{.99473} - 1.73 - .1} = 1.0402301$$

Percent body fat (%Fat):

$$\%Fat = \frac{495}{BD} - 450 = \frac{495}{1.0402301} - 450 = 25.9\ \%$$

Follow-up percent body fat: %

II. What I learned from the underwater weighing procedure.

Describe the experience of being weighed underwater. Do you feel that the results of the test were accurate?

Weight Management

CHAPTER 5

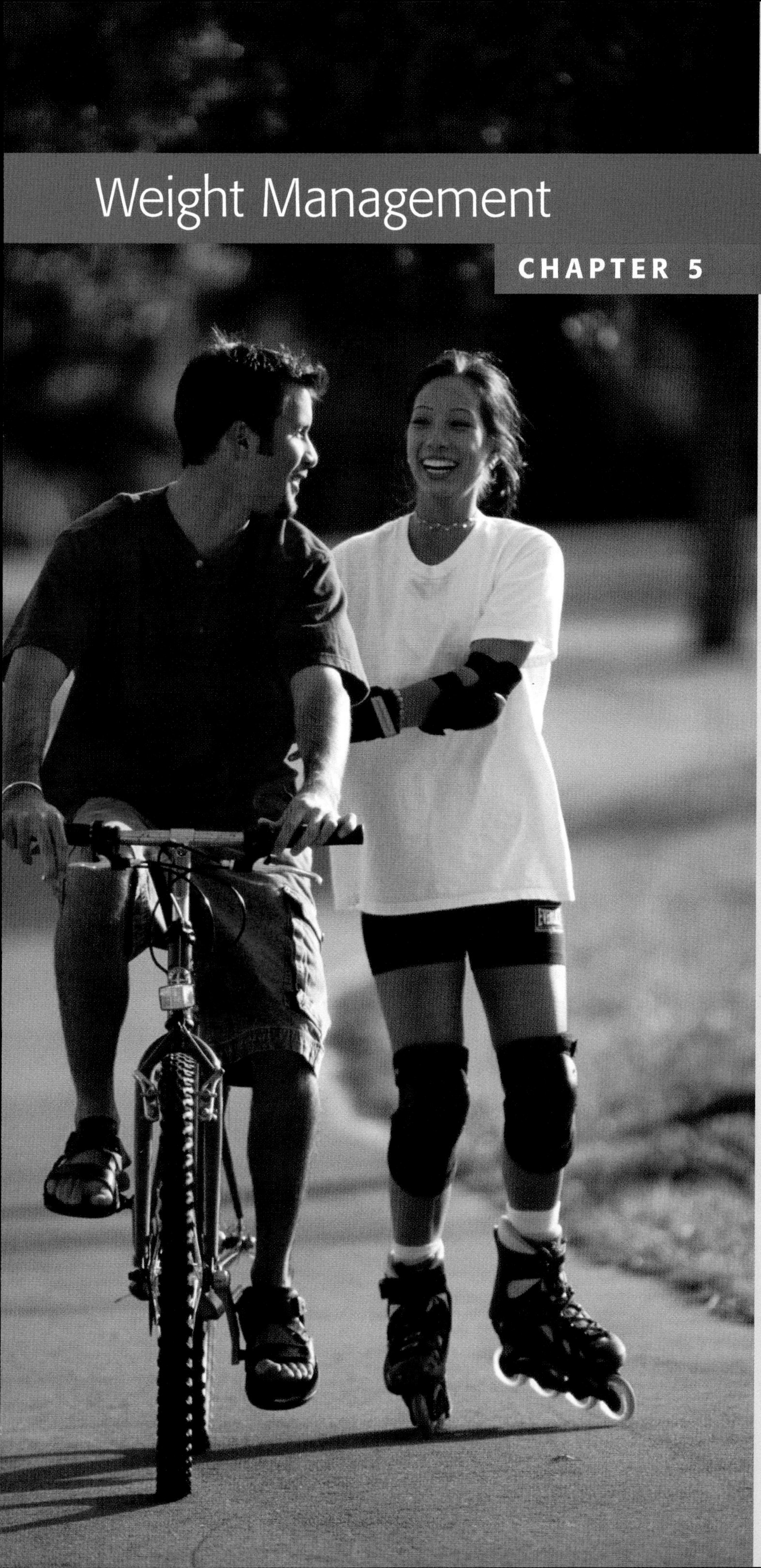

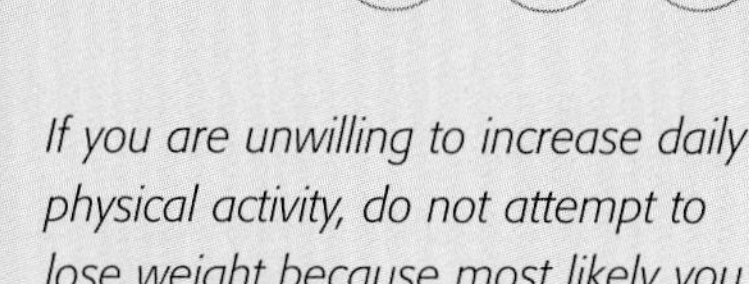

If you are unwilling to increase daily physical activity, do not attempt to lose weight because most likely you won't be able to keep it off.

OBJECTIVES

- Describe the health consequences of obesity.
- Expose some popular fad diets and myths and fallacies regarding weight control.
- Describe eating disorders and their associated medical problems and behavior patterns, and outline the need for professional help in treating these conditions.
- Explain the physiology of weight loss, including setpoint theory and the effects of diet on basal metabolic rate.
- Explain the role of a lifetime exercise program as the key to a successful weight loss and weight maintenance program.
- Be able to implement a physiologically sound weight reduction and weight maintenance program.
- Describe behavior modification techniques that help support adherence to a lifetime weight maintenance program.

Thomson™ NOW! go to www.thomsonedu.com/login to:

- Check your progress in your exercise log.
- Check how well you understand the chapter's concepts.

Photo © Bill Losh/Getty Images

Obesity is a health hazard of epidemic proportions in most developed countries around the world. According to the World Health Organization, an estimated 35 percent of the adult population in industrialized nations is obese. **Obesity** has been defined as a body mass index (BMI) of 30 or higher. The obesity level is the point at which excess body fat can lead to serious health problems.

The number of people who are obese and overweight in the United States has increased dramatically in the past few years, a direct result of physical inactivity and poor dietary habits. The average weight of American adults between the ages of 20 and 74 has increased by 25 pounds or more since 1965 (see Figure 5.1). More than one-half of all adults in the United States do not achieve the minimum recommended amount of physical activity (see Figure 1.6, page 7). In 2004, American women consumed 335 more calories daily than they did 20 years ago, and men an additional 170 calories per day.[1]

Approximately 65 percent of U.S. adults age 20 and older are **overweight** (have a BMI greater than 25), and 30 percent are obese[2] (see Figure 5.2). More than 120 million people are overweight and 30 million are obese. Between 1960 and 2002, the overall (men and women combined) prevalence of adult obesity increased from about 13 percent to 30 percent. Most of this increase occurred in the 1990s.

As illustrated in Figure 5.3, the obesity epidemic continues to escalate. Before 1990, not a single state reported an obesity rate above 15 percent of the state's total population (includes both adults and children). By the year 2005, all states reported a rate above 15 percent, 17 states had an obesity rate equal to or greater than 25 percent, and three states had reached a rate above 30 percent.

In the last decade alone, the average weight of American adults increased by about 15 pounds. The prevalence of obesity is even higher in ethnic groups, especially African Americans and Hispanic Americans. Further, as the nation continues to evolve into a more mechanized and automated society (relying on escalators, elevators, remote controls, computers, electronic mail, cell phones, and automatic-sensor doors), the amount of required daily physical activity continues to decrease. We are being lulled into a high-risk sedentary lifestyle.

About 44 percent of all women and 29 percent of all men are on a diet at any given moment.[3] People spend about $40 billion yearly attempting to lose weight, with more than $10 billion going to memberships in weight reduction centers and another $30 billion to diet food sales. Furthermore, the total cost attributable to treating obesity-related diseases is estimated at $100 billion per year.[4]

Excessive body weight and physical inactivity are the second leading cause of preventable death in the United States, causing more than 112,000 deaths each year.[5] Furthermore, obesity is more prevalent than smoking (19 percent), poverty (14 percent), and problem drinking (6 percent).[6] Obesity and unhealthy lifestyle habits are the most critical public health problems that we face in the 21st century.

Excessive body weight and obesity are associated with poor health status and are risk factors for many physical ailments, including cardiovascular disease and cancer. Evidence indicates that health risks associated with increased body weight start at a BMI over 25 and are enhanced greatly at a BMI over 30.

FIGURE 5.1 Average weight of Americans between 1963–1965 and 1999–2002.

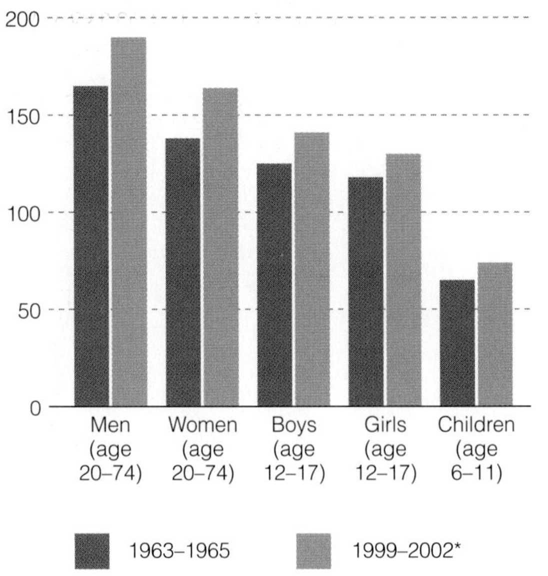

*Adults are about an inch taller and children about half an inch taller as compared with the early 1960s. The height difference accounts for about 3 to 6 extra pounds.

Source: "It's gaining on us." *UC Berkeley Wellness Letter,* May 2005.

FIGURE 5.2 Percentage of the adult population that is overweight (BMI ≥ 25) and obese (BMI ≥ 30) and in the United States.

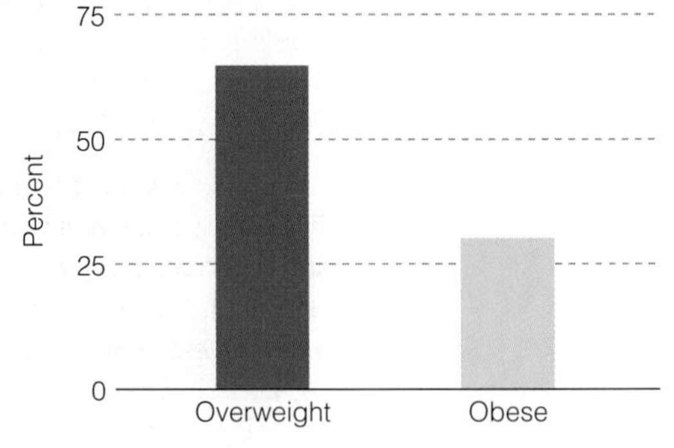

FIGURE 5.3 Obesity trends in the United States 1985–2005 based on BMI ≥ 30 or 30 pounds overweight.

Percentages of the total number of people in the respective state who are obese.

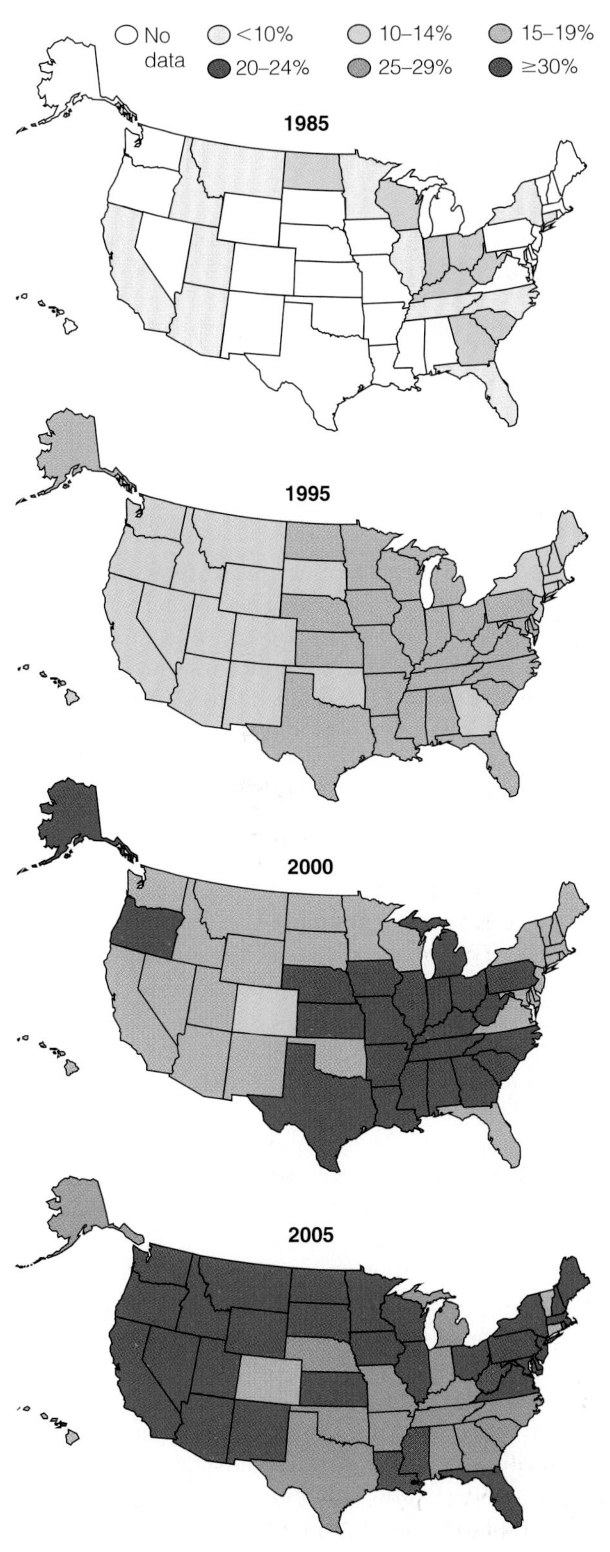

Source: Obesity Trends among U.S. Adults between 1985 and 2005. (Atlanta: Centers for Disease Control and Prevention, 2006).

HEALTH CONSEQUENCES
OF EXCESSIVE BODY WEIGHT

Being overweight or obese increases the risk for

- high blood pressure
- elevated blood lipids (high blood cholesterol and triglycerides)
- type 2 (non-insulin-dependent) diabetes
- insulin resistance, glucose intolerance
- coronary heart disease
- angina pectoris
- congestive heart failure
- stroke
- gallbladder disease
- gout
- osteoarthritis
- obstructive sleep apnea and respiratory problems
- some types of cancer (endometrial, breast, prostate, and colon)
- complications of pregnancy (gestational diabetes, gestational hypertension, preeclampsia, and complications during C-sections)
- poor female reproductive health (menstrual irregularities, infertility, irregular ovulation)
- bladder control problems (stress incontinence)
- psychological disorders (depression, eating disorders, distorted body image, discrimination, and low self-esteem)
- shortened life expectancy
- decreased quality of life

Source: Centers for Disease Control and Prevention, downloaded September 30, 2006.

The American Heart Association has identified obesity as one of the six major risk factors for coronary heart disease. Estimates also indicate that 14 percent of all cancer deaths in men and 20 percent in women are related to current overweight and obesity patterns in the United States.[7] Furthermore, excessive body weight is implicated in psychological maladjustment and a higher accidental death rate. Extremely obese people have a lower mental health–related quality of life.

Overweight Versus Obesity

Overweight and obesity are not the same thing. Many overweight people (people who weigh about 10 to 20 pounds over the recommended weight) are not obese. Although a few pounds of excess weight may not be harmful to most people, this is not always the case. People with excessive body fat who have type 2 diabetes and

Obesity A chronic disease characterized by body mass index (BMI) 30 or higher.

Overweight Excess weight characterized by a body mass index (BMI) greater than 25 but less than 30.

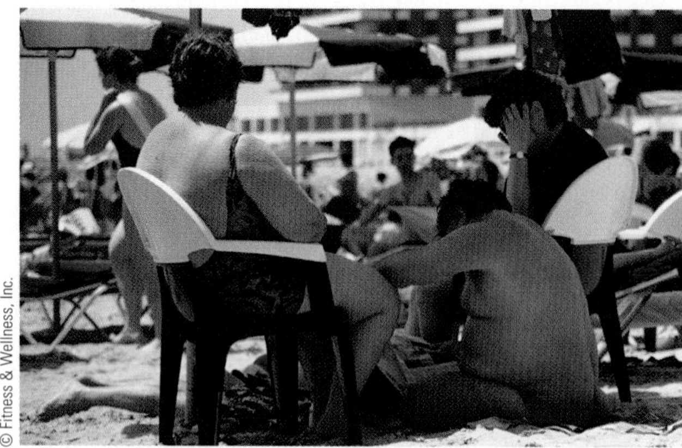

Obesity is a health hazard of epidemic proportions in industrialized nations.

other cardiovascular risk factors (elevated blood lipids, high blood pressure, physical inactivity, and poor eating habits) benefit from losing weight. People who have a few extra pounds of weight but are otherwise healthy and physically active, exercise regularly, and eat a healthy diet may not be at higher risk for early death. Such is not the case, however, with obese individuals.

Research indicates that individuals who are 30 or more pounds overweight during middle age (30 to 49 years of age) lose about 7 years of life, whereas being 10 to 30 pounds overweight decreases the lifespan by about 3 years.[8] These decreases are similar to those seen with tobacco use. Severe obesity (BMI greater than 45) at a young age, nonetheless, may cut up to 20 years off one's life.[9]

Although the loss of years of life is significant, the decreased life expectancy doesn't even begin to address the loss in quality of life and increased illness and disability throughout the years. Even a modest reduction of 5 to 10 percent can reduce the risk for chronic diseases including heart disease, high blood pressure, high cholesterol, and diabetes.[10]

A primary objective to achieve overall physical fitness and enhanced quality of life is to attain recommended body composition. Individuals at recommended body weight are able to participate in a wide variety of moderate-to-vigorous activities without functional limitations. These people have the freedom to enjoy most of life's recreational activities to their fullest potential. Excessive body weight does not afford an individual the fitness level to enjoy many lifetime activities such as basketball, soccer, racquetball, surfing, mountain cycling, or mountain climbing. Maintaining high fitness and recommended body weight gives a person a degree of independence throughout life that most people in developed nations no longer enjoy.

Scientific evidence also recognizes problems with being underweight. Although the social pressure to be thin has declined slightly in recent years, the pressure to attain model-like thinness is still with us and contributes to the gradual increase in the number of people who develop eating disorders (anorexia nervosa and bulimia, discussed under "Eating Disorders" on pages 136–140).

Extreme weight loss can lead to medical conditions such as heart damage, gastrointestinal problems, shrinkage of internal organs, abnormalities of the immune system, disorders of the reproductive system, loss of muscle tissue, damage to the nervous system, and even death. About 14 percent of people in the United States are underweight.

Critical Thinking

Do you consider yourself overweight? If so, how long have you had a weight problem, what attempts have you made to lose weight, and what has worked best for you?

Tolerable Weight

Many people want to lose weight so they will look better. That's a noteworthy goal. The problem, however, is that they have a distorted image of what they would really look like if they were to reduce to what they think is their ideal weight. Hereditary factors play a big role, and only a small fraction of the population has the genes for a "perfect body."

The media have the greatest influence on people's perception of what constitutes "ideal" body weight. Most people consult fashion, fitness, and beauty magazines to determine what they should look like. The "ideal" body shapes, physiques, and proportions illustrated in these magazines are rare and are achieved mainly through airbrushing and medical reconstruction.[11] Many individuals, primarily young women, go to extremes in an attempt to achieve these unrealistic figures. Failure to attain a "perfect body" may lead to eating disorders in some individuals.

When people set their own target weight, they should be realistic. Attaining the "Excellent" percent of body fat shown in Table 4.8 (page 120) is extremely difficult for some. It is even more difficult to maintain over time, unless the person makes a commitment to a vigorous lifetime exercise program and permanent dietary changes. Few people are willing to do that. The "Moderate" percent body fat category may be more realistic for many people.

The question you should ask yourself is: Am I happy with my weight? Part of enjoying a higher quality of life is being happy with yourself. If you are not, you either need to do something about it or learn to live with it.

If your percent of body fat is higher than those in the Moderate category of Table 4.8 (page 120), you should try to reduce it and stay in this category, for health reasons. This is the category that seems to pose no detriment to health.

If you are in the Moderate category but would like to reduce your percent of body fat further, you need to ask yourself a second question: How badly do I want it? Do I want it badly enough to implement lifetime exercise and dietary changes? If you are not willing to change, you should stop worrying about your weight and deem the Moderate category "tolerable" for you.

The Weight Loss Dilemma

Yo-yo dieting carries as great a health risk as being overweight and remaining overweight in the first place. Epidemiological data show that frequent fluctuations in weight (up or down) markedly increase the risk of dying from cardiovascular disease.

Based on the findings that constant losses and regains can be hazardous to health, quick-fix diets should be replaced by a slow but permanent weight loss program (as described under "Losing Weight the Sound and Sensible Way," page 148). Individuals reap the benefits of recommended body weight when they get to that weight and stay there throughout life.

Unfortunately, only about 10 percent of all people who begin a traditional weight loss program without exercise are able to lose the desired weight. Worse, only 5 in 100 are able to keep the weight off. The body is highly resistant to permanent weight changes through caloric restrictions alone.

Traditional diets have failed because few of them incorporate lifetime changes in food selection and an overall increase in physical activity and exercise as fundamental to successful weight loss and weight maintenance. When the diet stops, weight gain begins. The $40 billion diet industry tries to capitalize on the false idea that a person can lose weight quickly without considering the consequences of fast weight loss or the importance of lifetime behavioral changes to ensure proper weight loss and maintenance.

In addition, various studies indicate that most people, especially obese people, underestimate their energy intake. Those who try to lose weight but apparently fail to do so are often described as "diet-resistant." One study found that, while on a "diet," a group of obese individuals with a self-reported history of diet resistance underreported their average daily caloric intake by almost 50 percent (1,028 self-reported versus 2,081 actual calories—see Figure 5.4).[12] These individuals also overestimated their amount of daily physical activity by about 25 percent (1,022 self-reported versus 771 actual calories). These differences represent an additional 1,304 calories of energy per day unaccounted for by the subjects in the study. The findings indicate that failing to lose weight often is related to misreports of actual food intake and level of physical activity.

FIGURE 5.4 Differences between self-reported and actual daily caloric intake and exercise in obese individuals attempting to lose weight.

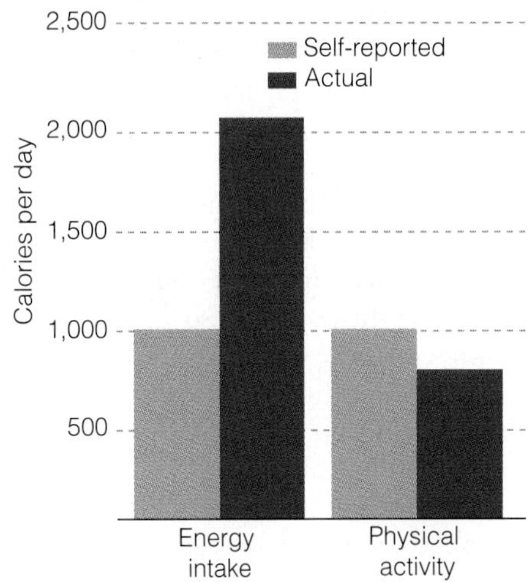

Source: S. W. Lichtman et al., "Discrepancy Between Self-Reported and Actual Caloric Intake and Exercise in Obese Subjects," *New England Journal of Medicine* 327 (1992): 1893–1898.

Diet Crazes

Capitalizing on hopes that the latest diet to hit the market will really work this time, fad diets continue to appeal to people of all shapes and sizes. These diets may work for a while, but their success is usually short-lived. Regarding the effectiveness of these diets, Dr. Kelly Brownell, a foremost researcher in the field of weight management, has stated: "When I get the latest diet fad, I imagine a trick birthday cake candle that keeps lighting up and we have to keep blowing it out."

Fad diets deceive people and claim that dieters will lose weight by following all instructions. Most diets are very low in calories and deprive the body of certain nutrients, generating a metabolic imbalance. Under these conditions, a lot of the weight lost is in the form of water and protein, and not fat. Most fad diets create a nutritional deficiency, which can be detrimental to health.

On a crash diet, close to half the weight loss is in lean (protein) tissue. When the body uses protein instead of a combination of fats and carbohydrates as a source of energy, weight is lost as much as 10 times faster. This is because a gram of protein produces half the amount of energy that fat does. In the case of muscle protein, one-fifth of protein is mixed with four-fifths water. Therefore, each pound of muscle yields only one-tenth the amount of energy of a pound of fat. As a result, most of the weight lost is in the form of water, which on the scale, of course, looks good.

Yo-yo dieting Constantly losing and gaining weight.

Low-Carb Diets

Among the most popular diets on the market in recent years were the low-carbohydrate/high-protein (LCHP) diet plans. Although they vary slightly, low-carb diets, in general, limit the intake of carbohydrate-rich foods—bread, potatoes, rice, pasta, cereals, crackers, juices, sodas, sweets (candy, cake, cookies), and even fruits and vegetables. Dieters are allowed to eat all the protein-rich foods they desire, including steak, ham, chicken, fish, bacon, eggs, nuts, cheese, tofu, high-fat salad dressings, butter, and small amounts of a few fruits and vegetables. Typically, these diets also are high in fat content. Examples of these diets are the Atkins Diet, The Zone, Protein Power, the Scarsdale Diet, The Carb Addict's Diet, South Beach Diet, and Sugar Busters.

During digestion, carbohydrates are converted into glucose, a basic fuel used by every cell in the body. As blood glucose rises, the pancreas releases insulin. Insulin is a hormone that facilitates the entry of glucose into the cells, thereby lowering the glucose level in the bloodstream. A rapid rise in glucose also causes a rapid spike in insulin, which is followed by a rapid removal and drop in blood glucose that leaves you hungry again. A slower rise in blood glucose is desirable because the level is kept constant longer, delaying the onset of hunger. If the cells don't need the glucose for normal cell functions or to fuel physical activity, and if cellular glucose stores are already full, glucose is converted to, and stored as, body fat.

Not all carbohydrates cause a similar rise in blood glucose. The rise in glucose is based on the speed of digestion, which depends on a number of factors, including the size of the food particles. Small-particle carbohydrates break down rapidly and cause a quick, sharp rise in blood glucose. Thus, to gauge a food's effect on blood glucose, carbohydrates are classified by their **glycemic index.**

A high glycemic index signifies a food that causes a quick rise in blood glucose. At the top of the 100-point scale is glucose itself. This index is not directly related to simple and complex carbohydrates, and the glycemic values are not always what one might expect. Rather, the index is based on the actual laboratory-measured speed of absorption. Processed foods generally have a high glycemic index, whereas high-fiber foods tend to have a lower index (see Table 5.1). Other factors that affect the index are the amount of carbohydrate, fat, and protein in the food; how refined the ingredients are; and whether the food was cooked.

The body functions best when blood sugar remains at a constant level. Although this is best accomplished by consuming foods with a low glycemic index (nuts, apples, oranges, low-fat yogurt), a person does not have to eliminate all high–glycemic index foods (sugar, potatoes, bread, white rice, soda drinks) from the diet. Foods with a high glycemic index along with some protein are useful to replenish depleted glycogen stores following prolonged or exhaustive aerobic exercise. Combining high– with low–glycemic index items or with some fat and protein brings down the average index.

TABLE 5.1 Approximate Glycemic Index of Selected Foods (index may vary according to variety, food preparation, and food brand)

Item	Index	Item	Index
All-Bran cereal	46	Honey	58
Apples	40	Milk, chocolate	43
Bagel, white	72	Milk, skim	32
Banana	56	Milk, whole	30
Bread, French	95	Jelly beans	80
Bread, wheat	69	Oatmeal	54
Bread, white	69	Oranges	40
Carrots, boiled (Australia)	41	Pasta, white	50
		Pasta, wheat	42
Carrots, boiled (Canada)	92	Peanuts	20
		Peas	50
Carrots, raw	47	Pizza, cheese	60
Cherries	20	Potato, baked	56–100
Colas	65	Potato, French fries	75
Corn, sweet	55		
Corn Flakes	83	Potato, sweet	51
Doughnut	76	Rice, white	45–70
Frosted Flakes	55	Sugar, table	65
Fruit cocktail	55	Watermelon	72
Gatorade	78	Yogurt, low-fat	30
Glucose	100		

Regular consumption of high-glycemic foods by themselves may increase the risk of cardiovascular disease, especially in people at risk for diabetes. A person does not need to plan the diet around the index itself as many popular diet programs indicate. The glycemic index deals with single foods eaten alone. Most people eat high glycemic index foods in combination with other foods as a part of a meal. In combination, these foods have a lower effect on blood sugar. Even people at risk of diabetes or with the disease can use high-glycemic foods in moderation.

Low-glycemic foods may also aid in weight loss and weight maintenance. As blood sugar levels drop between snacks and meals, hunger increases. Keeping blood sugar levels constant by including low-glycemic foods in the diet helps stave off hunger, appetite, and overeating (see Figure 5.5).

Proponents of LCHP diets claim that if a person eats fewer carbohydrates and more protein, the pancreas will produce less insulin, and as insulin drops, the body will turn to its own fat deposits for energy. There is no scientific proof, however, that high levels of insulin lead to weight gain. None of the authors of these diets published any studies validating their claims. Yet, these authors base their diets on the faulty premise that high insulin leads to obesity. We know the opposite to

FIGURE 5.5 Effects of high- and low-glycemic carbohydrate intake on blood glucose levels.

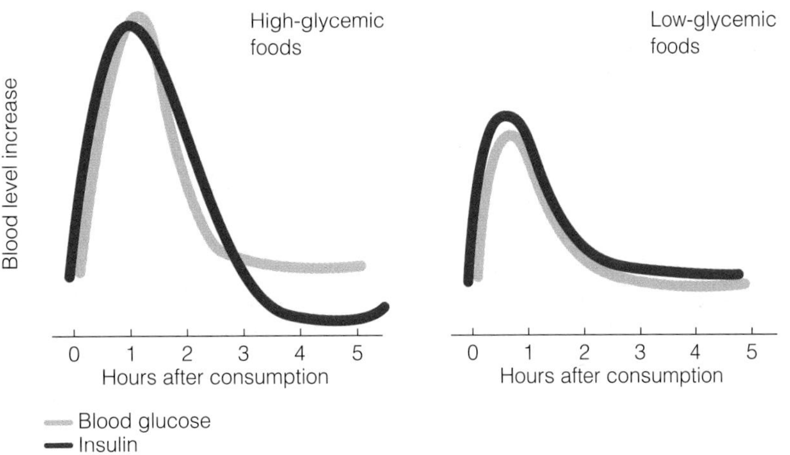

ARE LOW-CARB/HIGH-PROTEIN DIETS MORE EFFECTIVE?

A few studies suggest that, at least over the short-term, low-carb/high-protein (LCHP) diets are more effective in producing weight loss then carbohydrate-based diets. These results are preliminary and controversial. In LCHP diets:

- A large amount of weight loss is water and muscle protein, not body fat. Some of this weight is quickly regained when regular dietary habits are resumed.
- Few people are able to stay with LCHP diets for more than a few weeks at a time. The majority stop dieting before the targeted program completion.
- LCHP dieters are rarely found in a national weight loss registry of people who have lost 30 pounds and kept them off for a minimum of 6 years.
- Food choices are severely restricted in LCHP diets. With less variety, individuals tend to eat less (800 to 1,200 calories/day) and thus lose more weight.
- LCHP diets may promote heart disease, cancer, and increase the risk for osteoporosis.
- LCHP diets are fundamentally high in fat (about 60 percent fat calories).
- LCHP diets are not recommended for people with diabetes, high blood pressure, heart disease, or kidney disease.
- LCHP diets do not promote long-term healthy eating patterns.

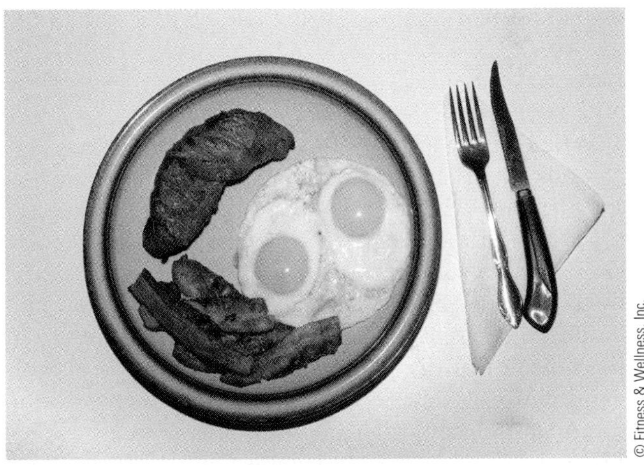

Low-carbohydrate/high-protein diets create nutritional deficiencies and contribute to the development of cardiovascular disease, cancer, and osteoporosis.

be true: Excessive body fat causes insulin levels to rise, thereby increasing the risk for developing diabetes.

The reason for rapid weight loss in LCHP dieting is that a low carbohydrate intake forces the liver to produce glucose. The source for most of this glucose is body proteins—your lean body mass, including muscle. As indicated earlier, protein is mostly water; thus, weight is lost rapidly. When a person terminates the diet, the body rebuilds some of the protein tissue and quickly regains some weight.

A study in the *New England Journal of Medicine* indicated that individuals on an LCHP (Atkins) diet for 12 months lost about twice as much weight as those on a low-fat diet at the midpoint of the study.[13] The effectiveness of the diet, however, seemed to dwindle over time. At 12 months into the diet, participants in the LCHP diet had regained more weight than those on the low-fat diet plan.

Years of research will be required to determine the extent to which adhering over the long-term to LCHP

Glycemic index A measure that is used to rate the plasma glucose response of carbohydrate-containing foods with the response produced by the same amount of carbohydrate from a standard source, usually glucose or white bread.

HOW TO RECOGNIZE FAD DIETS

Fad diets have characteristics in common. These diets typically

- are nutritionally unbalanced.
- rely primarily on a single food (for example grapefruit).
- are based on testimonials.
- were developed according to "confidential research."
- are based on a "scientific breakthrough."
- promote rapid and "painless" weight loss.
- promise miraculous results.
- restrict food selection.
- are based on pseudo claims that excessive weight is related to a specific condition such as insulin resistance, combinations or timing of nutrient intake, food allergies, hormone imbalances, certain foods (fruits for example).
- require the use of selected products.
- use liquid formulas instead of foods.
- misrepresent salespeople as individuals qualified to provide nutrition counseling.
- fail to provide information on risks associated with weight loss and of the diet use.
- do not involve physical activity.
- do not encourage healthy behavioral changes.
- are not supported by the scientific community or national health organizations.
- fail to provide information for weight maintenance upon completion of diet phase.

diets increases the risk for heart disease, cancer, and kidney or bone damage. Low-carb diets are contrary to the nutrition advice of most national leading health organizations (which recommend a diet lower in saturated fat and trans fats, and high in complex carbohydrates). Without fruits, vegetables, and whole grains, high-protein diets lack many vitamins, minerals, antioxidants, phytonutrients, and fiber—all dietary factors that protect against an array of ailments and diseases.

The major risk associated with long-term adherence to LCHP diets could be the increased risk of heart disease because high-protein foods are also high in fat content (see Chapter 11). A low carbohydrate intake also produces a loss of vitamin B, calcium, and potassium. Potential bone loss can accentuate the risk for osteoporosis. Side effects commonly associated with these diets include weakness, nausea, bad breath, constipation, irritability, lightheadedness, and fatigue. Long-term adherence to an LCHP diet also can increase the risk of cancer. Phytonutrients found in fruits, vegetables, and whole grains protect against certain types of cancer. If you choose to go on an LCHP diet for longer than a few weeks, let your physician know so he or she may monitor your blood lipids, bone density, and kidney function.

The benefit of adding extra protein to a weight loss program may be related to the hunger-suppressing effect of protein. Data suggest that protein curbs hunger more effectively than carbohydrates or fat. Dieters feel less hungry when caloric intake from protein is increased to about 30 percent of total calories and fat intake is cut to about to 20 percent (while carbohydrate intake is kept constant at 50 percent of total calories). Thus, if you struggle with frequent hunger pangs, try to include 10 to 15 grams of lean protein with each meal. This amount of protein is the equivalent of one and a half ounces of lean meat (beef, fowl, or fish), two tablespoons of natural peanut butter, or eight ounces of plain low-fat yogurt.

Combo Diets

In addition to the low-carb diets, "combo diets" such as the Schwarzbein and Suzanne Sommers diets are popular. The Schwarzbein diet claims that eating proteins and nonstarchy carbohydrates together will keep the food from being stored as fat. The Suzanne Sommers diet doesn't allow you to eat proteins within 3 hours after eating carbohydrates and, if eating fruits, the dieter must wait at least 20 minutes before eating other carbohydrate foods. Both of these diets allow consumption of high-protein/high-fat food items, which can increase the risk for heart disease.

The reason many of these diets succeed is that they restrict a large number of foods. Thus, people tend to eat less food overall. With the extraordinary variety of foods available to us, it is unrealistic to think that people will adhere to these diets for very long. People eventually get tired of eating the same thing day in and day out and start eating less, leading to weight loss. If they happen to achieve the lower weight but do not make permanent dietary changes, they regain the weight quickly once they go back to their previous eating habits.

A few diets recommend exercise along with caloric restrictions—the best method for weight reduction, of course. People who adhere to these programs will succeed, so the diet has achieved its purpose. Unfortunately, if the people do not change their food selection and activity level permanently, they gain back the weight once they discontinue dieting and exercise.

If people only accepted that no magic foods will provide all of the necessary nutrients, that a person has to eat a variety of foods to be well-nourished, dieters would be more successful and the diet industry would go broke. Also, let's not forget that we eat for pleasure and for health. Two of the most essential components of a wellness lifestyle are healthy eating and regular physical activity, and they provide the best weight-management program available today.

Eating Disorders

Eating disorders are medical illnesses that involve crucial disturbances in eating behaviors thought to stem from some combination of environmental pressures. These disorders are characterized by an intense fear of becoming fat, which does not disappear even when the

Behavior Modification Planning

CALCIUM AND WEIGHT MAINTENANCE

Initial research stated that eating calcium-rich foods—especially from dairy products—may help control or reduce body weight. Women with a high calcium intake were found to gain less weight and body fat than those with a lower intake. Furthermore, women on low-calcium diets more than double the risk of becoming overweight. The data also indicate that even in the absence of caloric restriction, obese women with high dietary calcium intake (the equivalent of 3 to 4 cups of milk per day) lose body fat and weight. And dieters who consume calcium-rich dairy foods lose more fat and less lean body mass than those who consume less dairy products. Researchers believe that

- calcium regulates fat storage inside the cell.
- calcium helps the body break down fat or cause fat cells to produce less fat.
- high calcium intake converts more calories into heat rather than fat.
- adequate calcium intake contributes to a decrease in intra-abdominal (visceral) fat.

The data in women also seem to indicate that calcium from dairy sources is more effective in attenuating weight and fat gain and accelerating fat loss than calcium obtained from other sources. Most likely other nutrients found in dairy products may enhance the weight-regulating action of calcium.

More recent data in a 12-year weight change study in men, however, do not support the theory that an increase in calcium intake or dairy foods leads to lower long-term weight gain in men.

Although additional research is needed, the best recommendation at this point is that if you are attempting to lose or maintain weight loss, do not eliminate dairy foods from your diet. Substitute nonfat (skim milk) or low-fat dairy products for other drinks and foods in your diet to enhance nutrition, and possibly, to help you manage weight.

Sources: M. B. Zemel, "Role of Dietary Calcium and Dairy Products in Modulating Adiposity" *Lipids* 38, no. 2 (2003): 139–146; "A Nice Surprise from Calcium," *University of California Berkeley Wellness Letter,* 19, no. 11 (August 2003): 1; S. N. Rajpathak et al., "Calcium and Dairy Intakes in Relation to Long-term Weight Gain in US Men," *The American Journal of Clinical Nutrition* 83, no. 3 (2006): 559–566.

Try It

If you limit dairy products in your regular diet or while on a negative caloric balance, record in your Online Journal or class notebook what effects such a practice might have on your weight management and overall health. What is one thing you could change in your diet to increase your intake of dairy products?

person is losing weight in extreme amounts. The two most common types of eating disorders are anorexia nervosa and bulimia nervosa. A third condition, binge-eating disorder, or compulsive overeating, also is recognized as an eating disorder.

Most people who have eating disorders are afflicted by significant family and social problems. They may lack fulfillment in many areas of their lives. The eating disorder then becomes the coping mechanism to avoid dealing with these problems. Taking control over their own body weight helps them believe that they are restoring some sense of control over their lives.

Anorexia nervosa and bulimia nervosa are common in industrialized nations where society encourages low-calorie diets and thinness. The female role in society has changed rapidly, which makes women more susceptible to eating disorders. Although frequently seen in young women, the disorder is most prevalent among individuals between the ages of 25 and 50. Surveys, nonetheless, indicate that as many as 40 percent of college-age women are struggling with an eating disorder.

Eating disorders are not limited to women. Every one in 10 cases occurs in men. But because the men's role and body image are viewed differently in our society, these cases often go unreported.

Although genetics may play a role in the development of eating disorders, most cases are environmentally related. Individuals who have clinical depression

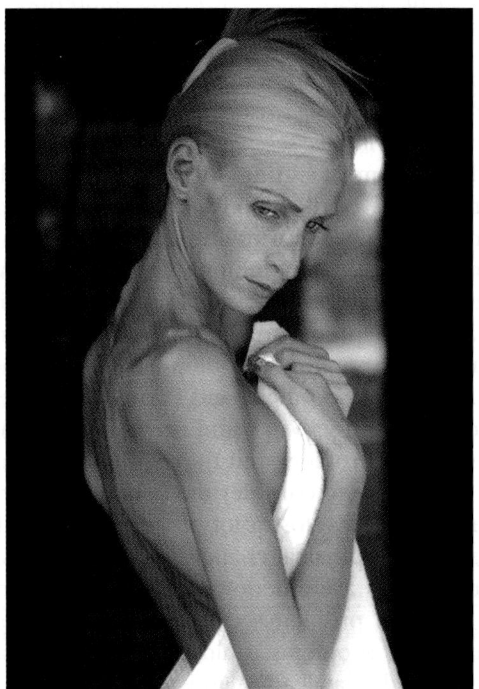

Society's unrealistic view of what constitutes recommended weight and "ideal" body image contributes to the development of eating disorders.

Treatment

Treatment for eating disorders is available on most school campuses through the school's counseling center or the health center. Local hospitals also offer treatment for these conditions. Many communities have support groups, frequently led by professional personnel and often free of charge. All information and the individual's identity are kept confidential so the person need not fear embarrassment or repercussion when seeking professional help.

FIGURE 5.6 Components of total daily energy requirement

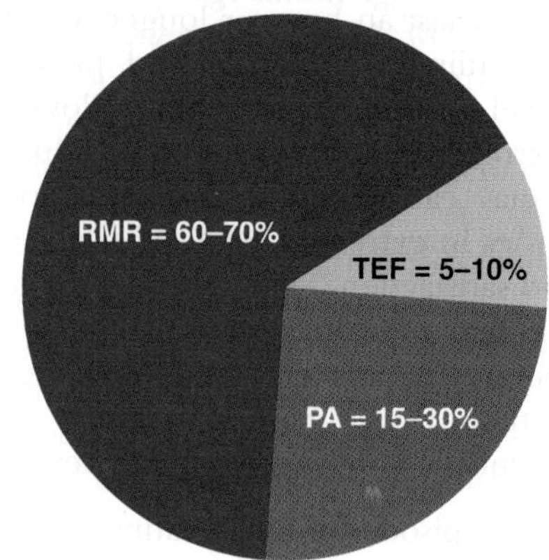

RMR = resting metabolic rate
TEF = thermic effect of food
PA = physical activity

The Physiology of Weight Loss

Traditional concepts related to weight control have centered on three assumptions:

1. Balancing food intake against output allows a person to achieve recommended weight.
2. All fat people simply eat too much.
3. The human body doesn't care how much (or little) fat it stores.

Although these statements contain some truth, they are open to much debate and research. We now know that the causes of obesity are complex, involving a combination of genetics, behavior, and lifestyle factors.

Energy-Balancing Equation

The principle embodied in the **energy-balancing equation** is simple: As long as caloric input equals caloric output, the person will not gain or lose weight. If caloric intake exceeds output, the person gains weight; when output exceeds input, the person loses weight. If daily energy requirements could be determined accurately, caloric intake could be balanced against output. This is not always the case, though, because genetic and lifestyle-related individual differences determine the number of calories required to maintain or lose body weight.

Table 5.3 (page 149) offers general guidelines to determine the **estimated energy requirement (EER)** in calories per day according to lifestyle patterns. This is an estimated figure and (as discussed under "Losing Weight the Sound and Sensible Way," page 148) serves only as a starting point from which individual adjustments have to be made.

The total daily energy requirement has three basic components (see Figure 5.6):

1. resting metabolic rate (RMR)
2. the thermic effect of food (TEF)
3. physical activity (PA)

The **resting metabolic rate (RMR)**—the energy requirement to maintain the body's vital processes in the resting state—accounts for approximately 60 percent to 70 percent of the total daily energy requirement. The thermic effect of food—the energy required to digest, absorb, and store food—accounts for about 5 percent to 10 percent of the total daily requirement. Physical activity accounts for 15 percent to 30 percent of the daily total requirement.

One pound of fat is the equivalent of 3,500 calories. If a person's estimated energy requirement is 2,500 calories and that person were to decrease intake by 500 calories per day, it should result in a loss of 1 pound of fat in 7 days ($500 \times 7 = 3{,}500$). But research has shown—and many people have experienced—that even when dieters carefully balance caloric input against caloric output, weight loss does not always result as predicted. Furthermore, two people with similar measured caloric intake and output seldom lose weight at the same rate.

The most common explanation for individual differences in weight loss and weight gain has been the variation in human metabolism from one person to another. We are all familiar with people who can eat "all day long" and not gain an ounce of weight while others cannot even "dream about food" without gaining weight. Because experts did not believe that human metabolism alone could account for such extreme differences, they developed other theories that might better explain these individual variations.

Setpoint Theory

Results of several research studies point toward a **weight-regulating mechanism (WRM)** that has a **setpoint** for controlling both appetite and the amount of fat stored. Setpoint is hypothesized to work like a thermostat for body fat, maintaining fairly constant body weight, because it "knows" at all times the exact amount of adipose tissue stored in the fat cells. Some people have high settings; others have low settings.

If body weight decreases (as in dieting), the setpoint senses this change and triggers the WRM to increase the person's appetite or make the body conserve energy to maintain the "set" weight. The opposite also may be true. Some people have a hard time gaining weight. In this case, the WRM decreases appetite or causes the body to waste energy to maintain the lower weight.

Every person has his or her own certain body fat percentage (as established by the setpoint) that the body attempts to maintain. The genetic instinct to survive tells the body that fat storage is vital, and therefore it sets an acceptable fat level. This level may remain somewhat constant or may climb gradually because of poor lifestyle habits.

For instance, under strict calorie reduction, the body may make extreme metabolic adjustments in an effort to maintain its setpoint for fat. The **basal metabolic rate (BMR),** the lowest level of caloric intake necessary to sustain life, may drop dramatically when operating under a consistent negative caloric balance, and that person's weight loss may plateau for days or even weeks. A low metabolic rate compounds a person's problems in maintaining recommended body weight.

These findings were substantiated by research conducted at Rockefeller University in New York.[16] The authors showed that the body resists maintaining altered weight. Obese and lifetime non-obese individuals were used in the investigation. Following a 10 percent weight loss, the body, in an attempt to regain the lost weight, compensated by burning up to 15 percent fewer calories than expected for the new reduced weight (after accounting for the 10 percent loss). The effects were similar in the obese and non-obese participants. These results imply that after a 10 percent weight loss, a person would have to eat even less or exercise even more to compensate for the estimated 15 percent slowdown (a difference of about 200 to 300 calories).

In this same study, when the participants were allowed to increase their weight to 10 percent above their "normal" body (pre-weight loss) weight, the body burned 10 to 15 percent *more* calories than expected—attempting to waste energy and maintain the pre-set weight. This is another indication that the body is highly resistant to weight changes unless additional lifestyle changes are incorporated to ensure successful weight management. (These methods are discussed under "Losing Weight the Sound and Sensible Way," page 148.)

Critical Thinking

Do you see a difference in the amount of food that you are now able to eat compared with the amount that you ate in your mid- to late-teen years? If so, to what do you attribute these differences? What actions are you taking to account for the difference?

Dietary restriction alone will not lower the setpoint, even though the person may lose weight and fat. When the dieter goes back to the normal or even below-normal caloric intake (at which the weight may have been stable for a long time), he or she quickly regains the lost fat as the body strives to regain a comfortable fat store.

An Example

Let's use a practical illustration. A person would like to lose some body fat and assumes that his or her current, stable body weight has been reached at an average daily caloric intake of 1,800 calories (no weight gain or loss occurs at this daily intake). In an attempt to lose weight rapidly, this person now goes on a **very low-calorie diet** (defined as 800 calories per day or less), or, even worse, a near-fasting diet. This immediately activates the body's survival mechanism and readjusts the metabolism to a lower caloric balance. After a few weeks of dieting at the 800-calories-per-day level, the body now can maintain its normal functions at 1,300 calories per day. This new figure (1,300) represents a drop of 500 calories per day in the metabolic rate.

Having lost the desired weight, the person terminates the diet but realizes that the original intake of 1,800 calories per day will have to be lower to maintain the new lower weight. To adjust to the new lower body weight, the person restricts intake to about 1,600 calories per day. The individual is surprised to find that, even at this lower daily intake (200 fewer calories), the weight comes back at a rate of 1 pound every 1 to 2 weeks. After the diet is over, this new lowered metabolic rate may take several months to kick back up to its normal level.

Based on this explanation, individuals clearly should not go on very low-calorie diets. This will slow the resting metabolic rate and also will deprive the

Energy-balancing equation A principle holding that as long as caloric input equals caloric output, the person will not gain or lose weight. If caloric intake exceeds output, the person gains weight; when output exceeds input, the person loses weight.

Estimated energy requirement (EER) The average dietary energy (caloric) intake that is predicted to maintain energy balance in a healthy adult of defined age, gender, weight, height, and level of physical activity, consistent with good health.

Resting metabolic rate (RMR) The energy requirement to maintain the body's vital processes in the resting state.

Weight-regulating mechanism (WRM) A feature of the hypothalamus of the brain that controls how much the body should weigh.

Setpoint Weight control theory that the body has an established weight and strongly attempts to maintain that weight.

Basal metabolic rate (BMR) The lowest level of oxygen consumption necessary to sustain life.

Very low-calorie diet A diet that allows an energy intake (consumption) of only 800 calories or less per day.

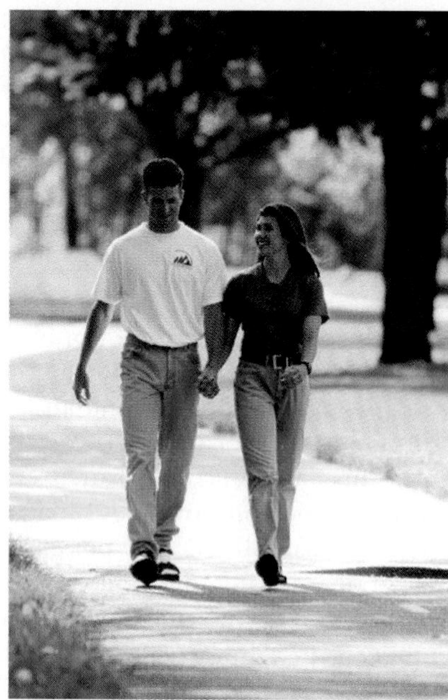

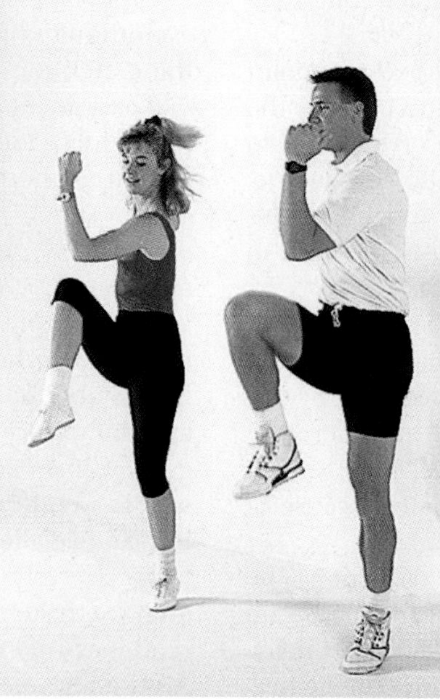

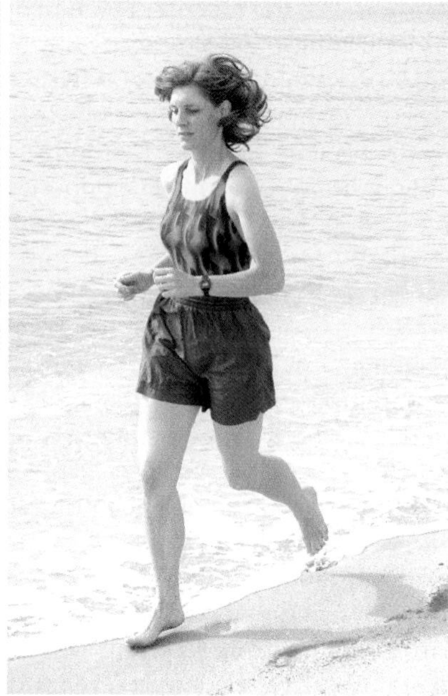

Exercising with other people and in different places helps people maintain exercise regularity.

body of basic daily nutrients required for normal function. Very low-calorie diets should be used only in conjunction with dietary supplements and under proper medical supervision.[17] Furthermore, people who use very low-calorie diets are not as effective in keeping the weight off once the diet is terminated.

Recommendation

Daily caloric intakes of 1,200 to 1,500 calories provide the necessary nutrients if they are distributed properly over the basic food groups (meeting the daily recommended amounts from each group). Of course, the individual will have to learn which foods meet the requirements and yet are low in fat and sugar.

Under no circumstances should a person go on a diet that calls for a level of 1,200 calories or less for women or 1,500 calories or less for men. Weight (fat) is gained over months and years, not overnight. Likewise, weight loss should be gradual, not abrupt.

A second way in which the setpoint may work is by keeping track of the nutrients and calories consumed daily. It is thought that the body, like a cash register, records the daily food intake and that the brain will not feel satisfied until the calories and nutrients have been "registered."

This setpoint for calories and nutrients seems to operate even when people participate in moderately intense exercise. Some evidence suggests that people do not become hungrier with moderate physical activity. Therefore, people can choose to lose weight either by going hungry or by combining a sensible calorie-restricted diet with an increase in daily physical activity. Burning more calories through physical activity helps to lower body fat.

Lowering the Setpoint

The most common question regarding the setpoint is how to lower it so the body will feel comfortable at a reduced fat percentage. These factors seem to affect the setpoint directly by lowering the fat thermostat:

1. Exercise.
2. A diet high in complex carbohydrates.
3. Nicotine.
4. Amphetamines.

The last two are more destructive than the extra fat weight, so they are not reasonable alternatives (as far as the extra strain on the heart is concerned, smoking one pack of cigarettes per day is said to be the equivalent of carrying 50 to 75 pounds of excess body fat). A diet high in fats and refined carbohydrates, near-fasting diets, and perhaps even artificial sweeteners seem to raise the setpoint. Therefore, the only practical and sensible way to lower the setpoint and lose fat weight is a combination of exercise and a diet high in complex carbohydrates and only moderate amounts of fat.

Because of the effects of proper food management on the body's setpoint, most of the successful dieter's effort should be spent in re-forming eating habits, increasing the intake of complex carbohydrates and high-fiber foods, and decreasing the consumption of processed foods that are high in refined carbohydrates (sugars) and fats. This change in eating habits will

Behavior Modification Planning

EATING RIGHT WHEN ON THE RUN

Current lifestyles often require people to be on the run. We don't seem to have time to eat right, but fortunately it doesn't have to be that way. If you are on the run, it is even more critical to make healthy choices to keep up with a challenging schedule. Look at the following food choices for eating on the run:

Water
Whole-grain cereal and skim milk
Whole-grain bread and bagels
Whole-grain bread with peanut butter
Non-fat or low-fat yogurt
Fresh fruits
Frozen fresh fruit (grapes, cherries, banana slices)
Dried fruits
Raw vegetables (carrots, red peppers, cucumbers, radishes, cauliflower, asparagus)
Crackers
Pretzels
Bread sticks
Low-fat cheese sticks
Granola bars
Snack-size cereal boxes
Nuts
Trail mix
Plain popcorn
Vegetable soups

Try It

In your Online Journal or class notebook, plan your fast-meal menus for the upcoming week. It may require extra shopping and some food preparation (for instance, cutting vegetables to place in snack plastic bags). At the end of the week, evaluate how many days you had a "healthy eating on the run day." What did you learn from the experience?

bring about a decrease in total daily caloric intake. Because 1 gram of carbohydrates provides only 4 calories, as opposed to 9 calories per gram of fat, you could eat twice the volume of food (by weight) when substituting carbohydrates for fat. Some fat, however, is recommended in the diet—preferably polyunsaturated and monounsaturated fats. These so-called good fats do more than help protect the heart; they help delay hunger pangs.

A "diet" should not be viewed as a temporary tool to aid in weight loss but, instead, as a permanent change in eating behaviors to ensure weight management and better health. The role of increased physical activity also must be considered, because successful weight loss, maintenance, and recommended body composition are seldom attained without a moderate reduction in caloric intake combined with a regular exercise program.

FIGURE 5.7 Outcome of three forms of diet on fat loss.

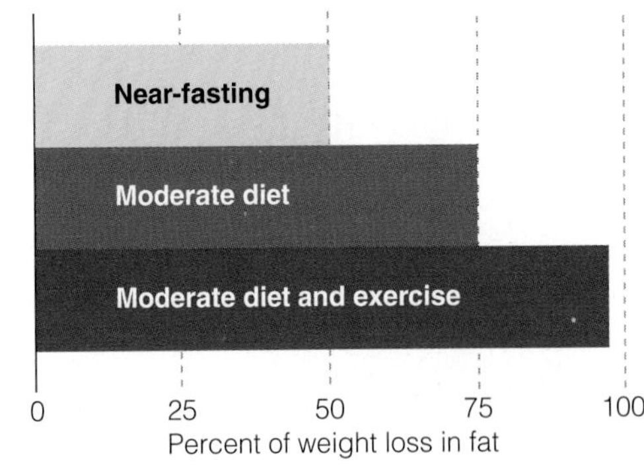

Adapted from R. J. Shephard, *Alive Man: The Physiology of Physical Activity* (Springfield, IL: Charles C. Thomas, 1975), 484–488.

Diet and Metabolism

Fat can be lost by selecting the proper foods, exercising, or restricting calories. However, when dieters try to lose weight by dietary restrictions alone, they also lose lean body mass (muscle protein, along with vital organ protein). The amount of lean body mass lost depends entirely on caloric limitation. When people go on a near-fasting diet, up to half of the weight loss is lean body mass and the other half is actual fat loss (see Figure 5.7).[18] When diet is combined with exercise, close to 100 percent of the weight loss is in the form of fat, and lean tissue actually may increase. Loss of lean body mass is never good, because it weakens the organs and muscles and slows metabolism. Large losses in lean tissue can cause disturbances in heart function and damage to other organs. Equally important is not to overindulge (binge) following a very low-calorie diet, as this may cause changes in metabolic rate and electrolyte balance, which could trigger fatal cardiac arrhythmias.

Contrary to some beliefs, aging is not the main reason for the lower metabolic rate. It is not so much that metabolism slows down as that people slow down. As people age, they tend to rely more on the amenities of life (remote controls, cell phones, intercoms, single-level homes, riding lawnmowers) that lull a person into sedentary living.

Basal metabolism also is related to lean body weight. More lean tissue yields a higher metabolic rate. As a consequence of sedentary living and less physical activity, the lean component decreases and fat tissue increases. The human body requires a certain amount of oxygen per pound of lean body mass. Given that fat is considered metabolically inert from the point of view of caloric use, the lean tissue uses most of the oxygen, even at rest. As muscle and organ mass (lean body mass) decrease, so do the energy requirements at rest.

FIGURE 5.8 Body composition changes as a result of frequent dieting without exercise.

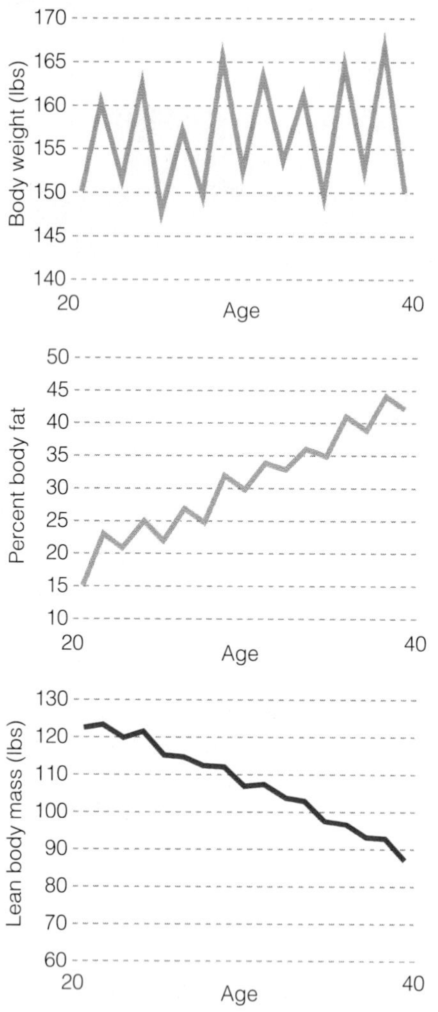

Diets with caloric intakes below 1,200 to 1,500 calories cannot guarantee the retention of lean body mass. Even at this intake level, some loss is inevitable unless the diet is combined with exercise. Despite the claims of many diets that they do not alter the lean component, the simple truth is that, regardless of what nutrients may be added to the diet, severe caloric restrictions *always* prompt the loss of lean tissue. Sadly, many people go on very low-calorie diets constantly. Every time they do, their metabolic rate slows as more lean tissue is lost.

People in their 40s and older who weigh the same as they did when they were 20 tend to think they are at recommended body weight. During this span of 20 years or more, though, they may have dieted many times without participating in an exercise program. After they terminate each diet, they regain the weight, and much of that gain is additional body fat. Maybe at age 20 they weighed 150 pounds, of which only 15 percent was fat. Now at age 40, even though they still weigh 150 pounds, they might be 30 percent fat (see Figure 5.8). At recommended body weight, they wonder why they are eating very little and still having trouble staying at that weight.

Exercise: The Key to Weight Management

A more effective way to tilt the energy-balancing equation in your favor is by burning calories through physical activity. Research shows that the combination of diet and exercise leads to greater weight loss. Further, exercise seems to be the best predictor of long-term maintenance of weight loss.[19]

Exercise seems to exert control over how much a person weighs. On the average, starting at age 25, the typical American gains 1 to 2 pounds of weight per year. A 1-pound weight gain represents a simple energy surplus of under 10 calories per day. The additional weight accumulated in middle age comes from people becoming less physically active and increasing caloric intake. Dr. Jack Wilmore, a leading exercise physiologist and expert weight management researcher, stated:

> Physical inactivity is certainly a major, if not the primary, cause of obesity in the United States today. A certain minimal level of activity might be necessary for us to accurately balance our caloric intake to our caloric expenditure. With too little activity, we appear to lose the fine control we normally have to maintain this incredible balance. This fine balance amounts to less than 10 calories per day, or the equivalent of one potato chip.[20]

Exercise enhances the rate of weight loss and is vital in maintaining the lost weight. Not only will exercise maintain lean tissue, but advocates of the setpoint theory say that exercise resets the fat thermostat to a new, lower level. This change may be rapid, or it may take time.

Although a few individuals lose weight by participating in 30 minutes of exercise per day, many overweight people need 60 to 90 minutes of daily physical activity to effectively manage body weight (the 30 minutes of exercise are included as part of the 60 to 90 minutes of physical activity).

Accumulating 30 minutes of moderate-intensity activity per day provides substantial health benefits. From a weight management point of view, however, the Institute of Medicine of the National Academy of Sciences recommends that people accumulate 60 minutes of moderate-intensity physical activity most days of the week.[21] The evidence shows that people who maintain recommended weight typically accumulate an hour or more of daily physical activity.

As illustrated in Figure 5.9, greater weight loss is achieved by combining a diet with an exercise program.

FIGURE 5.9 The roles of diet and exercise in weight loss.

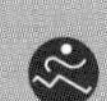

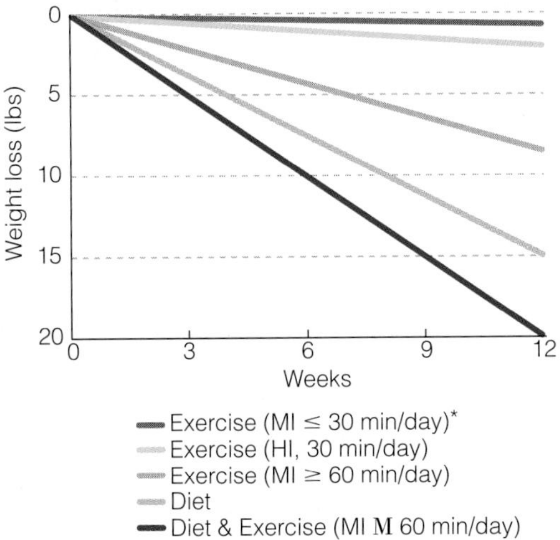

Based on data from American College of Sports Medicine, "Position Stand: Appropriate Intervention Strategies for Weight Loss and Prevention for Weight Regain for Adults," *Medicine and Science in Sports and Exercise* 33 (2001): 2145–2156.

FIGURE 5.10 Effects of different amounts of daily energy expenditure on weight maintenance following a weight reduction program.

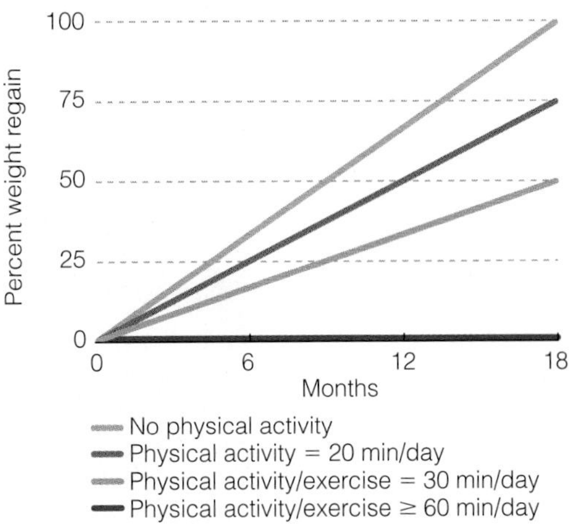

Based on data from American College of Sports Medicine, "Position Stand: Appropriate Intervention Strategies for Weight Loss and Prevention for Weight Regain for Adults," *Medicine and Science in Sports and Exercise* 33 (2001): 2145–2156.

Of even greater significance, however, only individuals who remain physically active for 60 or more minutes per day are able to keep the weight off (see Figure 5.10).

Further, data from the National Weight Control Registry (http://www.nwcr.ws/) indicate that individuals who have lost at least 30 pounds and kept them off for a minimum of 6 years typically accumulate 90 minutes of daily activity. Those who are less active gradually regain the lost weight. Individuals who completely stop physical activity regain almost 100 percent of the weight within 18 months of discontinuing the weight loss program (see Figure 5.10). Thus, if weight management is *not* a consideration, 30 minutes of daily activity provides health benefits. *To prevent weight gain, 60 minutes of daily activity are recommended; to maintain substantial weight loss, 90 minutes may be required.*

If a person is trying to lose weight, a combination of aerobic and strength-training exercises works best. Aerobic exercise is the best to offset the setpoint, and the continuity and duration of these types of activities cause many calories to be burned in the process. The role of aerobic exercise in successful lifetime weight management cannot be overestimated. Strength training is critical in helping maintain lean body mass. Unfortunately, of those individuals who are attempting to lose weight, only 19 percent of women and 22 percent of men decrease their caloric intake and exercise above an average of 25 or more minutes per day.[22]

The number of calories burned during a typical hour-long strength-training session is much less than during an hour of aerobic exercise. Because of the high in-

Behavior Modification Planning

PHYSICAL ACTIVITY GUIDELINES FOR WEIGHT MANAGEMENT

The following physical activity guidelines are recommended to effectively manage body weight:

- 30 minutes of physical activity on most days of the week if you do not have difficulty maintaining body weight (more minutes and/or higher intensity if you choose to reach a high level of physical fitness).
- 60 minutes of daily activity if you want to prevent weight gain.
- Between 60 and 90 minutes each day if you are trying to lose weight or attempting to keep weight off following extensive weight loss (30 pounds of weight loss or more). Be sure to include some high-intensity/low impact activities at least twice a week in your program.

Try It

In your Behavior Change Planner Progress Tracker, Online Journal, or class notebook, record how many minutes of daily physical activity you accumulate on a regular basis and record your thoughts on how effectively your activity has helped you manage your body weight. Is there one thing you could do today to increase your physical activity?

Behavior Modification Planning

WEIGHT-MAINTENANCE BENEFITS OF LIFETIME AEROBIC EXERCISE

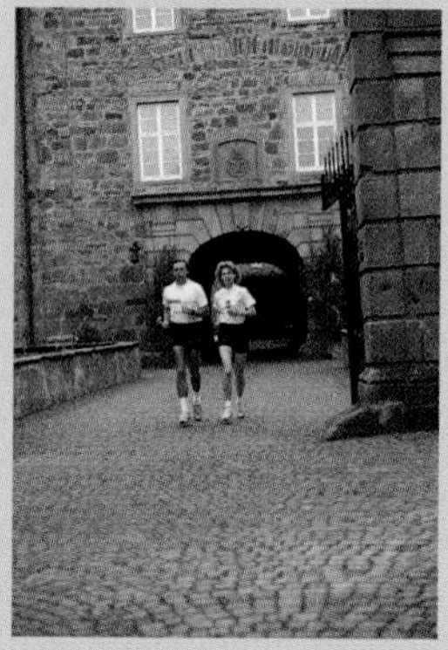

The authors of this book have been jogging together a minimum of 15 miles per week (3 miles/5 times per week) for the past 30 years. Without considering the additional energy expenditure from their regular strength-training program and their many other sport and recreational activities, the energy cost of this regular jogging program over 30 years has been approximately 2,340,000 calories (15 miles × 100 calories/mile × 52 weeks × 30 years), or the equivalent of 668 pounds of fat (2,340,000 ÷ 3,500). In essence, without this 30-minute workout 5 times per week, the authors would weigh 810 and 784 pounds respectively!

Try It

Ask yourself whether a regular aerobic exercise program is part of your long-term gratification and health enhancement program. If the answer is no, are you ready to change your behavior? Use the Behavior Change Planner to help you answer the question.

tensity of strength training, the person needs frequent rest intervals to recover from each set of exercises. The average person actually lifts weights only 10 to 12 minutes during each hour of exercise. In the long run, however, the person enjoys the benefits of gains in lean tissue. Guidelines for developing aerobic and strength-training programs are given in Chapters 6 and 7.

Weight loss might be more rapid if aerobic exercise is combined with a strength-training program. Although the increase in BMR (basal metabolic rate) through increased muscle mass is being debated in the literature and merits further research, data indicate that each additional pound of muscle tissue raises the BMR in the range of 6 to 35 calories per day.[23]

To examine the effects of even a small increase in BMR on long-term body weight, let's use a low estimate of 10 calories per pound of muscle per day. For an individual who adds 3 pounds of muscle tissue as a result of strength training, the increase in BMR would be 30 calories per day (10 × 3). Such an increase would burn an additional 10,950 calories per year (30 × 365), or the equivalent of 3.1 pounds of fat (10,950 ÷ 3,500). This increase in BMR would more than offset the typical adult weight gain of 1 to 2 pounds per year.

This figure of 10,950 calories per year does not include the actual energy cost of the strength-training workout. If we use an energy expenditure of only 150 calories per strength-training session, done twice per week, over a year's time it would represent 15,600 calories (150 × 2 × 52), or the equivalent of another 4.5 pounds of fat (15,600 ÷ 3,500).

In addition, although the amounts seem small, the previous calculations do not account for the increase in metabolic rate following the strength-training workout (the time it takes the body to return to its pre-workout resting rate—about 2 hours). Depending on the training volume (see Chapter 7, pages 221–222), this recovery energy expenditure ranges from 20 to 100 calories following each strength-training workout.[24] All these "apparently small" changes make a big difference in the long run.

Although size (inches) and percent body fat both decrease when sedentary individuals begin an exercise program, body weight often remains the same or may even increase during the first couple of weeks of the program. Exercise helps to increase muscle tissue, connective tissue, blood volume (as much as 500 ml, or the equivalent of 1 pound, following the first week of aerobic exercise), enzymes and other structures within the cell, and glycogen (which binds water). All of these changes lead to a higher functional capacity of the human body. With exercise, most of the weight loss becomes apparent after a few weeks of training, when the lean component has stabilized.

We know that a negative caloric balance of 3,500 calories does not always result in a loss of exactly 1 pound of fat, but the role of exercise in achieving a negative balance by burning additional calories is significant in weight reduction and maintenance programs. Sadly, some individuals claim that the number of calories burned during exercise is hardly worth the effort. They think that cutting their daily intake by 300 calories is easier than participating in some sort of exercise that would burn the same amount of calories. The problem is that the willpower to cut those 300 calories lasts only a few weeks, and then the person goes back to the old eating patterns.

If a person gets into the habit of exercising regularly, say 3 times a week, jogging 3 miles per exercise session (about 300 calories burned), this represents 900 calories in 1 week, about 3,600 calories in one month, or 46,800 calories per year. This minimal amount of exercise represents as many as 13.5 extra pounds of fat in one year, 27 in two, and so on.

We tend to forget that our weight creeps up gradually over the years, not just overnight. Hardly worth the effort? And we have not even taken into consideration the increase in lean tissue, possible resetting of the setpoint, benefits to the cardiovascular system, and, most important, the improved quality of life. Fundamental reasons for overfatness and obesity, few

TABLE 5.2 Comparison of Energy Expenditure Between 30–40 Minutes of Low-Intensity Versus High-Intensity Exercise

Exercise Intensity	Total Energy Expenditure (Calories)	Percent Calories From Fat	Total Fat Calories	Percent Calories From CHO*	Total CHO Calories	Calories Burned Per Minute	Calories Per Pound Per Minute
Low Intensity	200	50%	100	50%	100	6.67	0.045
High Intensity	400	30%	120	70%	280	13.5	0.090

* CHO = Carbohydrates

could argue, are sedentary living and lack of a regular exercise program.

In terms of preventing disease, many of the health benefits that people seek by losing weight are reaped through exercise alone, even without weight loss. Exercise offers protection against premature morbidity and mortality for everyone, including people who already have risk factors for disease.

Low-Intensity Versus High-Intensity Exercise for Weight Loss

Some individuals promote low-intensity exercise over high-intensity for weight-loss purposes. Compared with high-intensity, a greater proportion of calories burned during low-intensity exercise are derived from fat. The lower the intensity of exercise, the higher the percentage of fat utilization as an energy source. In theory, if you are trying to lose fat, this principle makes sense, but in reality it is misleading. The bottom line when you are trying to lose weight is to burn more calories. When your daily caloric expenditure exceeds your intake, you lose weight. The more calories you burn, the more fat you lose.

During low-intensity exercise, up to 50 percent of the calories burned may be derived from fat (the other 50 percent from glucose [carbohydrates]). With intense exercise, only 30 to 40 percent of the caloric expenditure comes from fat. Overall, however, you can burn twice as many calories during high-intensity exercise and, subsequently, more fat as well.

Let's look at a practical illustration (also see Table 5.2). If you exercise for 30–40 minutes at moderate intensity and burn 200 calories, about 100 of those calories (50 percent) would come from fat. If you exercise at high intensity during those same 30–40 minutes, you can burn 400 calories with 120 to 160 of the calories (30 to 40 percent) coming from fat. Thus, even though it is true that the percentage of fat used is greater during low-intensity exercise, the overall amount of fat used is still less during low-intensity exercise. Plus, if you were to exercise at a low intensity, you would have to do so twice as long to burn the same amount of calories. Another benefit is that the metabolic rate remains at a slightly higher level longer after high-intensity exercise, so you continue to burn a few extra calories following exercise.

Moreover, high-intensity exercise by itself seems to trigger more fat loss than low-intensity exercise. Research conducted at Laval University in Quebec, Canada, showed that subjects who performed a high-intensity intermittent-training program lost more body fat than participants in a low- to moderate-intensity continuous aerobic endurance group.[25] Even more surprisingly, this finding occurred despite the fact that the high-intensity group burned fewer total calories per exercise session. The results support the notion that vigorous exercise is more conducive to weight loss than low- to moderate-intensity exercise.

Before you start high-intensity exercise sessions, a word of caution is in order: Be sure that it is medically safe for you to participate in such activities and that you build up gradually to that level. If you are cleared to participate in high-intensity exercise, do not attempt to do too much too quickly, because you may incur injuries and become discouraged. You must allow your body a proper conditioning period of 8 to 12 weeks, or even longer for people with a moderate-to-serious weight problem. High intensity also does not mean high impact. High-impact activities are the most common cause of exercise-related injuries. Additional information on these topics is presented in Chapter 6.

The previous discussion on high- versus low-intensity exercise does not mean that low intensity is ineffective. Low-intensity exercise provides substantial health benefits, and people who initiate exercise programs are more willing to participate and stay with low-intensity programs. Low-intensity exercise does promote weight loss, but it is not as effective. You will have to exercise longer to obtain the same results.

Healthy Weight Gain

"Skinny" people, too, should realize that the only healthy way to gain weight is through exercise (mainly strength-training exercises) and a slight increase in caloric intake. Attempting to gain weight by overeating alone will raise the fat component and not the lean component—which is not the path to better health. Exercise is the best solution to weight (fat) reduction and weight (lean) gain alike.

A strength-training program such as the one outlined in Chapter 7 is the best approach to add body weight. The training program should include at least two exercises of one to three sets for each major body part. Each set should consist of about 8 to 12 repetitions maximum.

Even though the metabolic cost of synthesizing a pound of muscle tissue is still unclear, consuming an estimated 500 additional calories per day is recommended to gain an average of 1 pound of muscle tissue per week. Your diet should include a daily total intake of about 1.5 grams of protein per kilogram of body weight. If your daily protein intake already exceeds 1.5 grams per day, the extra 500 calories should be primarily in the form of complex carbohydrates. The higher caloric intake must be accompanied by a strength-training program; otherwise, the increase in body weight will be in the form of fat, not muscle tissue (Lab 5C can be used to monitor your caloric intake for healthy weight gain). Additional information on nutrition to optimize muscle growth and strength development is provided in Chapter 7 under the section "Dietary Guidelines for Strength Development," page 223.

Weight Loss Myths

Cellulite and **spot reducing** are mythical concepts. **Cellulite** is nothing but enlarged fat cells that bulge out from accumulated body fat.

Doing several sets of daily sit-ups will not get rid of fat in the midsection of the body. When fat comes off, it does so throughout the entire body, not just the exercised area. The greatest proportion of fat may come off the biggest fat deposits, but the caloric output of a few sets of sit-ups has practically no effect on reducing total body fat. A person has to exercise much longer to see results.

Other touted means toward quick weight loss, such as rubberized sweatsuits, steam baths, and mechanical vibrators, are misleading. When a person wears a sweatsuit or steps into a sauna, the weight lost is not fat but merely a significant amount of water. Sure, it looks nice when you step on the scale immediately afterward, but this represents a false loss of weight. As soon as you replace body fluids, you gain back the weight quickly.

Wearing rubberized sweatsuits hastens the rate of body fluid that is lost—fluid that is vital during prolonged exercise—and raises core temperature at the same time. This combination puts a person in danger of dehydration, which impairs cellular function and, in extreme cases, can even cause death.

Similarly, mechanical vibrators are worthless in a weight-control program. Vibrating belts and turning rollers may feel good, but they require no effort whatsoever. Fat cannot be shaken off. It is lost primarily by burning it in muscle tissue.

Losing Weight the Sound and Sensible Way

Dieting never has been fun and never will be. People who are overweight and are serious about losing weight, however, have to include regular exercise in their lives along with proper food management and a sensible reduction in caloric intake.

Because excessive body fat is a risk factor for cardiovascular disease, some precautions are in order. Depending on the extent of the weight problem, a medical examination and possibly a stress ECG (see "Abnormal Electrocardiograms" in Chapter 11) may be a good idea before undertaking the exercise program. Consult a physician in this regard.

Significantly overweight individuals may have to choose activities in which they will not have to support their own body weight but that still will be effective in burning calories. Injuries to joints and muscles are common in excessively overweight individuals who participate in weight-bearing exercises such as walking, jogging, and aerobics.

Swimming may not be a good weight loss exercise either. More body fat makes a person more buoyant, and many people are not at the skill level required to swim fast enough to get the best training effect, thus limiting the number of calories burned as well as the benefits to the cardiorespiratory system.

During the initial stages of exercise, better alternatives include riding a bicycle (either road or stationary), walking in a shallow pool, doing water aerobics, or running in place in deep water (treading water). The latter forms of water exercise are gaining popularity and have proven to be effective in reducing weight without fear of injuries.

How long should each exercise session last? The amount of exercise needed to lose weight and maintain the weight loss is different from the amount of exercise needed to improve fitness. For health fitness, accumulating 30 minutes of physical activity on most days of the week is recommended. To develop and maintain cardiorespiratory fitness, 20 to 60 minutes of exercise at the recommended target rate, three to five times per week, is suggested (see Chapter 6). For successful weight loss, however, 60 to 90 minutes of physical activity on most days of the week is recommended.

A person should not try to do too much too fast. Unconditioned beginners should start with about 15 minutes of aerobic activity 3 times a week, and during the next 3 to 4 weeks gradually increase the duration by approximately 5 minutes per week and the frequency by 1 day per week.

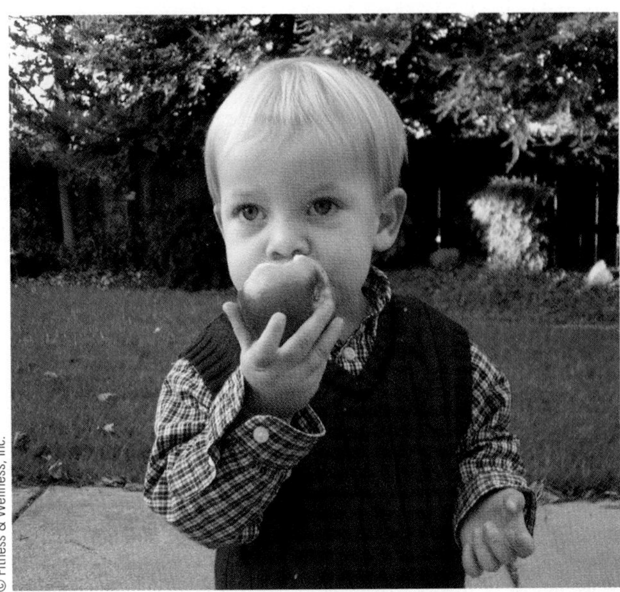

The establishment of healthy eating patterns starts at a young age.

One final benefit of long-duration exercise for weight control is that fat-burning enzymes increase with aerobic training. Fat is lost primarily by burning it in muscle. Therefore, as the concentration of the enzymes increases, so does the ability to burn fat.

In addition to exercise and food management, a sensible reduction in caloric intake and careful monitoring of this intake are recommended. Most research finds that a negative caloric balance is required to lose weight because:

1. Most people underestimate their caloric intake and are eating more than they should be eating.
2. Developing new behaviors takes time, and most people have trouble changing and adjusting to new eating habits.
3. Many individuals are in such poor physical condition that they take a long time to increase their activity level enough to offset the setpoint and burn enough calories to aid in losing body fat.
4. Most successful dieters carefully monitor their daily caloric intake.
5. A few people simply will not alter their food selection. For those who will not (which will increase their risk for chronic diseases), the only solution to lose weight successfully is a large increase in physical activity, a negative caloric balance, or a combination of the two.

Perhaps the only exception to a decrease in caloric intake for weight loss purposes is in people who already are eating too few calories. A nutrient analysis (see Chapter 3) often reveals that long-term dieters are not consuming enough calories. These people actually need to increase their daily caloric intake and combine it with an exercise program to get their metabolism to kick back up to a normal level.

TABLE 5.3 Estimated Energy Requirement (EER) Based on Age, Body Weight, and Height

Men	EER = 662 − (9.53 × Age) + (15.91 × BW) + (539 × HT)
Women	EER = 354 − (6.91 × Age) + (9.36 × BW) + (726 × HT)

Note. Includes activities of independent living only and no moderate physical activity or exercise.
BW = body weight in kilograms (divide BW in pounds by 2.2046),
HT = height in meters (multiply HT in inches by .0254).

You also must learn to make wise food choices. Think in terms of long-term benefits (weight management) instead of instant gratification (unhealthy eating and subsequent weight gain). Making healthful choices allows you to eat more food, eat more nutritious food, and ingest fewer calories. For example, instead of eating a high-fat, 700-calorie scone, you could eat as much as 1 orange, 1 cup of grapes, a hard-boiled egg, 2 slices of whole-wheat toast, 2 teaspoons of jam, ½ cup of honey-sweetened oatmeal, and 1 glass of skim milk (see Figure 5.11).

You can estimate your daily energy (caloric) requirement by consulting Tables 5.3 and 5.4 and completing Lab 5A. Given that this is only an estimated value, individual adjustments related to many of the factors discussed in this chapter may be necessary to establish a more precise value. Nevertheless, the estimated value does offer beginning guidelines for weight control or reduction.

The estimated energy requirement (EER) without additional planned activity and exercise is based on age, total body weight, and gender. Individuals who hold jobs that require a lot of walking or heavy manual labor burn more calories during the day than those who have sedentary jobs (such as working behind a desk). To estimate your EER, refer to Table 5.3. For example, the EER computation for a 20-year-old man, 71 inches tall, who weighs 160 pounds, would be as follows:

1. Body weight in kilograms = 72.6 kg (160 lbs ÷ 2.2046)
   Height in meters = 1.8 mts (71 × 0.0254)
2. EER = 662 − (9.53 × Age) + (15.91 × BW) + (539 × Ht)
   EER = 662 − (9.53 × 20) + (15.91 × 72.6) + (539 × 1.8)
   EER = 662 − 190.6 + 1155 + 970
   EER = 2,596 calories/day

Spot reducing Fallacious theory proposing that exercising a specific body part will result in significant fat reduction in that area.

Cellulite Term frequently used in reference to fat deposits that "bulge out"; these deposits are nothing but enlarged fat cells from excessive accumulation of body fat.

FIGURE 5.11 Making Wise Food Choices.

These illustrations provide a comparison of how much more food you can eat when you make healthy choices. You also get more vitamins, minerals, phytochemicals, antioxidants, and fiber by making healthy choices.

Breakfast

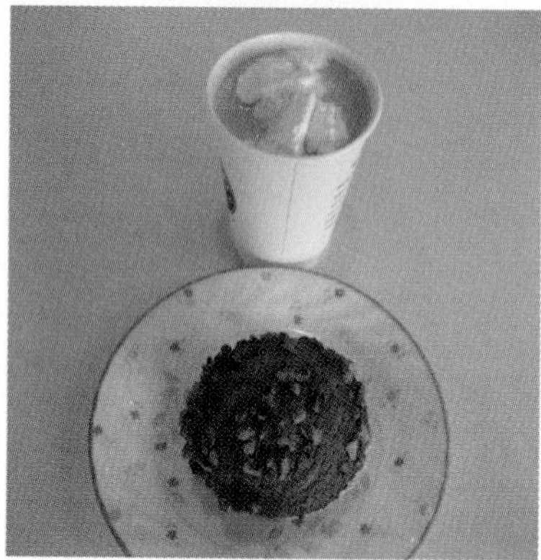

1 banana nut muffin, 1 cafe mocha
Calories: 940
Percent fat calories: 48%

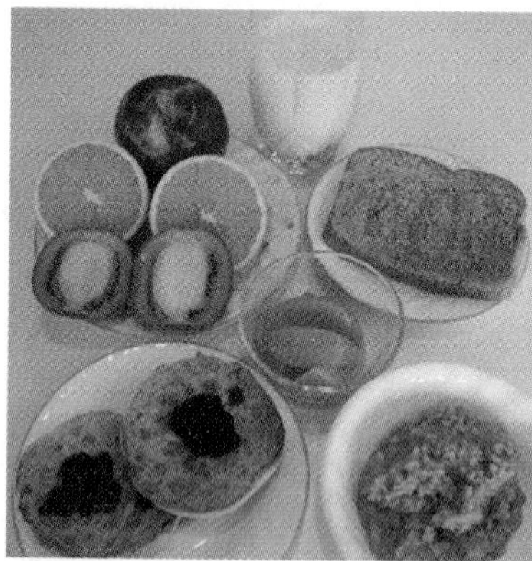

1 cup oatmeal, 1 English muffin with jelly, 1 slice whole wheat bread with honey, ½ cup peaches, 1 kiwi fruit, 1 orange, 1 apple, 1 cup skim milk
Calories: 900
Percent fat calories: 5%

Lunch

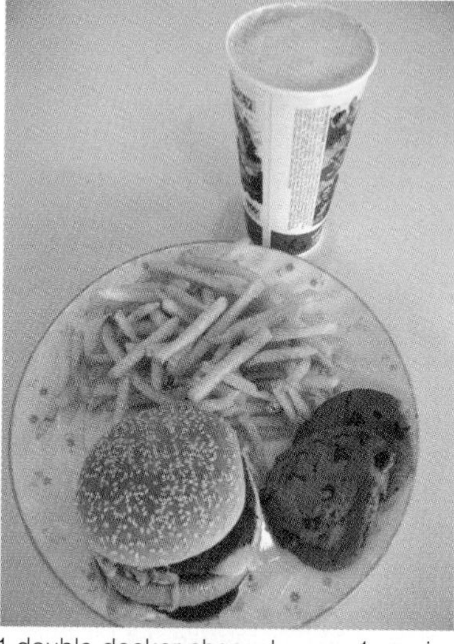

1 double-decker cheeseburger, 1 serving medium French fries, 2 chocolate chip cookies, 1 medium strawberry milkshake
Calories: 1790
Percent fat calories: 37%

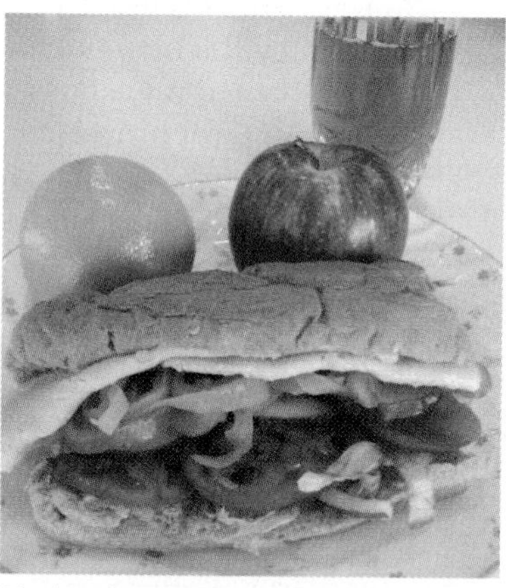

6-inch turkey breast/vegetable sandwich, 1 apple, 1 orange, 1 cup sweetened green tea
Calories: 500
Percent fat calories: 10%

Dinner

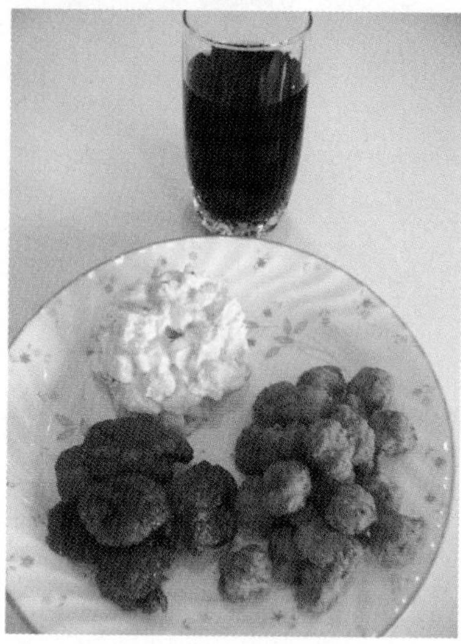

6 oz. popcorn chicken, 3 oz. barbecue chicken wings, 1 cup potato salad, 1 12-oz. cola drink
Calories: 1250
Percent fat calories: 42%

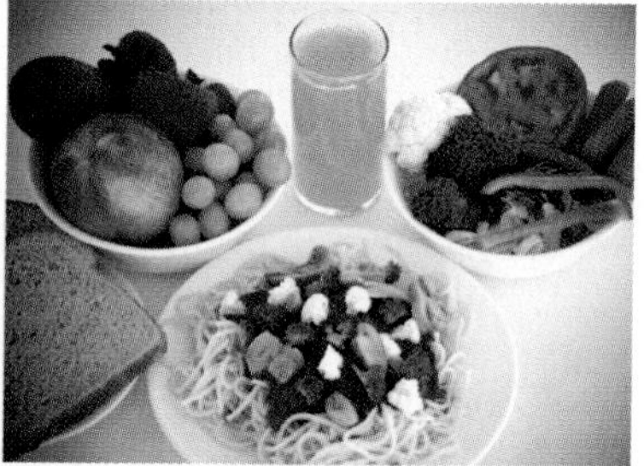

2 cups spaghetti with tomato sauce and vegetables, a 2-cup salad bowl with two tablespoons Italian dressing, 2 slices whole wheat bread, 1 cup grapes, 3 large strawberries, 1 kiwi fruit, 1 peach, 1 12-oz. fruit juice drink
Calories: 1240
Percent fat calories: 14%

Thus, the EER to maintain body weight for this individual would be 2,596 calories per day.

To determine the average number of calories you burn daily as a result of exercise, figure out the total number of minutes you exercise weekly, then figure the daily average exercise time. For instance, a person cycling at 10 miles per hour five times a week, 60 minutes each time, exercises 300 minutes per week (5 × 60). The average daily exercise time, therefore, is 42 minutes (300 ÷ 7, rounded off to the lowest unit).

Next, from Table 5.4, find the energy expenditure for the activity (or activities) chosen for the exercise program. In the case of cycling (10 miles per hour), the expenditure is .05 calories per pound of body weight per

TABLE 5.4 Caloric Expenditure of Selected Physical Activities

Activity*	Cal/lb/min	Activity*	Cal/lb/min
Aerobics		7.0 min/mile	0.102
Moderate	0.065	6.0 min/mile	0.114
Vigorous	0.095	Deep water**	0.100
Step aerobics	0.070	Skating (moderate)	0.038
Archery	0.030	Skiing	
Badminton		Downhill	0.060
Recreation	0.038	Level (5 mph)	0.078
Competition	0.065	Soccer	0.059
Baseball	0.031	Stairmaster	
Basketball		Moderate	0.070
Moderate	0.046	Vigorous	0.090
Competition	0.063	Stationary Cycling	
Bowling	0.030	Moderate	0.055
Calisthenics	0.033	Vigorous	0.070
Cycling (on a level surface)		Strength Training	0.050
5.5 mph	0.033	Swimming (crawl)	
10.0 mph	0.050	20 yds/min	0.031
13.0 mph	0.071	25 yds/min	0.040
Dance		45 yds/min	0.057
Moderate	0.030	50 yds/min	0.070
Vigorous	0.055	Table Tennis	0.030
Golf	0.030	Tennis	
Gymnastics		Moderate	0.045
Light	0.030	Competition	0.064
Heavy	0.056	Volleyball	0.030
Handball	0.064	Walking	
Hiking	0.040	4.5 mph	0.045
Judo/Karate	0.086	Shallow pool	0.090
Racquetball	0.065	Water Aerobics	
Rope Jumping	0.060	Moderate	0.050
Rowing (vigorous)	0.090	Vigorous	0.070
Running (on a level surface)		Wrestling	0.085
11.0 min/mile	0.070		
8.5 min/mile	0.090		

* Values are for actual time engaged in the activity.
** Treading water

Adapted from:

P. E. Allsen, J. M. Harrison, and B. Vance, *Fitness for Life: An Individualized Approach* (Dubuque, IA: Wm. C. Brown, 1989).

C. A. Bucher and W. E. Prentice, *Fitness for College and Life* (St. Louis: Times Mirror/Mosby College Publishing, 1989).

C. F. Consolazio, R. E. Johnson, and L. J. Pecora, *Physiological Measurements of Metabolic Functions in Man* (New York: McGraw-Hill, 1963).

R. V. Hockey, *Physical Fitness: The Pathway to Healthful Living* (St. Louis: Times Mirror/Mosby College Publishing, 1989).

W. W. K. Hoeger et al., Research conducted at Boise State University, 1986–1993.

minute of activity (cal/lb/min). With a body weight of 160 pounds, this man would burn 8 calories each minute (body weight × .05, or 160 × .05). In 42 minutes he would burn approximately 336 calories (42 × 8).

Now you can obtain the daily energy requirement, with exercise, needed to maintain body weight. To do this, add the EER obtained from Table 5.3 and the average calories burned through exercise. In our example, it is 2,932 calories (2,596 + 336).

If a negative caloric balance is recommended to lose weight, this person has to consume fewer than 2,932 calories daily to achieve the objective. Because of the many factors that play a role in weight control, this 2,932-calorie value is only an estimated daily requirement. Furthermore, we cannot predict that you will lose exactly 1 pound of fat in 1 week if you cut your daily intake by 500 calories (500 × 7 = 3,500 calories, or the equivalent of 1 pound of fat).

The daily energy requirement figure is only a target guideline for weight control. Periodic readjustments are necessary because individuals differ, and the daily requirement changes as you lose weight and modify your exercise habits.

To determine the target caloric intake to lose weight, multiply your current weight by 5 and subtract this amount from the total daily energy requirement (2,932 in our example) with exercise. For our example, this would mean 2,132 calories per day to lose weight (160 × 5 = 800 and 2,932 − 800 = 2,132 calories).

This final caloric intake to lose weight should never be below 1,200 calories for women and 1,500 for men. If distributed properly over the various food groups, these figures are the lowest caloric intakes that provide the necessary nutrients the body needs. In terms of percentages of total calories, the daily distribution should be approximately 60 percent carbohydrates (mostly complex carbohydrates), less than 30 percent fat, and about 12 percent protein.

Many experts believe that a person can take off weight more efficiently by reducing the amount of daily fat intake to about 20 percent of the total daily caloric intake. Because 1 gram of fat supplies more than twice the amount of calories that carbohydrates and protein do, the tendency when someone eats less fat is to consume fewer calories. With fat intake at 20 percent of total calories, the individual will have sufficient fat in the diet to feel satisfied and avoid frequent hunger pangs.

Further, it takes only 3 to 5 percent of ingested calories to store fat as fat, whereas it takes approximately 25 percent of ingested calories to convert carbohydrates to fat. Some evidence indicates that if people eat the same number of calories as carbohydrate or as fat, those on the fat diet will store more fat. Long-term successful weight loss and weight management programs are low in fat content.

Many people have trouble adhering to a low-fat-calorie diet. During times of weight loss, however, you are strongly encouraged to do so. Refer to Table 5.5 to aid you in determining the grams of fat at 20 percent of the total calories for selected energy intakes. Also, use the form provided in Lab 3B, Figure 3B.1 (Chapter 3) to monitor your daily fat intake. For weight maintenance, individuals who have been successful in main-

TABLE 5.5 Grams of Fat at 10%, 20%, and 30% of Total Calories for Selected Energy Intakes

	Grams of Fat		
Caloric Intake	10%	20%	30%
1,200	13	27	40
1,300	14	29	43
1,400	16	31	47
1,500	17	33	50
1,600	18	36	53
1,700	19	38	57
1,800	20	40	60
1,900	21	42	63
2,000	22	44	67
2,100	23	47	70
2,200	24	49	73
2,300	26	51	77
2,400	27	53	80
2,500	28	56	83
2,600	29	58	87
2,700	30	60	90
2,800	31	62	93
2,900	32	64	97
3,000	33	67	100

taining an average weight loss of 30 pounds for more than 6 years are consuming about 24 percent of calories from fat, 56 percent from carbohydrates, and 20 percent from protein.[26]

The time of day when a person eats food also may play a part in weight reduction. When a person is attempting to lose weight, intake should consist of a minimum of 25 percent of the total daily calories for breakfast, 50 percent for lunch, and 25 percent or less at dinner. Also, while trying to lose weight, try not to eat within 3 hours of going to bed. This is the time of day when your metabolism is slowest. Your caloric intake is less likely to be used for energy and more likely to be stored as fat.

Breakfast, in particular, is a critical meal. Many people skip breakfast because it's the easiest meal to skip. Evidence indicates that people who skip breakfast are hungrier later in the day and end up consuming more total daily calories than those who eat breakfast. Furthermore, regular breakfast eaters have less of a weight problem, lose weight more effectively, and have less difficulty maintaining the weight loss.

If most of the daily calories are consumed during one meal (as in the typical evening meal), the body may perceive that something is wrong and will slow the metabolism so it can store more calories in the form of fat. Also, eating most of the calories during one meal causes a person to go hungry the rest of the day, making it more difficult to adhere to the diet.

Consuming most of the calories earlier in the day seems helpful in losing weight and also in managing atherosclerosis. The time of day when most of the fats and cholesterol are consumed can influence blood lipids and coronary heart disease. Peak digestion time following a heavy meal is about seven hours after that meal. If most lipids are consumed during the evening meal, digestion peaks while the person is sound asleep, when the metabolism is at its lowest rate. Consequently, the body may not metabolize fats and cholesterol as well, leading to a higher blood lipid count and increasing the risk for atherosclerosis and coronary heart disease.

Before you proceed to develop a thorough weight loss program, take a moment to identify, in Lab 5A, your current stage of change as it pertains to your recommended body weight. If applicable—that is, if you are not at recommended weight—list also the processes and techniques for change that you will use to accomplish your goal. In Lab 5A you also outline your exercise program for weight management.

Behavior Modification Planning

HEALTHY BREAKFAST CHOICES

Breakfast is the most important meal of the day. Skipping breakfast makes you hungrier later in the day and leads to overconsumption and greater caloric intake throughout the rest of the day. Regular breakfast eaters have less of a weight problem, lose weight more effectively, have less difficulty maintaining lost weight, and live longer. Skipping breakfast also temporarily raises LDL (bad) cholesterol and lowers insulin sensitivity, changes that may increase the risk for heart disease and diabetes. Here are some healthy breakfast food choices:

Fresh fruit
Low-fat or skim milk
Low-fat yogurt
Whole-grain cereal
Whole-grain bread or bagel with fat-free cream cheese and slices of red or green pepper
Hummus over a whole-grain bagel
Peanut butter with whole-grain bread or bagel
Low-fat cottage cheese with fruit
Oatmeal
Reduced-fat cheese
Egg Beaters with salsa
An occasional egg

Try It

Select a healthy breakfast choice each day for the next 7 days. Evaluate how you feel the rest of the morning. What effect did eating breakfast have on your activities of daily living and daily caloric intake? Be sure to record your food choices, how you felt, and what activities you engaged in.

Monitoring Your Diet with Daily Food Logs

To help you monitor and adhere to a weight loss program, use the daily food logs provided in Lab 5B. If the goal is to maintain or increase body weight, use Lab 5C.

Evidence indicates that people who monitor daily caloric intake are more successful at weight loss than those who don't self-monitor. Before using the forms in Lab 5B, make a master copy for your files so you can make future copies as needed. Guidelines are provided for 1,200-, 1,500-, 1,800-, and 2,000-calorie diet plans. These plans have been developed based on the MyPyramid and the Dietary Guidelines for Americans to meet the Recommended Dietary Allowances.[27] The objective is to meet (not exceed) the number of servings allowed for each diet plan. Each time you eat a serving of a certain food, record it in the appropriate box.

To lose weight, you should use the diet plan that most closely approximates your target caloric intake. The plan is based on the following caloric allowances for these food groups:

- Grains: 80 calories per serving.
- Fruits: 60 calories per serving.
- Vegetables: 25 calories per serving.
- Milk (use low-fat products): 120 calories per serving.
- Meat and beans: Use low-fat (300 calories per serving) frozen entrees or an equivalent amount if you prepare your own main dish (see the following discussion).

As you start your diet plan, pay particular attention to food serving sizes. Take care with cup and glass sizes. A standard cup is 8 ounces, but most glasses nowadays contain between 12 and 16 ounces. If you drink 12 ounces of fruit juice, in essence you are getting two servings of fruit because a standard serving is $\frac{3}{4}$ cup of juice.

Read food labels carefully to compare the caloric value of the serving listed on the label with the caloric guidelines provided above. Here are some examples:

- One slice of standard white bread has about 80 calories. A plain bagel may have 200 to 350 calories. Although it is low in fat, a 350-calorie bagel is equivalent to almost 4 servings in the grains group.
- The standard serving size listed on the food label for most cereals is 1 cup. As you read the nutrition information, however, you will find that for the same cup of cereal, one type of cereal has 120 calories and another cereal has 200 calories. Because a standard serving in the grains group is 80 calories, the first cereal would be $1\frac{1}{2}$ servings and the second one $2\frac{1}{2}$ servings.
- A medium-size fruit is usually considered to be 1 serving. A large fruit could provide as many as 2 or more servings.
- In the milk group, 1 serving represents 120 calories. A cup of whole milk has about 160 calories, compared with a cup of skim milk, which contains 88 calories. A cup of whole milk, therefore, would provide $1\frac{1}{3}$ servings in this food group.

Using Low-Fat Entrees

To be more accurate with caloric intake and to simplify meal preparation, use commercially prepared low-fat frozen entrees as the main dish for lunch and dinner meals (only one entree per meal for the 1,200-calorie diet plan, see Lab 5B). Look for entrees that provide about 300 calories and no more than 6 grams of fat per entree. These two entrees can be used as selections for the meat and beans group and will provide most of your daily protein requirement. Along with each entree, supplement the meal with some of your servings from the other food groups. This diet plan has been used successfully in weight loss research programs.[28] If you choose not to use these low-fat entrees, prepare a similar meal using 3 ounces (cooked) of lean meat, poultry, or fish with additional vegetables, rice, or pasta that will provide 300 calories with fewer than 6 grams of fat per dish.

In your daily logs, be sure to record the precise amount in each serving. You also can run a computerized nutrient analysis to verify your caloric intake and food distribution pattern (percent of total calories from carbohydrate, fat, and protein).

Behavior Modification and Adherence to a Weight Management Program

Achieving and maintaining recommended body composition is certainly possible, but it does require desire and commitment. If weight management is to become a priority, people must realize that they have to transform their behavior to some extent.

Modifying old habits and developing new, positive behaviors take time. Individuals who apply the management techniques provided in the Behavior Modification Planning box (pages 154–155) are more successful at changing detrimental behavior and adhering to a positive lifetime weight-control program. In developing a retraining program, you are not expected to incorporate all of the strategies given but should note the ones that apply to you. The form provided in Lab 5E will allow you to evaluate and monitor your own weight management behaviors.

Behavior Modification Planning

WEIGHT LOSS STRATEGIES

1. *Make a commitment to change.* The first necessary ingredient is the desire to modify your behavior. You have to stop precontemplating or contemplating change and get going! You must accept that you have a problem and decide by yourself whether you really want to change. Sincere commitment increases your chances for success.
2. *Set realistic goals.* The weight problem developed over several years. Similarly, new lifetime eating and exercise habits take time to develop. A realistic long-term goal also will include short-term objectives that allow for regular evaluation and help maintain motivation and renewed commitment to attain the long-term goal.
3. *Incorporate exercise into the program.* Choosing enjoyable activities, places, times, equipment, and people to work out with will help you adhere to an exercise program. (See Chapters 6, 7, 8, and 9.)
4. *Differentiate hunger and appetite.* Hunger is the actual physical need for food. Appetite is a desire for food, usually triggered by factors such as stress, habit, boredom, depression, availability of food, or just the thought of food itself. Developing and sticking to a regular meal pattern will help control hunger.
5. *Eat less fat.* Each gram of fat provides 9 calories, and protein and carbohydrates provide only 4. In essence, you can eat more food on a low-fat diet because you consume fewer calories with each meal. Most of your fat intake should come from unsaturated sources.
6. *Pay attention to calories.* Just because food is labeled "low-fat" does not mean you can eat as much as you want. When reading food labels—and when eating—don't just look at the fat content. Pay attention to calories as well. Many low-fat foods are high in calories.
7. *Cut unnecessary items from your diet.* Substituting water for a daily can of soda would cut 51,100 (140 × 365) calories yearly from the diet—the equivalent of 14.6 (51,000 ÷ 3,500) pounds of fat.
8. *Maintain a daily intake of calcium-rich foods,* especially low-fat or non-fat dairy products.
9. *Add foods to your diet that reduce cravings.* such as eggs; small amounts of red meat, fish, poultry, tofu, oils, fats; and nonstarchy vegetables such as lettuce, green beans, peppers, asparagus, broccoli, mushrooms, and Brussels sprouts. Also increasing the intake of low-glycemic carbohydrates with your meals helps you go longer before you feel hungry again.
10. *Avoid automatic eating.* Many people associate certain daily activities with eating, for example, cooking, watching television, or reading. Most foods consumed in these situations lack nutritional value or are high in sugar and fat.
11. *Stay busy.* People tend to eat more when they sit around and do nothing. Occupying the mind and body with activities not associated with eating helps take away the desire to eat. Some options are walking; cycling; playing sports; gardening; sewing; or visiting a library, a museum, or a park. You also might develop other skills and interests not associated with food.
12. *Plan meals and shop sensibly.* Always shop on a full stomach, because hungry shoppers tend to buy unhealthy foods impulsively—and then snack on the way home. Always use a shopping list, which should include whole-grain breads and cereals, fruits and vegetables, low-fat milk and dairy products, lean meats, fish, and poultry.
13. *Cook wisely:*
    - Use less fat and fewer refined foods in food preparation.
    - Trim all visible fat from meats and remove skin from poultry before cooking.
    - Skim the fat off gravies and soups.
    - Bake, broil, boil, or steam instead of frying.
    - Sparingly use butter, cream, mayonnaise, and salad dressings.
    - Avoid coconut oil, palm oil, and cocoa butter.
    - Prepare plenty of foods that contain fiber.
    - Include whole-grain breads and cereals, vegetables, and legumes in most meals.
    - Eat fruits for dessert.
    - Stay away from soda pop, fruit juices, and fruit-flavored drinks.
    - Use less sugar, and cut down on other refined carbohydrates, such as corn syrup, malt sugar, dextrose, and fructose.
    - Drink plenty of water—at least six glasses a day.
14. Do not serve more food than you should eat. Measure the food in portions and keep serving dishes away from the table. Do not force yourself or anyone else to "clean the plate" after they are satisfied (including children after they already have had a healthy, nutritious serving).
15. Try "junior size" instead of "super size." People who are served larger portions eat more, whether they are hungry or not. Use smaller plates, bowls, cups, and glasses. Try eating half as much food as you commonly eat. Watch for portion sizes at restaurants as well: Supersized foods create supersized people.
16. Eat out infrequently. The more often people eat out, the more body fat they have. People who eat out six or more times per week consume an average of about 300 extra calories per day and 30 percent more fat than those who eat out less often.
17. Eat slowly and at the table only. Eating on the run promotes overeating because the body doesn't have enough time to "register" consumption and people overeat before the body perceives the fullness signal. Eating at the table encourages people to take time out to eat and deters snacking between meals. After eating, do not sit around the table but, rather, clean up and put away the food to avoid snacking.
18. Avoid social binges. Social gatherings tend to entice self-defeating behavior. Use visual imagery to plan

Behavior Modification Planning

ahead. Do not feel pressured to eat or drink and don't rationalize in these situations. Choose low-calorie foods and entertain yourself with other activities, such as dancing and talking.

19. Do not place unhealthy foods within easy reach. Ideally, avoid bringing high-calorie, high-sugar, or high-fat foods into the house. If they are there already, store them where they are hard to get to or see—perhaps the garage or basement.
20. Avoid evening food raids. Most people do really well during the day but then "lose it" at night. Take control. Stop and think. To avoid excessive nighttime snacking, stay busy after your evening meal. Go for a short walk; floss and brush your teeth, and get to bed earlier. Even better, close the kitchen after dinner and try not to eat anything 3 hours prior to going to sleep.
21. Practice stress management techniques (discussed in Chapter 10). Many people snack and increase their food consumption in stressful situations.
22. Get support. People who receive support from friends, relatives, and formal support groups are much more likely to lose and maintain weight loss than those without such support. The more support you receive, the better off you will be.
23. Monitor changes and reward accomplishments. Being able to exercise without interruption for 15, 20, 30, or 60 minutes; swimming a certain distance; running a mile—all these accomplishments deserve recognition. Create rewards that are not related to eating: new clothing, a tennis racquet, a bicycle, exercise shoes, or something else that is special and you would not have acquired otherwise.
24. Prepare for slip-ups. Most people will slip and occasionally splurge. Do not despair and give up. Reevaluate and continue with your efforts. An occasional slip won't make much difference in the long run.
25. Think positive. Avoid negative thoughts about how difficult changing past behaviors might be. Instead, think of the benefits you will reap, such as feeling, looking, and functioning better, plus enjoying better health and improving the quality of life. Avoid negative environments and unsupportive people.

Try It

In your Online Journal or class notebook, answer the following questions: How many of the above strategies do you use to help you maintain recommended body weight? Do you feel that any of these strategies specifically help you manage body weight more effectively? If so, explain why.

Critical Thinking

What behavioral strategies have you used to properly manage your body weight? How do you think those strategies would work for others?

The Simple Truth

There is no quick and easy way to take off excess body fat and keep it off for good. Weight management is accomplished by making a lifetime commitment to physical activity and proper food selection. When taking part in a weight (fat) reduction program, people also have to decrease their caloric intake moderately, be physically active, and implement strategies to modify unhealthy eating behaviors.

During the process, relapses into past negative behaviors are almost inevitable. The three most common reasons for relapse are:

1. stress-related factors (such as major life changes, depression, job changes, illness),
2. social reasons (entertaining, eating out, business travel), and
3. self-enticing behaviors (placing yourself in a situation to see how much you can get away with: "One small taste won't hurt" leads to "I'll eat just one slice" and finally to "I haven't done well, so I might as well eat some more").

Making mistakes is human and does not necessarily mean failure. Failure comes to those who give up and do not build upon previous experiences and thereby develop skills that will prevent self-defeating behaviors in the future. Where there's a will, there's a way, and those who persist will reap the rewards.

Assess Your Behavior

Thomson NOW! *Log on to www.thomsonedu.com/login to track your progress in your exercise log and update your pedometer log if you are tracking your steps.*

1. Are you satisfied with your current body composition (including body weight) and quality of life? If not, are you willing to do something about it; and if so, what do you plan to do to properly resolve the problem?
2. Are physical activity, aerobic exercise, and strength training a regular part of your lifetime weight management program?
3. Do you weigh yourself regularly and make adjustments in energy intake and physical activity habits if your weight starts to slip upward?
4. Do you exercise portion control, watch your overall fat intake, and plan ahead before you eat out or attend social functions that entice overeating?

Assess Your Knowledge

Thomson NOW! *Log on to www.thomsonedu.com/login to assess your understanding of this chapter's topics by taking the Student Practice Test and exploring the modules recommended in your Personalized Study Plan.*

1. During the last decade, the rate of obesity in the United States has
   a. been on the decline.
   b. increased at an alarming rate.
   c. increased slightly.
   d. remained steady.
   e. increased in men and decreased in women.
2. Obesity is defined as a body mass index equal to or above
   a. 10.
   b. 25.
   c. 30.
   d. 45.
   e. 50.
3. Obesity increases the risk for
   a. hypertension.
   b. congestive heart failure.
   c. atherosclerosis.
   d. type 2 diabetes.
   e. all of the above.
4. Tolerable weight is a body weight
   a. that is not ideal but one that you can live with.
   b. that will tolerate the increased risk of chronic diseases.
   c. with a BMI range between 25 and 30.
   d. that meets both ideal values for percent body weight and BMI.
   e. All are correct choices.
5. When the body uses protein instead of a combination of fats and carbohydrates as a source of energy,
   a. weight loss is very slow.
   b. a large amount of weight loss is in the form of water.
   c. muscle turns into fat.
   d. fat is lost very rapidly.
   e. fat cannot be lost.
6. Eating disorders
   a. are characterized by an intense fear of becoming fat.
   b. are physical and emotional conditions.
   c. almost always require professional help for successful treatment of the disease.
   d. are common in societies that encourage thinness.
   e. All are correct choices.
7. The mechanism that seems to regulate how much a person weighs is known as
   a. setpoint.
   b. weight factor.
   c. basal metabolic rate.
   d. metabolism.
   e. energy-balancing equation.
8. The key to maintaining weight loss successfully is
   a. frequent dieting.
   b. very low-calorie diets when "normal" dieting doesn't work.
   c. a lifetime physical activity program.
   d. regular high protein/low carbohydrate meals.
   e. All are correct choices.

9. The daily amount of physical activity recommended for weight loss purposes is
   a. 15 to 20 minutes.
   b. 20 to 30 minutes.
   c. 30 to 60 minutes.
   d. 60 to 90 minutes.
   e. Any amount is sufficient as long as it is done daily.

10. A daily energy expenditure of 300 calories through physical activity is the equivalent of approximately _______ pounds of fat per year.
   a. 12
   b. 15
   c. 22
   d. 27
   e. 31

Correct answers can be found at the back of the book.

Media Menu

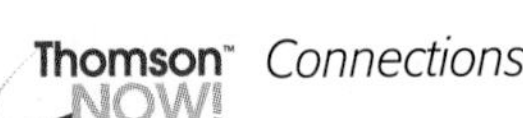

Connections

- Check your progress in your exercise log.
- Check how well you understand the chapter's concepts.

Internet Connections

Shape Up America!

This excellent fitness and weight management site is endorsed by former U.S. Surgeon General C. Everett Koop, M.D.
http://www.shapeup.org

Eating Disorders

This award-winning site, by MentalHelp Net, features links describing symptoms, possible causes, consequences, treatment, online resources, organizations, online support, and research.
http://eatingdisorders.mentalhelp.net

Mayo Clinic Food & Nutrition Center

This site features a wealth of reliable nutrition information including information on different food pyramids and the benefits and dangers of herbs, vitamins, and mineral supplements.
http://www.mayoclinic.com/health/food-and-nutrition/NU99999

Count Your Calories Because Your Calories Count

This interactive site, sponsored by Wake Forest University Baptist Medical Center, features a four-step assessment of your diet—"How's Your Diet?," "Fit or Not Quiz," "Calorie Counter," and "Drive-Through Diet."
http://www.bgsm.edu/nutrition/in.html

Notes

1. "Wellness Facts," *University of California at Berkeley Wellness Letter* (Palm Coast, FL: The Editors, May 2004).
2. Centers for Disease Control and Prevention, "Age-Adjusted Prevalence of Overweight and Obesity Among U.S. Adults, Age 20 Years and Over," http://www.cdc.gov/nchs/products/pubs/pubd/hestats/obese/obesefig1.gif (Atlanta, GA: Centers for Disease Control and Prevention. Accessed July 18, 2006).
3. M. K. Serdula et al., "Prevalence of Attempting Weight Loss and Strategies for Controlling Weight," *Journal of the American Medical Association* 282 (1999): 1353–1358.
4. A. M. Wolf and G. A. Colditz, "Current Estimates of the Economic Cost of Obesity in the United States," *Obesity Research* 6 (1998): 97–106.
5. A. H. Mokdad, J. S. Marks, D. F. Stroup, and J. L. Gerberding, "Actual Causes of Death in the United States, 2000," *Journal of the American Medical Association* 291 (2004): 1238–1241.
6. R. Sturm and K. B. Wells, "Does Obesity Contribute as Much to Morbidity as Poverty or Smoking?" *Public Health* 115 (2001): 229–235.
7. E. E. Calle et. al., "Overweight, Obesity, and Mortality from Cancer in a Prospectively Studied Cohort of U.S. Adults," *New England Journal of Medicine* 348 (2003): 1625–1638.
8. A. Peeters et al., "Obesity in Adulthood and Its Consequences for Life Expectancy: A Life-Table Analysis," *Annals of Internal Medicine* 138 (2003): 2432.
9. K. R. Fontaine et al., "Years of Life Lost Due to Obesity," *Journal of the American Medical Association* 289 (2003): 187–193.
10. R. R. Wing, E. Venditti, J. M. Jakicic, B. A. Polley, and W. Lang, "Lifestyle Intervention in Overweight Individuals with a Family History of Diabetes," *Diabetes Care* 21 (1998): 350–359.
11. S. Thomsen, "A Steady Diet of Images," *BYU Magazine* 57, no. 3 (2003): 20–21.
12. S. Lichtman et al., "Discrepancy between Self-Reported and Actual Caloric Intake and Exercise in Obese Subjects," *New England Journal of Medicine* 327 (1992): 1893–1898.
13. G. D. Foster et al., "A Randomized Trial of a Low-Carbohydrate Diet for Obesity," *New England Journal of Medicine* 348 (2003): 2082–2090.
14. American Psychiatric Association, *Diagnostic and Statistical Manual of Mental Disorders* (Washington, DC: APA, 1994).
15. See note 14.

16. R. L. Leibel, M. Rosenbaum, and J. Hirsh, "Changes in Energy Expenditure Resulting from Altered Body Weight," *New England Journal of Medicine* 332 (1995): 621–628.
17. American College of Sports Medicine, "Position Stand: Appropriate Intervention Strategies for Weight Loss and Prevention for Weight Regain for Adults," *Medicine and Science in Sports and Exercise* 33 (2001): 2145–2156.
18. R. J. Shepard, *Alive Man: The Physiology of Physical Activity* (Springfield, IL: Charles C Thomas, 1975): 484–488.
19. W. C. Miller, D. M. Koceja, and E. J. Hamilton, "A Meta-Analysis of the Past 25 Years of Weight Loss Research Using Diet, Exercise, or Diet Plus Exercise Intervention," *International Journal of Obesity* 21 (1997): 941–947.
20. J. H. Wilmore, "Exercise, Obesity, and Weight Control," *Physical Activity and Fitness Research Digest* (Washington, DC: President's Council on Physical Fitness & Sports, 1994).
21. National Academy of Sciences, Institute of Medicine, *Dietary Reference Intakes for Energy, Carbohydrates, Fiber, Fat, Protein and Amino Acids (Macronutrients)* (Washington, DC: National Academy Press, 2002).
22. See note 3.
23. E. T. Poehlman et al., "Effects of Endurance and Resistance Training on Total Daily Energy Expenditure in Young Women: A Controlled Randomized Trial," *Journal of Clinical Endocrinology and Metabolism* 87 (2002): 1004–1009; L. M. Van Etten et al., "Effect of an 18-wk Weight-training Program on Energy Expenditure and Physical Activity," *Journal of Applied Physiology* 82 (1997): 298-304; W. W. Campbell, M. C. Crim, V. R. Young, and W. J. Evans, "Increased Energy Requirements and Changes in Body Composition with Resistance Training in Older Adults," *American Journal of Clinical Nutrition* 60 (1994): 167–175; Z. Wang et al., "Resting Energy Expenditure: Systematic Organization and Critique of Prediction Methods," *Obesity Research* 9 (2001): 331–336.
24. American College of Sports Medicine, *ACSM's Guidelines for Exercise Testing and Prescription* (Baltimore: Williams & Wilkins, 2006).
25. A. Tremblay, J. A. Simoneau, and C. Bouchard. "Impact of Exercise Intensity on Body Fatness and Skeletal Muscle Metabolism," *Metabolism* 43 (1994): 814–818.
26. M. L. Klem, R. R. Wing, M. T. McGuire, H. M. Seagle, and J. O. Hill, "A Descriptive Study of Individuals Successful at Long-Term Maintenance of Substantial Weight Loss," *American Journal of Clinical Nutrition* 66 (1997): 239–246.
27. National Academy of Sciences, Institute of Medicine, *Dietary Reference Intakes for Energy, Carbohydrates, Fiber, Fat, Protein and Amino Acids (Macronutrients)* (Washington, DC: National Academy Press, 2002); U.S. Department of Health and Human Services, Department of Agriculture, *Dietary Guidelines for Americans 2005* (Washington, DC: DHHS, 2005).
28. W. W. K. Hoeger, C. Harris, E. M. Long, and D. R. Hopkins, "Four-Week Supplementation with a Natural Dietary Compound Produces Favorable Changes in Body Composition," *Advances in Therapy* 15, no. 5 (1998): 305–313; W. W. K. Hoeger, C. Harris, E. M. Long, R. L. Kjorstad, M. Welch, T. L. Hafner, and D. R. Hopkins, "Dietary Supplementation with Chromium Picolinate/L-Carnitine Complex in Combination with Diet and Exercise Enhances Body Composition," *Journal of the American Nutraceutical Association* 2, no. 2 (1999): 40–45.

Suggested Readings

ACSM's Health and Fitness Journal, Vol. 9, Issue 1, January/February 2005.

American College of Sports Medicine. "Effective Weight Management." *ACSM Fit Society Page* (http://acsm.org/health+fitness/fit_society.htm), Summer 2004.

American College of Sports Medicine. "Position Stand: Appropriate Intervention Strategies for Weight Loss and Prevention for Weight Regain for Adults." *Medicine and Science in Sports and Exercise* 33 (2001): 2145–2156.

American Diabetes Association and American Dietetic Association. *Exchange Lists for Meal Planning.* Chicago: American Dietetic Association and American Diabetes Association, 1995.

Brownell, K. *The Learn Program for Weight Control.* Dallas: American Health Publishing, 1997.

Clarkson, P. M. "The Skinny on Weight Loss Supplements and Drugs: Winning the War against Fat." *ACSM's Health and Fitness Journal* (1998): 18.

Mokdad, A. H., et al. "The Spread of the Obesity Epidemic in the United States, 1991–1998." *Journal of the American Medical Association* 282 (1999): 1519–1522.

National Academy of Sciences, Institute of Medicine. *Dietary Reference Intakes for Energy, Carbohydrates, Fiber, Fat, Protein and Amino Acids (Macronutrients).* Washington, DC: National Academy Press, 2002.

National Institutes of Health. *Clinical Guidelines on the Identification, Evaluation, and Treatment of Overweight and Obesity in Adults* (NIH Publication No. 98-4083). Washington, DC: NIH, 1998.

Lab 5A Daily Caloric Requirement and Exercise Plan

Name: | Date: | Grade:

Instructor: | Course: | Section:

Necessary Lab Equipment
Tables 5.3 (page 149) and 5.4 (page 151).

Instructions
Complete all of the sections provided in this lab.

Objective
To estimate your daily caloric requirement for weight maintenance or reduction and to select fitness activities for your exercise program.

I. Computation Form for Daily Caloric Requirement and Weight Loss if Necessary

A. Current body weight in pounds . . . .

B. Caloric requirement per pound of body weight (use Table 5.3) . . . .

C. Estimated daily energy requirement without exercise to maintain body weight (A × B) . . . .

D. Selected physical activity (e.g., jogging)[a] . . . .

E. Number of exercise sessions per week . . . .

F. Duration of exercise session (in minutes) . . . .

G. Total weekly exercise time in minutes (E × F) . . . .

H. Average daily exercise time in minutes (G ÷ 7) . . . .

I. Caloric expenditure per pound per minute (cal/lb/min) of physical activity (use Table 5.4) . . . .

J. Total calories burned per minute of physical activity (A × I) . . . .

K. Average daily calories burned as a result of the exercise program (H × J) . . . .

L. Total daily energy requirement with exercise to maintain body weight (C + K) . . . .

Stop here if no weight loss is required, otherwise proceed to items M and N.

M. Number of calories to subtract from daily requirement to achieve a negative caloric balance (multiply current body weight by 5) . . . .

N. Target caloric intake to lose weight (L − M)[b] . . . .

[a] If more than one physical activity is selected, you will need to estimate the average daily calories burned as a result of each additional activity (steps D through K) and add all of these figures to L above.

[b] This figure should never be below 1,200 calories for women or 1,500 calories for men. See Lab 5B for the 1,200-, 1,500-, 1,800-, and 2,000-calorie diet plans.

II. Stage of Change

1. Using Figure 2.5 (page 49) and Table 2.3 (page 49), identify your current stage of change regarding **recommended body weight:**
2. If weight loss is recommended, how much weight do you need to lose? Is it a realistic goal?
3. Based on the processes and techniques of change discussed in Chapter 2, indicate what you can do to help yourself implement a weight management program.

III. Exercise Program Selection

1. How much effort are you willing to put into maintaining recommended weight or reaching your weight loss goal?

2. Indicate your feelings about participating in an exercise program.

3. Will you commit to participate in a combined aerobic and strength-training program?[c] Yes No

   If your answer is "Yes," proceed to the next question; if you answered "No," please review Chapters 3, 4, and 5 again and read Chapters 6, 7, 8, and 9.

4. List aerobic activities you enjoy or may enjoy doing.

5. Select one or two aerobic activities in which you will participate regularly.

6. List facilities available to you where you can carry out the aerobic and strength-training programs.

7. Indicate days and times you will set aside for your aerobic and strength-training program (5 to 6 days per week should be devoted to aerobic exercise and 1 to 3 nonconsecutive days per week to strength training).

   Monday:

   Tuesday:

   Wednesday:

   Thursday:

   Friday:

   Saturday:

   Sunday: A complete day of rest once a week is recommended to allow your body to fully recover from exercise.

[c] Flexibility programs are necessary for injury prevention, adequate fitness, and good health but do not help with weight loss. Stretching exercises can be conducted regularly during the cool-down phase of your aerobic and strength-training programs (see Chapter 7).

Behavior Modification

Briefly describe whether you think you can meet the goals of your aerobic and strength training programs. What obstacles will you have to overcome and how will you overcome them?

Lab 5B Calorie-Restricted Diet Plans

Name: Date: Grade:

Instructor: Course: Section:

Necessary Lab Equipment
None required.

Objective
To help you implement a calorie-restricted diet plan according to your target caloric intake obtained in Lab 5A.

Lab Preparation
Read Chapter 5 prior to this lab and make additional copies (as needed) of your selected diet plan.

1,200 Calorie Diet Plan

Instructions:
The objective of the diet plan is to meet (not exceed) the number of servings allowed for the food groups listed. Each time that you eat a particular food, record it in the space provided for each group along with the amount you ate. Refer to the Food Guide Pyramid (Figure 3.1, page 63) to find out what counts as one serving for each group listed. Instead of the meat, poultry, fish, dry beans, eggs, and nuts group, you are allowed to have a commercially available low-fat frozen entree for your main meal (this entree should provide no more than 300 calories and less than 6 grams of fat). You can make additional copies of this form as needed.

Meat & Beans: 1 low-fat frozen entree
Milk: 2 servings
Fruits: 2 servings
Veggies: 3 servings
Grains: 6 servings

Bread, Cereal, Rice, Pasta Group (80 calories/serving): 6 servings

1
2
3
4
5
6

Vegetable Group (25 calories/serving): 3 servings

1
2
3

Fruit Group (60 calories/serving): 2 servings

1
2

Milk Group (120 calories/serving, use low-fat milk and milk products): 2 servings

1
2

Low-fat Frozen Entree (300 calories and less than 6 grams of fat): 1 serving

1

Today's physical activity: Intensity: Duration: min Number of steps:

1,500 Calorie Diet Plan

Instructions:

The objective of the diet plan is to meet (not exceed) the number of servings allowed for the food groups listed. Each time that you eat a particular food, record it in the space provided for each group along with the amount you ate. Refer to the Food Guide Pyramid (Figure 3.1, page 63) to find out what counts as one serving for each group listed. Instead of the meat, poultry, fish, dry beans, eggs, and nuts group, you are allowed to have two commercially available low-fat frozen entrees for your main meal (these entrees should provide no more than 300 calories and less than 6 grams of fat). You can make additional copies of this form as needed.

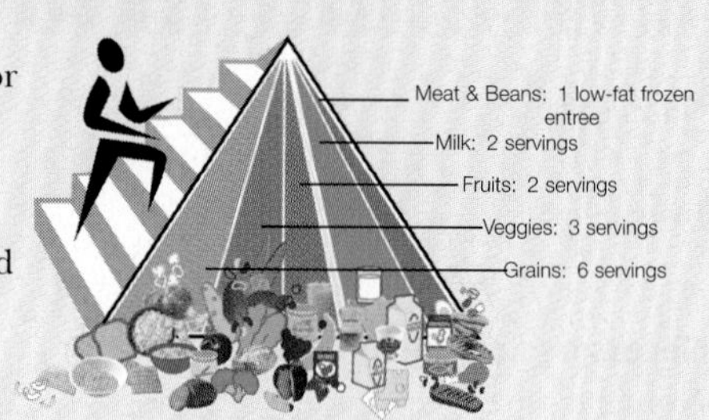

Bread, Cereal, Rice, Pasta Group (80 calories/serving): 6 servings

1

2

3

4

5

6

Vegetable Group (25 calories/serving): 3 servings

1

2

3

Fruit Group (60 calories/serving): 2 servings

1

2

Milk Group (120 calories/serving, use low-fat milk and milk products): 2 servings

1

2

Two Low-fat Frozen Entrees (300 calories and less than 6 grams of fat): 2 servings

1

2

Today's physical activity: ______ Intensity: ______ Duration: ______ min Number of steps: ______

1,800 Calorie Diet Plan

Instructions:

The objective of the diet plan is to meet (not exceed) the number of servings allowed for the food groups listed. Each time that you eat a particular food, record it in the space provided for each group along with the amount you ate. Refer to the Food Guide Pyramid (Figure 3.1, page 63) to find out what counts as one serving for each group listed. Instead of the meat, poultry, fish, dry beans, eggs, and nuts group, you are allowed to have two commercially available low-fat frozen entrees for your main meal (these entrees should provide no more than 300 calories and less than 6 grams of fat). You can make additional copies of this form as needed.

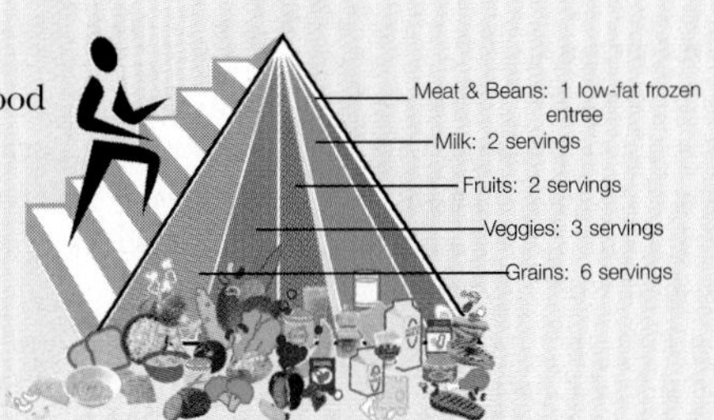

Bread, Cereal, Rice, Pasta Group (80 calories/serving): 8 servings

1

2

3

4

5

6

7

8

Vegetable Group (25 calories/serving): 5 servings

1

2

3

4

5

Fruit Group (60 calories/serving): 3 servings

1

2

3

Milk Group (120 calories/serving, use low-fat milk and milk products): 2 servings

1

2

Two Low-fat Frozen Entrees (300 calories and less than 6 grams of fat): 2 servings

1

2

Today's physical activity: ______ Intensity: ______ Duration: ______ min Number of steps: ______

2,000 Calorie Diet Plan

Instructions:

The objective of the diet plan is to meet (not exceed) the number of servings allowed for the food groups listed. Each time that you eat a particular food, record it in the space provided for each group along with the amount you ate. Refer to the Food Guide Pyramid (Figure 3.1, page 63) to find out what counts as one serving for each group listed. Instead of the meat, poultry, fish, dry beans, eggs, and nuts group, you are allowed to have two commercially available low-fat frozen entrees for your main meal (these entrees should provide no more than 300 calories and less than 6 grams of fat). You can make additional copies of this form as needed.

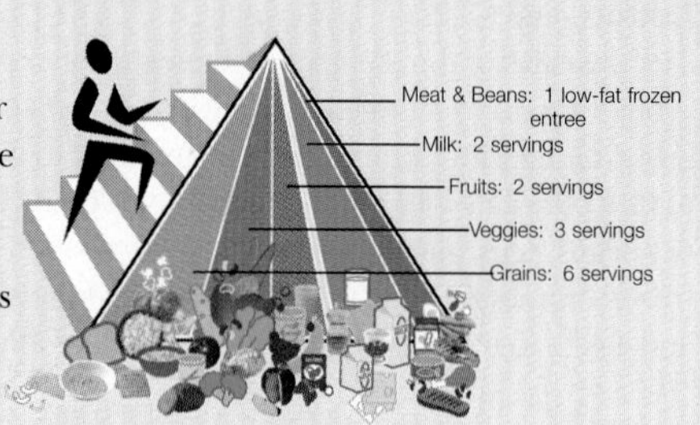

Bread, Cereal, Rice, Pasta Group (80 calories/serving): 10 servings

1

2

3

4

5

6

7

8

9

10

Vegetable Group (25 calories/serving): 5 servings

1

2

3

4

5

Fruit Group (60 calories/serving): 4 servings

1

2

3

4

Milk Group (120 calories/serving, use low-fat milk and milk products): 2 servings

1

2

Two Low-fat Frozen Entrees (300 calories and less than 6 grams of fat): 2 servings

1

2

Today's physical activity: ______ Intensity: ______ Duration: ______ min Number of steps: ______

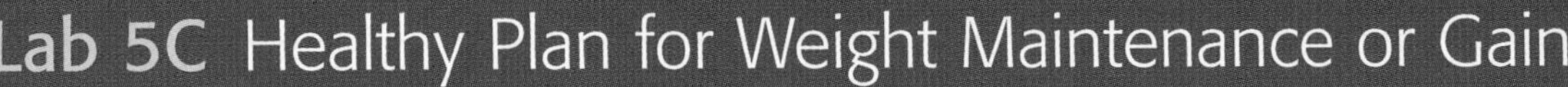

Lab 5C Healthy Plan for Weight Maintenance or Gain

Name:		Date:		Grade:	
Instructor:		Course:		Section:	

Necessary Lab Equipment
None.

Lab Preparation
Read Chapters 3, 4, and 5 prior to this lab.

Objective
To design a sample daily healthy diet plan to maintain current body weight or increase body weight.

I. Daily Caloric Requirement

A. Current body weight in pounds . . . .

B. Current percent body fat . . . .

C. Current body composition classification (Table 4.8, page 120) . . . .

D. Total daily energy requirement with exercise to maintain body weight (use item L from Lab 5A). Use this figure and stop further computations if the goal is to maintain body weight . . . .

E. Target body weight to increase body weight . . . .

F. Number of additional daily calories to increase body weight (combine this increased caloric intake with a strength-training program, see Chapter 7) . . . .

G. Total daily energy (caloric) requirement with exercise to increase body weight (D + 500) . . . .

II. Strength-Training Program

For weight gain purposes, indicate three days during the week and the time when you will engage in a strength-training program.

III. Healthy Diet Plan

Design a sample healthy daily diet plan according to the total daily energy requirement computed in D (maintenance) or G (weight gain) above. Using Appendix A, list all individual food items that you can consume on that day, along with their caloric, carbohydrate, fat, protein content. Be sure that the diet meets the recommended number of servings from the five food groups.

Breakfast

	Food item	Serving Size	Calories	Carbohydrates (gr)	Fat (gr)	Protein (gr)
1.						
2.						
3.						
4.						
5.						

Breakfast

	Food item	Serving Size	Calories	Carbohydrates (gr)	Fat (gr)	Protein (gr)
6.						
7.						
8.						

Lunch

	Food item	Serving Size	Calories	Carbohydrates (gr)	Fat (gr)	Protein (gr)
1.						
2.						
3.						
4.						
5.						
6.						
7.						
8.						

Snack

	Food item	Serving Size	Calories	Carbohydrates (gr)	Fat (gr)	Protein (gr)
1.						

Dinner

	Food item	Serving Size	Calories	Carbohydrates (gr)	Fat (gr)	Protein (gr)
1.						
2.						
3.						
4.						
5.						
6.						
7.						
8.						
		Totals:				

IV. Percent of Macronutrients

Determine the percent of total calories that are derived from carbohydrates, fat, and protein.

A. Total calories = ______

B. Grams of carbohydrates ______ × 4 ÷ ______ (total calories) = ______ %

C. Grams of fat ______ × 9 ÷ ______ (total calories) = ______ %

D. Grams of protein ______ × 4 ÷ ______ (total calories) = ______ %

E. Body weight (BW) in kilograms (BW in pounds divided by 2.2046) = ______ kg

F. Grams of protein per kilogram of body weight ______ (grams of protein) ÷ ______ (BW in kg) = ______ gr/kg

G. Please summarize your diet and protein intake to either maintain or gain weight.

____

____

Lab 5D Weight Management: Measuring Progress

Name: | Date: | Grade:

Instructor: | Course: | Section:

Necessary Lab Equipment
None.

Lab Preparation
Read Chapters 2, 3, 4, and 5 prior to this lab.

Objective
To prepare and monitor behavioral changes for weight management.

I. Please answer all of the following:

1. State your own feelings regarding your current body weight, your target body composition, and a completion date for this goal.

Completion date:

2. Do you have an eating disorder? If so, express your feelings about it. Can your instructor help you find professional advice so that you can work toward resolving this problem?

3. Is your present diet adequate according to the nutrient analysis? Yes No

4. State dietary changes necessary to achieve a balanced diet and/or to lose weight (increase or decrease caloric intake, decrease fat intake, increase intake of complex carbohydrates, etc.). List specific foods that will help you improve in areas where you may have deficiencies and food items to avoid or consume in moderation to help you achieve better nutrition.

Changes to make:

Foods that will help:

Foods to avoid:

II. Behavior Modification Progress Form

Instructions: Read the section on tips for behavior modification and adherence to a weight management program (pages 154–155). On a weekly or bi-weekly basis, go through the list of strategies and provide a "Yes" or "No" answer to each statement. If you are able to answer "Yes" to most questions, you have been successful in implementing positive weight management behaviors. (Make additional copies of this page as needed.)

Strategy	**Date**					
1. I have made a commitment to change.						
2. I set realistic goals.						
3. I exercise regularly.						
4. I have healthy eating patterns.						
5. I exercise control over my appetite.						
6. I am consuming less fat in my diet.						
7. I pay attention to the number of calories in food.						
8. I have eliminated unnecessary food items from my diet.						
9. I use craving-reducing foods in my diet.						
10. I avoid automatic eating.						
11. I stay busy.						
12. I plan meals ahead of time.						
13. I cook wisely.						
14. I do not serve more food than I should eat.						
15. I use portion control in my diet.						
16. I eat slowly and at the table only.						
17. I avoid social binges.						
18. I avoid food raids.						
19. I do not eat out more than once per week. When I do, I eat low-fat meals.						
20. I practice stress management.						
21. I have a strong support group.						
22. I monitor behavior changes.						
23. I prepare for lapses/relapses.						
24. I reward my accomplishments.						
25. I think positive.						

Cardiorespiratory Endurance

CHAPTER 6

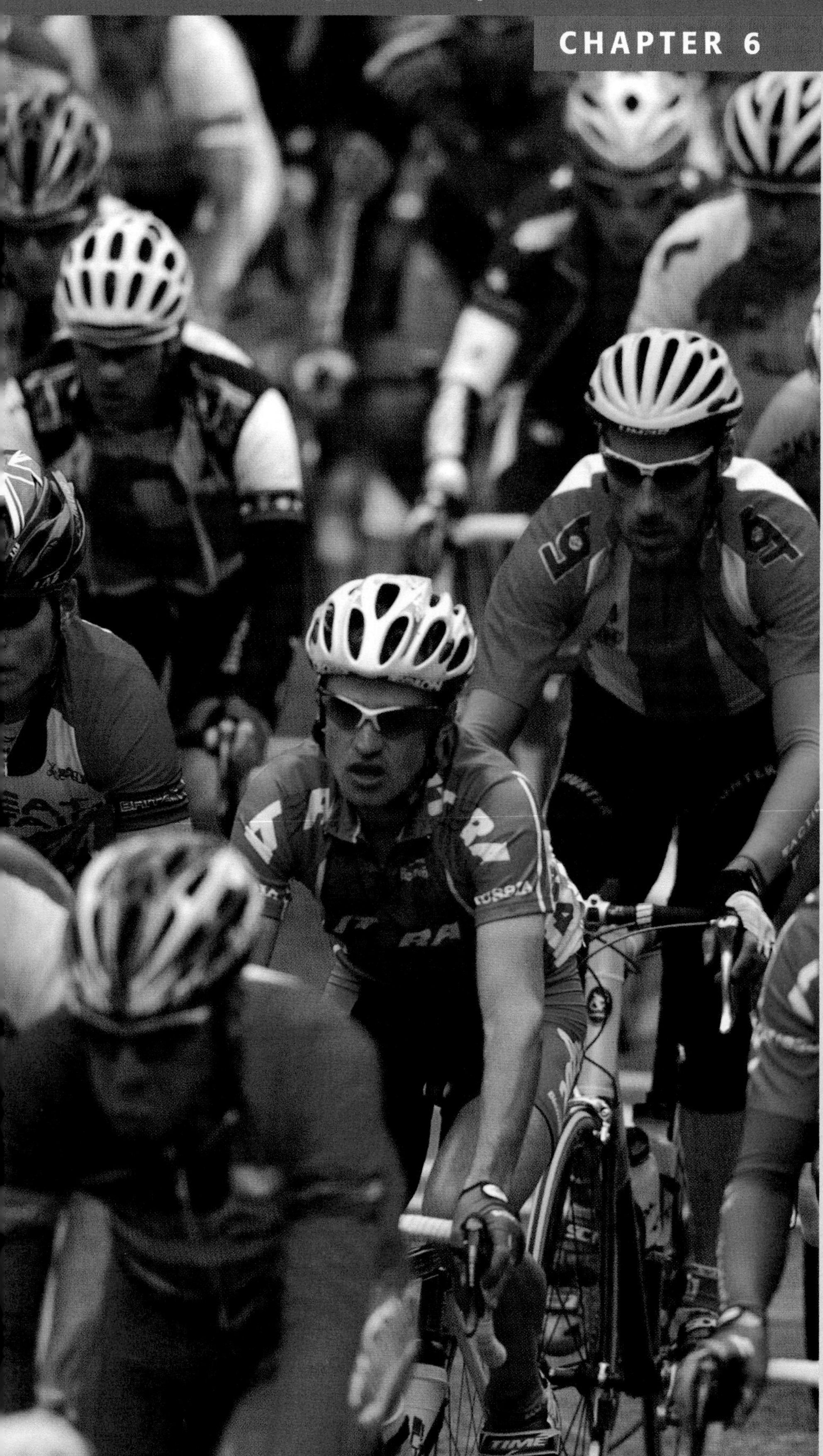

Exercise is the closest thing we'll ever get to the miracle pill that people seek. It brings weight loss, appetite control, improved mood and self-esteem, an energy kick, and longer life by decreasing the risk of heart disease, diabetes, stroke, osteoporosis, and chronic disabilities.[1]

OBJECTIVES

- Define cardiorespiratory endurance and describe the benefits of cardiorespiratory endurance training in maintaining health and well-being.
- Define aerobic and anaerobic exercise and give examples.
- Be able to assess cardiorespiratory fitness through five different test protocols.
- Be able to interpret the results of cardiorespiratory endurance assessments according to health fitness and physical fitness standards.
- Be able to estimate oxygen uptake and caloric expenditure from walking and jogging.
- Determine your readiness to start an exercise program.
- Explain the principles that govern cardiorespiratory exercise prescription: intensity, mode, duration, and frequency.
- Learn some ways to foster adherence to exercise.

ThomsonNOW! Go to www.thomsonedu.com/login to:

- Assess your cardiorespiratory fitness level.
- Maintain a log of your fitness activities.
- Check how well you understand the chapter's concepts.

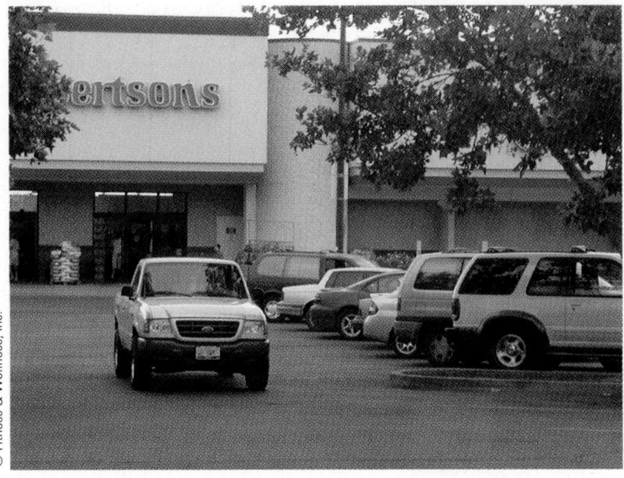

© Fitness & Wellness, Inc.

The epitome of physical inactivity: driving around a parking lot for several minutes in search of a parking spot 20 yards closer to the store's entrance.

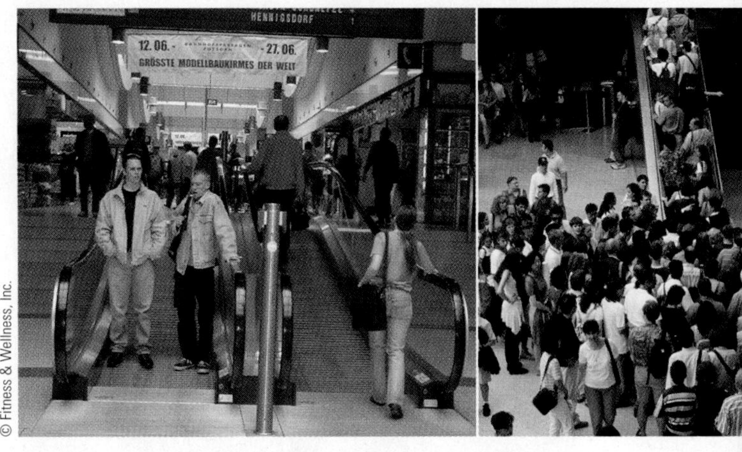

© Fitness & Wellness, Inc.

Advances in modern technology have almost completely eliminated the need for physical activity, significantly enhancing the deterioration rate of the human body.

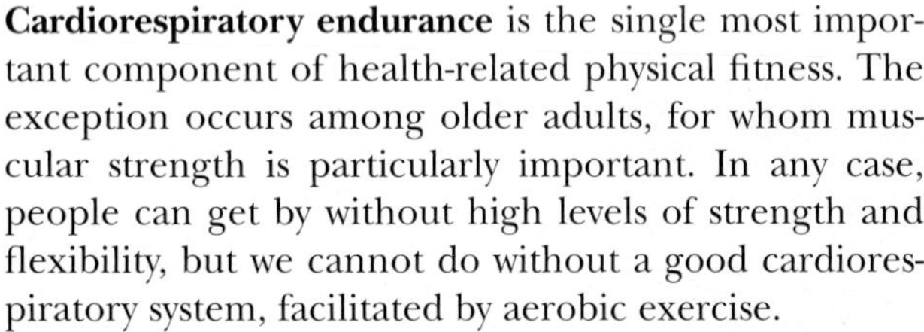

Cardiorespiratory endurance is the single most important component of health-related physical fitness. The exception occurs among older adults, for whom muscular strength is particularly important. In any case, people can get by without high levels of strength and flexibility, but we cannot do without a good cardiorespiratory system, facilitated by aerobic exercise.

Aerobic exercise is especially important in preventing cardiovascular disease. A poorly conditioned heart, which has to pump more often just to keep a person alive, is subject to more wear and tear than a well-conditioned heart. In situations that place strenuous demands on the heart, such as doing yard work, lifting heavy objects or weights, or running to catch a bus, the unconditioned heart may not be able to sustain the strain. Regular participation in cardiorespiratory endurance activities also helps a person achieve and maintain recommended body weight—the fourth component of health-related physical fitness.

Physical activity, unfortunately, is no longer a natural part of our existence. Technological developments have driven most people in developed countries into sedentary lifestyles. For instance, when many people go to a store only a couple of blocks away, most drive their automobiles and then spend a couple of minutes driving around the parking lot to find a spot 20 yards closer to the store's entrance. They do not even have to carry the groceries to the car—a store employee usually offers to do this for them.

Similarly, during a visit to a multilevel shopping mall, almost everyone chooses to take the escalator instead of the stairs (which tend to be inaccessible). Automobiles, elevators, escalators, telephones, intercoms, remote controls, electric garage door openers—all are modern-day commodities that minimize the amount of movement and effort required of the human body.

One of the most harmful effects of modern-day technology is an increase in chronic conditions related to a lack of physical activity. These **hypokinetic diseases** include hypertension, heart disease, chronic low-back pain, and obesity. (The term "hypo" means low or little, and "kinetic" implies motion.) Lack of adequate physical activity is a fact of modern life that most people can avoid no longer. To enjoy modern-day conveniences and still expect to live life to its fullest, however, one has to make a personalized lifetime exercise program a part of daily living.

Basic Cardiorespiratory Physiology: A Quick Survey

Before we begin to overhaul our bodies with an exercise program, we should understand the mechanisms that we propose to alter and survey the ways by which to measure how well we perform them. Cardiorespiratory endurance is a measure of how the pulmonary (lungs), cardiovascular (heart and blood vessels), and muscular systems work together during aerobic activities. As a person breathes, part of the oxygen in the air is taken up by the **alveoli** in the lungs. As blood passes through the alveoli, oxygen is picked up by **hemoglobin** and transported in the blood to the heart. The heart then is responsible for pumping the oxygenated blood through the circulatory system to all organs and tissues of the body.

At the cellular level, oxygen is used to convert food substrates (primarily carbohydrates and fats) through aerobic metabolism into **adenosine triphosphate (ATP).** This compound provides the energy for physical activity, body functions, and maintenance of a constant internal equilibrium. During physical exertion, more ATP is needed to perform the activity. As a result, the lungs, heart, and blood vessels have to deliver more oxygen to the muscle cells to supply the required energy.

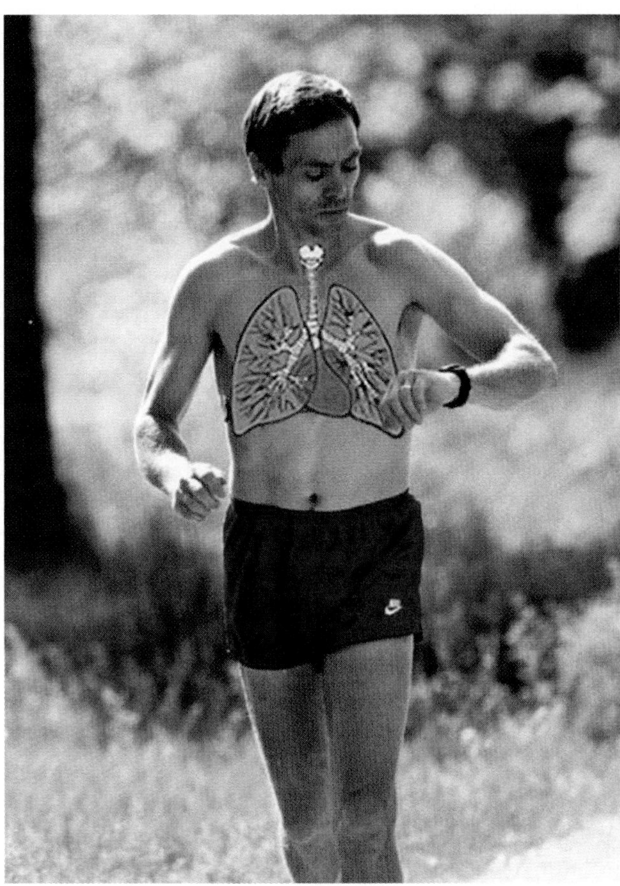

Cardiorespiratory endurance refers to the ability of the lungs, heart, and blood vessels to deliver adequate amounts of oxygen to the cells to meet the demands of prolonged physical activity.

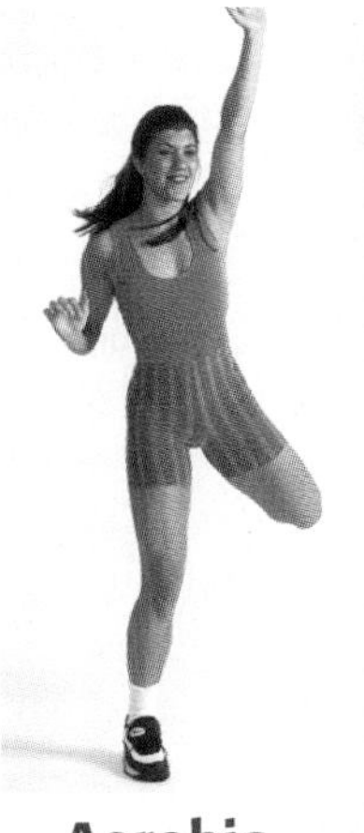

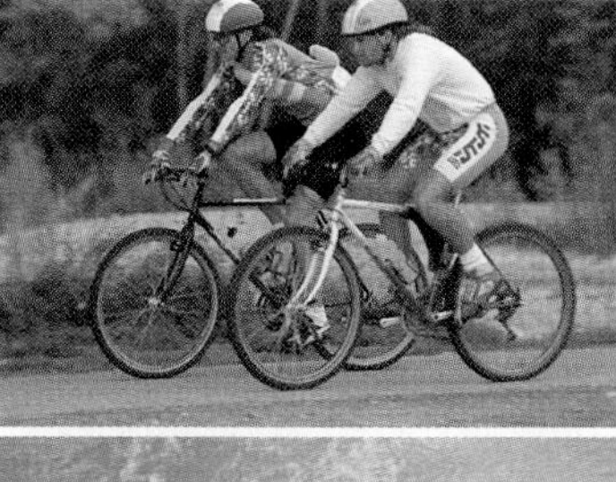

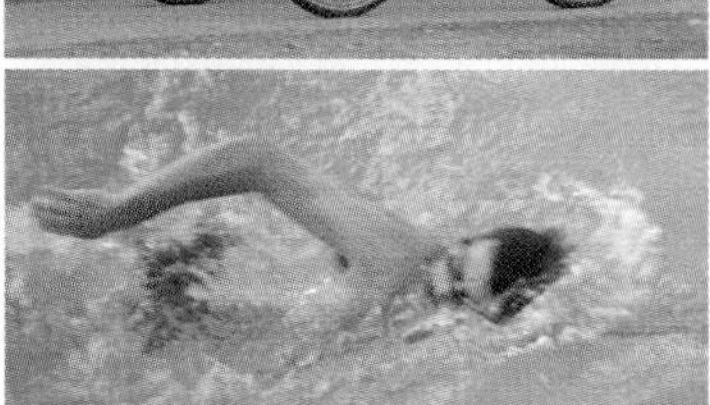

Photos © Fitness & Wellness, Inc.

Aerobic Activities

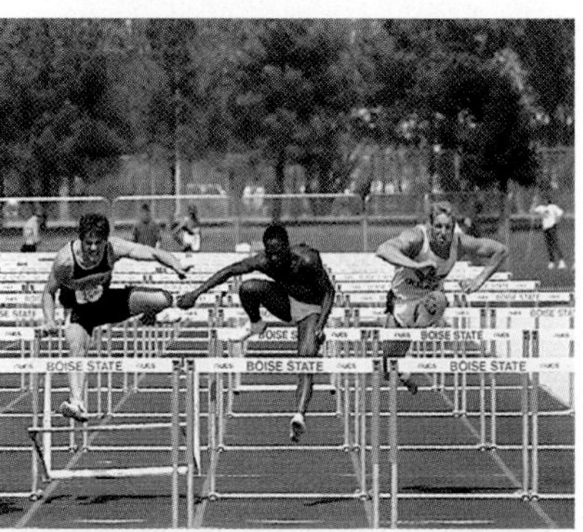

© Fitness & Wellness, Inc.

Anaerobic Activities

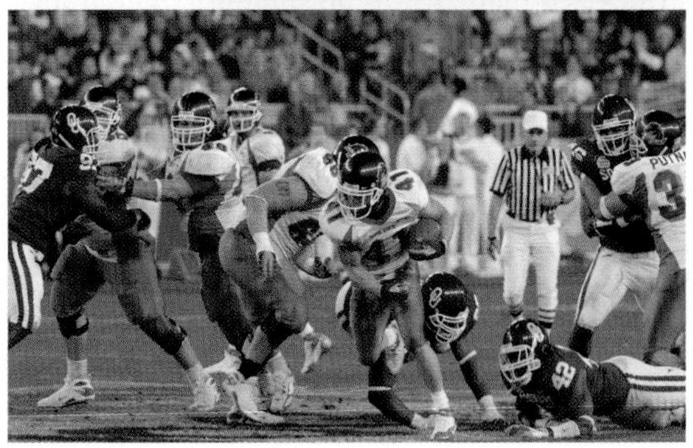

John Kelly © Boise State University, 2007

During prolonged exercise, an individual with a high level of cardiorespiratory endurance is able to deliver the required amount of oxygen to the tissues with relative ease. In contrast, the cardiorespiratory system of a person with a low level of endurance has to work much harder, the heart has to work at a higher rate, less oxygen is delivered to the tissues and, consequently, the individual fatigues faster. Hence, a higher capacity to deliver and utilize oxygen—called **oxygen uptake** or **VO_2**—indicates a more efficient cardiorespiratory system. Measuring oxygen uptake, therefore, is an important way by which to evaluate our cardiorespiratory health.

Aerobic and Anaerobic Exercise

Cardiorespiratory endurance activities often are called **aerobic** exercises. Examples are walking, jogging, swimming, cycling, cross-country skiing, water aerobics, rope skipping, and aerobics. By contrast, the intensity of **anaerobic** exercise is so high that oxygen cannot be de-

Cardiorespiratory endurance The ability of the lungs, heart, and blood vessels to deliver adequate amounts of oxygen to the cells to meet the demands of prolonged physical activity.

Hypokinetic diseases "Hypo" denotes "lack of"; therefore, lack of physical activity.

Alveoli Air sacs in the lungs where oxygen is taken up and carbon dioxide (produced by the body) is released from the blood.

Hemoglobin Iron-containing compound, found in red blood cells, that transports oxygen.

Adenosine triphosphate (ATP) A high-energy chemical compound that the body uses for immediate energy.

Oxygen uptake (VO_2) The amount of oxygen the human body uses.

Aerobic Describes exercise that requires oxygen to produce the necessary energy (ATP) to carry out the activity.

Anaerobic Describes exercise that does not require oxygen to produce the necessary energy (ATP) to carry out the activity.

TABLE 6.1 Average Resting and Maximal Cardiac Output, Stroke Volume, and Heart Rate for Sedentary, Trained, and Highly Trained Males*

	Resting			Maximal		
	Cardiac Output (l/min)	Stroke Volume (ml)	Heart Rate (bpm)	Cardiac Output (l/min)	Stroke Volume (ml)	Heart Rate (bpm)
Sedentary	5–6	68	74	20	100	200
Trained	5–6	90	56	30	150	200
Highly Trained	5–6	110	45	35	175	200

* Cardiac output and stroke volume in women are about 25 percent lower than in men.

livered and utilized to produce energy. Because energy production is limited in the absence of oxygen, anaerobic activities can be carried out for only short periods—2 to 3 minutes. The higher the intensity of the activity, the shorter the duration.

Good examples of anaerobic activities are the 100, 200, and 400 meters in track and field, the 100 meters in swimming, gymnastics routines, and strength training. Anaerobic activities do not contribute much to developing the cardiorespiratory system. Only aerobic activities will increase cardiorespiratory endurance. The basic guidelines for cardiorespiratory exercise prescription are set forth later in this chapter.

Critical Thinking

Your friend Joe is not physically active and doesn't exercise. He manages to keep his weight down by dieting and tells you that because he feels and looks good, he doesn't need to exercise. How do you respond to your friend?

Benefits of Aerobic Training

Everyone who participates in a cardiorespiratory or aerobic exercise program can expect a number of beneficial physiological adaptations from training. Among them are the following.

1. A higher **maximal oxygen uptake (VO_{2max}).** The amount of oxygen the body is able to use during exercise increases significantly. This allows the individual to exercise longer and more intensely before becoming fatigued. Depending on the initial fitness level, the increases in VO_{2max} range from 5 to 30 percent, although higher increases have been reported in people who have very low initial levels of fitness or who were significantly overweight prior to starting the aerobic exercise program.

2. An increase in the oxygen-carrying capacity of the blood. As a result of training, the red blood cell count goes up. Red blood cells contain hemoglobin, which transports oxygen in the blood.

3. A decrease in **resting heart rate (RHR)** and an increase in cardiac muscle strength. During resting conditions, the heart ejects between 5 and 6 liters of blood per minute (a liter is slightly larger than a quart). This amount of blood, also referred to as **cardiac output,** meets the body's energy demands in the resting state.

Like any other muscle, the heart responds to training by increasing in strength and size. As the heart gets stronger, the muscle can produce a more forceful contraction, which helps the heart to eject more blood with each beat. This **stroke volume** yields a lower heart rate. The lower heart rate also allows the heart to rest longer between beats. Average resting and maximal cardiac outputs, stroke volumes, and heart rates for sedentary, trained, and highly trained (elite) males are shown in Table 6.1.

Resting heart rates frequently decrease by 10 to 20 beats per minute (bpm) after only 6 to 8 weeks of training. A reduction of 20 bpm saves the heart about 10,483,200 beats per year. The average heart beats between 70 and 80 bpm. As seen in Table 6.1, resting heart rates in highly trained athletes are often around 45 bpm.

4. A lower heart rate at given **workloads.** When compared with untrained individuals, a trained person has a lower heart rate response to a given task because of greater efficiency of the cardiorespiratory system. Individuals are surprised to find that, following several weeks of training, a given workload (let's say a 10-minute mile) elicits a much lower heart rate response than their response when they first started training.

5. An increase in the number and size of the **mitochondria.** All energy necessary for cell function is produced in the mitochondria. As their size and numbers increase, so does their potential to produce energy for muscular work.

6. An increase in the number of functional **capillaries.** Capillaries allow for the exchange of oxygen and car-

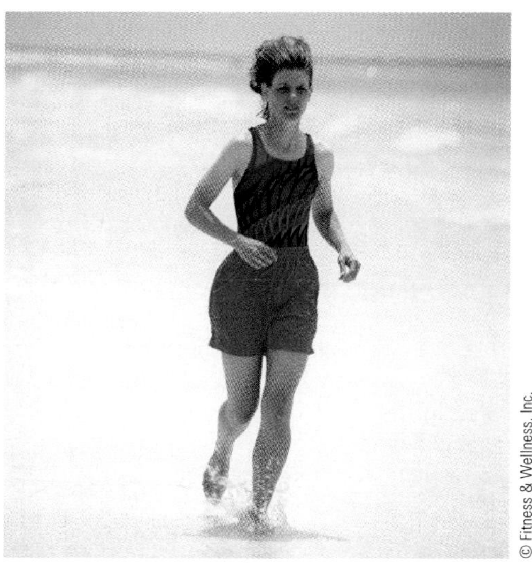

Aerobic fitness leads to better health and a higher quality of life.

bon dioxide between the blood and the cells. As more vessels open up, more gas exchange can take place, delaying the onset of fatigue during prolonged exercise. This increase in capillaries also speeds the rate at which waste products of cell metabolism can be removed. This increased capillarization also occurs in the heart, which enhances the oxygen delivery capacity to the heart muscle itself.

7. A faster **recovery time.** Trained individuals recover more rapidly after exercising. A fit system is able to more quickly restore any internal equilibrium disrupted during exercise.

8. Lower blood pressure and blood lipids. A regular aerobic exercise program leads to lower blood pressure (thereby reducing a major risk factor for stroke) and lower levels of fats (such as cholesterol and triglycerides), all of which have been linked to the formation of atherosclerotic plaque, which obstructs the arteries. This decreases the risk of coronary heart disease (see Chapter 11).

9. An increase in fat-burning enzymes. These enzymes are significant because fat is lost primarily by burning it in muscle. As the concentration of the enzymes increases, so does the ability to burn fat.

Physical Fitness Assessment

The assessment of physical fitness serves several purposes:

- To educate participants regarding their present fitness levels and compare them to health fitness and physical fitness standards.
- To motivate individuals to participate in exercise programs.
- To provide a starting point for individualized exercise prescription.
- To evaluate improvements in fitness achieved through exercise programs and adjust exercise prescription accordingly.
- To monitor changes in fitness throughout the years.

Responders Versus Nonresponders

Individuals who follow similar training programs show a wide variation in physiological responses. Heredity plays a crucial role in how each person responds to and improves after beginning an exercise program. Several studies have documented that following exercise training, most individuals, called **responders,** readily show improvements, but a few, **nonresponders,** exhibit small or no improvements at all. This concept is referred to as the **principle of individuality.**

After several months of aerobic training, VO_{2max} increases are between 15 and 20 percent, on the average, although individual responses can range from 0 percent (in a few selected cases) to more than 50 percent improvement, even when all participants follow exactly the same training program. Nonfit and low-fitness participants, however, should not label themselves nonre-

Maximal oxygen uptake (VO_{2max}) Maximum amount of oxygen the body is able to utilize per minute of physical activity, commonly expressed in ml/kg/min; the best indicator of cardiorespiratory or aerobic fitness.

Resting heart rate (RHR) Heart rate after a person has been sitting quietly for 15–20 minutes.

Cardiac output Amount of blood pumped by the heart in one minute.

Stroke volume Amount of blood pumped by the heart in one beat.

Workload Load (or intensity) placed on the body during physical activity.

Mitochondria Structures within the cells where energy transformations take place.

Capillaries Smallest blood vessels carrying oxygenated blood to the tissues in the body.

Recovery time Amount of time the body takes to return to resting levels after exercise.

Responders Individuals who exhibit improvements in fitness as a result of exercise training.

Nonresponders Individuals who exhibit small or no improvements in fitness, compared with others who undergo the same training program.

Principle of individuality Training concept holding that genetics plays a major role in individual responses to exercise training and these differences must be considered when designing exercise programs for different people.

Behavior Modification Planning

TIPS TO INCREASE DAILY PHYSICAL ACTIVITY

Adults need recess, too! There are 1440 minutes in every day. Schedule a minimum of 30 of these minutes for physical activity. With a little creativity and planning, even the person with the busiest schedule can make room for physical activity. For many folks, before or after work or meals is often an available time to cycle, walk, or play. Think about your weekly or daily schedule and look for or make opportunities to be more active. Every little bit helps. Consider the following suggestions:

- Walk, cycle, jog, skate, etc., to school, work, the store, or place of worship.
- Use a pedometer to count your daily steps.
- Walk while doing errands.
- Get on or off the bus several blocks away.
- Park the car farther away from your destination.
- At work, walk to nearby offices instead of sending e-mails or using the phone.
- Walk or stretch a few minutes every hour that you are at your desk.
- Take fitness breaks—walking or doing desk exercises—instead of taking cigarette breaks or coffee breaks.
- Incorporate activity into your lunch break (walk to the restaurant).
- Take the stairs instead of the elevator or escalator.
- Play with children, grandchildren, or pets. Everybody wins. If you find it too difficult to be active after work, try it before work.
- Do household tasks.
- Work in the yard or garden.
- Avoid labor-saving devices. Turn off the self-propelled option on your lawnmower or vacuum cleaner.
- Use leg power. Take small trips on foot to get your body moving.
- Exercise while watching TV (for example, use hand weights, stationary bicycle/treadmill/stairclimber, or stretch).
- Spend more time playing sports than sitting in front of the TV or the computer.
- Dance to music.
- Keep a pair of comfortable walking or running shoes in your car and office. You'll be ready for activity wherever you go!
- Make a Saturday morning walk a group habit.
- Learn a new sport or join a sports team.
- Avoid carts when golfing.
- When out of town, stay in hotels with fitness centers.

Source: Adapted from Centers for Disease Control and Prevention, Atlanta, 2005.

Try It

Keep a three-day log of all your activities. List the activities performed, time of day, and how long you were engaged in these activities. You may be surprised by your findings.

sponders based on the previous discussion. Nonresponders constitute less than 5 percent of exercise participants. Although additional research is necessary, lack of improvement in cardiorespiratory endurance among nonresponders might be related to low levels of leg strength. A lower body strength-training program has been shown to help these individuals improve VO_{2max} through aerobic exercise.[2]

Following your self-assessment of cardiorespiratory fitness, if your fitness level is less than adequate, do not let that discourage you, but do set a priority to be physically active every day. In addition to regular exercise, lifestyle behaviors—walking, taking stairs, cycling to work, parking farther from the office, doing household tasks, gardening, and doing yard work, for example—provide substantial benefits. In this regard, daily **physical activity** and **exercise** habits should be monitored in conjunction with fitness testing to evaluate adherence among nonresponders. After all, it is through increased daily activity that we reap the health benefits that improve our quality of life.

Assessment of Cardiorespiratory Endurance

Cardiorespiratory endurance, cardiorespiratory fitness, or aerobic capacity is determined by the maximal amount of oxygen the human body is able to utilize (the oxygen uptake) per minute of physical activity (VO_{2max}). This value can be expressed in liters per minute (l/min) or milliliters per kilogram per minute (ml/kg/min). The relative value in ml/kg/min is used most often because it considers total body mass (weight) in kilograms. When comparing two individuals with the same absolute value, the one with the lesser body mass will have a higher relative value, indicating that more oxygen is available to each kilogram (2.2 pounds) of body weight. Because all tissues and organs of the body need oxygen to function, higher oxygen consumption indicates a more efficient cardiorespiratory system.

Components of Oxygen Uptake (VO_2)

The amount of oxygen the body actually uses at rest or during submaximal (VO_2) or maximal (VO_{2max}) exercise is determined by the heart rate, the stroke volume, and the amount of oxygen removed from the vascular system (for use by all organs and tissues of the body, including the muscular system).

Heart Rate

Normal heart rate ranges from about 40 bpm during resting conditions in trained athletes to 200 bpm or higher during maximal exercise. The **maximal heart rate (MHR)** that a person can achieve starts to drop by about one beat per year beginning at about 12 years of age. Maximal heart rate in trained endurance athletes is sometimes slightly lower than in untrained individuals. This adaptation to training is thought to allow the heart more time to effectively fill with blood so as to produce a greater stroke volume.

Stroke Volume

Stroke volume ranges from 50 ml per beat (stroke) during resting conditions in untrained individuals to 200 ml at maximum in endurance-trained athletes (see Table 6.1). Following endurance training, stroke volume increases significantly. Some of the increase is the result of a stronger heart muscle, but it also is related to an increase in total blood volume and a greater filling capacity of the ventricles during the resting phase (diastole) of the cardiac cycle. As more blood enters the heart, more blood can be ejected with each heartbeat (systole). The increase in stroke volume is primarily responsible for the increase in VO_{2max} with endurance training.

Amount of Oxygen Removed from Blood

The amount of oxygen removed from the vascular system is known as the **arterial–venous oxygen difference ($a\text{-}\bar{v}O_2diff$).** The oxygen content in the arteries at sea level is typically 20 ml of oxygen per 100 cc of blood. (This value decreases at higher altitudes because of the drop in barometric pressure, which affects the amount of oxygen picked up by hemoglobin.) The oxygen content in the veins during a resting state is about 15 ml per 100 cc. Thus, the $a\text{-}\bar{v}O_2diff$—the amount of oxygen in the arteries minus the amount in the veins—at rest is 5 ml per 100 cc. The arterial value remains constant during both resting and exercise conditions, but during maximal exercise the venous oxygen content drops to about 5 ml per 100 cc, yielding an $a\text{-}\bar{v}O_2diff$ of 15 ml per 100 cc. The latter value may be slightly higher in endurance athletes.

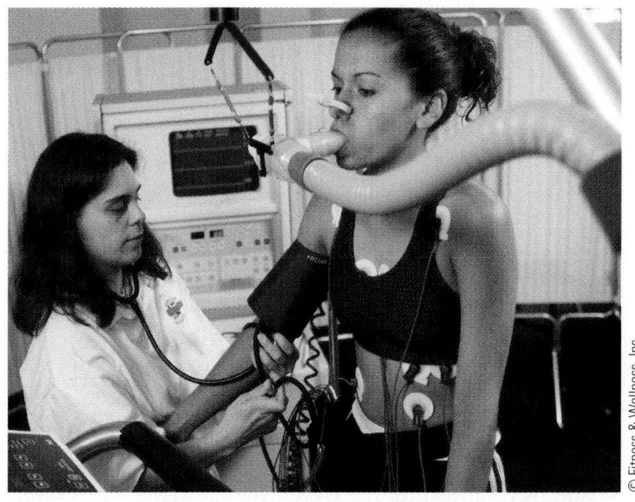
© Fitness & Wellness, Inc.

Oxygen uptake (VO_2), as determined through direct gas analysis.

These three factors are used to compute VO_2 using the following equation:

$$VO_2 \text{ in l/min} = (HR \times SV \times a\text{-}\bar{v}O_2diff) \div 100{,}000$$

where

HR = heart rate
SV = stroke volume

For example, the resting VO_2 (also known as "resting metabolic rate") of an individual with a resting heart rate of 76 bpm and a stroke volume of 79 ml would be

$$VO_2 \text{ in l/min} = (76 \times 79 \times 5) \div 100{,}000 = .3 \text{ l/min}$$

Likewise, the VO_{2max} of a person exercising maximally who achieves a heart rate of 190 bpm and a maximal stroke volume of 120 ml would be

$$VO_{2max} \text{ in l/min} = (190 \times 120 \times 15) \div 100{,}000 = 3.42 \text{ l/min}$$

To convert l/min to ml/kg/min, multiply the l/min value by 1,000 and divide by body weight in kilograms. In the above example, if the person weighs 70 kilograms, the VO_{2max} in ml/kg/min would be 48.9 ($3.42 \times 1000 \div 70$).

Physical activity Bodily movement produced by skeletal muscles; requires expenditure of energy and produces progressive health benefits. Examples include walking, taking the stairs, dancing, gardening, yard work, house cleaning, snow shoveling, washing the car, and all forms of structured exercise.

Exercise A type of physical activity that requires planned, structured, and repetitive bodily movement with the intent of improving or maintaining one or more components of physical fitness.

Maximal heart rate (MHR) Highest heart rate for a person, related primarily to age.

Arterial–venous oxygen difference ($a\text{-}\bar{v}O_2diff$) The amount of oxygen removed from the blood as determined by the difference in oxygen content between arterial and venous blood.

Critical Thinking

You can improve your relative VO_{2max} without engaging in an aerobic exercise program. How do you accomplish this? Would you benefit from doing so?

Because the actual measurement of the stroke volume and the $a\text{-}\bar{v}O_2diff$ is impractical in the fitness setting, VO_2 also is determined through gas (air) analysis. The person being tested breathes into a metabolic cart that measures the difference in oxygen content between the person's exhaled air and the atmosphere. The air we breathe contains 21 percent oxygen; thus, VO_2 can be assessed by establishing the difference between 21 percent and the percent of oxygen left in the air the person exhales, according to the total amount of air taken into the lungs. This type of equipment, however, is expensive. Consequently, several alternative methods of estimating VO_{2max} using limited equipment have been developed. These methods are discussed next.

VO_{2max} is affected by genetics, training, gender, age, and body composition. Although aerobic training can help people attain good or excellent cardiorespiratory fitness, only those with a strong genetic component are able to reach an "elite" level of aerobic capacity (60 to 80 ml/kg/min). Further, VO_{2max} is 15 to 30 percent higher in men. This is related to a greater hemoglobin content, lower body fat (see "Essential and Storage Fat" in Chapter 4), and larger heart size in men (a larger heart pumps more blood, and thus produces a greater stroke volume). VO_{2max} also decreases by about 1 percent per year starting at age 25. This decrease, however, is only 0.5 percent per year in physically active individuals.

Tests to Estimate VO_{2max}

Even though most cardiorespiratory endurance tests probably are safe to administer to apparently healthy individuals (those with no major coronary risk factors or symptoms), an exercise clearance questionnaire, such as found in Lab 6C, should be used as a minimum screening tool prior to exercise testing or participation. The American College of Sports Medicine (ACSM) also recommends that a physician be present for all maximal exercise tests on apparently healthy men 45 or older and women 55 or older.[3] A maximal test is any test that requires the participant's all-out or nearly all-out effort. For submaximal exercise tests, a physician should be present when testing higher risk/symptomatic individuals or diseased people, regardless of the participant's current age.

Five exercise tests used to assess cardiorespiratory fitness are introduced in this chapter: the 1.5-Mile Run Test, the 1.0-Mile Walk Test, the Step Test, the Astrand–Ryhming Test, and the 12-Minute Swim Test. The test procedures are explained in detail in Figures 6.1, 6.2, 6.3, 6.4, and 6.5, respectively.

Several tests are provided in this chapter so you may choose one test depending on time, equipment, and individual physical limitations. For example, people who can't jog or walk could take the bike (Astrand–Ryhming) or swim test. You may perform more than one of these tests, but because these are different tests and they estimate VO_{2max}, they will not necessarily yield the same results. Therefore, to make valid comparisons, you should take the same test when doing pre- and post-assessments. You may record the results of your test(s) in Lab 6A.

1.5-Mile Run Test

The 1.5-Mile Run Test is used most frequently to predict VO_{2max} according to the time the person takes to run or walk a 1.5-mile course (see Figure 6.1). VO_{2max} is estimated based on the time the person takes to cover the distance (see Table 6.2).

The only equipment necessary to conduct this test is a stopwatch and a track or premeasured 1.5-mile course. This perhaps is the easiest test to administer, but a note of caution is in order when conducting the test: Given that the objective is to cover the distance in the shortest time, it is considered a maximal exercise test. The 1.5-Mile Run Test should be limited to conditioned individuals who have been cleared for exercise. The test is not recommended for unconditioned beginners, men over age 45, and women over age 55 without proper medical clearance, symptomatic individuals, and those with known disease or risk factors for coronary heart disease. A program of at least 6 weeks of aerobic training is recommended before unconditioned individuals take this test.

1.0-Mile Walk Test

The 1.0-Mile Walk Test can be used by individuals who are unable to run because of low fitness levels or injuries. All that is required is a brisk 1.0-mile walk that will elicit an exercise heart rate of at least 120 beats per minute at the end of the test.

You will need to know how to take your heart rate by counting your pulse. You can do this by gently placing the middle and index fingers over the radial artery on the wrist (inside the wrist on the side of the thumb) or over the carotid artery in the neck just below the jaw, next to the voice box. You should not use the thumb to check the pulse because it has a strong pulse of its own, which can make you miscount. When checking the carotid pulse, do not press too hard, because it may cause a reflex action that slows the heart. Some exercise leaders recommend that when you check the pulse over the carotid artery, the hand on the same side of the neck (left hand over left carotid artery) be used to avoid excessive pressure on the artery. With minimum

FIGURE 6.1 Procedure for the 1.5-Mile Run Test.

1. Make sure you qualify for this test. This test is contraindicated for unconditioned beginners, individuals with symptoms of heart disease, and those with known heart disease or risk factors.
2. Select the testing site. Find a school track (each lap is one-fourth of a mile) or a premeasured 1.5-mile course.
3. Have a stopwatch available to determine your time.
4. Conduct a few warm-up exercises prior to the test. Do some stretching exercises, some walking, and slow jogging.
5. Initiate the test and try to cover the distance in the fastest time possible (walking or jogging). Time yourself during the run to see how fast you have covered the distance. If any unusual symptoms arise during the test, do not continue. Stop immediately and retake the test after another 6 weeks of aerobic training.
6. At the end of the test, cool down by walking or jogging slowly for another 3 to 5 minutes. Do not sit or lie down after the test.
7. According to your performance time, look up your estimated maximal oxygen uptake (VO_{2max}) in Table 6.2.

Example: A 20-year-old female runs the 1.5-mile course in 12 minutes and 40 seconds. Table 6.2 shows a VO_{2max} of 39.8 ml/kg/min for a time of 12:40. According to Table 6.8, this VO_{2max} would place her in the "good" cardiorespiratory fitness category.

TABLE 6.2 Estimated Maximal Oxygen Uptake (VO_{2max}) for the 1.5-Mile Run Test

Time	VO_{2max} (ml/kg/min)	Time	VO_{2max} (ml/kg/min)	Time	VO_{2max} (ml/kg/min)
6:10	80.0	10:40	48.0	15:10	33.1
6:20	79.0	10:50	47.4	15:20	32.7
6:30	77.9	11:00	46.6	15:30	32.2
6:40	76.7	11:10	45.8	15:40	31.8
6:50	75.5	11:20	45.1	15:50	31.4
7:00	74.0	11:30	44.4	16:00	30.9
7:10	72.6	11:40	43.7	16:10	30.5
7:20	71.3	11:50	43.2	16:20	30.2
7:30	69.9	12:00	42.3	16:30	29.8
7:40	68.3	12:10	41.7	16:40	29.5
7:50	66.8	12:20	41.0	16:50	29.1
8:00	65.2	12:30	40.4	17:00	28.9
8:10	63.9	12:40	39.8	17:10	28.5
8:20	62.5	12:50	39.2	17:20	28.3
8:30	61.2	13:00	38.6	17:30	28.0
8:40	60.2	13:10	38.1	17:40	27.7
8:50	59.1	13:20	37.8	17:50	27.4
9:00	58.1	13:30	37.2	18:00	27.1
9:10	56.9	13:40	36.8	18:10	26.8
9:20	55.9	13:50	36.3	18:20	26.6
9:30	54.7	14:00	35.9	18:30	26.3
9:40	53.5	14:10	35.5	18:40	26.0
9:50	52.3	14:20	35.1	18:50	25.7
10:00	51.1	14:30	34.7	19:00	25.4
10:10	50.4	14:40	34.3		
10:20	49.5	14:50	34.0		
10:30	48.6	15:00	33.6		

Source: Adapted from K. H. Cooper, "A Means of Assessing Maximal Oxygen Intake," in *Journal of the American Medical Association*, 203 (1968): 201–204; M. L. Pollock, J. H. Wilmore, and S. M. Fox III, *Health and Fitness Through Physical Activity*, (New York: John Wiley & Sons, 1978); and J. H. Wilmore and D. L. Costill, *Training for Sport and Activity* (Dubuque, IA: Wm. C. Brown Publishers, 1988).

experience, however, you can be accurate using either hand as long as you apply only gentle pressure. If available, heart rate monitors can be used to increase the accuracy of heart rate assessment.

VO_{2max} is estimated according to a prediction equation that requires the following data: 1.0-mile walk time, exercise heart rate at the end of the walk, gender, and body weight in pounds. The procedure for this test and the equation are given in Figure 6.2.

Step Test

The Step Test requires little time and equipment and can be administered to almost anyone, because a submaximal workload is used to estimate VO_{2max}. Symptomatic and diseased individuals should not take this test. Significantly overweight individuals and those with joint problems in the lower extremities may have difficulty performing the test.

The actual test takes only 3 minutes. A 15-second recovery heart rate is taken between 5 and 20 seconds following the test (see Figure 6.3 and Table 6.3). The required equipment consists of a bench or gymnasium bleacher 16¼ inches high, a stopwatch, and a metronome.

You also will need to know how to take your heart rate by counting your pulse (explained under the 1.0-Mile Walk Test). Once people learn to take their own heart rate, a large group of people can be tested at once, using gymnasium bleachers for the steps.

Astrand–Ryhming Test

Because of its simplicity and practicality, the Astrand–Ryhming Test is one of the most popular tests used to estimate VO_{2max} in the laboratory setting. The test is conducted on a bicycle ergometer, and, similar to the Step Test, it requires only submaximal workloads and little time to administer.

The cautions given for the Step Test also apply to the Astrand–Ryhming Test. Nevertheless, because the participant does not have to support his or her own body weight while riding the bicycle, overweight individuals and those with limited joint problems in the lower extremities can take this test.

The bicycle ergometer to be used for this test should allow for the regulation of workloads (see the test procedure in Figure 6.4, page 180). Besides the bicycle ergometer, a stopwatch and an additional technician to monitor the heart rate are needed to conduct the test.

FIGURE 6.2 Procedure for the 1.0-Mile Walk Test.

1. Select the testing site. Use a 440-yard track (4 laps to a mile) or a premeasured 1.0-mile course.
2. Determine your body weight in pounds prior to the test.
3. Have a stopwatch available to determine total walking time and exercise heart rate.
4. Walk the 1.0-mile course at a brisk pace (the exercise heart rate at the end of the test should be above 120 beats per minute).
5. At the end of the 1.0-mile walk, check your walking time and immediately count your pulse for 10 seconds. Multiply the 10-second pulse count by 6 to obtain the exercise heart rate in beats per minute.
6. Convert the walking time from minutes and seconds to minute units. Because each minute has 60 seconds, divide the seconds by 60 to obtain the fraction of a minute. For instance, a walking time of 12 minutes and 15 seconds would equal 12 + (15 ÷ 60), or 12.25 minutes.
7. To obtain the estimated maximal oxygen uptake (VO_{2max}) in ml/kg/min, plug your values in the following equation:
   $VO_{2max} = 88.768 - (0.0957 \times W) + (8.892 \times G) - (1.4537 \times T) - (0.1194 \times HR)$

Where:

W = Weight in pounds
G = Gender (use 0 for women and 1 for men)
T = Total time for the one-mile walk in minutes (see item 6)
HR = Exercise heart rate in beats per minute at the end of the 1.0-mile walk

Example: A 19-year-old female who weighs 140 pounds completed the 1.0-mile walk in 14 minutes 39 seconds with an exercise heart rate of 148 beats per minute. Her estimated VO_{2max} would be:

W = 140 lbs
G = 0 (female gender = 0)
T = 14:39 = 14 + (39 ÷ 60) = 14.65 min
HR = 148 bpm
$VO_{2max} = 88.768 - (0.0957 \times 140) + (8.892 \times 0) - (1.4537 \times 14.65) - (0.1194 \times 148)$
$VO_{2max} = 36.4$ ml/kg/min

Source: F. A. Dolgener, L. D. Hensley, J. J. Marsh, and J. K. Fjelstul, "Validation of the Rockport Fitness Walking Test in College Males and Females," *Research Quarterly for Exercise and Sport* 65 (1994): 152–158.

FIGURE 6.3 Procedure for the Step Test.

1. Conduct the test with a bench or gymnasium bleacher 16¼ inches high.
2. Perform the stepping cycle to a four-step cadence (up-up-down-down). Men should perform 24 complete step-ups per minute, regulated with a metronome set at 96 beats per minute. Women perform 22 step-ups per minute, or 88 beats per minute on the metronome.
3. Allow a brief practice period of 5 to 10 seconds to familiarize yourself with the stepping cadence.
4. Begin the test and perform the step-ups for exactly 3 minutes.
5. Upon completing the 3 minutes, remain standing and take your heart rate for a 15-second interval from 5 to 20 seconds into recovery. Convert recovery heart rate to beats per minute (multiply 15-second heart rate by 4).
6. Maximal oxygen uptake (VO_{2max}) in ml/kg/min is estimated according to the following equations:
   Men:
   $VO_{2max} = 111.33 - (0.42 \times \text{recovery heart rate in bpm})$
   Women:
   $VO_{2max} = 65.81 - (0.1847 \times \text{recovery heart rate in bpm})$

Example: The recovery 15-second heart rate for a male following the 3-minute step test is found to be 39 beats. His VO_{2max} is estimated as follows:

15-second heart rate = 39 beats
Minute heart rate = 39 × 4 = 156 bpm
$VO_{2max} = 111.33 - (0.42 \times 156) = 45.81$ ml/kg/min
VO_{2max} also can be obtained according to recovery heart rates in Table 6.3.

Source: From W. D. McArdle et al., *Exercise Physiology: Energy, Nutrition, and Human Performance* (Philadelphia: Lea & Febiger, 1986).

The heart rate is taken every minute for 6 minutes. At the end of the test, the heart rate should be in the range given for each workload in Table 6.5 (page 181), generally between 120 and 170 bpm.

When administering the test to older people, good judgment is essential. Low workloads should be used, because if the higher heart rates (around 150 to 170 bpm) are reached, these individuals could be working near or at their maximal capacity, making this an unsafe test without adequate medical supervision. When testing older people, choose workloads so the final exercise heart rates do not exceed 130 to 140 bpm.

12-Minute Swim Test

Similar to the 1.5-Mile Run Test, the 12-Minute Swim Test is considered a maximal exercise test, and the same precautions apply. The objective is to swim as far as possible during the 12-Minute Swim Test (Figure 6.5, page 182).

TABLE 6.3 Predicted Maximal Oxygen Uptake for the Step Test

15-Sec Heart Rate	Heart Rate (bpm)	VO_{2max} (ml/kg/min) Men	Women
30	120	60.9	43.6
31	124	59.3	42.9
32	128	57.6	42.2
33	132	55.9	41.4
34	136	54.2	40.7
35	140	52.5	40.0
36	144	50.9	39.2
37	148	49.2	38.5
38	152	47.5	37.7
39	156	45.8	37.0
40	160	44.1	36.3
41	164	42.5	35.5
42	168	40.8	34.8
43	172	39.1	34.0
44	176	37.4	33.3
45	180	35.7	32.6
46	184	34.1	31.8
47	188	32.4	31.1
48	192	30.7	30.3
49	196	29.0	29.6
50	200	27.3	28.9

Unlike land-based tests, predicting VO_{2max} through a swimming test is difficult. A swimming test is practical only for those who are planning to take part in a swimming program or who cannot perform any of the other tests. Differences in skill level, swimming conditioning, and body composition greatly affect the energy requirements (oxygen uptake) of swimming.

Unskilled and unconditioned swimmers can expect lower cardiorespiratory fitness ratings than the ratings obtained with a land-based test. A skilled swimmer is able to swim more efficiently and expend much less energy than an unskilled swimmer. Improper breathing patterns cause premature fatigue. Overweight individuals are more buoyant in the water, and the larger surface area (body size) produces more friction against movement in the water medium.

Lack of conditioning affects swimming test results as well. An unconditioned skilled swimmer who is in good cardiorespiratory shape because of a regular jogging program will not perform as effectively in a swimming test. Swimming conditioning is important for adequate performance on this test.

Because of these limitations, VO_{2max} cannot be estimated for a swimming test and the fitness categories given in Table 6.7 (page 182) are only estimated ratings.

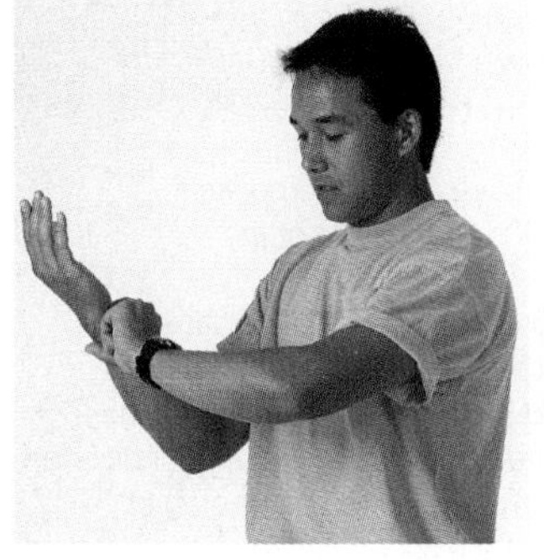

Pulse taken at the radial artery.

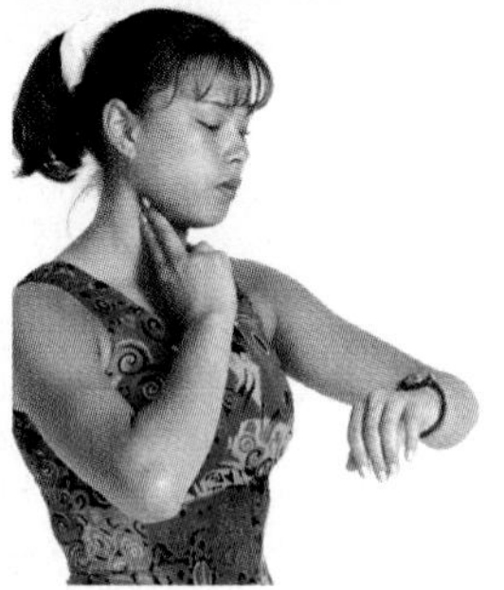

Pulse taken at the carotid artery.

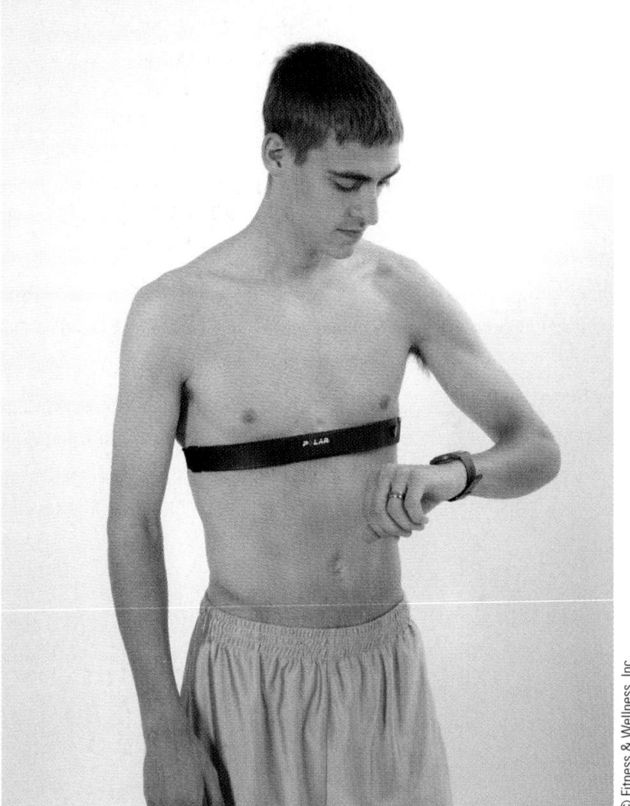

Heart rate monitors increase the accuracy of heart rate assessment.

Critical Thinking

Should fitness testing be a part of a fitness program? Why or why not? Does preparticipation fitness testing have benefits, or should fitness testing be done at a later date?

FIGURE 6.4 Procedure for the Astrand–Ryhming Test.

1. Adjust the bike seat so the knees are almost completely extended as the foot goes through the bottom of the pedaling cycle.
2. During the test, keep the speed constant at 50 revolutions per minute. Test duration is 6 minutes.
3. Select the appropriate workload for the bike based on gender, age, weight, health, and estimated fitness level. For unconditioned individuals: women, use 300 kpm (kilopounds per meter) or 450 kpm; men, 300 kpm or 600 kpm. Conditioned adults: women, 450 kpm or 600 kpm; men, 600 kpm or 900 kpm.*
4. Ride the bike for 6 minutes and check the heart rate every minute, during the last 15 seconds of each minute. Determine heart rate by recording the time it takes to count 30 pulse beats and then converting to beats per minute using Table 6.4.
5. Average the final two heart rates (5th and 6th minutes). If these two heart rates are not within 5 beats per minute of each other, continue the test for another few minutes until this is accomplished. If the heart rate continues to climb significantly after the 6th minute, stop the test and rest for 15 to 20 minutes. You may then retest, preferably at a lower workload. The final average heart rate should also fall between the ranges given for each workload in Table 6.5 (men: 300 kpm = 120 to 140 beats per minute; 600 kpm = 120 to 170 beats per minute).
6. Based on the average heart rate of the final 2 minutes and your workload, look up the maximal oxygen uptake (VO_{2max}) in Table 6.5 (for example: men: 600 kpm and average heart rate = 145, VO_{2max} = 2.4 liters/minute).
7. Correct VO_{2max} using the correction factors found in Table 6.6 (if VO_{2max} = 2.4 and age 35, correction factor = .870. Multiply 2.4 × .870 and final corrected VO_{2max} = 2.09 liters/minute).
8. To obtain VO_{2max} in ml/kg/min, multiply the VO_{2max} by 1,000 (to convert liters to milliliters) and divide by body weight in kilograms (to obtain kilograms, divide your body weight in pounds by 2.2046).

Example: Corrected VO_{2max} = 2.09 liters/minute
Body weight = 132 pounds ÷ 2.2046 = 60 kilograms

$$VO_{2max} \text{ in ml/kg/min} = \frac{2.09 \times 1{,}000}{60} = 34.8 \text{ ml/kg/min}$$

*On the Monarch bicycle ergometer, at a speed of 50 revolutions per minute, a load of 1 kp = 300 kpm, 1.5 kp = 450, 2 kp = 600 kpm, and so forth, with increases of 150 kpm to each half kp.

TABLE 6.4 Conversion of Time for 30 Pulse Beats to Pulse Rate per Minute

Sec.	bpm	Sec.	bpm	Sec.	bpm	Sec.	bpm	Sec.	bpm	Sec.	bpm
22.0	82	19.6	92	17.2	105	14.8	122	12.4	145	10.0	180
21.9	82	19.5	92	17.1	105	14.7	122	12.3	146	9.9	182
21.8	83	19.4	93	17.0	106	14.6	123	12.2	148	9.8	184
21.7	83	19.3	93	16.9	107	14.5	124	12.1	149	9.7	186
21.6	83	19.2	94	16.8	107	14.4	125	12.0	150	9.6	188
21.5	84	19.1	94	16.7	108	14.3	126	11.9	151	9.5	189
21.4	84	19.0	95	16.6	108	14.2	127	11.8	153	9.4	191
21.3	85	18.9	95	16.5	109	14.1	128	11.7	154	9.3	194
21.2	85	18.8	96	16.4	110	14.0	129	11.6	155	9.2	196
21.1	85	18.7	96	16.3	110	13.9	129	11.5	157	9.1	198
21.0	86	18.6	97	16.2	111	13.8	130	11.4	158	9.0	200
20.9	86	18.5	97	16.1	112	13.7	131	11.3	159	8.9	202
20.8	87	18.4	98	16.0	113	13.6	132	11.2	161	8.8	205
20.7	87	18.3	98	15.9	113	13.5	133	11.1	162	8.7	207
20.6	87	18.2	99	15.8	114	13.4	134	11.0	164	8.6	209
20.5	88	18.1	99	15.7	115	13.3	135	10.9	165	8.5	212
20.4	88	18.0	100	15.6	115	13.2	136	10.8	167	8.4	214
20.3	89	17.9	101	15.5	116	13.1	137	10.7	168	8.3	217
20.2	89	17.8	101	15.4	117	13.0	138	10.6	170	8.2	220
20.1	90	17.7	102	15.3	118	12.9	140	10.5	171	8.1	222
20.0	90	17.6	102	15.2	118	12.8	141	10.4	173	8.0	225
19.9	90	17.5	103	15.1	119	12.7	142	10.3	175		
19.8	91	17.4	103	15.0	120	12.6	143	10.2	176		
19.7	91	17.3	104	14.9	121	12.5	144	10.1	178		

TABLE 6.5 Maximal Oxygen Uptake (VO_{2max}) Estimates for the Astrand–Ryhming Test

	Men					Women				
	Workload					Workload				
Heart Rate	300	600	900	1200	1500	300	450	600	750	900
120	2.2	3.4	4.8			2.6	3.4	4.1	4.8	
121	2.2	3.4	4.7			2.5	3.3	4.0	4.8	
122	2.2	3.4	4.6			2.5	3.2	3.9	4.7	
123	2.1	3.4	4.6			2.4	3.1	3.9	4.6	
124	2.1	3.3	4.5	6.0		2.4	3.1	3.8	4.5	
125	2.0	3.2	4.4	5.9		2.3	3.0	3.7	4.4	
126	2.0	3.2	4.4	5.8		2.3	3.0	3.6	4.3	
127	2.0	3.1	4.3	5.7		2.2	2.9	3.5	4.2	
128	2.0	3.1	4.2	5.6		2.2	2.8	3.5	4.2	4.8
129	1.9	3.0	4.2	5.6		2.2	2.8	3.4	4.1	4.8
130	1.9	3.0	4.1	5.5		2.1	2.7	3.4	4.0	4.7
131	1.9	2.9	4.0	5.4		2.1	2.7	3.4	4.0	4.6
132	1.8	2.9	4.0	5.3		2.0	2.7	3.3	3.9	4.5
133	1.8	2.8	3.9	5.3		2.0	2.6	3.2	3.8	4.4
134	1.8	2.8	3.9	5.2		2.0	2.6	3.2	3.8	4.4
135	1.7	2.8	3.8	5.1		2.0	2.6	3.1	3.7	4.3
136	1.7	2.7	3.8	5.0		1.9	2.5	3.1	3.6	4.2
137	1.7	2.7	3.7	5.0		1.9	2.5	3.0	3.6	4.2
138	1.6	2.7	3.7	4.9		1.8	2.4	3.0	3.5	4.1
139	1.6	2.6	3.6	4.8		1.8	2.4	2.9	3.5	4.0
140	1.6	2.6	3.6	4.8	6.0	1.8	2.4	2.8	3.4	4.0
141		2.6	3.5	4.7	5.9	1.8	2.3	2.8	3.4	3.9
142		2.5	3.5	4.6	5.8	1.7	2.3	2.8	3.3	3.9
143		2.5	3.4	4.6	5.7	1.7	2.2	2.7	3.3	3.8
144		2.5	3.4	4.5	5.7	1.7	2.2	2.7	3.2	3.8
145		2.4	3.4	4.5	5.6	1.6	2.2	2.7	3.2	3.7
146		2.4	3.3	4.4	5.6	1.6	2.2	2.6	3.2	3.7
147		2.4	3.3	4.4	5.5	1.6	2.1	2.6	3.1	3.6
148		2.4	3.2	4.3	5.4	1.6	2.1	2.6	3.1	3.6
149		2.3	3.2	4.3	5.4		2.1	2.6	3.0	3.5
150		2.3	3.2	4.2	5.3		2.0	2.5	3.0	3.5
151		2.3	3.1	4.2	5.2		2.0	2.5	3.0	3.4
152		2.3	3.1	4.1	5.2		2.0	2.5	2.9	3.4
153		2.2	3.0	4.1	5.1		2.0	2.4	2.9	3.3
154		2.2	3.0	4.0	5.1		2.0	2.4	2.8	3.3
155		2.2	3.0	4.0	5.0		1.9	2.4	2.8	3.2
156		2.2	2.9	4.0	5.0		1.9	2.3	2.8	3.2
157		2.1	2.9	3.9	4.9		1.9	2.3	2.7	3.2
158		2.1	2.9	3.9	4.9		1.8	2.3	2.7	3.1
159		2.1	2.8	3.8	4.8		1.8	2.2	2.7	3.1
160		2.1	2.8	3.8	4.8		1.8	2.2	2.6	3.0
161		2.0	2.8	3.7	4.7		1.8	2.2	2.6	3.0
162		2.0	2.8	3.7	4.6		1.8	2.2	2.6	3.0
163		2.0	2.8	3.7	4.6		1.7	2.2	2.6	2.9
164		2.0	2.7	3.6	4.5		1.7	2.1	2.5	2.9
165		2.0	2.7	3.6	4.5		1.7	2.1	2.5	2.9
166		1.9	2.7	3.6	4.5		1.7	2.1	2.5	2.8
167		1.9	2.6	3.5	4.4		1.6	2.1	2.4	2.8
168		1.9	2.6	3.5	4.4		1.6	2.0	2.4	2.8
169		1.9	2.6	3.5	4.3		1.6	2.0	2.4	2.8
170		1.8	2.6	3.4	4.3		1.6	2.0	2.4	2.7

From Astrand, I. *Acta Physiologica Scandinavica* 49 (1960). Supplementum 169: 45–60.

TABLE 6.6 Age-Based Correction Factors for Maximal Oxygen Uptake

Age	Correction Factor	Age	Correction Factor	Age	Correction Factor
14	1.11	32	.909	50	.750
15	1.10	33	.896	51	.742
16	1.09	34	.883	52	.734
17	1.08	35	.870	53	.726
18	1.07	36	.862	54	.718
19	1.06	37	.854	55	.710
20	1.05	38	.846	56	.704
21	1.04	39	.838	57	.698
22	1.03	40	.830	58	.692
23	1.02	41	.820	59	.686
24	1.01	42	.810	60	.680
25	1.00	43	.800	61	.674
26	.987	44	.790	62	.668
27	.974	45	.780	63	.662
28	.961	46	.774	64	.656
29	.948	47	.768	65	.650
30	.935	48	.762		
31	.922	49	.756		

Adapted from Astrand, I. *Acta Physiologica Scandinavica* 49 (1960). Supplementum 169: 45–60.

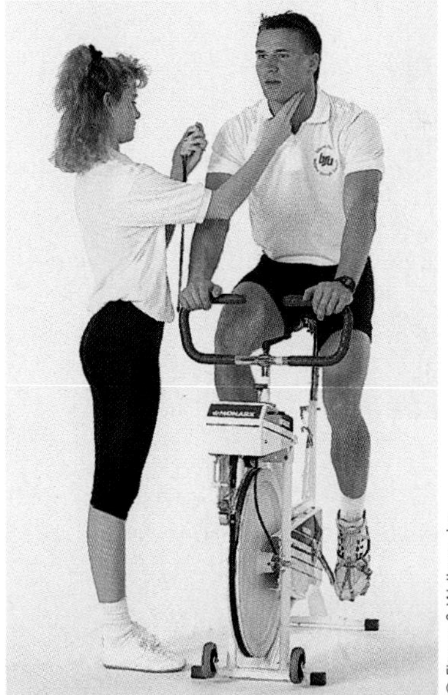

Monitoring heart rate on the carotid artery during the Astrand–Ryhming Test.

Interpreting the Results of Your Maximal Oxygen Uptake

After obtaining your VO_{2max}, you can determine your current level of cardiorespiratory fitness by consulting Table 6.8 (page 182). Locate the VO_{2max} in your age category, and on the top row you will find your present level of cardiorespiratory fitness. For example, a 19-year-old male with a VO_{2max} of 35 ml/kg/min would be classified in the "Average" cardiorespiratory fitness category. After you initiate your personal cardiorespiratory

FIGURE 6.5 Procedure for the 12-Minute Swim Test.

1. Enlist a friend to time the test. The only other requisites are a stopwatch and a swimming pool. Do not attempt to do this test in an unsupervised pool.
2. Warm up by swimming slowly and doing a few stretching exercises before taking the test.
3. Start the test and swim as many laps as possible in 12 minutes. Pace yourself throughout the test and do not swim to the point of complete exhaustion.
4. After completing the test, cool down by swimming another 2 or 3 minutes at a slower pace.
5. Determine the total distance you swam during the test and look up your fitness category in Table 6.7.

TABLE 6.7 12-Minute Swim Test Fitness Categories

Distance (yards)	Fitness Category
≥700	Excellent
500–700	Good
400–500	Average
200–400	Fair
≤200	Poor

Adapted from K. H. Cooper, *The Aerobics Program for Total Well-Being* (New York: Bantam Books, 1982).

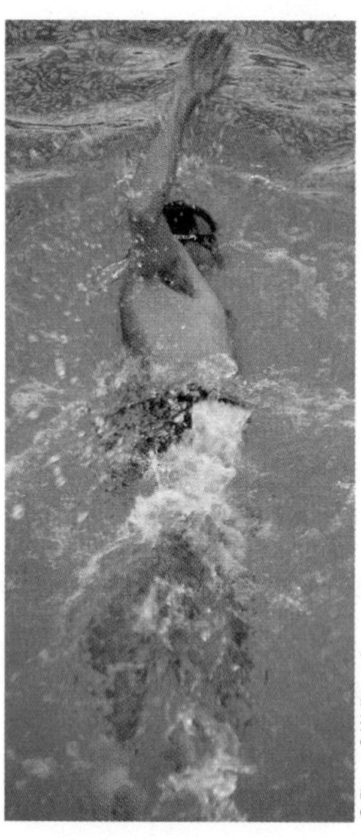

Only those with swimming skill and proper conditioning should take the 12-minute swimming test.

TABLE 6.8 Cardiorespiratory Fitness Category According to Maximal Oxygen Uptake (VO_{2max})

		FITNESS CLASSIFICATION (based on VO_{2max} in ml/kg/min)				
Gender	Age	Poor	Fair	Average	Good	Excellent
Men	<29	<24.9	25–33.9	34–43.9	44–52.9	>53
	30–39	<22.9	23–30.9	31–41.9	42–49.9	>50
	40–49	<19.9	20–26.9	27–38.9	39–44.9	>45
	50–59	<17.9	18–24.9	25–37.9	38–42.9	>43
	60–69	<15.9	16–22.9	23–35.9	36–40.9	>41
	≥70	≤12.9	13–20.9	21–32.9	33–37.9	≥38
Women	<29	<23.9	24–30.9	31–38.9	39–48.9	>49
	30–39	<19.9	20–27.9	28–36.9	37–44.9	>45
	40–49	<16.9	17–24.9	25–34.9	35–41.9	>42
	50–59	<14.9	15–21.9	22–33.9	34–39.9	>40
	60–69	<12.9	13–20.9	21–32.9	33–36.9	>37
	≥70	≤11.9	12–19.9	20–30.9	31–34.9	≥35

☐ Health fitness standard ■ High physical fitness standard

See the Chapter 1 discussion on health fitness versus physical fitness.

exercise program (see Lab 6D), you may wish to retest yourself periodically to evaluate your progress.

Predicting Oxygen Uptake and Caloric Expenditure from Walking and Jogging

As indicated earlier in the chapter, oxygen uptake can be expressed in liters per minute (l/min) or milliliters per kilogram per minute (ml/kg/min). The latter is used to classify individuals into the various cardiorespiratory fitness categories (see Table 6.8).

Oxygen uptake expressed in l/min is valuable in determining the caloric expenditure of physical activity. The human body burns about 5 calories for each liter of oxygen consumed. During aerobic exercise the average person trains between 50 and 75 percent of maximal oxygen uptake.

A person with a maximal oxygen uptake of 3.5 l/min who trains at 60 percent of maximum uses 2.1 (3.5 × .60) liters of oxygen per minute of physical activity. This indicates that 10.5 calories are burned each minute of exercise (2.1 × 5). If the activity is carried out for 30 minutes, 315 calories (10.5 × 30) have been burned.

For individuals concerned about weight management, these computations are valuable in determining energy expenditure. Because a pound of body fat represents 3,500 calories, this individual would have to exercise for a total of 333 minutes (3,500 ÷ 10.5) to burn the equivalent of a pound of body fat. At 30 minutes per exercise session, approximately 11 sessions would be required to expend the 3,500 calories.

Applying the principle of 5 calories burned per liter of oxygen consumed, you can determine with reasonable accuracy your own caloric output for walking and jogging. Table 6.9 contains the oxygen requirement (uptake) for walking speeds between 50 and 100 meters per minute and for jogging speeds in excess of 80 meters per minute.

TABLE 6.9 Oxygen Requirement Estimates for Selected Walking and Jogging Speeds

Walking		Jogging			
Speed (m/min)	VO_2 (ml/kg/min)	Speed (m/min)	VO_2 (ml/kg/min)	Speed (m/min)	VO_2 (ml/kg/min)
50	8.5	80	19.5	210	45.5
52	8.7	85	20.5	215	46.5
54	8.9	90	21.5	220	47.5
56	9.1	95	22.5	225	48.5
58	9.3	100	23.5	230	49.5
60	9.5	105	24.5	235	50.5
62	9.7	110	25.5	240	51.5
64	9.9	115	26.5	245	52.5
66	10.1	120	27.5	250	53.5
68	10.3	125	28.5	255	54.5
70	10.5	130	29.5	260	55.5
72	10.7	135	30.5	265	56.5
74	10.9	140	31.5	270	57.5
76	11.1	145	32.5	275	58.5
78	11.3	150	33.5	280	59.5
80	11.5	155	34.5		
82	11.7	160	35.5		
84	11.9	165	36.5		
86	12.1	170	37.5		
88	12.3	175	38.5		
90	12.5	180	39.5		
92	12.7	185	40.5		
94	12.9	190	41.5		
96	13.1	195	42.5		
98	13.3	200	43.5		
100	13.5	205	44.5		

m/min = meters per minute
ml/kg/min = milliliers per kilogram per minute

Table developed using the metabolic calculations contained in *Guidelines for Exercise Testing and Exercise Prescription,* by the American College of Sports Medicine (Baltimore: Williams & Wilkins, 2006).

There is a transition period from walking to jogging for speeds in the range of 80 to 134 meters per minute. Consequently, the person must be truly jogging at these lower speeds to use the estimated oxygen uptakes for jogging in Table 6.9. Because these uptakes are expressed in ml/kg/min, you will need to convert this figure to l/min to predict caloric output. This is done by multiplying the oxygen uptake in ml/kg/min by your body weight in kilograms (kg) and then dividing by 1,000.

For example, let's estimate the caloric cost for an individual who weighs 145.5 pounds and runs 3 miles in 21 minutes. Each mile is about 1,600 meters, or four laps around a 400-meter (440-yard) track. Three miles then would be 4,800 meters (1,600 × 3). Therefore, 3 miles (4,800 meters) in 21 minutes represents a pace of 228.6 meters per minute (4,800 ÷ 21).

Table 6.9 indicates an oxygen requirement (uptake) of about 49.5 ml/kg/min for a speed of 228.6 meters per minute. A weight of 145.5 pounds equals 66 kilograms (145.5 ÷ 2.2046). The oxygen uptake in l/min now can be calculated by multiplying the value in ml/kg/min by body weight in kg and dividing by 1,000. In our example, it is (49.5 × 66) ÷ 1,000 = 3.3 l/min. This oxygen uptake in 21 minutes represents a total of 347 calories (3.3 × 5 × 21).

In Lab 6B you have an opportunity to determine your own oxygen uptake and caloric expenditure for walking and jogging. Using your oxygen uptake information in conjunction with exercise heart rates allows you to estimate your caloric expenditure for almost any activity, as long as the heart rate ranges from 110 to 180 beats per minute.

To make an accurate estimate, you have to be skilled in assessing exercise heart rate. You may also use a heart rate monitor to increase the accuracy of the exercise heart rate assessment. Also, as your level of fitness improves, you will need to reassess your exercise heart rate because it will drop (given the same workload) with improved physical condition.

Principles of Cardiorespiratory Exercise Prescription

Before proceeding with the principles of exercise prescription, you should ask yourself if you are willing to give exercise a try. A low percentage of the U.S. population is truly committed to exercise. Further, more than half of the people who start exercising drop out during the first 3 to 6 months of the program. Sports psychologists are trying to find out why some people exercise habitually and many do not. All of the benefits of exercise cannot help unless people commit to a lifetime program of physical activity.

Readiness for Exercise

The first step is to answer the question: Am I ready to start an exercise program? The information provided in Lab 6C can help you answer this question. You are evaluated in four categories: mastery (self-control), attitude, health, and commitment. The higher you score in any category—mastery, for example—the more important that reason is for you to exercise.

Scores can vary from 4 to 16. A score of 12 or above is a strong indicator that the factor is important to you, whereas 8 or below is low. If you score 12 or more points in each category, your chances of initiating and sticking to an exercise program are good. If you do not score at least 12 points each in any three categories, your chances of succeeding at exercise may be slim. You need to be better informed about the benefits of exercise, and a retraining process might be helpful. More tips on how you can become committed to exercise are provided in "Getting Started and Adhering to a Lifetime Exercise Program" (page 191).

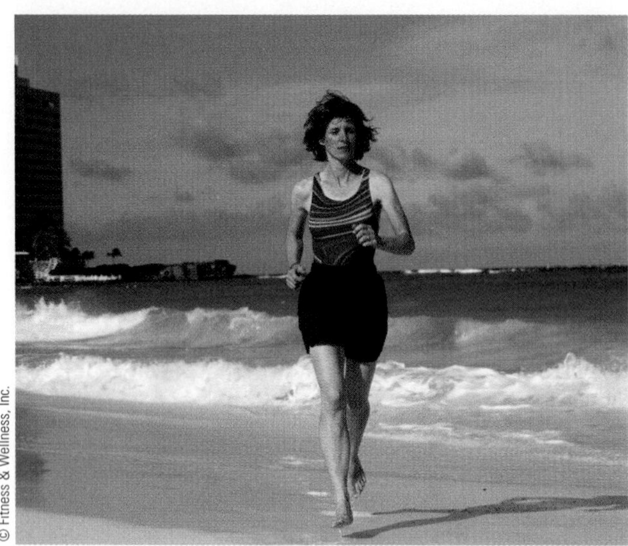

Aerobic exercise promotes cardiorespiratory development and helps decrease the risk for disease.

Next you will have to decide positively that you will try. Using Lab 6C, you can list the advantages and disadvantages of incorporating exercise into your lifestyle. Your list might include advantages such as:

- It will make me feel better.
- I will lose weight.
- I will have more energy.
- It will lower my risk for chronic diseases.

Your list of disadvantages might include the following:

- I don't want to take the time.
- I'm too out of shape.
- There's no good place to exercise.
- I don't have the willpower to do it.

When your reasons for exercising outweigh your reasons for not exercising, you will find it easier to try. In Lab 6C you will also determine your stage of change for aerobic exercise. Using the information learned in Chapter 2, you can outline specific processes and techniques for change (also see "Personal Fitness Programming: An Example" in Chapter 9, page 310).

Guidelines for Cardiorespiratory Exercise Prescription

In spite of the release of the U.S. Surgeon General's statement on physical activity and health more than a decade ago (see Chapter 1, page 5) and the overwhelming evidence validating the benefits of exercise on health and longevity, only about 19 percent of adults in the United States meet minimum recommendations of the ACSM for the improvement and maintenance of cardiorespiratory fitness.[4]

Most people are not familiar with the basic principles of cardiorespiratory exercise prescription. Thus, although they exercise regularly, they do not reap significant improvements in cardiorespiratory endurance.

To develop the cardiorespiratory system, the heart muscle has to be overloaded like any other muscle in the human body. Just as the biceps muscle in the upper arm is developed through strength-training exercises, the heart muscle has to be exercised to increase in size, strength, and efficiency. To better understand how the cardiorespiratory system can be developed, you have to be familiar with the four variables that govern exercise prescription: intensity, mode, duration, and frequency.[5] The acronym **FITT** is sometimes used to describe these variables: *F*requency, *I*ntensity, *T*ype (mode), and *T*ime (duration).

First, however, you should be aware that the ACSM recommends that apparently healthy men over age 45 and women over age 55 get a diagnostic exercise stress test prior to **vigorous exercise.**[6] The ACSM has defined vigorous exercise as an exercise intensity above 60 percent of maximal capacity. For individuals initiating an exercise program, this intensity is the equivalent of exercise that provides a "substantial challenge" to the participant or one that cannot be maintained for 20 continuous minutes.

Intensity of Exercise

When trying to develop the cardiorespiratory system, many people ignore **intensity** of exercise. For muscles to develop, they have to be overloaded to a given point. The training stimulus to develop the biceps muscle, for example, can be accomplished with arm curl-up exercises with increasing weights. Likewise, the cardiorespiratory system is stimulated by making the heart pump faster for a specified period.

Health and cardiorespiratory fitness benefits result when the heart is working between 40 and 85 percent of **heart rate reserve (HRR)** combined with an appropriate duration and frequency of training.[7] Health benefits are achieved when training at a lower exercise intensity (40 to 60 percent) for a longer time. Larger and faster improvements in cardiorespiratory fitness (VO_{2max}), however, are achieved primarily through higher-intensity programs.

Unconditioned people and older adults should start at a 40 to 50 percent training intensity. Active and fit people can train at higher intensities. Increases in VO_{2max} are accelerated when the heart is working closer to 85 percent of heart rate reserve (HRR). For this reason, after several weeks of progressive training at lower intensities, exercise can be performed between 60 and 85 percent training intensity.

FIGURE 6.6 Recommended cardiorespiratory or aerobic training pattern.

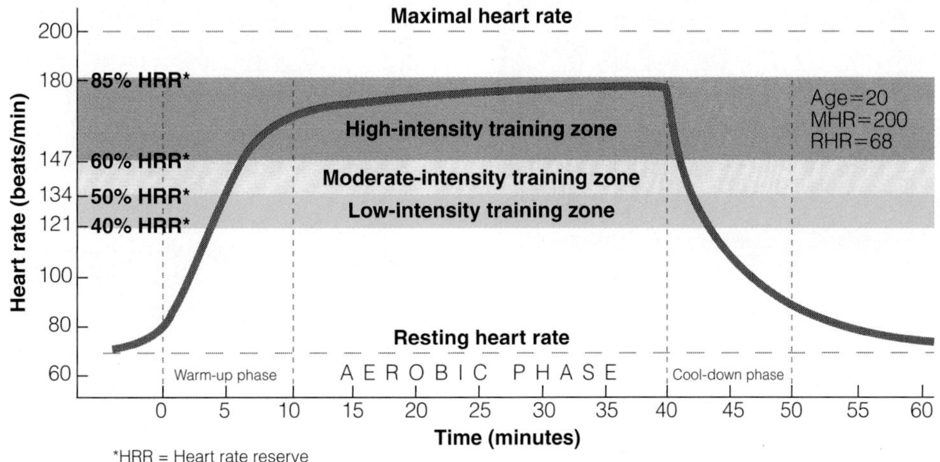

Exercise training above 85 percent is recommended only for healthy, performance-oriented individuals and competitive athletes. For most people, training above 85 percent is discouraged to avoid potential cardiovascular problems associated with high-intensity exercise. As intensity increases, exercise adherence decreases and the risk of orthopedic injuries increases.

Intensity of exercise can be calculated easily, and training can be monitored by checking your pulse. To determine the intensity of exercise or **cardiorespiratory training zone** according to heart rate reserve, follow these steps:

1. Estimate your maximal heart rate (MHR) according to the following formula:
   MHR = 220 minus age (220 − age)
2. Check your resting heart rate (RHR) some time after you have been sitting quietly for 15 to 20 minutes. You may take your pulse for 30 seconds and multiply by 2, or take it for a full minute. As explained on page 176, you can check your pulse on the wrist by placing two or three fingers over the radial artery or in the neck, using the carotid artery.
3. Determine the heart rate reserve (HRR) by subtracting the resting heart rate from the maximal heart rate (HRR = MHR − RHR).
4. Calculate the training intensities (TI) at 40, 50, 60, and 85 percent. Multiply the heart rate reserve by the respective .40, .50, .60, and .85, and then add the resting heart rate to all four of these figures (for example, 85% TI = HRR × .85 + RHR).
   Example. The 40, 50, 60, and 85 percent training intensities for a 20-year-old with a resting heart rate of 68 beats per minute (bpm) would be as follows:
   MHR: 220 − 20 = 200 bpm
   RHR: = 68 bpm
   HRR: 200 − 68 = 132 beats
   40% TI = (132 × .40) + 68 = 121 bpm
   50% TI = (132 × .50) + 68 = 134 bpm
   60% TI = (132 × .60) + 68 = 147 bpm
   85% TI = (132 × .85) + 68 = 180 bpm
   Low-intensity cardiorespiratory training zone: 121 to 134 bpm
   Moderate-intensity cardiorespiratory training zone: 134 to 147 bpm
   High-intensity (vigorous) cardiorespiratory training zone: 147 to 180 bpm

When you exercise to accelerate cardiorespiratory development, your goal is to maintain your heart rate between the 60 and 85 percent training intensities (see Figure 6.6). If you have been physically inactive, start at 40 to 50 percent intensity and gradually increase to 60 percent during the first 6 to 8 weeks of the exercise pro-

---

FITT An acronym used to describe the four cardiorespiratory exercise prescription variables: Frequency, Intensity, Type (mode), and Time (duration).

Vigorous exercise Cardiorespiratory exercise that requires an intensity level above 60 percent of maximal capacity.

Intensity In cardiorespiratory exercise, how hard a person has to exercise to improve or maintain fitness.

Heart rate reserve (HRR) The difference between maximal heart rate and resting heart rate.

Cardiorespiratory training zone Recommended training intensity range, in terms of exercise heart rate, to obtain adequate cardiorespiratory endurance development.

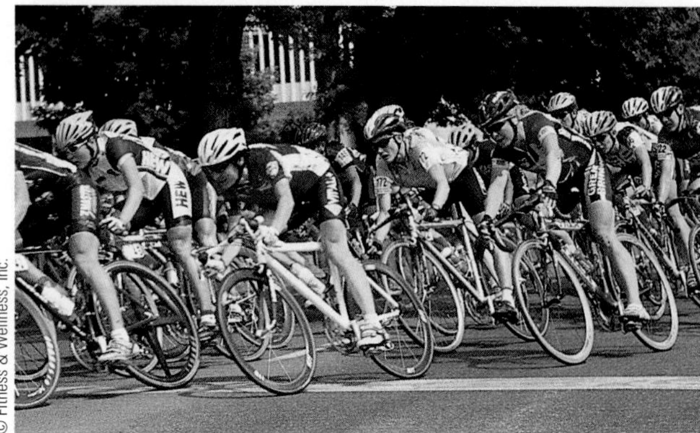

High-intensity exercise is required to achieve the high physical fitness standard (excellent category) for cardiorespiratory endurance.

FIGURE 6.7 Rate of perceived exertion (RPE) scale.

6	
7	Very, very light
8	
9	Very light
10	
11	Fairly light
12	
13	Somewhat hard
14	
15	Hard
16	
17	Very Hard
18	
19	Very, very hard
20	

From G. Borg, "Perceived Exertion: A Note on History and Methods," *Medicine and Science in Sports and Exercise,* 5 (1983): 90–93.

gram. After that, you may exercise between 60 and 85 percent training intensity.

Following a few weeks of training, you may have a considerably lower resting heart rate (10 to 20 beats fewer in 8 to 12 weeks). Therefore, you should recompute your target zone periodically. You can compute your own cardiorespiratory training zone using Lab 6D, or you can use the ThomsonNOW online resources available with this book to obtain a printout of your personalized cardiorespiratory exercise prescription (see Figure 9.5, page 312). You also can use ThomsonNOW to create and regularly update an exercise log to keep a record of your activity program (see Figure 9.6, page 313). Once you have reached an ideal level of cardiorespiratory endurance, continued training in the 60 to 85 percent range will allow you to maintain your fitness level.

Monitoring Exercise Heart Rate

During the first few weeks of an exercise program, you should monitor your exercise heart rate regularly to make sure you are training in the proper zone. Wait until you are about 5 minutes into the aerobic phase of your exercise session before taking your first reading. When you check your heart rate, count your pulse for 10 seconds, then multiply by 6 to get the per-minute pulse rate. The exercise heart rate will remain at the same level for about 15 seconds after you stop aerobic exercise, then drop rapidly. Do not hesitate to stop during your exercise bout to check your pulse. If the rate is too low, increase the intensity of exercise. If the rate is too high, slow down.

When determining the training intensity for your own program, you need to consider your personal fitness goals. Individuals who exercise at around the 50 percent training intensity will reap significant health benefits—in particular, improvements in the metabolic profile (see "Health Fitness Standards" in Chapter 1, page 14). Training at this lower percentage, however, may place you in only the "average" (moderate fitness) category (see Table 6.8 on page 182). Exercising at this lower intensity does lower the risk for cardiovascular mortality (the health fitness standard), but will not allow you to achieve a "good" or "excellent" cardiorespiratory fitness rating (the physical fitness standard). The latter ratings are obtained by exercising closer to the 85 percent threshold.

Rate of Perceived Exertion

Because many people do not check their heart rate during exercise, an alternative method of prescribing intensity of exercise was created using the **rate of perceived exertion (RPE)** scale. Using the scale in Figure 6.7, a person subjectively rates the perceived exertion or difficulty of exercise when training in the appropriate target zone. The exercise heart rate then is associated with the corresponding RPE value.

For example, if the training intensity requires a heart rate between 150 and 170 bpm, the person may associate this with training between "hard" and "very hard." Some individuals perceive less exertion than others when training in the correct zone. Therefore, you have to associate your own inner perception of the task with the phrases given on the scale. You then may proceed to exercise at that rate of perceived exertion.

For young people, the numbers on the scale also can be used in reference to exercise heart rates. If you multiply each number by 10, it will approximate the exercise heart rate at the perceived exertion phase. For example, when you are exercising "somewhat hard,"

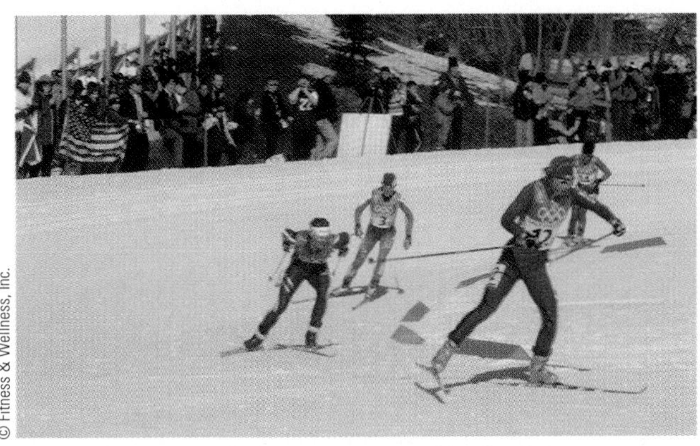

Cross-country skiing requires more oxygen and energy than most other aerobic activities.

your heart rate will be around 130 bpm (13 × 10). When you exercise "hard," the heart rate will be about 150 bpm.

You must be sure to cross-check your target zone with your perceived exertion during the first weeks of your exercise program. To help you develop this association, you should regularly keep a record of your activities, using the form provided in Figure 6.10 (page 196). After several weeks of training, you should be able to predict your exercise heart rate just by your own perceived exertion of the intensity of exercise.

Whether you monitor the intensity of exercise by checking your pulse or through rate of perceived exertion, you should be aware that changes in normal exercise conditions will affect the training zone. For example, exercising on a hot, humid day or at high altitude increases the heart rate response to a given task, requiring adjustments in the intensity of your exercise.

Mode of Exercise

The **mode,** or type, of exercise that develops the cardiorespiratory system has to be aerobic in nature. Once you have established your cardiorespiratory training zone, any activity or combination of activities that will get your heart rate up to that training zone and keep it there for as long as you exercise will give you adequate development. Examples of these activities are walking, jogging, stair climbing, elliptical activity, aerobics, swimming, water aerobics, cross-country skiing, rope skipping, cycling, racquetball, and stationary running or cycling.

Aerobic exercise has to involve the major muscle groups of the body, and it has to be rhythmic and continuous. As the amount of muscle mass involved during exercise increases, so do the demands on the cardiorespiratory system. The activity you choose should be based on your personal preferences, what you most enjoy doing, and your physical limitations. Low-impact activities greatly reduce the risk for injuries. Most injuries to beginners result from high-impact activities. Also, general strength conditioning (see Chapter 7) is recommended prior to initiating an aerobic exercise program for individuals who have been inactive. Strength conditioning can significantly reduce the incidence of injuries.

The amount of strength or flexibility you develop through various activities differs. In terms of cardiorespiratory development, though, the heart doesn't know whether you are walking, swimming, or cycling. All the heart knows is that it has to pump at a certain rate, and as long as that rate is in the desired range, your cardiorespiratory fitness will improve. From a health fitness point of view, training in the lower end of the cardiorespiratory zone will yield optimal health benefits. The closer the heart rate is to the higher end of the cardiorespiratory training zone, however, the greater will be the improvements in VO_{2max} (high physical fitness).

Because of the specificity of training, to ascertain changes in fitness, it is recommended that you use the same mode of exercise for training and testing. If your primary mode of training is cycling, it is recommended that you assess VO_{2max} using a bicycle test. For joggers, a field or treadmill running test is best. Swimmers should use a swim test.

Duration of Exercise

The general recommendation is that a person exercise between 20 and 60 minutes per session. For people who have been successful at losing weight, however, up to 90 minutes of moderate-intensity activity daily may be required to prevent weight regain.

The duration of exercise is based on how intensely a person trains. The variables are inversely related. If the training is done at around 85 percent, a session of 20 to 30 minutes is sufficient. At about 50 percent intensity, the person should train between 30 and 60 minutes. As mentioned under "Intensity of Exercise," unconditioned people and older adults should train at lower percentages and, therefore, the activity should be carried out over a longer time.

Although the recommended guideline is 20 to 30 minutes of aerobic exercise per session, accumulating 30 minutes or more of moderate-intensity physical activity throughout the day does provide substantial health benefits. Three 10-minute exercise sessions per day (separated by at least 4 hours), at approximately 70 percent of maximal heart rate, have been shown to produce training benefits.[8] Although the increases in VO_{2max} with the latter program were not as

Rate of perceived exertion (RPE) A perception scale to monitor or interpret the intensity of aerobic exercise.

Mode Form or type of exercise.

large (57 percent) as those found in a group performing a continuous 30-minute bout of exercise per day, the researchers concluded that moderate-intensity physical activity, conducted for 10 minutes three times per day, benefits the cardiorespiratory system significantly.

Results of this study are meaningful because people often mention lack of time as the reason they do not take part in an exercise program. Many think they have to exercise at least 20 continuous minutes to get any benefits at all. Even though a duration of 20 to 30 high-intensity minutes is ideal, short, intermittent exercise bouts are beneficial to the cardiorespiratory system.

From a weight management point of view, the recommendation to prevent weight gain is for people to accumulate 60 minutes of moderate-intensity physical activity most days of the week,[9] whereas 60 to 90 minutes of daily moderate-intensity activity is necessary to prevent weight regain.[10] These recommendations are based on evidence that people who maintain healthy weight typically accumulate between 1 and 1½ hours of physical activity daily. The duration of exercise should be increased gradually to avoid undue fatigue and exercise-related injuries.

If lack of time is a concern, you should exercise at a high intensity for 30 minutes, which can burn as many calories as 60 minutes of moderate intensity (also see "Low-Intensity Versus High-Intensity Exercise for Weight Loss," Chapter 5), but only 19 percent of adults in the United States typically exercise at a high intensity level. Novice and overweight exercisers also need proper conditioning prior to high-intensity exercise to avoid injuries or cardiovascular-related problems.

Exercise sessions always should be preceded by a 5- to 10-minute **warm-up** and be followed by a 10-minute **cool-down** period (see Figure 6.6). The purpose of the warm-up is to aid in the transition from rest to exercise. A good warm-up increases extensibility of the muscles and connective tissue, extends joint range of motion, and enhances muscular activity. A warm-up consists of general calisthenics, mild stretching exercises, and walking/jogging/cycling for a few minutes at a lower intensity than the actual target zone. The concluding phase of the warm-up is a gradual increase in exercise intensity to the lower end of the target training zone.

In the cool-down, the intensity of exercise is decreased gradually to help the body return to near resting levels, followed by stretching and relaxation activities. Stopping abruptly causes blood to pool in the exercised body parts, diminishing the return of blood to the heart. Less blood return can cause a sudden drop in blood pressure, dizziness and faintness, or it can bring on cardiac abnormalities. The cool-down phase also helps dissipate body heat and aid in removing the lactic acid produced during high-intensity exercise.

Behavior Modification Planning

TIPS FOR PEOPLE WHO HAVE BEEN INACTIVE FOR A WHILE

- Take the sensible approach by starting slowly.
- Begin by choosing moderate-intensity activities you enjoy the most. By choosing activities you enjoy, you'll be more likely to stick with them.
- Gradually build up the time spent exercising by adding a few minutes every few days or so until you can comfortably perform a minimum recommended amount of exercise (20 minutes per day).
- As the minimum amount becomes easier, gradually increase either the length of time exercising or increase the intensity of the activity, or both.
- Vary your activities, both for interest and to broaden the range of benefits.
- Explore new physical activities.
- Reward and acknowledge your efforts.

Source: Adapted from: Centers for Disease Control and Prevention, Atlanta, 2005.

Try It

Fill out the cardiorespiratory exercise prescription in Lab 6D either in your text or online. In your Online Journal or class notebook, describe how well you implement the above suggestions.

Frequency of Exercise

The recommended exercise **frequency** for aerobic exercise is three to five days per week. Initially, only three weekly training sessions of 15 to 20 minutes are recommended to avoid musculo-skeletal injuries. You may then increase the frequency so that by the fourth or fifth week you are exercising five times per week for 20 minutes per session in the appropriate heart rate target zone (see Lab 6D and Figure 9.5 on page 312). Thereafter, progressively continue to increase frequency, duration, and intensity of exercise until you have accomplished your goals.

When exercising at 60 to 85 percent of HRR, three 20- to 30-minute exercise sessions per week, on nonconsecutive days, are sufficient to improve (in the early stages) or maintain VO_{2max}. When training at lower intensities, exercising 30 to 60 minutes more than three days per week is required. If training is conducted more than five days a week, further improvements in VO_{2max} are minimal. Although endurance athletes often train six or seven days per week (often twice per day), their training programs are designed to increase training mileage to endure long-distance races (6 to 100 miles) at a high percentage of VO_{2max}. This is called the **anaerobic threshold.**

For individuals on a weight loss program, the recommendation is 60 to 90 minutes of low-intensity to moderate-intensity activity on most days of the week. Longer exercise sessions increase caloric expenditure for faster weight reduction (see Chapter 5, "Exercise: The Key to Weight Management," page 144).

Although three exercise sessions per week will maintain cardiorespiratory fitness, the importance of regular physical activity in preventing disease and enhancing quality of life has been pointed out clearly by the ACSM, by the U.S. Centers for Disease Control and Prevention, and by the President's Council on Physical Fitness and Sports.[11] These organizations advocate at least 30 minutes of moderate-intensity physical activity almost daily. This routine has been promoted as an effective way to improve health.

These recommendations subsequently were upheld by the U.S. Surgeon General in the 1996 "Report on Physical Activity and Health."[12] The Surgeon General's report states that people can improve their health and quality of life substantially by including moderate amounts of physical activity on most, preferably all, days of the week. Further, it states that no one, including older adults, is too old to enjoy the benefits of regular physical activity.

If you want to enjoy better health and fitness, physical activity must be pursued regularly. According to Dr. William Haskell of Stanford University: "Most of the health-related benefits of exercise are relatively short-term, so people should think of exercise as medication and take it on a daily basis."[13] Many of the benefits of exercise and activity diminish within 2 weeks of substantially decreased physical activity. These benefits are completely lost within 2 to 8 months of inactivity.[14]

To sum up: Ideally, a person should engage in physical activity six or seven times per week. Based on the previous discussion, to reap both the high-fitness and health-fitness benefits of exercise, a person should exercise a minimum of three times per week in the appropriate target zone for high fitness maintenance and three or four additional times per week in moderate-intensity activities (see Figure 6.8). Depending on the intensity of the activity and the health/fitness goals, all exercise sessions should last between 20 and 60 minutes. For adequate weight management purposes, additional daily physical activity, up to 90 minutes, may be necessary. A summary of the cardiorespiratory exercise prescription guidelines according to the ACSM is provided in Figure 6.9.

FIGURE 6.8 Cardiorespiratory exercise prescription guidelines.

Activity:	Aerobic (examples: walking, jogging, cycling, swimming, aerobics, racquetball, soccer, stair climbing)
Intensity:	40/50%–85% of heart rate reserve
Duration:	20–60 minutes of continuous aerobic activity
Frequency:	3 to 5 days per week

Source: American College of Sports Medicine, *ACSM's Guidelines for Exercise Testing and Prescription* (Philadelphia: Lippincott Williams & Wilkins, 2006).

Fitness Benefits of Aerobic Activities

The contributions of different aerobic activities to the health-related components of fitness vary. Although an accurate assessment of the contributions to each fitness component is difficult to establish, a summary of likely benefits of several activities is provided in Table 6.10 (page 191). Instead of a single rating or number, ranges are given for some of the categories. The benefits derived are based on the person's effort while participating in the activity.

The nature of the activity often dictates the potential aerobic development. For example, jogging is much more strenuous than walking. The effort during exercise also affects the amount of physiological development. During a low-impact aerobics routine, accentuating all movements (instead of just going through the motions) increases training benefits by orders of magnitude.

Table 6.10 indicates a starting fitness level for each aerobic activity. Attempting to participate in high-intensity activities without proper conditioning often leads to injuries, not to mention discouragement. Beginners should start with low-intensity activities that carry a minimum risk for injuries.

In some cases, such as high-impact aerobics and rope skipping, the risk for orthopedic injuries remains high even if the participants are adequately conditioned. These activities should be supplemental only and are not recommended as the sole mode of exercise. Most exercise-related injuries occur as a result of high-impact activities, not high intensity of exercise.

Warm-up Starting a workout slowly.

Cool-down Tapering off an exercise session slowly.

Frequency Number of times per week a person engages in exercise.

Anaerobic threshold The highest percentage of the VO_{2max} at which an individual can exercise (maximal steady state) for an extended time without accumulating significant amounts of lactic acid (accumulation of lactic acid forces an individual to slow down the exercise intensity or stop altogether).

FIGURE 6.9 The Physical Activity Pyramid 

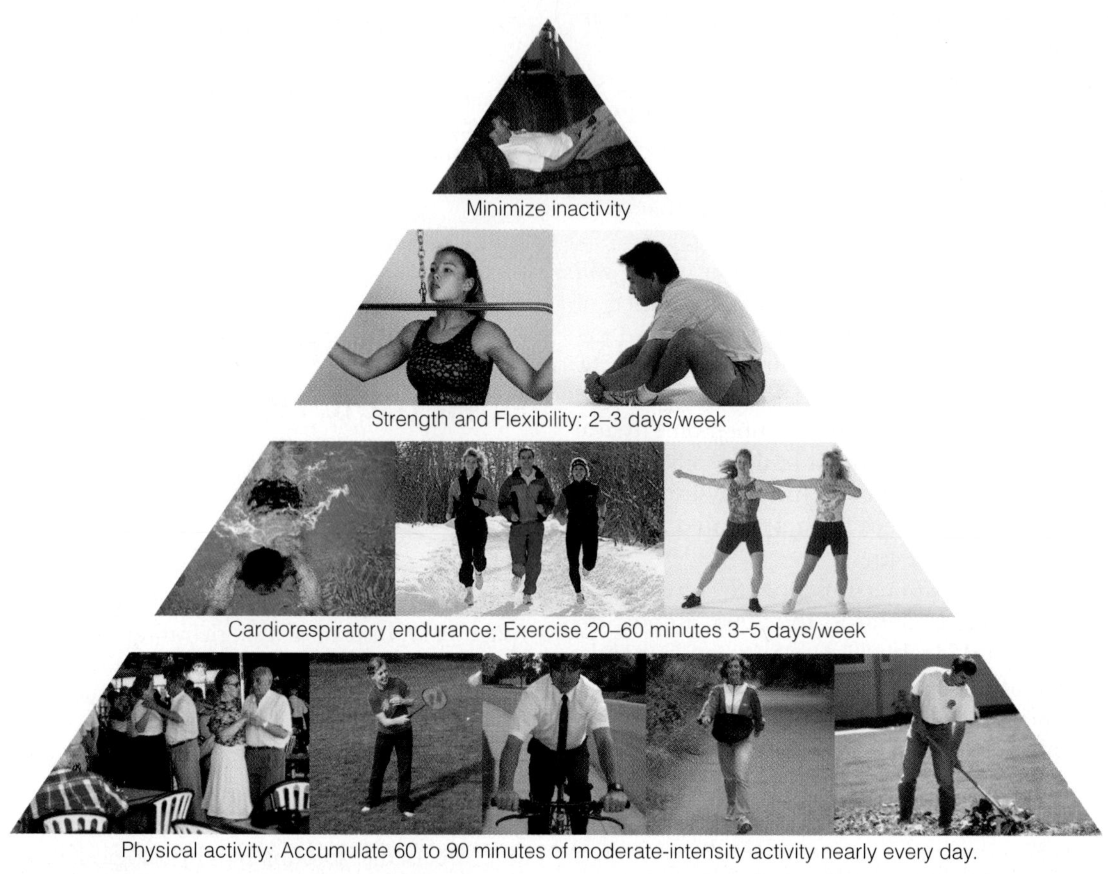

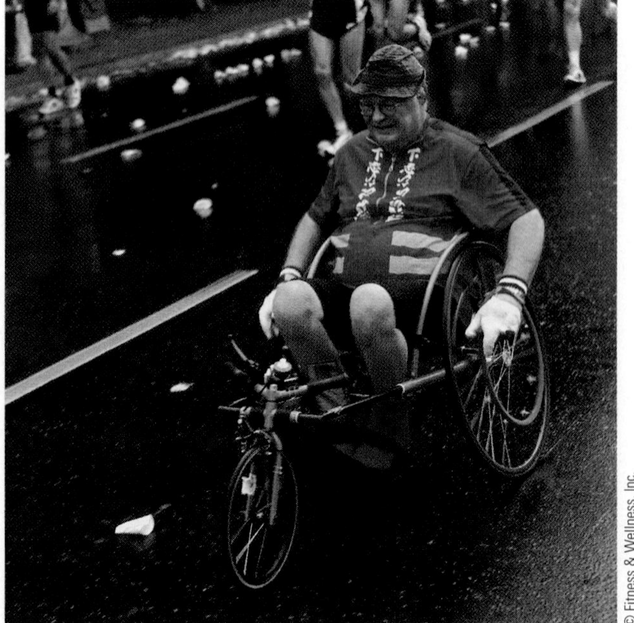

Physically challenged people can participate and derive health and fitness benefits through a high-intensity exercise program.

Physicians who work with cardiac patients frequently use METs as an alternative method of prescribing exercise intensity. One **MET** (short for metabolic equivalent) represents the rate of energy expenditure at rest, that is, 3.5 ml/kg/min. METs are used to measure the intensity of physical activity and exercise in multiples of the resting metabolic rate. At an intensity level of 10 METs, the activity requires a tenfold increase in the resting energy requirement (or approximately 35 ml/kg/min). MET levels for a given activity vary according to the effort expended. The MET range for various activities is included in Table 6.10. The harder a person exercises, the higher the MET level.

The effectiveness of various aerobic activities in weight management also is provided in Table 6.10. As a general rule, the greater the muscle mass involved in exercise, the better the results. Rhythmic and continuous activities that involve large amounts of muscle mass are most effective in burning calories.

Higher-intensity activities increase caloric expenditure as well. Exercising longer, however, compensates for lower intensities. If carried out long enough (45 to 60 minutes five or six times per week), even walking is a good exercise mode for weight management. Addi-

TABLE 6.10 Ratings for Selected Aerobic Activities

Activity	Recommended Starting Fitness Level[1]	Injury Risk[2]	Potential Cardiorespiratory Endurance Development (VO_{2max})[3,5]	Upper Body Strength Development[3]	Lower Body Strength Development[3]	Upper Body Flexibility Development[3]	Lower Body Flexibility Development[3]	Weight Control[3]	MET Level[4,5,6]	Caloric Expenditure (cal/hour)[5,6]
Aerobics										
High-Impact Aerobics	A	H	3–4	2	4	3	2	4	6–12	450–900
Moderate-Impact Aerobics	I	M	2–4	2	3	3	2	3	6–12	450–900
Low-Impact Aerobics	B	L	2–4	2	3	3	2	3	5–10	375–750
Step Aerobics	I	M	2–4	2	3–4	3	2	3–4	5–12	375–900
Cross-Country Skiing	B	M	4–5	4	4	2	2	4–5	10–16	750–1,200
Cross-Training	I	M	3–5	2–3	3–4	2–3	1–2	3–5	6–15	450–1,125
Cycling										
Road	I	M	2–5	1	4	1	1	3	6–12	450–900
Stationary	B	L	2–4	1	4	1	1	3	6–10	450–750
Hiking	B	L	2–4	1	3	1	1	3	6–10	450–750
In-Line Skating	I	M	1–4	2	4	2	2	3	6–10	450–750
Jogging	I	M	3–5	1	3	1	1	5	6–15	450–1,125
Jogging, Deep Water	A	L	3–5	2	2	1	1	5	8–15	600–1,125
Racquet Sports	I	M	2–4	3	3	3	2	3	6–10	450–750
Rope Skipping	I	H	3–5	2	4	1	2	3–5	8–15	600–1,125
Rowing	B	L	3–5	4	2	3	1	4	8–14	600–1,050
Spinning	I	L	4–5	1	4	1	1	4	8–15	600–1,125
Stair Climbing	B	L	3–5	1	4	1	1	4–5	8–15	600–1,125
Swimming (front crawl)	B	L	3–5	4	2	3	1	3	6–12	450–900
Walking	B	L	1–2	1	2	1	1	3	4–6	300–450
Walking, Water, Chest-Deep	I	L	2–4	2	3	1	1	3	6–10	450–750
Water Aerobics	B	L	2–4	3	3	3	2	3	6–12	450–900

[1] B = Beginner, I = Intermediate, A = Advanced
[2] L = Low, M = Moderate, H = High
[3] l = Low, 2 = Fair, 3 = Average, 4 = Good, 5 = Excellent
[4] One MET represents the rate of energy expenditure at rest (3.5 ml/kg/min). Each additional MET is a multiple of the resting value. For example, 5 METs represents an energy expenditure equivalent to five times the resting value, or about 17.5 ml/kg/min.
[5] Varies according to the person's effort (intensity) during exercise.
[6] Varies according to body weight.

tional information on a comprehensive weight management program is given in Chapter 5.

Critical Thinking

Mary started an exercise program last year as a means to lose weight and enhance her body image. She now runs more than 6 miles every day, works out regularly on stair-climbers and elliptical machines, strength-trains daily, participates in step-aerobics three times per week, and plays tennis or racquetball twice a week. Evaluate her program and make suggestions for improvements.

Getting Started and Adhering to a Lifetime Exercise Program

Following the guidelines provided in Lab 6D, you may proceed to initiate your own cardiorespiratory endurance program. If you have not been exercising regularly, you might begin by attempting to train five or six times a week for 30 minutes at a time. You might find

MET Short for metabolic equivalent, the rate of energy expenditure at rest; 1 MET is the equivalent of a VO_2 of 3.5 ml/kg/min.

Behavior Modification Planning

TIPS TO ENHANCE EXERCISE COMPLIANCE

1. Set aside a regular time for exercise. If you don't plan ahead, it is a lot easier to skip. On a weekly basis, using red ink, schedule your exercise time into your day planner. Next, hold your exercise hour "sacred." Give exercise priority equal to the most important school or business activity of the day.

   If you are too busy, attempt to accumulate 30 to 60 minutes of daily activity by doing separate 10-minute sessions throughout the day. Try reading the mail while you walk, taking stairs instead of elevators, walking the dog, or riding the stationary bike as you watch the evening news.
2. Exercise early in the day, when you will be less tired and the chances of something interfering with your workout are minimal; thus, you will be less likely to skip your exercise session.
3. Select aerobic activities you enjoy. Exercise should be as much fun as your favorite hobby. If you pick an activity you don't enjoy, you will be unmotivated and less likely to keep exercising. Don't be afraid to try out a new activity, even if that means learning new skills.
4. Combine different activities. You can train by doing two or three different activities the same week. This cross-training may reduce the monotony of repeating the same activity every day. Try lifetime sports. Many endurance sports, such as racquetball, basketball, soccer, badminton, roller skating, cross-country skiing, and body surfing (paddling the board), provide a nice break from regular workouts.
5. Use the proper clothing and equipment for exercise. A poor pair of shoes, for example, can make you more prone to injury, discouraging you from the beginning.
6. Find a friend or group of friends to exercise with. Social interaction will make exercise more fulfilling. Besides, exercise is harder to skip if someone is waiting to go with you.
7. Set goals and share them with others. Quitting is tougher when someone else knows what you are trying to accomplish. When you reach a targeted goal, reward yourself with a new pair of shoes or a jogging suit.
8. Purchase a pedometer (step counter) and build up to 10,000 steps per day. These 10,000 steps may include all forms of daily physical activity combined. Pedometers motivate people toward activity because they track daily activity, provide feedback on activity level, and remind the participant to enhance daily activity.
9. Don't become a chronic exerciser. Overexercising can lead to chronic fatigue and injuries. Exercise should be enjoyable, and in the process you should stop and smell the roses.
10. Exercise in different places and facilities. This will add variety to your workouts.
11. Exercise to music. People who listen to fast-tempo music tend to exercise more vigorously and longer. Using headphones when exercising outdoors, however, can be dangerous. Even indoors, it is preferable not to use headphones so you still can be aware of your surroundings.
12. Keep a regular record of your activities. Keeping a record allows you to monitor your progress and compare it against previous months and years (see Figure 6.10, page 196).
13. Conduct periodic assessments. Improving to a higher fitness category is often a reward in itself, and creating your own rewards is even more motivating.
14. Listen to your body. If you experience pain or unusual discomfort, stop exercising. Pain and aches are an indication of potential injury. If you do suffer an injury, don't return to your regular workouts until you are fully recovered. You may cross-train using activities that don't aggravate your injury (for instance, swimming instead of jogging).
15. If a health problem arises, see a physician. When in doubt, it's better to be safe than sorry.

Try It

The most difficult challenge about exercise is to keep going once you start. The above behavioral change tips will enhance your chances for exercise adherence. In your Online Journal or class notebook, describe which suggestions were most useful in helping you stick to your exercise program and why they are so effective for you.

this discouraging, however, and drop out before getting too far, because you will probably develop some muscle soreness and stiffness and possibly incur minor injuries. Muscle soreness and stiffness and the risk for injuries can be lessened or eliminated by increasing the intensity, duration, and frequency of exercise progressively, as outlined in Lab 6D.

Once you have determined your exercise prescription, the difficult part begins: starting and sticking to a lifetime exercise program. Although you may be motivated after reading the benefits to be gained from physical activity, lifelong dedication and perseverance are necessary to reap and maintain good fitness.

The first few weeks probably will be the most difficult for you, but where there's a will, there's a way. Once you begin to see positive changes, it won't be as hard. Soon you will develop a habit of exercising that will be deeply satisfying and will bring about a sense of self-accomplishment. The suggestions provided in the accompanying Behavior Modification Planning box have been used successfully to help change behavior and adhere to a lifetime exercise program.

A Lifetime Commitment to Fitness

The benefits of fitness can be maintained only through a regular lifetime program. Exercise is not like putting money in the bank. It doesn't help much to exercise 4 or 5 hours on Saturday and not do anything else the rest of the week. If anything, exercising only once a week is not safe for unconditioned adults.

The time involved in losing the benefits of exercise varies among the different components of physical fitness and also depends on the person's condition before the interruption. In regard to cardiorespiratory endurance, it has been estimated that 4 weeks of aerobic training are completely reversed in 2 consecutive weeks of physical inactivity. But if you have been exercising regularly for months or years, 2 weeks of inactivity won't hurt you as much as it will someone who has exercised only a few weeks. As a rule, after 48 to 72 hours of aerobic inactivity, the cardiorespiratory system starts to lose some of its capacity.

To maintain fitness, you should keep up a regular exercise program, even during vacations. If you have to interrupt your program for reasons beyond your control, you should not attempt to resume training at the same level you left off but, rather, build up gradually again.

Even the greatest athletes on earth, if they were to stop exercising, would be, after just a few years, at about the same risk for disease as someone who never has done any physical activity. Staying with a physical fitness program long enough brings about positive physiological and psychological changes. Once you are there, you will not want to have it any other way.

Assess Your Behavior

Thomson NOW! *Log on to www.thomsonedu.com/login to update your exercise log to include all your physical activity (climbing stairs, walking around campus, etc.) Be sure to update your pedometer log as well.*

1. Do you consciously attempt to incorporate as much physical activity as possible in your activities of daily living (by walking, taking stairs, cycling, participating in sports and recreational activities)?
2. Are you accumulating at least 30 minutes of moderate-intensity physical activity on most days of the week?
3. Is aerobic exercise in the appropriate target zone a priority in your life a minimum of three times per week for at least 20 minutes per exercise session?
4. Do you own a pedometer and do you accumulate 10,000 or more steps on most days of the week?
5. Have you evaluated your aerobic fitness and do you meet at least the health-fitness category?

Assess Your Knowledge

Thomson NOW! *Log on to www.thomsonedu.com/login to assess your understanding of this chapter's topics by taking the Student Practice Test and exploring the modules recommended in your Personalized Study Plan.*

1. Cardiorespiratory endurance is determined by
   a. the amount of oxygen the body is able to utilize per minute of physical activity.
   b. the length of time it takes the heart rate to return to 120 bpm following the 1.5-mile run test.
   c. the difference between the maximal heart rate and the resting heart rate.
   d. the product of the heart rate and blood pressure at rest versus exercise.
   e. the time it takes a person to reach a heart rate between 120 and 170 bpm during the Astrand–Ryhming test.
2. Which of the following is *not* a benefit of aerobic training?
   a. a higher VO_{2max}
   b. an increase in red blood cell count
   c. a decrease in resting heart rate
   d. an increase in heart rate at a given workload
   e. an increase in functional capillaries
3. The oxygen uptake for a person with an exercise heart rate of 130, a stroke volume of 100, and an $a\text{-}\bar{v}O_2diff$ of 10 is
   a. 130,000 ml/kg/min.
   b. 1,300 l/min.
   c. 1.3 l/min.
   d. 130 ml/kg/min.
   e. 13 ml/kg/min.

4. The oxygen uptake in ml/kg/min for a person with a VO_2 of 2.0 l/min who weighs 60 kilograms is
   a. 120.
   b. 26.5.
   c. 33.3.
   d. 30.
   e. 120,000.
5. The step test estimates VO_{2max} according to
   a. how long a person is able to sustain the proper step test cadence.
   b. the lowest heart rate achieved during the test.
   c. the recovery heart rate following the test.
   d. the difference between the maximal heart rate achieved and the resting heart rate.
   e. the exercise heart rate and the total stepping time.
6. An "excellent" cardiorespiratory fitness rating, in ml/kg/min, for young male adults is about
   a. 10.
   b. 20.
   c. 30.
   d. 40.
   e. 50.
7. How many minutes would a person training at 2 l/min have to exercise to burn the equivalent of one pound of fat?
   a. 700
   b. 350
   c. 120
   d. 60
   e. 20
8. The high-intensity cardiorespiratory training zone for a 22-year-old individual with a resting heart rate of 68 bpm is
   a. 120 to 148.
   b. 132 to 156.
   c. 138 to 164.
   d. 146 to 179.
   e. 154 to 188.
9. Which of the following activities does *not* contribute to the development of cardiorespiratory endurance?
   a. low-impact aerobics
   b. jogging
   c. 400-yard dash
   d. racquetball
   e. All of these activities contribute to its development.
10. The recommended duration for each cardiorespiratory training session is
   a. 10 to 20 minutes.
   b. 15 to 30 minutes.
   c. 20 to 60 minutes.
   d. 45 to 70 minutes.
   e. 60 to 120 minutes.

Correct answers can be found at the back of the book.

Media Menu

ThomsonNOW! *Connections*

- Assess your cardiorespiratory fitness level.
- Maintain a log of all your fitness activities.
- Check how well you understand the chapter's concepts.

Internet Connections

FitFacts

This site features information about a variety of cardiovascular forms of exercise, including walking, running, jumping rope, swimming, spinning, cross-training, interval training, and others.
http://www.acefitness.org/default.aspx

Fitness Fundamentals: Guidelines for Personal Exercise Programs

This site, developed by the President's Council on Physical Fitness and Sports, features information about starting an exercise program, including tips on how to select the right kinds of exercise to improve cardiovascular health, flexibility, and muscle strength and endurance.
http://www.hoptechno.com/book11.htm

Exercise Physiology: The Methods and Mechanisms Underlying Performance

This site features information on the principles of training, gender differences in performance and training, cardiovascular benefits, and much more.
http://home.hia.no/~stephens/exphys.htm

Check Your Physical Activity and Heart IQ

This site, sponsored by the National Heart, Lung, and Blood Institute, provides a true/false quiz to assess what you know about how physical activity affects your heart. The answers provided will uncover exercise myths and give you information on ways to improve your heart health.
http://www.nhlbi.nih.gov/health/public/heart/obesity/pa_iq_ab.htm

Notes

1. H. Atkinson, "Exercise for Longer Life: The Physician's Perspective," *HealthNews* 7, no. 3 (1997): 3.
2. R. B. O'Hara et al., "Increased Volume Resistance Training: Effects upon Predicted Aerobic Fitness in a Select Group of Air Force Men," *ACSM's Health and Fitness Journal* 8, no. 4 (2004): 16–25.
3. American College of Sports Medicine, *ACSM's Guidelines for Exercise Testing and Prescription* (Philadelphia: Lippincott Williams & Wilkins, 2006).
4. U.S. Department of Health and Human Services, Centers for Disease Control and Prevention, National Center for Health Statistics, *Physical Activity Among Adults: United States, 2000,* no. 15 (May 14, 2003).
5. American College of Sports Medicine, "Position Stand: The Recommended Quantity and Quality of Exercise for Developing and Maintaining Cardiorespiratory and Muscular Fitness, and Flexibility in Healthy Adults," *Medicine and Science in Sports and Exercise* 30 (1998): 975–991.
6. See note 3, ACSM.
7. See note 3, ACSM.
8. R. F. DeBusk, U. Stenestrand, M. Sheehan, and W. L. Haskell, "Training Effects of Long Versus Short Bouts of Exercise in Healthy Subjects," *American Journal of Cardiology* 65 (1990): 1010–1013.
9. National Academy of Sciences, Institute of Medicine, *Dietary Reference Intakes for Energy, Carbohydrates, Fiber, Fat, Protein and Amino Acids (Macronutrients)* (Washington, DC: National Academy Press, 2002).
10. U.S. Department of Health and Human Services, Department of Agriculture, *Dietary Guidelines for Americans 2005* (Washington, DC: DHHS, 2005).
11. "Summary Statement: Workshop on Physical Activity and Public Health," *Sports Medicine Bulletin* 28 (1993): 7.
12. U.S. Department of Health and Human Services, *Physical Activity and Health: A Report of the Surgeon General* (Atlanta: Centers for Disease Control and Prevention, National Center for Chronic Disease Prevention and Health Promotion, 1996).
13. "Scanning Sports," *Physician and Sportsmedicine* 21, no. 11 (1993): 34.
14. See note 3, ACSM.

Suggested Readings

ACSM's Guidelines for Exercise Testing and Prescription (Philadelphia: Lippincott Williams & Wilkins, 2006).

ACSM's Resource Manual for Guidelines for Exercise Testing and Prescription (Philadelphia: Lippincott Williams & Wilkins, 2006).

Akalan, C., L. Kravitz, and R. Robergs. "VO_{2max}: Essentials of the Most Widely Used Test in Exercise Physiology." *ACSM's Health & Fitness Journal* 8, no. 3 (2004): 5–9.

Borg, G. "Perceived Exertion: A Note on History and Methods." *Medicine and Science in Sports and Exercise 5* (1993): 90–93.

Hoeger, W. W. K., and S. A. Hoeger. *Lifetime Fitness & Wellness: A Personalized Program* (Belmont, CA: Wadsworth/Thomson Learning, 2007).

Karvonen, M. J., E. Kentala, and O. Mustala. "The Effects of Training on the Heart Rate, a Longitudinal Study." *Annales Medicinae Experimetalis et Biologiae Fenniae* 35 (1957): 307–315.

McArdle, W. D., F. I. Katch, and V. L. Katch. *Exercise Physiology: Energy, Nutrition, and Human Performance* (Philadelphia: Lippincott Williams & Wilkins, 2004).

Nieman, D. C. *Exercise Testing and Prescription: A Health-Related Approach* (Boston: McGraw-Hill, 2003).

Wilmore, J. H., and D. L. Costill. *Physiology of Sport and Exercise* (Champaign, IL: Human Kinetics, 2004).

FIGURE 6.10 Cardiorespiratory exercise record form.

Name: ______________________ Date: __________ Course: __________ Section: __________ Gender: ______ Age: ______

Month

Date	Body Weight	Exercise Heart Rate	Type of Activity	Distance In Miles	Time Minutes	RPE*	Daily Steps
1							
2							
3							
4							
5							
6							
7							
8							
9							
10							
11							
12							
13							
14							
15							
16							
17							
18							
19							
20							
21							
22							
23							
24							
25							
26							
27							
28							
29							
30							
31							
			Total				

*Rate of perceived exertion.

Month

Date	Body Weight	Exercise Heart Rate	Type of Activity	Distance In Miles	Time Minutes	RPE*	Daily Steps
1							
2							
3							
4							
5							
6							
7							
8							
9							
10							
11							
12							
13							
14							
15							
16							
17							
18							
19							
20							
21							
22							
23							
24							
25							
26							
27							
28							
29							
30							
31							
			Total				

*Rate of perceived exertion.

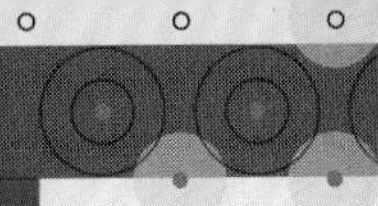

Lab 6B Caloric Expenditure and Exercise Heart Rate

Name:		**Date:**		**Grade:**	
Instructor:		**Course:**		**Section:**	

Necessary Lab Equipment

A school track (or premeasured course) and a stopwatch. Each student also should bring a watch with a second hand.

Objective

To monitor exercise heart rate and determine the caloric cost of physical activity based on exercise heart rate.

Lab Preparation

Wear exercise clothing, including jogging shoes. Do not engage in vigorous physical activity prior to this lab. Read the information on predicting oxygen uptake and caloric expenditure in this chapter, pages 182–183.

Procedure

1. **Cardiorespiratory Training Zone.** Look up your cardiovascular training zone at 60 percent and 85 percent of heart rate reserve in Lab 6D. Record this information in beats per minute (bpm) and in 10-second pulse counts in the blank spaces provided below.

		Beats/minute	**10-sec count**
60% intensity	=		
85% intensity	=		

2. **Resting Heart Rate (HR) and Body Weight (BW).** Determine your resting HR prior to exercise and your body weight in kilograms (divide pounds by 2.2046).

Resting HR: ______ bpm

BW: ______ lbs ÷ 2.2046 = ______ kg

3. **Walking HR, Oxygen Uptake (VO_2), and Caloric Expenditure.** Walk two laps around a 400-meter (440-yard) track at an average speed of 75 to 100 meters per minute. Try to maintain a constant speed around the track. You can monitor your speed by starting the walk at the beginning of the 100-meter straightway and making sure you have walked at least 75 meters and no more than 100 meters in one minute. As soon as you complete the two laps (800 meters), notice the time required to walk this distance and immediately check your exercise HR by taking a 10-second pulse count. Record this information in the spaces provided below. Do not record the time until after you have checked your pulse. Exercise HR will remain at the same rate for about 15 seconds following cessation of exercise. Therefore, you need to check your pulse as soon as you finish the walk, after noticing the 800-meter walk time.

10-sec. pulse count: ______ beats (from question 1 above)

800-meter time: ______ min ______ sec

HR in bpm = 10-sec pulse count × 6

HR in bpm = ______ × 6 = ______ bpm

800-meter time in minutes = min + (sec ÷ 60)

800-meter time in minutes = ______ + (______ ÷ 60) = ______ min

Speed in meters per minute (mts/min) = 800 ÷ 800-meter time in min

Speed in mts/min = 800 ÷ ______ = ______ mts/min

VO_2 in ml/kg/min at this walking speed (Use Table 6.9, page 183) = ______ ml/kg/min

VO_2 in l/min = VO_2 in ml/kg/min × BW in kg ÷ 1,000

VO_2 in l/min = ______ × ______ ÷ 1,000 = ______ l/min

Caloric expenditure for 800-meter walk = VO_2 in l/min × 5 × 800-meter time in min

Caloric expenditure for 800-meter walk = ______ × 5 × ______ = ______ calories

4. **Slow-Jogging HR, VO_2, and Caloric Expenditure.** Slowly jog 800 meters (two laps) around the track. Try to maintain the same slow-jogging pace throughout the two laps. Do NOT jog fast or sprint. This is not a speed test and is intended to be a slow jog only. As soon as you complete the 800 meters, notice the time required to complete the distance and check your exercise HR immediately by taking another 10-second pulse count. Record this information below.

10-sec pulse count: ______ beats

800-meter time: ______ min ______ sec.

HR in bpm = 10-sec pulse count × 6

HR in bpm = ______ × 6 = ______ bpm

800-meter time in minutes = min + (sec ÷ 60)

800-meter time in minutes = ______ + (______ ÷ 60) = ______ min

Speed in mts/min = 800 ÷ 800-meter time in min

Speed in mts/min = 800 ÷ ______ = ______ mts/min.

VO_2 in ml/kg/min at this slow-jogging speed (Use Table 6.9, page 183) = ______ ml/kg/min

VO_2 in l/min = VO_2 in ml/kg/min × BW in kg ÷ 1,000

VO_2 in l/min = ______ × ______ ÷ 1,000 = ______ l/min

Caloric expenditure for 800-meter slow jog = VO_2 in l/min × 5 × 800-meter time in min

Caloric expenditure for 800-meter slow jog = ______ × 5 × ______ = ______ calories

5. **Fast-Jogging HR, VO_2, Caloric Expenditure, and Recovery HR.** Jog another 800 meters at a faster speed around the track. Again try to maintain the same jogging pace throughout the two laps. Do NOT sprint. Your HR should not exceed 180 bpm on this test. As soon as you complete the 800 meters, notice your time for the two laps and check your 10-second pulse count. Record this information below. You also should check your 2- and 5-minute recovery HRs after the run and record these rates below.

10-sec pulse count: ______ beats

800-meter time: ______ min ______ sec

HR in bpm = 10-sec pulse count × 6

HR in bpm = ______ × 6 = ______ bpm

800-meter time in minutes = min + (sec ÷ 60)

800-meter time in minutes = ______ + (______ ÷ 60) = ______ min

Speed in mts/min = 800 ÷ 800-meter time in min

Speed in mts/min = 800 ÷ ______ = ______ mts/min

VO_2 in ml/kg/min at this fast-jogging speed (Use Table 6.9, page 183) = ______ ml/kg/min

VO_2 in l/min = VO_2 in ml/kg/min × BW in kg ÷ 1,000

VO_2 in l/min = ______ × ______ ÷ 1,000 = ______ l/min

Caloric expenditure for 800-meter fast jog = VO_2 in l/min × 5 × 800-meter time in min

Caloric expenditure for 800-meter fast jog = ______ × 5 × ______ = ______ calories

Recovery HRs

	10-sec count	bpm
2 minutes		
5 minutes*		

6. **Resting, Exercise, and Recovery HRs.** Plot your resting, exercise, and recovery HRs on the graph provided below.

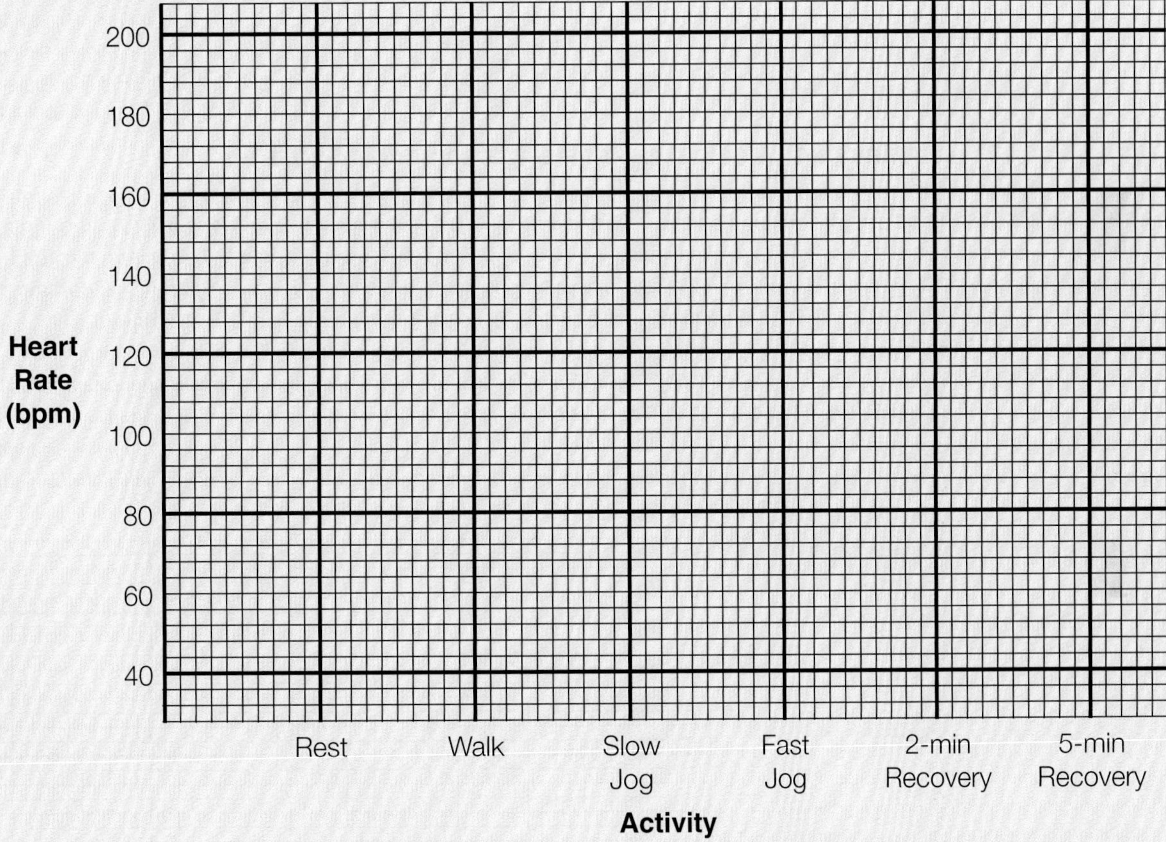

7. **Training Exercise HR and Equivalent Caloric Expenditure.** This part of the lab should be completed outside your regular lab time, during the next 2 or 3 days prior to turning in the assignment. According to the previous exercise HRs (items 3, 4, and 5), try to select a walking or jogging speed that will allow you to maintain your exercise HR in the appropriate cardiorespiratory training zone. Using a 400-meter track, walk or jog for 20 minutes at the selected speed and again try to maintain a constant speed throughout the exercise time. At the end of the 20 minutes, check your 10-second pulse count and estimate the distance covered in meters. Record this information below and estimate the VO_2 and caloric expenditure.

10-sec pulse count: ______ beats

HR in bpm = 10-sec pulse count × 6

HR in bpm = ______ × 6 = ______ bpm

Approximate distance covered in 20 minutes: ______ meters

* Your 5-minute recovery HR should be below 120 bpm. If it is above 120, you most likely have overexerted yourself and, therefore, need to decrease the intensity of exercise (and/or duration when exercising for long periods of time). If your 5-minute recovery HR is still above 120 after decreasing the intensity of exercise, you should consult a physician regarding this condition.

Speed in mts/min = distance in meters ÷ 20 minutes

Speed in mts/min = ______ ÷ 20 = ______ mts/min

VO_2 at this speed (see Table 6.9, page 183) = ______ ml/kg/min

VO_2 in l/min = VO_2 in ml/kg/min × BW in kg ÷ 1,000

VO_2 in l/min = ______ × ______ ÷ 1,000 = ______ l/min

Caloric expenditure for 20-min walk/jog = VO_2 in l/min × 5 × 20 min

Caloric expenditure for 20-min walk/jog = ______ × 5 × 20 = ______ calories

Using the previous information, how many calories would you have burned if you had maintained this pace for:

10 minutes (VO_2 in l/min × 5 × 10) = ______ × 5 × 10 = ______ calories

30 minutes (VO_2 in l/min × 5 × 30) = ______ × 5 × 30 = ______ calories

60 minutes (VO_2 in l/min × 5 × 60) = ______ × 5 × 60 = ______ calories

PREDICTING CALORIC EXPENDITURE ACCORDING TO EXERCISE HR

Research indicates that there is a linear relationship between HR and VO_2, as long as the HR ranges from about 110 to 180 bpm. If you obtain two exercise HRs in this range and the equivalent oxygen uptakes (in l/min), you can easily predict your VO_2 and caloric expenditure for any given HR in the specified range. Plot your two exercise HRs and the corresponding VO_2 values on the graph provided below. Next, draw a line between these two points on the graph and extend the line to 110 and 180 bpm. You now may look up the VO_2 for any HR by finding the desired HR on the Y axis, then going across to the reference line and straight down to the X axis, where you will find the corresponding VO_2 in l/min. To obtain the caloric expenditure in calories per minute, simply multiply the VO_2 by 5. You also may predict your maximal VO_2 (in l/min) by extending the line up to your estimated maximal HR. The maximal HR is estimated by subtracting your age from 220. To convert the maximal VO_2 to ml/kg/min, multiply the l/min value by 1,000 and divide by body weight in kilograms.

Using the results from your lab and the graph below, indicate the VO_2 in l/min and the caloric expenditure at the following HRs:

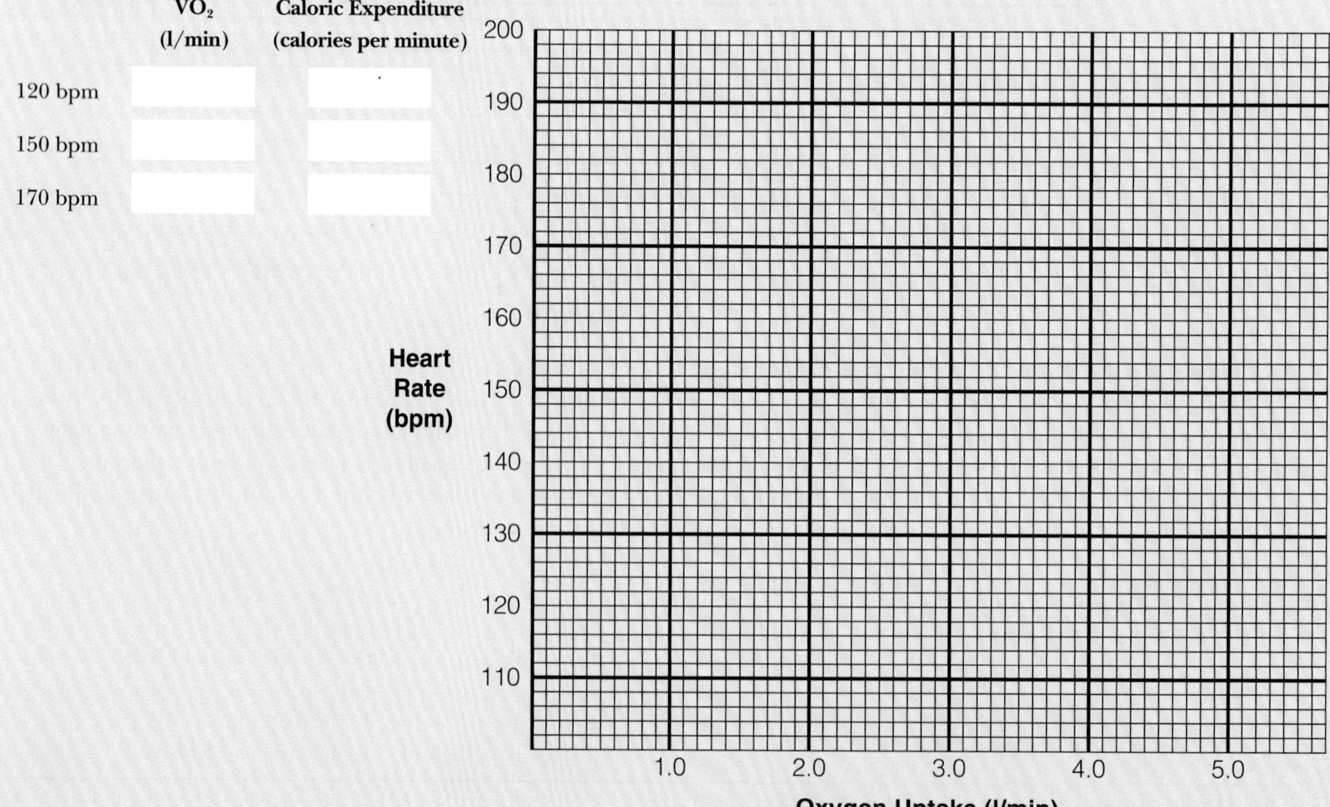

Lab 6C Exercise Readiness Questionnaire

Name: Sarah L. Kemball | Date: | Grade:

Instructor: Nola Sapienza | Course: | Section:

Necessary Lab Equipment
None required.

Objective
To determine your preparedness to start an exercise program.

Instructions
Read each statement carefully and circle the number that best describes your feelings in each statement. Please be completely honest with your answers. Interpret the results of this questionnaire using the guidelines provided on the next page.

I.	Strongly Agree	Mildly Agree	Mildly Disagree	Strongly Disagree
1. I can walk, ride a bike (or a wheelchair), swim, or walk in a shallow pool.	4 (circled)	3	2	1
2. I enjoy exercise.	4	3 (circled)	2	1
3. I believe exercise can help decrease the risk for disease and premature mortality.	4 (circled)	3	2	1
4. I believe exercise contributes to better health.	4 (circled)	3	2	1
5. I have previously participated in an exercise program.	4 (circled)	3	2	1
6. I have experienced the feeling of being physically fit.	4 (circled)	3	2	1
7. I can envision myself exercising.	4	3 (circled)	2	1
8. I am contemplating an exercise program.	4	3 (circled)	2	1
9. I am willing to stop contemplating and give exercise a try for a few weeks.	4	3 (circled)	2	1
10. I am willing to set aside time at least three times a week for exercise.	4	3 (circled)	2	1
11. I can find a place to exercise (the streets, a park, a YMCA, a health club).	4	3 (circled)	2	1
12. I can find other people who would like to exercise with me.	4	3 (circled)	2	1
13. I will exercise when I am moody, fatigued, and even when the weather is bad.	4	3	2 (circled)	1
14. I am willing to spend a small amount of money for adequate exercise clothing (shoes, shorts, leotards, swimsuit).	4	3 (circled)	2	1
15. If I have any doubts about my present state of health, I will see a physician before beginning an exercise program.	4	3 (circled)	2	1
16. Exercise will make me feel better and improve my quality of life.	4 (circled)	3	2	1

Scoring Your Test:

This questionnaire allows you to examine your readiness for exercise. You have been evaluated in four categories: mastery (self-control), attitude, health, and commitment. Mastery indicates that you can be in control of your exercise program. Attitude examines your mental disposition toward exercise. Health provides evidence of the wellness benefits of exercise. Commitment shows dedication and resolution to carry out the exercise program. Write the number you circled after each statement in the corresponding spaces below. Add the scores on each line to get your totals. Scores can vary from 4 to 16. A score of 12 and above is a strong indicator that that factor is important to you, and 8 and below is low. If you score 12 or more points in each category, your chances of initiating and adhering to an exercise program are good. If you fail to score at least 12 points in three categories, your chances of succeeding at exercise may be slim. You need to be better informed about the benefits of exercise, and a retraining process may be required.

Mastery:	1.	4	+	5.	4	+	6.	4	+	9.	3	= 17
Attitude:	2.	3	+	7.	3	+	8.	3	+	13.	2	= 11
Health:	3.	4	+	4.	4	+	15.	3	+	16.	4	= 15
Commitment:	10.	3	+	11.	3	+	12.	3	+	14.	3	= 12

II. Stage of Change for Cardiorespiratory Endurance Exercise

Using Figure 2.5 (page 49) and Table 2.3 (page 49), identify your current stage of change in regard to participation in a cardiorespiratory endurance exercise program:

III. Advantages and Disadvantages for Adding Aerobic Exercise to Your Lifestyle

Advantages: ______________________________

Disadvantages: ______________________________

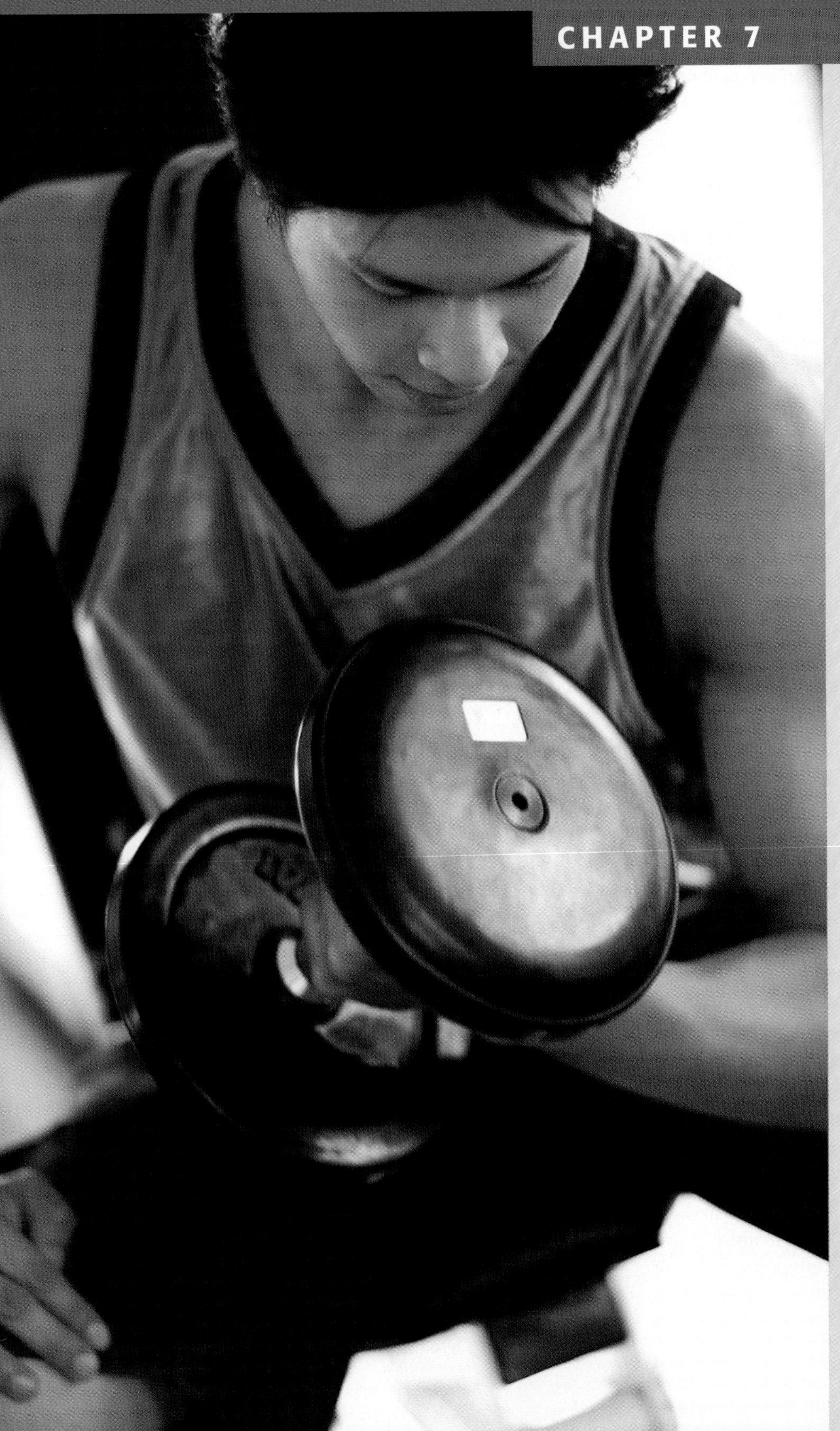

Muscular Strength and Endurance

CHAPTER 7

OBJECTIVES

- Explain the importance of adequate strength levels in maintaining good health and well-being.
- Clarify misconceptions about strength fitness.
- Define muscular strength and muscular endurance.
- Be able to assess muscular strength and endurance and learn to interpret test results according to health fitness and physical fitness standards.
- Identify the factors that affect strength.
- Understand the principles of overload and specificity of training for strength development.
- Become acquainted with two distinct strength-training programs—core strength training and Pilates.

ThomsonNOW! Go to www.thomsonedu.com/login to:

- Chart your achievements for strength tests.
- Check how well you understand the chapter's concepts.

Photo © Simon Marcus/Corbis

The need for strength is not confined to highly trained athletes, fitness enthusiasts, and individuals who have jobs that require heavy muscular work. In fact, a well-planned strength-training program leads to increased muscle strength and endurance, muscle tone, tendon and ligament strength, and bone density—all of which help to improve and maintain everyday functional physical capacity. The benefits of **strength training** or resistance training on health and well-being are well-documented.

Benefits of Strength Training

Strength is a basic health-related fitness component and is an important wellness component for optimal performance in daily activities such as sitting, walking, running, lifting and carrying objects, doing housework, and enjoying recreational activities. Strength also is of great value in improving posture, personal appearance, and self-image; in developing sports skills; in promoting stability of joints and in meeting certain emergencies in life.

From a health standpoint, increasing strength helps to increase or maintain muscle and a higher resting metabolic rate, encourages weight loss and maintenance, lessens the risk for injury, prevents osteoporosis, reduces chronic low-back pain, alleviates arthritic pain, aids in childbearing, improves cholesterol levels, promotes psychological well-being, and also may help to lower the risk of high blood pressure and diabetes.

Furthermore, with time, the heart rate and blood pressure response to lifting a heavy resistance (a weight) decreases. This adaptation reduces the demands on the cardiovascular system when performing activities such as carrying a child, the groceries, or a suitcase.

Regular strength training can also help control blood sugar. Much of the blood glucose from food consumption goes to the muscles, where it is stored as glycogen. When muscles are not used, muscle cells become insulin-resistant and glucose cannot enter the cells, thereby increasing the risk for diabetes. Following 16 weeks of strength training, a group of diabetic men and women improved their blood sugar control, gained strength, increased lean body mass, lost body fat, and lowered blood pressure.[1]

Muscular Strength and Aging

In the older adult population, muscular strength may be the most important health-related component of physical fitness. Though proper cardiorespiratory endurance is necessary to help maintain a healthy heart, good strength contributes more to independent living than any other fitness component. Older adults with good strength levels can successfully perform most **activities of daily living.**

A common occurrence as people age is **sarcopenia,** the loss of lean body mass, strength, and function. How much of this loss is related to the aging process itself or to actual physical inactivity and faulty nutrition is unknown. And whereas thinning of the bones from osteoporosis renders the bones prone to fractures, the gradual loss of muscle mass and ensuing frailty are what lead to falls and subsequent loss of function in older adults. Strength training helps to slow the age-related loss of muscle function. Protein deficiency, seen in some older adults, also contributes to loss of lean tissue.

More than anything else, older adults want to enjoy good health and to function independently. Many of them, however, are confined to nursing homes because they lack sufficient strength to move about. They cannot walk very far, and many have to be helped in and out of beds, chairs, and tubs.

A strength-training program can enhance quality of life tremendously, and nearly everyone can benefit from it. Only people with advanced heart disease are advised to refrain from strength training. Inactive adults between the ages of 56 and 86 who participated in a 12-week strength-training program increased their lean body mass by about 3 pounds, lost about 4 pounds of fat, and increased their resting metabolic rate by almost 7 percent.[2] In other research, leg strength improved by as much as 200 percent in previously inactive adults over age 90.[3] As strength improves, so does the ability to move about, the capacity for independent living, and enjoyment of life during the "golden years." More specifically, good strength enhances quality of life in that it

- improves balance and restores mobility,
- makes lifting and reaching easier,
- decreases the risk for injuries and falls, and
- stresses the bones and preserves bone mineral density, thereby decreasing the risk for osteoporosis.

Another benefit of maintaining a good strength level is its relationship to human **metabolism.** A primary outcome of a strength-training program is an increase in muscle mass or size (lean body mass), known as muscle **hypertrophy.**

Muscle tissue uses more energy than fatty tissue. That is, your body expends more calories to maintain muscle than to maintain fat. All other factors being equal, if two individuals both weigh 150 pounds but have different amounts of muscle mass, the one with more muscle mass will have a higher **resting metabolism** (also see "Exercise: The Key to Weight Management," pages 144–148). Even small increases in muscle mass have a long-term positive effect on metabolism.

Loss of lean tissue also is thought to be a primary reason for the decrease in metabolism as people grow older. Contrary to some beliefs, metabolism does not have to slow down significantly with aging. It is not so much that metabolism slows down. It's that we slow down. Lean body mass decreases with sedentary living, which, in turn, slows down the resting metabolic rate. Thus, if people continue eating at the same rate as they age, body fat increases.

Daily energy requirements decrease an average of 360 calories between age 26 and age 60.[4] Participating in a strength-training program can offset much of the decline and prevent and reduce excess body fat. One research study found an increase in resting metabolic rate of 35 calories per pound of muscle mass in older adults who participated in a strength-training program.[5]

Gender Differences

A common misconception about physical fitness concerns women in strength training. Because of the increase in muscle mass typically seen in men, some women think that a strength-training program will result in their developing large musculature.

Even though the quality of muscle in men and women is the same, endocrinological differences do not allow women to achieve the same amount of muscle hypertrophy (size) as men. Men also have more muscle fibers and, because of the sex-specific male hormones, each individual fiber has more potential for hypertrophy. On the average, following 6 months of training, women can achieve up to a 50 percent increase in strength but only a 10 percent increase in muscle size.

The idea that strength training allows women to develop muscle hypertrophy to the same extent as men do is as false as the notion that playing basketball will turn women into giants. Masculinity and femininity are established by genetic inheritance, not by the amount of physical activity. Variations in the extent of masculinity and femininity are determined by individual differences in hormonal secretions of androgen, testosterone, estrogen, and progesterone. Women with a bigger-than-average build often are inclined to participate in sports because of their natural physical advantage. As a result, many people have associated women's participation in sports and strength training with large muscle size.

As the number of females who participate in sports increased steadily during the last few years, the myth of strength training in women leading to large increases in muscle size abated somewhat. For example, per pound of body weight, female gymnasts are among the strongest athletes in the world. These athletes engage regularly in vigorous strength-training programs. Yet, female gymnasts have some of the most well-toned and graceful figures of all women.

In recent years, improved body appearance has become the rule rather than the exception for women who participate in strength-training programs. Some of the most attractive female movie stars also train with weights to further improve their personal image.

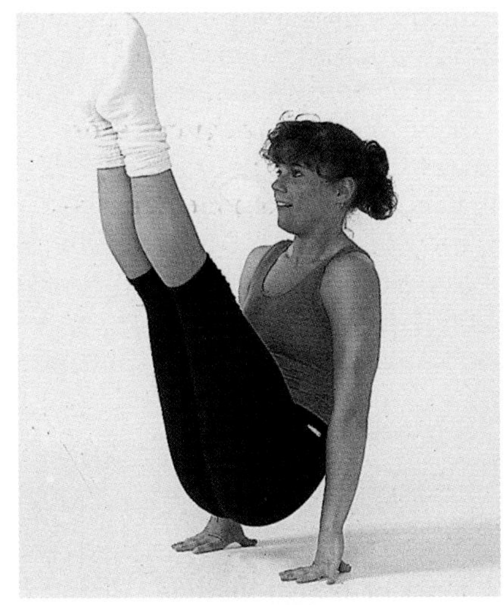

Female gymnast performs a strength skill.

Nonetheless, you may ask, "If weight training does not masculinize women, why do so many women body builders develop such heavy musculature?" In the sport of body building, the athletes follow intense training routines consisting of 2 or more hours of constant weight lifting with short rest intervals between sets. Many body-building training routines call for back-to-back exercises using the same muscle groups. The objective of this type of training is to pump extra blood into the muscles. This additional fluid makes the muscles appear much bigger than they do in a resting condition. Based on the intensity and the length of the training session, the muscles can remain filled with blood, appearing measurably larger for several hours after completing the training session. Performing such routines is a common practice before competitions. Therefore, in real life, these women are not as muscular as they seem when they are participating in a contest.

Strength training A program designed to improve muscular strength and/or endurance through a series of progressive resistance (weight) training exercises that overload the muscle system and cause physiological development.

Activities of daily living Everyday behaviors that people normally do to function in life (cross the street, carry groceries, lift objects, do laundry, sweep floors).

Sarcopenia Age-related loss of lean body mass, strength, and function.

Metabolism All energy and material transformations that occur within living cells; necessary to sustain life.

Hypertrophy An increase in the size of the cell, as in muscle hypertrophy.

Resting metabolism Amount of energy (expressed in milliliters of oxygen per minute or total calories per day) an individual requires during resting conditions to sustain proper body function.

FIGURE 7.1 Changes in body composition as a result of a combined aerobic and strength-training program.

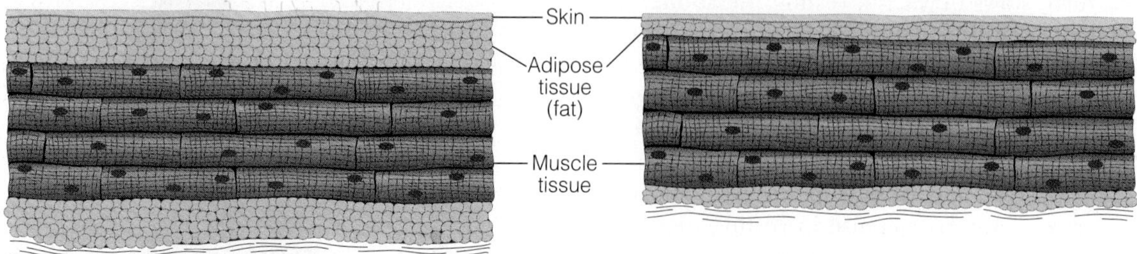

In the sport of body building (among others), a big point of controversy is the use of **anabolic steroids** and human growth hormones. These hormones produce detrimental and undesirable side effects in women (such as hypertension, fluid retention, decreased breast size, deepening of the voice, whiskers, and other atypical body hair growth), which some women deem tolerable. Anabolic steroid use in general—except for medical reasons and when carefully monitored by a physician—can lead to serious health consequences.

Critical Thinking

What role should strength training have in a fitness program? Should people be motivated for the health fitness benefits, or should they participate to enhance their body image? What are your feelings about individuals (male or female) with large body musculature?

Use of anabolic steroids by female body builders and female track-and-field athletes around the world is widespread. These athletes use anabolic steroids to remain competitive at the highest level. During the 2004 Olympic Games in Athens, Greece, two women shot putters, including the gold medal winner (later stripped of the medal), were expelled from the games for using steroids. Women who take steroids undoubtedly will build heavy musculature, and if they take them long enough, the steroids will produce masculinizing effects.

To prevent steroid use, the International Federation of Body Building instituted a mandatory steroid-testing program for women participating in the Miss Olympia contest. When drugs are not used to promote development, improved body image is the rule rather than the exception among women who participate in body building, strength training, and sports in general.

SELECTED DETRIMENTAL EFFECTS FROM USING ANABOLIC STEROIDS

- Liver tumors
- Hepatitis
- Hypertension
- Reduction of high-density lipoprotein (HDL) cholesterol
- Elevation of low-density lipoprotein (LDL) cholesterol
- Hyperinsulinism
- Impaired pituitary function
- Impaired thyroid function
- Mood swings
- Aggressive behavior
- Increased irritability
- Acne
- Fluid retention
- Decreased libido
- HIV infection (via injectable steroids)
- Prostate problems (men)
- Testicular atrophy (men)
- Reduced sperm count (men)
- Clitoral enlargement (women)
- Decreased breast size (women)
- Increased body and facial hair (nonreversible in women)
- Deepening of the voice (nonreversible in women)

Changes in Body Composition

A benefit of strength training, accentuated even more when combined with aerobic exercise, is a decrease in adipose or fatty tissue around muscle fibers themselves. This decrease is often greater than the amount of muscle hypertrophy (see Figure 7.1). Therefore, losing inches but not body weight is common.

Because muscle tissue is more dense than fatty tissue (and despite the fact that inches are lost during a combined strength-training and aerobic program), people, especially women, often become discouraged because they cannot see the results readily on the scale. They can offset this discouragement by determining body composition regularly to monitor their changes in percent body fat rather than simply measuring changes in total body weight (see Chapter 4).

Assessment of Muscular Strength and Endurance

Although muscular strength and endurance are interrelated, they do differ. **Muscular strength** is the ability to exert maximum force against resistance. **Muscular endurance** is the ability of a muscle to exert submaximal force repeatedly over time.

Muscular endurance (also referred to as "localized muscular endurance") depends to a large extent on muscular strength. Weak muscles cannot repeat an action several times or sustain it. Based upon these principles, strength tests and training programs have been designed to measure and develop absolute muscular strength, muscular endurance, or a combination of the two.

Muscular strength is usually determined by the maximal amount of resistance (weight)—**one repetition maximum,** or **1 RM**—an individual is able to lift in a single effort. Although this assessment yields a good measure of absolute strength, it does require considerable time, because the 1 RM is determined through trial and error. For example, strength of the chest muscles is frequently measured through the bench press exercise. If an individual has not trained with weights, he may try 100 pounds and lift this resistance easily. After adding 50 pounds, he fails to lift the resistance. Then he decreases resistance by 20 or 30 pounds. Finally, after several trials, the 1 RM is established.

Using this method, a true 1 RM might be difficult to obtain the first time an individual is tested, because fatigue becomes a factor. By the time the 1 RM is established, the person already has made several maximal or near-maximal attempts.

In contrast, muscular endurance typically is established by the number of repetitions an individual can perform against a submaximal resistance or by the length of time a given contraction can be sustained. For example: How many push-ups can an individual do? Or how many times can a 30-pound resistance be lifted? Or how long can a person hold a chin-up?

If time is a factor and only one test item can be done, the Hand Grip Strength Test, described in Figure 7.2, is commonly used to assess strength. This test, though, provides only a weak correlation with overall body strength. Two additional strength tests are provided in Figures 7.3 and 7.4. Lab 7A also offers you the opportunity to assess your own level of muscular strength or endurance with all three tests. You may take one or more of these tests according to your time and the facilities available.

In strength testing, several body sites should be assessed, because muscular strength and muscular endurance are both highly specific. A high degree of strength or endurance in one body part does not necessarily indicate similarity in other parts, so no single strength test provides a good assessment of overall body strength. Accordingly, exercises for the strength tests were selected to include the upper body, lower body, and abdominal regions.

Before taking the strength test, you should become familiar with the procedures for the respective tests. For safety reasons, always take at least one friend with you whenever you train with weights or undertake any type of strength assessment. Also, these are different tests, so to make valid comparisons, you should use the same

FIGURE 7.2 Procedure for the Hand Grip Strength Test.

1. Adjust the width of the dynamometer* so the middle bones of your fingers rest on the distant end of the dynamometer grip.
2. Use your dominant hand for this test. Place your elbow at a 90° angle and about 2 inches away from the body.
3. Now grip as hard as you can for a few seconds. Do not move any other body part as you perform the test (do not flex or extend the elbow, do not move the elbow away or toward the body, and do not lean forward or backward during the test).

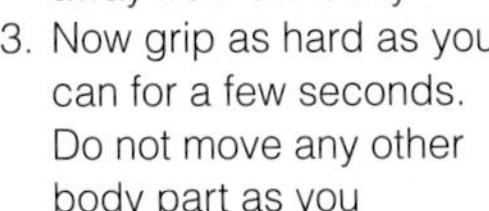

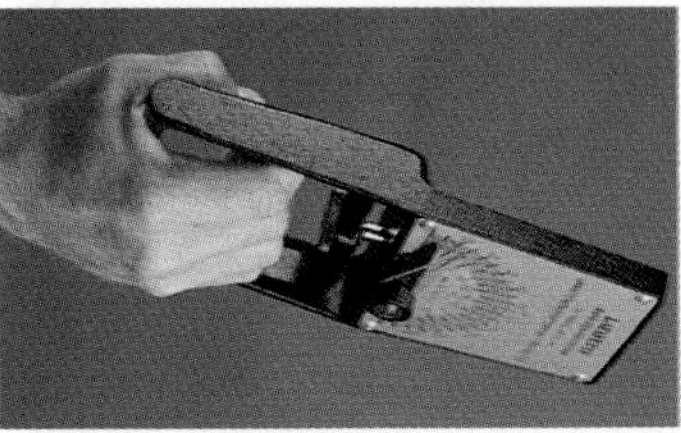

4. Record the dynamometer reading in pounds (if reading is in kilograms, multiply by 2.2046).
5. Three trials are allowed for this test. Use the highest reading for your final test score. Look up your percentile rank for this test in Table 7.1.
6. Based on your percentile rank, obtain the hand grip strength fitness category according to the following guidelines:

Percentile Rank	Fitness Category
≥90	Excellent
70–80	Good
50–60	Average
30–40	Fair
≤20	Poor

*A Lafayette 78010 dynamometer is recommended for this test (Lafayette Instruments Co., Sagamore and North 9th Street, Lafayette, IN 47903).

Anabolic steroids Synthetic versions of the male sex hormone testosterone, which promotes muscle development and hypertrophy.

Muscular strength The ability of a muscle to exert maximum force against resistance (for example, 1 repetition maximum [or 1 RM] on the bench press exercise).

Muscular endurance The ability of a muscle to exert submaximal force repeatedly over time.

One repetition maximum (1 RM) The maximum amount of resistance an individual is able to lift in a single effort.

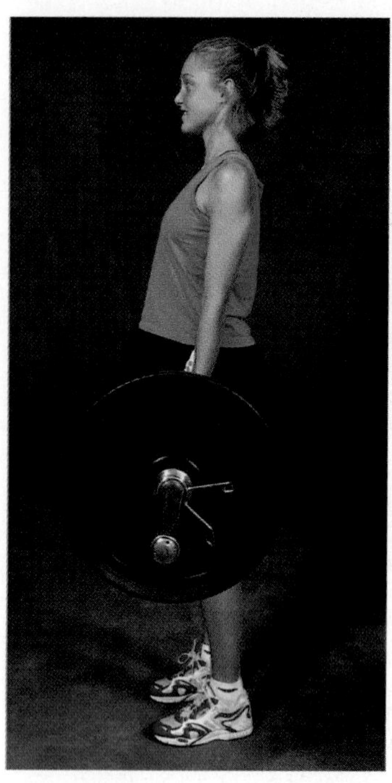

The maximal amount of resistance that an individual is able to lift in one single effort (1 repetition maximum or 1 RM) is a measure of absolute strength.

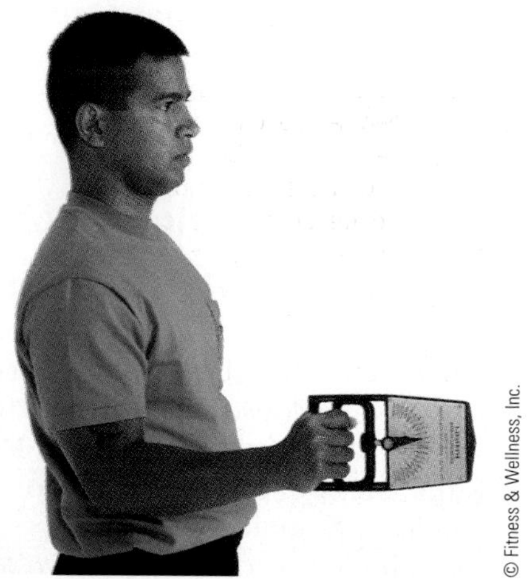

The hand grip tests strength.

TABLE 7.1 Scoring Table for Hand Grip Strength Test

Percentile Rank	Men	Women
99	153	101
95	145	94
90	141	91
80	139	86
70	132	80
60	124	78
50	122	74
40	114	71
30	110	66
20	100	64
10	91	60
5	76	58

High physical fitness standard

Health fitness standard

test for pre- and post-assessments. The following are your options.

Muscular Strength: Hand Grip Strength Test

As indicted previously, when time is a factor, the Hand Grip Test can be used to provide a rough estimate of strength. Unlike the next two tests, this is an isometric (static contraction, discussed later in the chapter) test. If the proper grip is used, no finger motion or body movement is visible during the test. The test procedure is given in Figure 7.2, and percentile ranks based on your results are provided in Table 7.1. You can record the results of this test in Lab 7A.

Changes in strength may be more difficult to evaluate with the Hand Grip Strength Test. Most strength-training programs are dynamic in nature (body segments are moved through a range of motion, discussed later in the chapter), whereas this test provides an isometric assessment. Further, grip strength exercises seldom are used in strength training, and increases in strength are specific to the body parts exercised. This test, however, can be used to supplement the following strength tests.

Muscular Endurance Test

Three exercises were selected to assess the endurance of the upper body, lower body, and mid-body muscle groups (see Figure 7.3). The advantage of the Muscular Endurance Test is that it does not require strength-training equipment—only a stopwatch, a metronome, a bench or gymnasium bleacher 16¼" high, a cardboard strip 3½" wide by 30" long, and a partner. A percentile rank is given for each exercise according to the number of repetitions performed (see Table 7.2, page 214). An overall endurance rating can be obtained by totaling the number of points obtained on each exercise. Record the results of this test in Lab 7A.

Muscular Strength and Endurance Test

In the Muscular Strength and Endurance Test, you will lift a submaximal resistance as many times as possible using the six strength-training exercises listed in Figure 7.4 (page 215). The resistance for each lift is determined according to selected percentages of body weight shown in Figure 7.4 and Lab 7A.

With this test, if an individual does only a few repetitions, the test will measure primarily absolute

FIGURE 7.3 Muscular Endurance Test.

Three exercises are conducted on this test: bench jumps, modified dips (men) or modified push-ups (women), and bent-leg curl-ups or abdominal crunches. All exercises should be conducted with the aid of a partner. The correct procedure for performing each exercise is as follows:

Bench-jump. Using a bench or gymnasium bleacher 16¼" high, attempt to jump up onto and down off of the bench as many times as possible in 1 minute. If you cannot jump the full minute, you may step up and down. A repetition is counted each time both feet return to the floor.

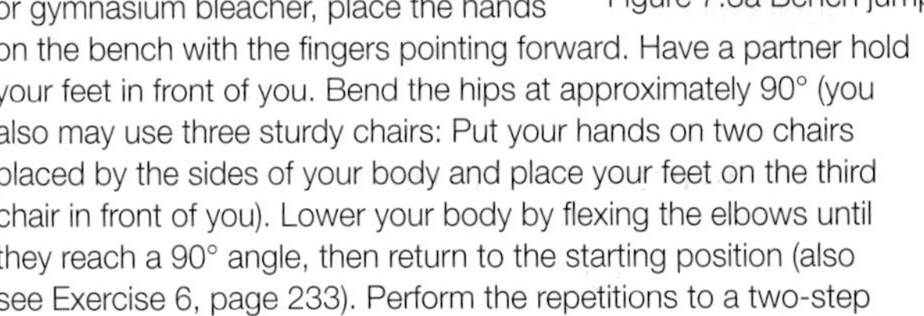

Figure 7.3a Bench jump

Modified dip. Men only: Using a bench or gymnasium bleacher, place the hands on the bench with the fingers pointing forward. Have a partner hold your feet in front of you. Bend the hips at approximately 90° (you also may use three sturdy chairs: Put your hands on two chairs placed by the sides of your body and place your feet on the third chair in front of you). Lower your body by flexing the elbows until they reach a 90° angle, then return to the starting position (also see Exercise 6, page 233). Perform the repetitions to a two-step cadence (down-up) regulated with a metronome set at 56 beats per minute. Perform as many continuous repetitions as possible. Do not count any more repetitions if you fail to follow the metronome cadence.

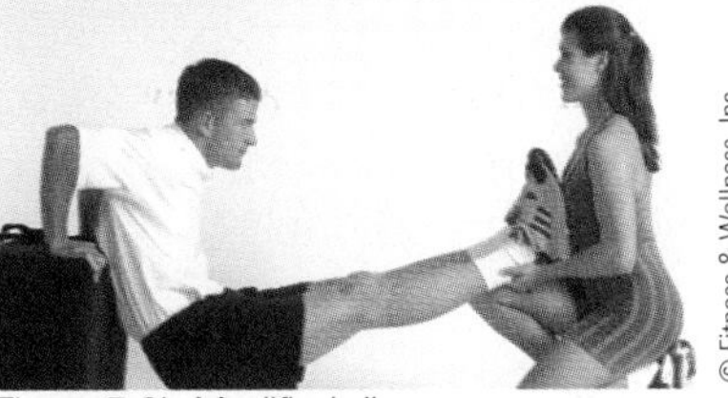

Figure 7.3b Modified dip

Modified push-up. Women: Lie down on the floor (face down), bend the knees (feet up in the air), and place the hands on the floor by the shoulders with the fingers pointing forward. The lower body will be supported at the knees (as opposed to the feet) throughout the test (see Figure 7.3c). The chest must touch the floor on each repetition. As with the modified-dip exercise (above), perform the repetitions to a two-step cadence (up-down) regulated with a metronome set at 56 beats per minute. Perform as many continuous repetitions as possible. Do not count any more repetitions if you fail to follow the metronome cadence.

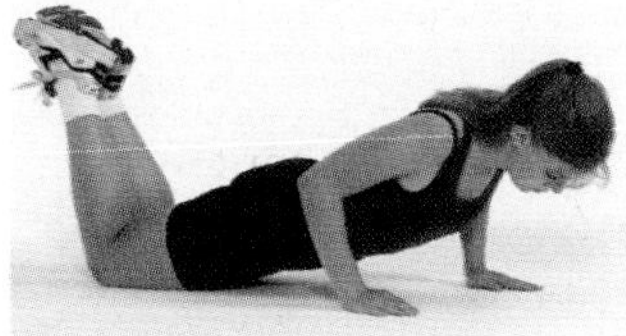

Figure 7.3c Modified push-up

Bent-leg curl-up. Lie down on the floor (face up) and bend both legs at the knees at approximately 100°. The feet should be on the floor, and you must hold them in place yourself throughout the test. Cross the arms in front of the chest, each hand on the opposite shoulder. Now raise the head off the floor, placing the chin against the chest. This is the starting and finishing position for each curl-up (see Figure 7.3d). **The back of the head may not come in contact with the floor, the hands cannot be removed from the shoulders, nor may the feet or hips be raised off the floor at any time during the test. The test is terminated if any of these four conditions occur.** When you curl up, the upper body must come to an upright position before going back down (see Figure 7.3e). The repetitions are performed to a two-step cadence (up-down) regulated with the metronome set at 40 beats per minute. For this exercise, you should allow a brief practice period of 5 to 10 seconds to familiarize yourself with the cadence (the *up* movement is initiated with the first beat, then you must wait for the next beat to initiate the *down* movement; one repetition is accomplished every two beats of the metronome). Count as many repetitions as you are able to perform following the proper cadence. The test is also terminated if you fail to maintain the appropriate cadence or if you accomplish 100 repetitions. Have your partner check the angle at the knees throughout the test to make sure to maintain the 100° angle as close as possible.

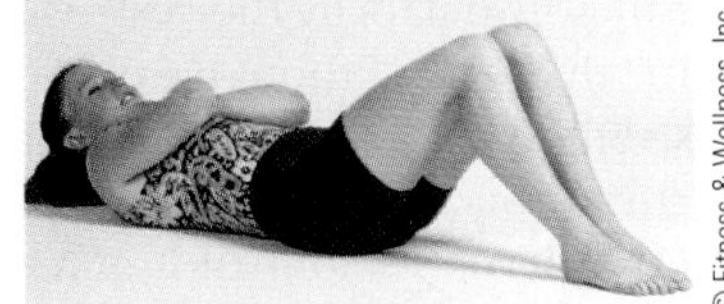

Figure 7.3d Bent-leg curl-up

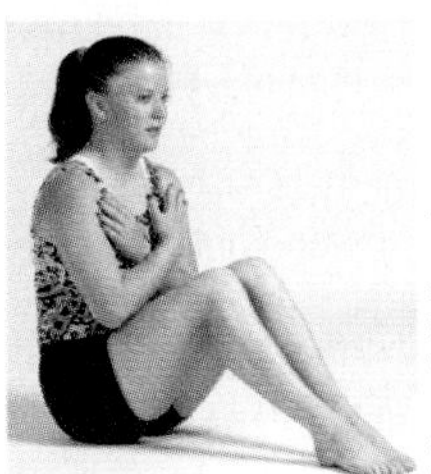

Figure 7.3e Bent-leg curl-up

Abdominal crunch. This test is recommended only for individuals who are unable to perform the bent-leg curl-up test because of susceptibility to low-back injury. Exercise form must be carefully monitored during the test. Several authors and researchers have indicated that proper form during this test is extremely difficult to control. Subjects often slide their bodies, bend their elbows, or shrug their shoulders during the test. Such actions facilitate the performance of the test and misrepresent the actual test results. Biomechanical factors also limit the ability to perform this test. Further, lack of spinal flexibility keeps some individuals from being able to move the full 3½" range of motion. Others are unable to keep their heels on the floor during the test. The validity of this test as an effective measure of abdominal strength or abdominal endurance has also been questioned through research.

Tape a 3½" × 30" strip of cardboard onto the floor. Lie down on the floor in a supine position (face up) with the knees bent at approximately 100° and the legs slightly apart. The feet should be on the floor, and you must hold them in place yourself throughout the test. Straighten out your arms and place them on the floor alongside the trunk with the palms down and the fingers fully extended. The fingertips of both hands should barely touch the closest edge of the cardboard (see Figure 7.3f). Bring the head off the floor until the chin is 1" to 2" away from your chest. Keep the head in this position during the entire test (do not move the head by flexing or extending the neck). You are now ready to begin the test.

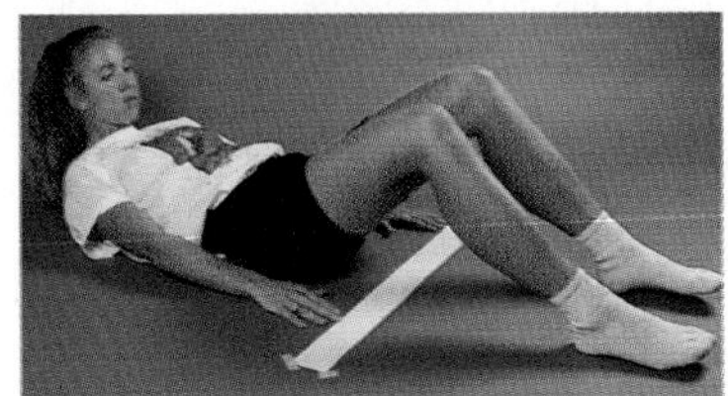

Figure 7.3f Abdominal crunch test

Perform the repetitions to a two-step cadence (up-down) regulated with a metronome set at 60 beats per minute. As you curl up, slide the fingers over the cardboard until the fingertips reach the far edge (3½") of the board (see Figure 7.3g), then return to the starting position.

Figure 7.3g Abdominal crunch test

Allow a brief practice period of 5 to 10 seconds to familiarize yourself with the cadence. Initiate the *up* movement with the first beat and the *down* movement with the next beat. Accomplish one repetition every two beats of the metronome. Count as many repetitions as you are able to perform following the proper cadence. You may not count a repetition if the fingertips fail to reach the distant edge of the cardboard.

Terminate the test if you (a) fail to maintain the appropriate cadence, (b) bend the elbows, (c) shrug the shoulders, (d) slide

FIGURE 7.3 Muscular Endurance Test. *(continued)*

the body, (e) lift heels off the floor, (f) raise the chin off the chest, (g) accomplish 100 repetitions, or (h) no longer can perform the test. Have your partner check the angle at the knees throughout the test to make sure that the 100° angle is maintained as closely as possible.

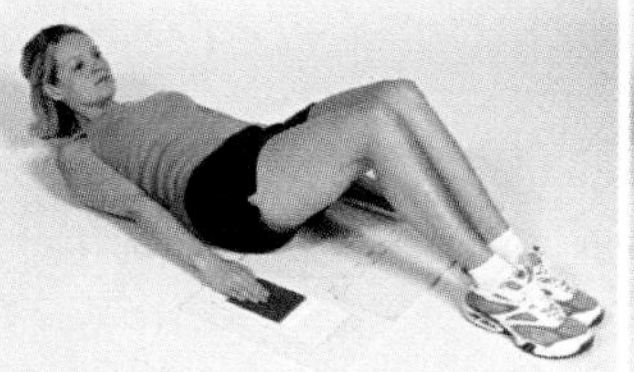

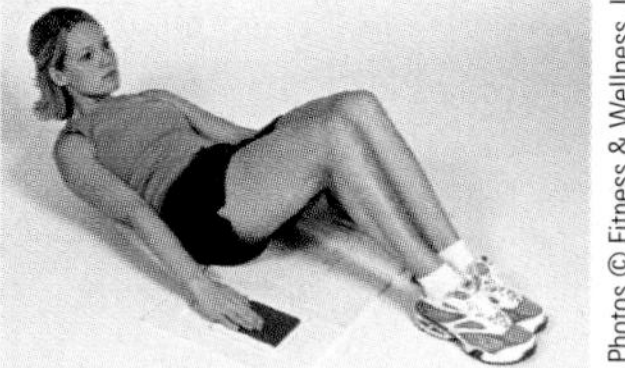

Photos © Fitness & Wellness, Inc.

Figure 7.3h Figure 7.3i

Abdominal crunch test performed with a Crunch-Ster Curl-Up Tester.

For this test you may also use a Crunch-Ster Curl-Up Tester, available from Novel Products.* An illustration of the test performed with this equipment is provided in Figures 7.3h and 7.3i.

According to the results, look up your percentile rank for each exercise in the far left column of Table 7.2 and determine your muscular endurance fitness category according to the following classification:

Average Score	Fitness Category	Points
≥90	Excellent	5
70–80	Good	4
50–60	Average	3
30–40	Fair	2
≤20	Poor	1

Look up the number of points assigned for each fitness category above. Total the number of points and determine your overall strength endurance fitness category according to the following ratings:

Total Points	Strength Endurance Category
≥13	Excellent
10–12	Good
7–9	Average
4–6	Fair
≤3	Poor

*Novel Products, Inc. Figure Finder Collection, P.O. Box 408, Rockton, IL 61072-0408. 1-800-323-5143, Fax 815-624-4866.

TABLE 7.2 Muscular Endurance Scoring Table

	Men				Women			
Percentile Rank	Bench Jumps	Modified Dips	Bent-Leg Curl-Ups	Abdominal Crunches	Bench Jumps	Modified Push-Ups	Bent-Leg Curl-Ups	Abdominal Crunches
99	66	54	100	100	58	95	100	100
95	63	50	81	100	54	70	100	100
90	62	38	65	100	52	50	97	69
80	58	32	51	66	48	41	77	49
70	57	30	44	45	44	38	57	37
60	56	27	31	38	42	33	45	34
50	54	26	28	33	39	30	37	31
40	51	23	25	29	38	28	28	27
30	48	20	22	26	36	25	22	24
20	47	17	17	22	32	21	17	21
10	40	11	10	18	28	18	9	15
5	34	7	3	16	26	15	4	0

High physical fitness standard — Health fitness standard

strength. For those who are able to do a lot of repetitions, the test will be an indicator of muscular endurance. If you are not familiar with the different lifts, illustrations are provided at the end of this chapter.

A strength/endurance rating is determined according to the maximum number of repetitions you are able to perform on each exercise. Fixed-resistance, strength units are necessary to administer all but the abdominal curls exercise on this test (see "Dynamic Training" on pages 217–219 for an explanation of fixed-resistance equipment).

A percentile rank for each exercise is given based on the number of repetitions performed (see Table 7.3). As with the muscular endurance test, an overall muscular strength/endurance rating is obtained by totaling the number of points obtained on each exercise.

If no fixed resistance equipment is available, you can still perform the test using different equipment. In that case, though, the percentile rankings and strength fitness categories may not be completely accurate because a certain resistance (for example, 50 pounds) is seldom the same on two different weight

FIGURE 7.4 Muscular Strength and Endurance Test.

1. Familiarize yourself with the six lifts used for this test: lat pull-down, leg extension, bench press, bent-leg curl-up or abdominal crunch,* leg curl, and arm curl. Graphic illustrations for each lift are given on pages 241, 243, 236, 232, 238, and 234, respectively. For the leg curl exercise, the knees should be flexed to 90°. A description and illustration of the bent-leg curl-up and the abdominal crunch exercises are provided in Figure 7.3. On the leg extension lift, maintain the trunk in an upright position.
2. Determine your body weight in pounds.
3. Determine the amount of resistance to be used on each lift. To obtain this number, multiply your body weight by the percent given below for each lift.

Lift	Percent of Body Weight	
	Men	**Women**
Lat Pull-Down	.70	.45
Leg Extension	.65	.50
Bench Press	.75	.45
Bent-Leg Curl-Up or Abdominal Crunch*	NA**	NA**
Leg Curl	.32	.25
Arm Curl	.35	.18

*The abdominal crunch exercise should be used only by individuals who suffer or are susceptible to low-back pain.
**NA = not applicable—see Figure 7.3

4. Perform the maximum continuous number of repetitions possible.
5. Based on the number of repetitions performed, look up the percentile rank for each lift in the left column of Table 7.3.
6. The individual strength fitness category is determined according to the following classification:

Percentile Rank	Fitness Category	Points
≥90	Excellent	5
70–80	Good	4
50–60	Average	3
30–40	Fair	2
≤20	Poor	1

7. Look up the number of points assigned for each fitness category under item 6 above. Total the number of points and determine you overall strength fitness category according to the following ratings:

Total Points	Strength Category
≥25	Excellent
19–24	Good
13–18	Average
7–12	Fair
≤6	Poor

8. Record your results in Lab 7A.

TABLE 7.3 Muscular Strength and Endurance Scoring Table

	Men							Women						
Percentile Rank	Lat Pull-Down	Leg Extension	Bench Press	Bent-Leg Curl-Up	Abdominal Crunch	Leg Curl	Arm Curl	Lat Pull-Down	Leg Extension	Bench Press	Bent-Leg Curl-Up	Abdominal Crunch	Leg Curl	Arm Curl
99	30	25	26	100	100	24	25	30	25	27	100	100	20	25
95	25	20	21	81	100	20	21	25	20	21	100	100	17	21
90	19	19	19	65	100	19	19	21	18	20	97	69	12	20
80	16	15	16	51	66	15	15	16	13	16	77	49	10	16
70	13	14	13	44	45	13	12	13	11	13	57	37	9	14
60	11	13	11	31	38	11	10	11	10	11	45	34	7	12
50	10	12	10	28	33	10	9	10	9	10	37	31	6	10
40	9	10	7	25	29	8	8	9	8	5	28	27	5	8
30	7	9	5	22	26	6	7	7	7	3	22	24	4	7
20	6	7	3	17	22	4	5	6	5	1	17	21	3	6
10	4	5	1	10	18	3	3	3	3	0	9	15	1	3
5	3	3	0	3	16	1	2	2	1	0	4	0	0	2

High physical fitness standard   Health fitness standard

machines (for example, Universal Gym versus Nautilus). The industry has no standard calibration procedure for strength equipment. Consequently, if you lift a certain resistance for a specific exercise (for example, bench press) on one machine, you may or may not be able to lift the same amount for this exercise on a different machine.

Even though the percentile ranks may not be valid when using different equipment, test results can be used to evaluate changes in fitness. For example, you may be able to do 7 repetitions during the initial test, but if you can perform 14 repetitions after 12 weeks of training, that's a measure of improvement. Results of the Muscular Strength and Endurance Test can be recorded in Lab 7A.

Strength-Training Prescription

The capacity of muscle cells to exert force increases and decreases according to the demands placed upon the muscular system. If muscle cells are overloaded beyond their normal use, such as in strength-training programs, the cells increase in size (hypertrophy) and strength. If the demands placed on the muscle cells decrease, such as in sedentary living or required rest because of illness or injury, the cells **atrophy** and lose strength. A good level of muscular strength is important to develop and maintain fitness, health, and total well-being.

Factors That Affect Strength

Several physiological factors combine to create muscle contraction and subsequent strength gains: neural stimulation, type of muscle fiber, overload, and specificity of training. Basic knowledge of these concepts is important to understand the principles involved in strength training.

Neural Stimulation

Within the neuromuscular system, single **motor neurons** branch and attach to multiple muscle fibers. The motor neuron and the fibers it innervates (supplies with nerves) form a **motor unit.** The number of fibers a motor neuron can innervate varies from just a few in muscles that require precise control (eye muscles, for example) to as many as 1,000 or more in large muscles that do not perform refined or precise movements.

Stimulation of a motor neuron causes the muscle fibers to contract maximally or not at all. Variations in the number of fibers innervated and the frequency of their stimulation determine the strength of the muscle contraction. As the number of fibers innervated and frequency of stimulation increase, so does the strength of the muscular contraction.

Types of Muscle Fiber

The human body has two basic types of muscle fibers: (a) slow-twitch or red fibers and (b) fast-twitch or white fibers. **Slow-twitch fibers** have a greater capacity for aerobic work. **Fast-twitch fibers** have a greater capacity for anaerobic work and produce more overall force. The latter are important for quick and powerful movements commonly used in strength-training activities.

The proportion of slow- and fast-twitch fibers is determined genetically, and consequently varies from one person to another. Nevertheless, training increases the functional capacity of both types of fiber and, more specifically, strength training increases their ability to exert force.

During muscular contraction, slow-twitch fibers always are recruited first. As the force and speed of muscle contraction increase, the relative importance of the fast-twitch fibers increases. To activate the fast-twitch fibers, an activity must be intense and powerful.

Overload

Strength gains are achieved in two ways:

1. Through increased ability of individual muscle fibers to generate a stronger contraction.
2. By recruiting a greater proportion of the total available fibers for each contraction.

These two factors combine in the **overload principle.** The demands placed on the muscle must be increased systematically and progressively over time, and the resistance must be of a magnitude significant enough to cause physiological adaptation. In simpler terms, just like all other organs and systems of the human body, to increase in physical capacity, muscles have to be taxed repeatedly beyond their accustomed loads. Because of this principle, strength training also is called *progressive resistance training.*

Several procedures can be used to overload in strength training:[6]

1. Increasing the resistance.
2. Increasing the number of repetitions.
3. Increasing or decreasing the speed of the normal repetition.
4. Decreasing the rest interval for endurance improvements (with lighter resistances) or lengthening the rest interval for strength gains (with higher resistances).
5. Increasing the volume (sum of the repetitions performed multiplied by the resistance used).
6. Using any combination of the above.

Specificity of Training

The principle of **specificity of training** holds that, for a muscle to increase in strength or endurance, the training program must be specific to obtain the desired effects (also see discussion on resistance on pages 219–220).

The principle of specificity also applies to activity or sport-specific development and is commonly referred to as **SAID training (specific adaptation to imposed demand).** The SAID principle implies that if an individual is attempting to improve specific sport skills, the strength-training exercises performed should resemble as closely as possible the movement patterns encountered in that particular activity or sport.

For example, a soccer player who wishes to become stronger and faster would emphasize exercises that will develop leg strength and power. In contrast, an individual recovering from a lower-limb fracture initially exercises to increase strength and stability, and subsequently muscle endurance. Additional information on the principle of specificity is provided in Chapter 9, "Sport-

Specific Conditioning," pages 307–308. Understanding all four concepts discussed thus far (neural stimulation, muscle fiber types, overload, and specificity) is required to design an effective strength-training program.

Principles Involved in Strength Training

Because muscular strength and endurance are important in developing and maintaining overall fitness and well-being, the principles necessary to develop a strength-training program have to be understood, just as in the prescription for cardiorespiratory endurance. These principles are mode, resistance, sets, frequency, and volume of training. The key factor in successful muscular strength development, however, is the individualization of the program according to these principles and the person's goals, as well as the magnitude of the individual's effort during training itself.[7]

Mode of Training

Two types of training methods are used to improve strength: isometric (static) and dynamic (previously called "isotonic"). In isometric training, muscle contractions produce little or no movement, such as pushing or pulling against an immovable object. In dynamic training, the muscle contractions produce movement, such as extending the knees with resistance on the ankles (leg extension). The specificity of training principle applies here, too. To increase isometric versus dynamic strength, an individual must use static instead of dynamic training to achieve the desired results.

Isometric Training

Isometric training does not require much equipment, and its popularity of several years ago has waned. Because strength gains with isometric training are specific to the angle of muscle contraction, this type of training is beneficial in a sport such as gymnastics, which requires regular static contractions during routines. As presented in Chapter 8, however, isometric training is a critical component of health conditioning programs for the back (see "Preventing and Rehabilitating Low-Back Pain," pages 267–272).

Dynamic Training

Dynamic training is the most popular mode for strength training. The primary advantage is that strength is gained through the full **range of motion.** Most daily activities are dynamic in nature. We are constantly lifting, pushing, and pulling objects, and strength is needed through a complete range of motion. Another advantage is that improvements are measured easily by the amount lifted.

Dynamic training consists of two action phases when an exercise is performed: **concentric** or **positive resistance,** and **eccentric** or **negative resistance.** In the concentric phase, the muscle shortens as it contracts to overcome the resistance. In the eccentric phase, the muscle lengthens to overcome the resistance. For example, during a bench press exercise, when the person lifts the resistance from the chest to full-arm

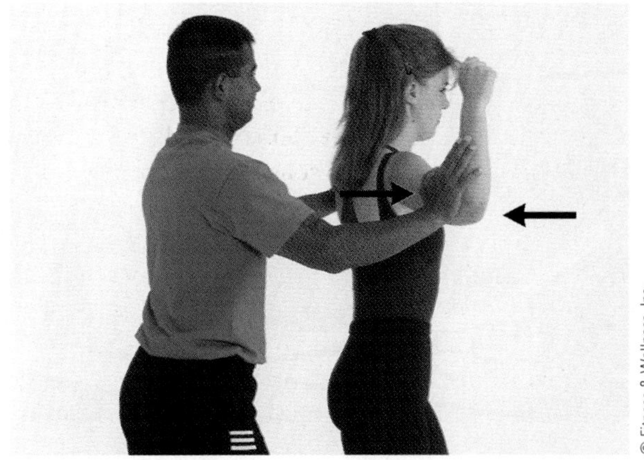

In isometric training, muscle contraction produces little or no movement.

Atrophy Decrease in the size of a cell.

Motor neurons Nerves connecting the central nervous system to the muscle.

Motor unit The combination of a motor neuron and the muscle fibers that neuron innervates.

Slow-twitch fibers Muscle fibers with greater aerobic potential and slow speed of contraction.

Fast-twitch fibers Muscle fibers with greater anaerobic potential and fast speed of contraction.

Overload principle Training concept that the demands placed on a system (cardiorespiratory or muscular) must be increased systematically and progressively over time to cause physiological adaptation (development or improvement).

Specificity of training Principle that training must be done with the specific muscle the person is attempting to improve.

Specific adaptation to imposed demand (SAID) training Training principle stating that, for improvements to occur in a specific activity, the exercises performed during a strength-training program should resemble as closely as possible the movement patterns encountered in that particular activity.

Isometric training Strength-training method referring to a muscle contraction that produces little or no movement, such as pushing or pulling against an immovable object.

Range of motion Entire arc of movement of a given joint.

Dynamic training Strength-training method referring to a muscle contraction with movement.

Concentric Describes shortening of a muscle during muscle contraction.

Positive resistance The lifting, pushing, or concentric phase of a repetition during a strength-training exercise.

Eccentric Describes lengthening of a muscle during muscle contraction.

Negative resistance The lowering or eccentric phase of a repetition during a strength-training exercise.

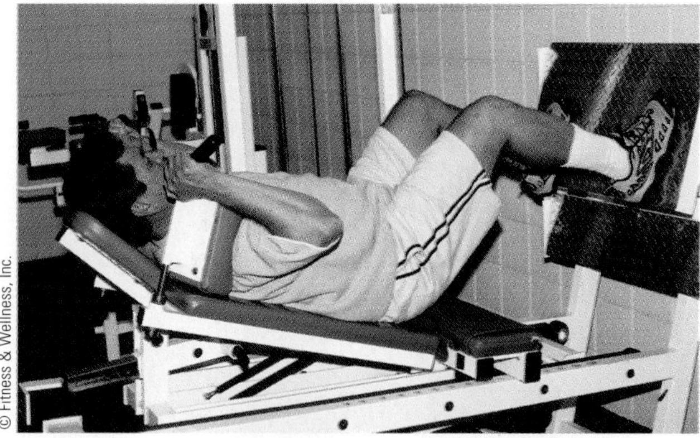

In dynamic training, muscle contraction produces movement in the respective joint.

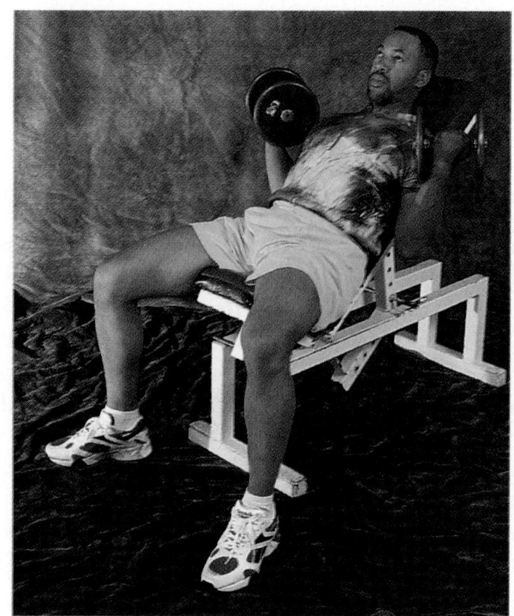

Strength training can be done using free weights.

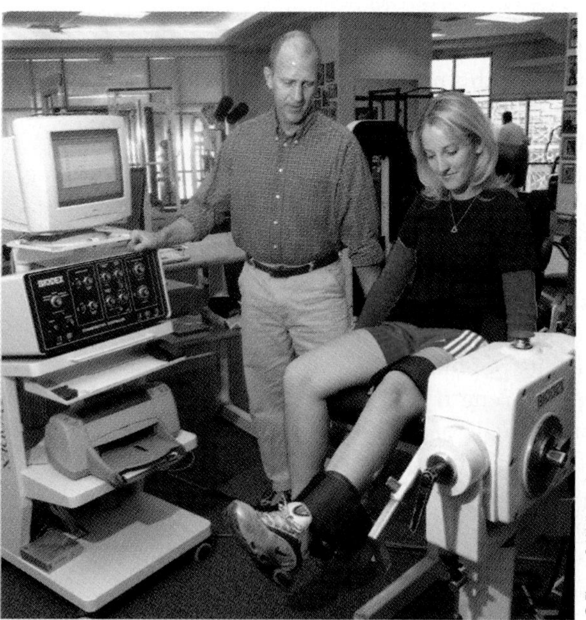

In isokinetic training, the speed of muscle contraction is constant.

extension, the triceps muscle on the back of the upper arm shortens to extend (straighten) the elbow. During the eccentric phase, the same triceps muscle is used to lower the weight during elbow flexion, but the muscle lengthens slowly to avoid dropping the resistance. Both motions work the same muscle against the same resistance.

Eccentric muscle contractions allow us to lower weights in a smooth, gradual, and controlled manner. Without eccentric contractions, weights would be suddenly dropped on the way down. Because the same muscles work when you lift and lower a resistance, always be sure to execute both actions in a controlled manner. Failure to do so diminishes the benefits of the training program and increases the risk for injuries. Eccentric contractions seem to be more effective in producing muscle hypertrophy but result in greater muscle soreness.[8]

Dynamic training programs can be conducted without weights; using exercise bands; and with **free weights, fixed-resistance** machines, **variable-resistance** machines, or isokinetic equipment. When you perform dynamic exercises without weights (for example, pull-ups and push-ups), with free weights, or with fixed-resistance machines, you move a constant resistance through a joint's full range of motion. The greatest resistance that can be lifted equals the maximum weight that can be moved at the weakest angle of the joint. This is because of changes in length of muscle and angle of pull as the joint moves through its range of motion. This type of training is also referred to as **dynamic constant external resistance** or **DCER.**

As strength training became more popular, new strength-training machines were developed. This technology brought about **isokinetic training** and variable-resistance training programs, which require special machines equipped with mechanical devices that provide differing amounts of resistance, with the intent of overloading the muscle group maximally through the entire range of motion. A distinction of isokinetic training is that the speed of the muscle contraction is kept constant because the machine provides resistance to match the user's force through the range of motion. The mode of training an individual selects depends mainly on the type of equipment available and the specific objective the training program is attempting to accomplish.

The benefits of isokinetic and variable-resistance training are similar to the other dynamic training methods. Theoretically, strength gains should be better because maximum resistance is applied at all angles. Research, however, has not shown this type of training to be more effective than other modes of dynamic training.

Free Weights Versus Machines in Dynamic Training

The most popular weight-training devices available during the first half of the 20th century were plate-loaded barbells (free weights). Strength-training machines were developed in the middle of the century but did not become popular until the 1970s. With subsequent technological improvements to these machines, a stirring debate arose over which of the two training modalities was better.

Free weights require that the individual balance the resistance through the entire lifting motion. Thus, one could logically assume that free weights are a better training modality because additional stabilizing muscles are needed to balance the resistance as it is moved through the range of motion. Research, however, has not shown any differences in strength development between the two exercise modalities.[9]

Although each modality has pros and cons, muscles do not know whether the source of a resistance is a barbell, a dumbbell, a Universal Gym machine, a Nautilus machine, or a simple cinder block. What determines the extent of a person's strength development is the quality of the program and the individual's effort during the training program itself—not the type of equipment used.

Advantages of Free Weights Following are the advantages of using free weights instead of machines in a strength-training program.

- *Cost:* Free weights are much less expensive than most exercise machines. On a limited budget, free weights are a better option.
- *Variety:* A bar and a few plates can be used to perform many exercises to strengthen most muscles in the body.
- *Portability:* Free weights can be easily moved from one area or station to another.
- *Balance:* Free weights require that a person balance the weight through the entire range of motion. This feature involves additional stabilizing muscles to keep the weight moving properly.
- *One size fits all:* People of almost all ages can use free weights. A drawback of machines is that individuals who are at the extremes in terms of height or limb length often do not fit into the machines. In particular, small women and adolescents are at a disadvantage.

Advantages of Machines Strength-training machines have the following advantages over free weights:

- *Safety:* Machines are safer because spotters are rarely needed to monitor exercises.
- *Selection:* A few exercises—such as hip flexion, hip abduction, leg curls, lat pull-downs, and neck exercises—can be performed only with machines.
- *Variable resistance:* Most machines provide variable resistance. Free weights provide only fixed resistance.
- *Isolation:* Individual muscles are better isolated with machines because stabilizing muscles are not used to balance the weight during the exercise.
- *Time:* Exercising with machines requires less time because the resistance is set quickly using a selector pin instead of having to manually change dumbbells or weight plates on both sides of a barbell.
- *Flexibility:* Most machines can provide resistance over a greater range of movement during the exercise, thereby contributing to more flexibility in the joints. For example, a barbell pullover exercise provides resistance over a range of 100 degrees, whereas a weight machine may allow for as much as 260 degrees.
- *Rehabilitation:* Machines are more useful during injury rehabilitation. A knee injury, for instance, is practically impossible to rehab using free weights, whereas, with a weight machine, small loads can be easily selected through a limited range of motion.
- *Skill acquisition:* Learning a new exercise movement—and performing it correctly—is faster because the machine controls the direction of the movement.

Resistance

Resistance in strength training is the equivalent of intensity in cardiorespiratory exercise prescription. To stimulate strength development, the general recommendation has been to use a resistance of approximately 80 percent of the maximum capacity (1 RM). For example, a person with a 1 RM of 150 pounds should work with about 120 pounds (150 × .80).

Free weights Barbells and dumbbells.

Fixed resistance Type of exercise in which a constant resistance is moved through a joint's full range of motion (dumbbells, barbells, machines using a constant resistance).

Variable resistance Training using special machines equipped with mechanical devices that provide differing amounts of resistance through the range of motion.

Dynamic constant external resistance (DCER) See fixed resistance.

Isokinetic training Strength-training method in which the speed of the muscle contraction is kept constant because the equipment (machine) provides an accommodating resistance to match the user's force (maximal) through the range of motion.

Resistance Amount of weight lifted.

TABLE 7.4 Number of Repetitions Performed at 80 Percent of the One Repetition Maximum (1 RM)

	Trained		Untrained	
Exercise	**Men**	**Women**	**Men**	**Women**
Leg press	19	22	15	12
Lat pulldown	12	10	10	10
Bench press	12	14	10	10
Leg extension	12	10	9	8
Sit-up*	12	12	8	7
Arm curl	11	7	8	6
Leg curl	7	5	6	6

* Sit-up exercise performed with weighted plates on the chest and feet held in place with an ankle strap.
SOURCE: W. W. K. Hoeger, D. R. Hopkins, S. L. Barette, and D. F. Hale, "Relationship Between Repetitions and Selected Percentages of One Repetition Maximum: A Comparison Between Untrained and Trained Males and Females," *Journal of Applied Sport Science Research* 4, no. 2 (1990): 47–51.

The number of repetitions that one can perform at 80 percent of the 1 RM varies among exercises (i.e., bench press, lat pull-down, leg curl—see Table 7.4). Data indicate that the total number of repetitions performed at a certain percentage of the 1 RM depends on the amount of muscle mass involved (bench press versus triceps extension) and whether it is a single or multi-joint exercise (leg press versus leg curl). In trained and untrained subjects alike, the number of repetitions is greater with larger muscle mass involvement and multi-joint exercises.[10]

Because of the time factor involved in constantly determining the 1 RM on each lift to ensure that the person is indeed working around 80 percent, the accepted rule for many years has been that individuals perform between 3 and 12 repetitions maximum (3 to 12 RM) for adequate strength gains. For example, if a person is training with a resistance of 120 pounds and cannot lift it more than 12 times—that is, the person reaches volitional fatigue at or before 12 repetitions—the training stimulus (weight used) is adequate for strength development. Once the person can lift the resistance more than 12 times, the resistance is increased by 5 to 10 pounds and the person again should build up to 12 repetitions. This is referred to as **progressive resistance training.**

Strength development, however, also can occur when working with less than 80 percent of the 1 RM. Although 3 to 12 RM is the most commonly prescribed resistance, benefits do accrue when working below 3 RM or above 12 RM.

At least in the health-fitness area, little evidence supports the notion that working with a given number of repetitions elicits specific or greater strength, endurance, or hypertrophy.[11] Although not precisely to the same extent, muscular strength and endurance are both increased when training within a reasonable amount of repetitions. Thus, the American College of Sports Medicine recommends a range between 3 RM and 20 RM. The individual may choose the number of repetitions based on personal preference.

Elite strength athletes typically work between 1 and 6 RM, but they often shuffle training with a different number of repetitions for selected periods (weeks) of time (see "Training Volume" on page 221). Body builders tend to work with moderate resistance levels (60 to 85 percent of the 1 RM) and perform 8 to 20 repetitions to near fatigue. A foremost objective of body building is to increase muscle size. Moderate resistance promotes blood flow to the muscles, "pumping up the muscles" (also known as "the pump"), which makes them look much larger than they do in a resting state.

From a general fitness point of view, working near a 10-repetition threshold seems to improve overall performance most effectively. We live in a dynamic world in which muscular strength and endurance are both required to lead an enjoyable life. Working around 10 RM produces good results in terms of strength, endurance, and hypertrophy.

Sets

In strength training, a **set** is the number of repetitions performed for a given exercise. For example, a person lifting 120 pounds eight times has performed one set of 8 repetitions ($1 \times 8 \times 120$). For general fitness, the recommendation is one to three sets per exercise. Some evidence suggests greater strength gains using multiple sets rather than a single set for a given exercise. Other research, however, concludes that similar increases in strength, endurance, and hypertrophy are derived between single- and multiple-set strength training; as long as the single set, or at least one of the multiple sets, is performed to volitional exhaustion (a heavy set).[12]

Because of the characteristics of muscle fiber, the number of sets the exerciser can do is limited. As the number of sets increases, so does the amount of muscle fatigue and subsequent recovery time. Therefore, strength gains may be lessened by performing too many sets. When time is a factor, single-set programs are preferable because they require less time and can enhance compliance with exercise.

A recommended program for beginners in their first year of training is one or two light warm-up sets per exercise, using about 50 percent of the 1 RM (no warm-up sets are necessary for subsequent exercises that use the same muscle group) followed by one to three sets to near fatigue per exercise. Maintaining a resistance and effort that will temporarily fatigue the muscle (volitional exhaustion) in the number of repetitions selected in at least one of the sets is crucial to achieve optimal progress. Because of the lower resistances used in body building, four to eight sets can be done for each exercise.

To avoid muscle soreness and stiffness, new participants ought to build up gradually to three sets of maximal repetitions. They can do this by performing only one set of each exercise with a lighter resistance on the first day, two sets of each exercise on the second day—the first light and the second with the required resistance to volitional exhaustion. If you choose to do so, you can increase to three sets on the third day—one light and two heavy. After that, a person should be able to perform all three heavy sets.

The time necessary to recover between sets depends mainly on the resistance used during each set. In strength training, the energy to lift heavy weights is derived primarily from the ATP–CP or phosphagen system (see Chapter 3, "Energy (ATP) Production," pages 90–91). Ten seconds of maximal exercise nearly depletes the CP stores in the exercised muscle(s). These stores are replenished in about 3 minutes of recovery.

Based on this principle, a rest period of up to 3 minutes between sets is necessary for people who are trying to maximize their strength gains. Individuals training for health-fitness purposes might allow 2 minutes of rest between sets. Body builders, who use lower resistances, should rest no more than 1 minute to maximize the "pumping" effect.

The exercise program will be more time-effective by alternating two or three exercises that require different muscle groups, called **circuit training.** In this way, an individual will not have to wait 2 to 3 minutes before proceeding to a new set on a different exercise. For example, the bench press, leg extension, and abdominal curl-up exercises may be combined so the person can go almost directly from one exercise set to the next.

Men and women alike should observe the guidelines given previously. Many women do not follow these guidelines. They erroneously believe that training with low resistances and many repetitions is best to enhance body composition and maximize energy expenditure. Unless a person is seeking to increase muscular endurance for a specific sport-related activity, the use of low resistances and high repetitions is not recommended to achieve optimal strength-fitness goals and maximize long-term energy expenditure (also see Chapter 5, "Exercise: The Key to Weight Management," pages 144–148).

Frequency

Strength training can be done either through a total body workout two or three times a week, or more frequently if using a split-body routine (upper body one day, lower body the next). After a maximum strength workout, the muscles should be rested for about 2 to 3 days to allow adequate recovery. If not completely recovered in 2 to 3 days, the person most likely is over-

FIGURE 7.5 Strength-training exercise prescription guidelines. 

Mode:	8 to 10 dynamic strength-training exercises involving the body's major muscle groups
Resistance:	Sufficient resistance to perform 3 to 20 repetitions to complete or near-complete fatigue (the number of repetitions is optional; you may use 3 to 6, 8 to 12, 12 to 15, or 16 to 20 repetitions)
Sets:	A minimum of 1 set
Frequency:	2 to 3 days per week on nonconsecutive days

Adapted from: American College of Sports Medicine, *Guidelines for Exercise Testing and Prescription* (Baltimore: Lippincott Williams & Wilkins, 2006).

training and therefore not reaping the full benefits of the program. In that case, the person should do fewer sets of exercises than in the previous workout. A summary of strength-training guidelines for health-fitness purposes is provided in Figure 7.5.

To achieve significant strength gains, a minimum of 8 weeks of consecutive training is necessary. After an individual has achieved a recommended strength level, from a health-fitness standpoint, one training session per week will be sufficient to maintain the new strength level. Highly trained athletes will have to train twice a week to maintain their strength level.

Frequency of strength training for body builders varies from person to person. Because they use moderate resistance, daily or even two-a-day workouts are common. The frequency depends on the amount of resistance, number of sets performed per session, and the person's ability to recover from the previous exercise bout (see Table 7.5). The latter often is dictated by level of conditioning.

Training Volume

Volume is the sum of all the repetitions performed multiplied by the resistances used during a strength-training session.[13] Volume frequently is used to quantify the amount of work performed in a given training session. For example, an individual who does 3 sets of 6 repetitions with 150 pounds has performed a training volume of 2,700 ($3 \times 6 \times 150$) for this exercise. The total training volume can be obtained by totaling the volume of all exercises performed.

The volume of training done in a strength-training session can be modified by changing the total number

Progressive resistance training A gradual increase of resistance over a period of time.

Set A fixed number of repetitions; one set of bench presses might be 10 repetitions.

Circuit training Alternating exercises by performing them in a sequence of three to six or more.

Volume (in strength training) The sum of all the repetitions performed multiplied by the resistances used during a strength-training session.

TABLE 7.5 Guidelines for Various Strength-Training Programs

Strength-Training Program	Resistance	Sets	Rest Between Sets*	Frequency (workouts per week)**
General fitness	3–20 reps max	1–3	2 min	2–3
Strength athletes	1–6 reps max	3–6	3 min	2–3
Body building	8–20 reps near max	3–8	up to 1 min	4–12

* Recovery between sets can be decreased by alternating exercises that use different muscle groups.
** Weekly training sessions can be increased by using a split-body routine.

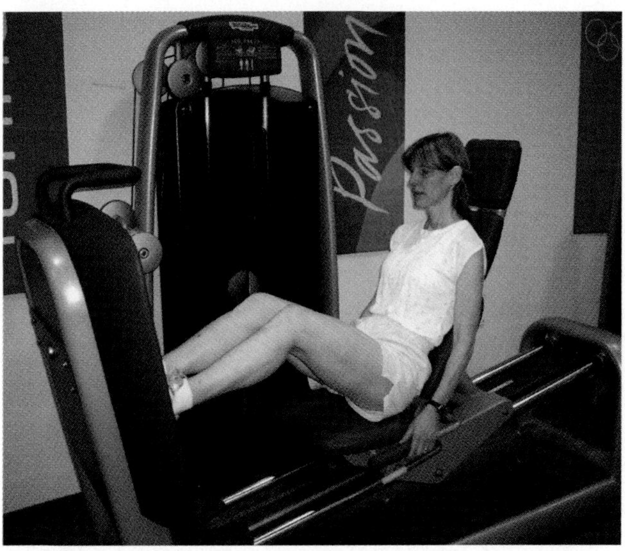

From a health-fitness standpoint, one strength-training session per week is sufficient to maintain strength.

of exercises performed—either by changing the number of sets done per exercise or the number of repetitions performed per set. Athletes typically use high training volumes and low intensities to achieve muscle hypertrophy, and low volumes and high intensities to increase strength and power.

Altering training volume and intensity is known as **periodization,** a training approach that athletes frequently use to achieve peak fitness and prevent **overtraining.** Periodization means cycling one's training objectives (hypertrophy, strength, and endurance), with each phase of the program lasting anywhere from 2 to 12 weeks. To prevent overtraining during periodization, the volume should not increase by more than 5 percent from one phase to the next.

Periodization now is becoming popular among fitness participants who want to achieve higher levels of fitness. A more thorough discussion on periodization is provided in Chapter 9 (pages 308–310).

Plyometrics

Strength, speed, and explosiveness are all crucial for success in athletics. All three of these factors are enhanced with a progressive resistance training program, but greater increases in speed and explosiveness are thought to be possible with **plyometric exercise.** The objective is to generate the greatest amount of force in the shortest time. A solid strength base is necessary before attempting plyometric exercises.

Plyometric training is popular in sports that require powerful movements, such as basketball, volleyball, sprinting, jumping, and gymnastics. A typical plyometric exercise involves jumping off and back onto a box, attempting to rebound as quickly as possible on each jump. Box heights are increased progressively from about 12 to 22 inches.

The bounding action attempts to take advantage of the stretch-recoil and stretch reflex characteristics of muscle. The rapid stretch applied to the muscle during contact with the ground is thought to augment muscle contraction, leading to more explosiveness. Plyometrics can be used, too, for strengthening upper body muscles. An example is doing push-ups so the extension of the arms is forceful enough to drive the hands (and body) completely off the floor during each repetition.

A drawback of plyometric training is its higher risk for injuries compared with conventional modes of progressive resistance training. For instance, the potential for injury in rebound exercise escalates with the increase in box height or the number of repetitions.

Strength Gains

A common question by many strength-training participants is: How quickly can strength gains be observed? Strength-training studies have revealed that most of the strength gains are seen in the first 8 weeks of training. The amount of improvement, however, is related to previous training status. Increases of 40 percent are seen in individuals with no previous strength-training experience, 16 percent in previously strength-trained people, and 10 percent in advanced individuals.[14] Adhering to a periodized strength-training program can yield further improvements (see "Periodization," Chapter 9, pages 308–310).

Critical Thinking

Your roommate started a strength-training program last year and has seen good results. He is now strength training on a nearly daily basis and taking performance-enhancing supplements hoping to accelerate results. What are your feelings about his program? What would you say (and not say) to him?

Strength-Training Exercises

The strength-training programs introduced on pages 231–252 provide a complete body workout. The major muscles of the human body referred to in the exercises are pointed out in Figure 7.6 (page 229) and with the exercises themselves.

Only a minimum of equipment is required for the first program, Strength-Training Exercises without Weights (Exercises 1 through 14). You can conduct this program in your own home. Your body weight is used as the primary resistance for most exercises. A few exercises call for a friend's help or some basic implements from around your house to provide greater resistance.

Strength-Training Exercises with Weights (Exercises 15 through 37) require machines (shown in the accompanying photographs). These exercises can be conducted on either fixed-resistance or variable-resistance equipment. Many of these exercises also can be performed with free weights. The first 13 of these exercises (15 to 27) are recommended to get a complete workout. You can do these exercises as circuit training. If time is a factor, as a minimum perform the first nine (15 through 23) exercises. Exercises 28 to 37 are supplemental or can replace some of the basic 13 (for instance, substitute Exercise 29 or 30 for 15; 31 for 16; 33 for 19; 34 for 24; 35 for 26; 32 for 27). Exercises 38 to 46 are stability ball exercises that can be used to complement your workout. Some of these exercises can also take the place of others that you use to strengthen similar muscle groups.

Selecting different exercises for a given muscle group is recommended between training sessions (for example, chest press for bench press). No evidence indicates that a given exercise is best for a given muscle group. Changing exercises works the specific muscle group through a different range of motion and may change the difficulty of the exercise. Alternating exercises is also beneficial to avoid the monotony of repeating the same training program each training session.

Dietary Guidelines for Strength Development

Individuals who wish to enhance muscle growth and strength during periods of intense strength training should increase protein intake from .8 grams per kilogram of body weight per day to about 1.5 grams per kilogram of body weight per day. An additional 500 daily calories are also recommended to optimize muscle mass gain. If protein intake is already at 1.5 grams per kilogram of body weight, the additional 500 calories should come primarily from complex carbohydrates to provide extra nutrients to the body and glucose for the working muscles.

The time of day when carbohydrates and protein are consumed in relation to the strength-training workout also plays a role in promoting muscle growth. Studies suggest that consuming a pre-exercise snack consisting of a combination of carbohydrates and protein is beneficial to muscle development. The carbohydrates supply energy for training, and the availability of amino acids (the building blocks of protein) in the blood during training enhances muscle-building. A peanut butter, turkey, or tuna sandwich, milk or yogurt and fruit, or nuts and fruit consumed 30 to 60 minutes before training are excellent choices for a pre-workout snack.

Consuming a carbohydrate/protein snack immediately following strength training and a second snack an hour thereafter further promotes muscle growth and strength development. Post-exercise carbohydrates help restore muscle glycogen depleted during training, and, in combination with protein, induce an increase in blood insulin and growth hormone levels. These hormones are essential to the muscle-building process.

Muscle fibers also absorb a greater amount of amino acids up to 48 hours following strength training. The first hour, nonetheless, seems to be the most critical. A higher level of circulating amino acids in the bloodstream immediately after training is believed to increase protein synthesis to a greater extent than amino acids made available later in the day. A ratio of 4-to-1 grams of carbohydrates to protein is recommended for a post-exercise snack—for example, a snack containing 40 grams of carbohydrates (160 calories) and 10 grams of protein (40 calories).

Core Strength Training

The trunk (spine) and pelvis are referred to as the "core" of the body. Core muscles include the abdominal muscles (rectus, transversus, and internal and external obliques), hip muscles (front and back), and spinal muscles (lower and upper back muscles). These muscle groups are responsible for maintaining the stability of the spine and pelvis.

Many of the major muscle groups of the legs, shoulders, and arms attach to the core. A strong core allows a person to perform activities of daily living with greater ease, improve sports performance through a more effective energy transfer from large to small body parts, and decrease the incidence of low-back pain.

Periodization A training approach that divides the season into cycles using a systematic variation in intensity and volume of training to enhance fitness and performance.

Overtraining An emotional, behavioral, and physical condition marked by increased fatigue, decreased performance, persistent muscle soreness, mood disturbances, and feelings of "staleness" or "burnout" as a result of excessive physical training.

Plyometric exercise Explosive jump training, incorporating speed and strength training to enhance explosiveness.

Core strength training also contributes to better posture and balance.

Interest in **core strength training** programs has increased recently. A major objective of core training is to exercise the abdominal and lower back muscles in unison. Furthermore, individuals should spend as much time training the back muscles as they do the abdominal muscles. Besides enhancing stability, core training improves dynamic balance, which is often required during physical activity and participation in sports.

Key core-training exercises include the abdominal crunch and bent-leg curl-up, reverse crunch, pelvic tilt, lateral bridge, prone bridge, leg press, seated back, lat pull-down, back extension, lateral trunk flexion, supine bridge, and pelvic clock (Exercises 4, 11, 12, 13, 14, 16, 20, 24, 36, and 37 in this chapter and Exercises 26 and 27 in Chapter 8, respectively). Stability ball exercises 38 through 46 are also used to strengthen the core.

When core training is used in athletic conditioning programs, athletes attempt to mimic the dynamic skills they use in their sport. To do so, they use special equipment such as balance boards, stability balls, and foam pads. Using this equipment allows the athletes to train the core while seeking balance and stability in a sport-specific manner.[15]

Behavior Modification Planning

HEALTHY STRENGTH TRAINING

- Make a progressive resistance strength-training program a priority in your weekly schedule.
- Strength-train at least once a week; even better, twice a week.
- Find a facility where you feel comfortable training and where you can get good professional guidance.
- Learn the proper technique for each exercise.
- Train with a friend or group of friends.
- Consume a pre-exercise snack consisting of a combination of carbohydrates and some protein about 30 to 60 minutes before each strength-training session.
- Use a minimum of 8 to 10 exercises that involve all major muscle groups of your body.
- Perform at least one set of each exercise to near muscular fatigue.
- To enhance protein synthesis, consume one post-exercise snack with a 4-to-l gram ratio of carbohydrates to protein immediately following strength training; and a second snack one hour thereafter.
- Allow at least 48 hours between strength-training sessions that involve the same muscle groups.

Try It

Attend the school's fitness or recreation center and have an instructor or fitness trainer help you design a progressive resistance strength-training program. Train twice a week for the next 4 weeks. Thereafter, evaluate the results and write down your feelings about the program.

Pilates Exercise System

Pilates exercises have become increasingly popular in recent years. Previously, Pilates training was used primarily by dancers, but now this exercise modality is embraced by a large number of fitness participants, rehab patients, models, actors, and even professional athletes. Pilates studios, college courses, and classes at health clubs are available nationwide.

The Pilates training system was originally developed in the 1920s by German physical therapist Joseph Pilates. He designed the exercises to help strengthen the body's core by developing pelvic stability and abdominal control, coupled with focused breathing patterns.

Pilates exercises are performed either on a mat (floor) or with specialized equipment to help increase strength and flexibility of deep postural muscles. The intent is to improve muscle tone and length (a limber body), instead of increasing muscle size (hypertrophy). Pilates mat classes focus on body stability and proper body mechanics. The exercises are performed in a slow, controlled, precise manner. When performed properly, these exercises require intense concentration. Initially, Pilates training should be conducted under the supervision of certified instructors with extensive Pilates teaching experience.

Fitness goals of Pilates programs include better flexibility, muscle tone, posture, spinal support, body balance, low-back health, sports performance, and mind–body awareness. Individuals with loose or unstable joints benefit from Pilates because the exercises are designed to enhance joint stability. The Pilates program also is used to help lose weight, increase lean tissue, and manage stress. Although Pilates programs are quite popular, more research is required to corroborate the benefits attributed to this training system.

Stability Exercise Balls

A stability exercise ball is a large flexible and inflatable ball used for exercises that combine the principles of Pilates with core strength training. Stability exercises are specifically designed to develop abdominal, hip, chest, and spinal muscles by addressing core stabilization while the exerciser maintains a balanced position over the ball. Particular emphasis is placed on correct movement and maintenance of proper body alignment to involve as much of the core as possible. Although the primary objective is core strength and stability, many stability exercises can be performed to strengthen other body areas as well.

Stability exercises are thought to be more effective than similar exercises on the ground. For example, just sitting on the ball requires the use of stabilizing core muscles (including the rectus abdominis and the external and internal obliques) to keep the body from falling off the ball. Traditional strength-training exercises are primarily for strength and power development and do not contribute as much to body balance.

When performing stability exercises, choose a ball size based on your height. Your thighs should be parallel to the floor when you sit on the ball. A slightly larger ball may be used if you suffer from back problems. Several stability ball exercises are provided on pages 249–252. For best results, have a trained specialist teach you the proper technique and watch your form while you learn the exercises. Individuals who have a weak muscular system or poor balance or who are over the age of 65 should perform stability exercises under the supervision of a qualified trainer.

Exercise Safety Guidelines

As you prepare to design your strength-training program, keep the following guidelines in mind:

• Select exercises that will involve all major muscle groups: chest, shoulders, back, legs, arms, hip, and trunk.

• Select exercises that will strengthen the core. Use controlled movements and start with light-to-moderate resistances (later, athletes may use explosive movements with heavier resistances).

• Never lift weights alone. Always have someone work out with you in case you need a spotter or help with an injury. When you use free weights, one to two spotters are recommended for certain exercises (for example, bench press, squats, overhead press).

• Prior to lifting weights, warm up properly by performing a light- to moderate-intensity aerobic activity (5 to 7 minutes) and some gentle stretches for a few minutes.

• Use proper lifting technique for each exercise. The correct lifting technique will involve only those muscles and joints intended for a specific exercise. Involving other muscles and joints to "cheat" during the exercise to complete a repetition or to be able to lift a greater resistance decreases the long-term effectiveness of the exercise and can lead to injury (such as arching the back during the push-up, squat, or bench press exercises).

Proper lifting technique also implies performing the exercises in a controlled manner and throughout the entire range of motion. Perform each repetition in a rhythmic manner and at a moderate speed. Avoid fast and jerky movements, and do not throw the entire body into the lifting motion. Do not arch the back when lifting a weight.

• Maintain proper body balance while lifting. Proper balance involves good posture, a stable body position, and correct seat and arm/leg settings on exercise machines. Loss of balance places undue strain on smaller muscles and leads to injuries because of the heavy resistances suddenly placed on them.

In the early stages of a program, first-time lifters often struggle with bar control and balance when using free weights. This problem is overcome quickly with practice following a few training sessions.

• Exercise larger muscle groups (such as those in the chest, back, and legs) before exercising smaller muscle groups (arms, abdominals, ankles, neck). For example, the bench press exercise works the chest, shoulders, and back of the upper arms (triceps), whereas the triceps extension works the back of the upper arms only.

• Exercise opposing muscle groups for a balanced workout. When you work the chest (bench press), also work the back (rowing torso). If you work the biceps (arm curl), also work the triceps (triceps extension).

• Breathe naturally. Inhale during the eccentric phase (bringing the weight down), and exhale during the concentric phase (lifting or pushing the weight up). Practice proper breathing with lighter weights when you are learning a new exercise.

• Avoid holding your breath while straining to lift a weight. Holding your breath increases the pressure inside the chest and abdominal cavity greatly, making it nearly impossible for the blood in the veins to return to the heart. Although rare, a sudden high intrathoracic pressure may lead to dizziness, a blackout, a stroke, a heart attack, or a hernia.

• Based on the program selected, allow adequate recovery time between sets of exercises (see Table 7.5, page 222).

• If you experience unusual discomfort or pain, discontinue training. The high tension loads used in strength training can exacerbate potential injuries. Discomfort and pain are signals to stop and determine what's wrong. Be sure to evaluate your condition properly before you continue training.

• Use common sense on days when you feel fatigued or when you are performing sets to complete fatigue. Excessive fatigue affects lifting technique, body balance,

---

Core strength training A program designed to strengthen the abdominal, hip, and spinal muscles (the core of the body).

Pilates A training program that uses exercises designed to help strengthen the body's core by developing pelvic stability and abdominal control; exercises are coupled with focused breathing patterns.

muscles involved, and range of motion—all of which increase the risk for injury. A spotter is recommended when sets are performed to complete fatigue. The spotter's help through the most difficult part of the repetition will relieve undue stress on muscles, ligaments, and tendons—and help ensure you perform the exercise correctly.

- At the end of each strength-training workout, stretch out for a few minutes to help your muscles return to their normal resting length and to minimize muscle soreness and risk for injury.

Setting Up Your Own Strength-Training Program

The same pre-exercise guidelines outlined for cardiorespiratory endurance training apply to strength training (see Lab 1C, "Clearance for Exercise Participation," on pages 29–30). If you have any concerns about your present health status or ability to participate safely in strength training, consult a physician before you start. Strength training is not advised for people with advanced heart disease.

Before you proceed to write your strength-training program, you should determine your stage of change for this fitness component in Lab 7B at the end of the chapter. Next, if you are prepared to do so, and depending on the facilities available, you can choose one of the training programs outlined in this chapter (use Lab 7B). Once you begin your strength-training program, you may use the form provided in Figure 7.7 (page 230) to keep a record of your training sessions.

You should base the resistance, number of repetitions, and sets you use with your program on your current strength-fitness level and the amount of time that you have for your strength workout. If you are training for reasons other than general health fitness, review Table 7.5, page 222, for a summary of the guidelines.

Assess Your Behavior

Thomson NOW! *Log on to www.thomsonedu.com/login to assess your muscular strength and endurance and to track your strength activities.*

1. Are your strength levels sufficient to perform tasks of daily living (climbing stairs, carrying a backpack, opening jars, doing housework, mowing the yard) without requiring additional assistance or feeling unusually fatigued?
2. Do you regularly participate in a strength-training program that includes all major muscle groups of the body and do you perform at least one set of each exercise to near fatigue?

Assess Your Knowledge

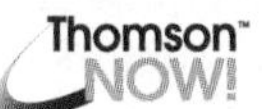

Log on to www.thomsonedu.com/login to assess your understanding of this chapter's topics by taking the Student Practice Test and exploring the modules recommended in your Personalized Study Plan.

1. The ability of a muscle to exert submaximal force repeatedly over time is known as
   a. muscular strength.
   b. plyometric training.
   c. muscular endurance.
   d. isokinetic training.
   e. isometric training.
2. In older adults, each additional pound of muscle tissue increases resting metabolism by
   a. 10 calories.
   b. 17 calories.
   c. 23 calories.
   d. 35 calories.
   e. 50 calories.
3. The Hand Grip Strength Test is an example of
   a. an isometric test.
   b. an isotonic test.
   c. a dynamic test.
   d. an isokinetic test.
   e. a plyometric test.
4. A 70 percentile rank places an individual in the ____________ fitness category.
   a. excellent
   b. good
   c. average
   d. fair
   e. poor

5. During an eccentric muscle contraction,
   a. the muscle shortens as it overcomes the resistance.
   b. there is little or no movement during the contraction.
   c. a joint has to move through the entire range of motion.
   d. the muscle lengthens as it contracts.
   e. the speed is kept constant throughout the range of motion.
6. The training concept stating that the demands placed on a system must be increased systematically and progressively over time to cause physiological adaptation is referred to as
   a. the overload principle.
   b. positive-resistance training.
   c. specificity of training.
   d. variable-resistance training.
   e. progressive resistance.
7. A set in strength training refers to
   a. the starting position for an exercise.
   b. the recovery time required between exercises.
   c. a given number of repetitions.
   d. the starting resistance used in an exercise.
   e. the sequence in which exercises are performed.
8. For health fitness, ACSM's recommendation is that a person should perform between
   a. 1 and 6 reps max.
   b. 4 and 10 reps max.
   c. 3 and 20 reps max.
   d. 8 and 12 reps max.
   e. 20 and 30 reps max.
9. Plyometric training frequently is used to help with performance in
   a. gymnastics.
   b. basketball.
   c. volleyball.
   d. sprinting.
   e. all of these sports.
10. The posterior deltoid, rhomboids, and trapezius muscles can be developed with the following exercise:
   a. bench press
   b. lat pull-down
   c. rotary torso
   d. squat
   e. rowing torso

Correct answers can be found at the back of the book.

Media Menu

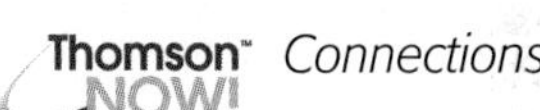

Connections

- Chart your achievements for strength tests.
- Check how well you understand the chapter's concepts.

Internet Connections

Muscle and Fitness

This comprehensive site features information on intermediate and advanced training techniques, with photographs and informative articles on the use of dietary supplements as well as the importance of mind–body activities to enhance your workout.
http://www.muscleandfitness.com/training/25

Strength Training Muscle Map & Explanation

This site provides an anatomical map of the body's muscles. Click on the muscle for exercises designed to specifically strengthen that muscle, complete with a video and safety information.
http://www.global-fitness.com/strength/s_musclemap.html

Sportspecific.com

Inside SportSpecific.com, you'll find more than 5,370 pages jam-packed with sports training programs, exercises, interviews, forums, and much more. The site includes sport-specific training programs, a sports nutrition section, animated sports training exercises, exercise spreadsheets for sets and reps, case studies, and a variety of articles.
http://www.sportspecific.com

Notes

1. C. Castaneda et al., "A Randomized Controlled Trial of Resistance Exercise Training to Improve Glycemic Control in Older Adults with Type 2 Diabetes," *Diabetes Care* 25 (2002): 2335–2341.
2. W. W. Campbell, M. C. Crim, V. R. Young, and W. J. Evans, "Increased Energy Requirements and Changes in Body Composition with Resistance Training in Older Adults," *American Journal of Clinical Nutrition* 60 (1994): 167–175.
3. W. J. Evans, "Exercise, Nutrition and Aging," *Journal of Nutrition* 122 (1992): 796–801.

4. P. E. Allsen, *Strength Training: Beginners, Body Builders and Athletes* (Dubuque, IA: Kendall/Hunt, 2003).
5. See note 2, Campbell et al.
6. American College of Sports Medicine, "Progression Models in Resistance Training for Healthy Adults," *Medicine and Science in Sports and Exercise* 34 (2002): 364–380.
7. J. K. Kraemer and N. A. Ratamess, "Fundamentals of Resistance Training: Progression and Exercise Prescription," *Medicine and Science in Sports and Exercise* 36 (2004): 674–688.
8. B. M. Hather, P. A. Tesch, P. Buchanan, and G. A. Dudley, "Influence of Eccentric Actions on Skeletal Muscle Adaptations to Resistance Training," *Acta Physiologica Scandinavica* 143 (1991): 177–185; C. B. Ebbeling and P. M. Clarkson, "Exercise-Induced Muscle Damage and Adaptation," *Sports Medicine* 7 (1989): 207–234.
9. S. P. Messier and M. Dill, "Alterations in Strength and Maximal Oxygen Uptake Consequent to Nautilus Circuit Weight Training," *Research Quarterly for Exercise and Sport* 56 (1985): 345–351; T. V. Pipes, "Variable Resistance Versus Constant Resistance Strength Training in Adult Males," *European Journal of Applied Physiology* 39 (1978): 27–35.
10. W. W. K. Hoeger, D. R. Hopkins, S. L. Barette, and D. F. Hale, "Relationship Between Repetitions and Selected Percentages of One Repetition Maximum: A Comparison Between Untrained and Trained Males and Females," *Journal of Applied Sport Science Research* 4, no. 2 (1990): 47–51.
11. American College of Sports Medicine, *ACSM's Guidelines for Exercise Testing and Prescription* (Baltimore: Williams & Wilkins, 2006).
12. See note 11, ACSM.
13. See note 6, ACSM.
14. See note 6, ACSM.
15. Gatorade Sports Science Institute, "Core Strength Training," *Sports Science Exchange Roundtable* 13, no. 1 (2002): 1–4.

Suggested Readings

American College of Sports Medicine. "Progression Models in Resistance Training for Healthy Adults." *Medicine and Science in Sports and Exercise* 34 (2002): 364–380.

Hesson, J. L. *Weight Training for Life*. Belmont, CA: Wadsworth/Thomson Learning, 2005.

Heyward, V. H. *Advanced Fitness Assessment and Exercise Prescription*. Champaign, IL: Human Kinetic Press, 2002.

Hoeger, W. W. K., and S. A. Hoeger. *Lifetime Physical Fitness and Wellness: A Personalized Program*. Belmont, CA: Wadsworth/Thomson Learning, 2005.

Kraemer, J. K., and N. A. Ratamess. "Fundamentals of Resistance Training: Progression and Exercise Prescription." *Medicine and Science in Sports and Exercise* 36 (2004): 674–688.

Liemohn, W., and G. Pariser. "Core Strength: Implications for Fitness and Low Back Pain." *ACSM's Health and Fitness Journal* 6, no. 5 (2002): 10–16.

Mannie, K. "Barbells Versus Machines: Balancing a Weighty Issue." *Coach and Athletic Director* 67 (1998): 6–7.

Volek, J. "Influence of Nutrition on Responses to Resistance Training." *Medicine and Science in Sports and Exercise* 36 (2004): 689–696.

Wescott, W. L., and T. R. Baechle. *Strength Training for Seniors*. Champaign, IL: Human Kinetic Press, 1999.

FIGURE 7.6 Major muscles of the human body.

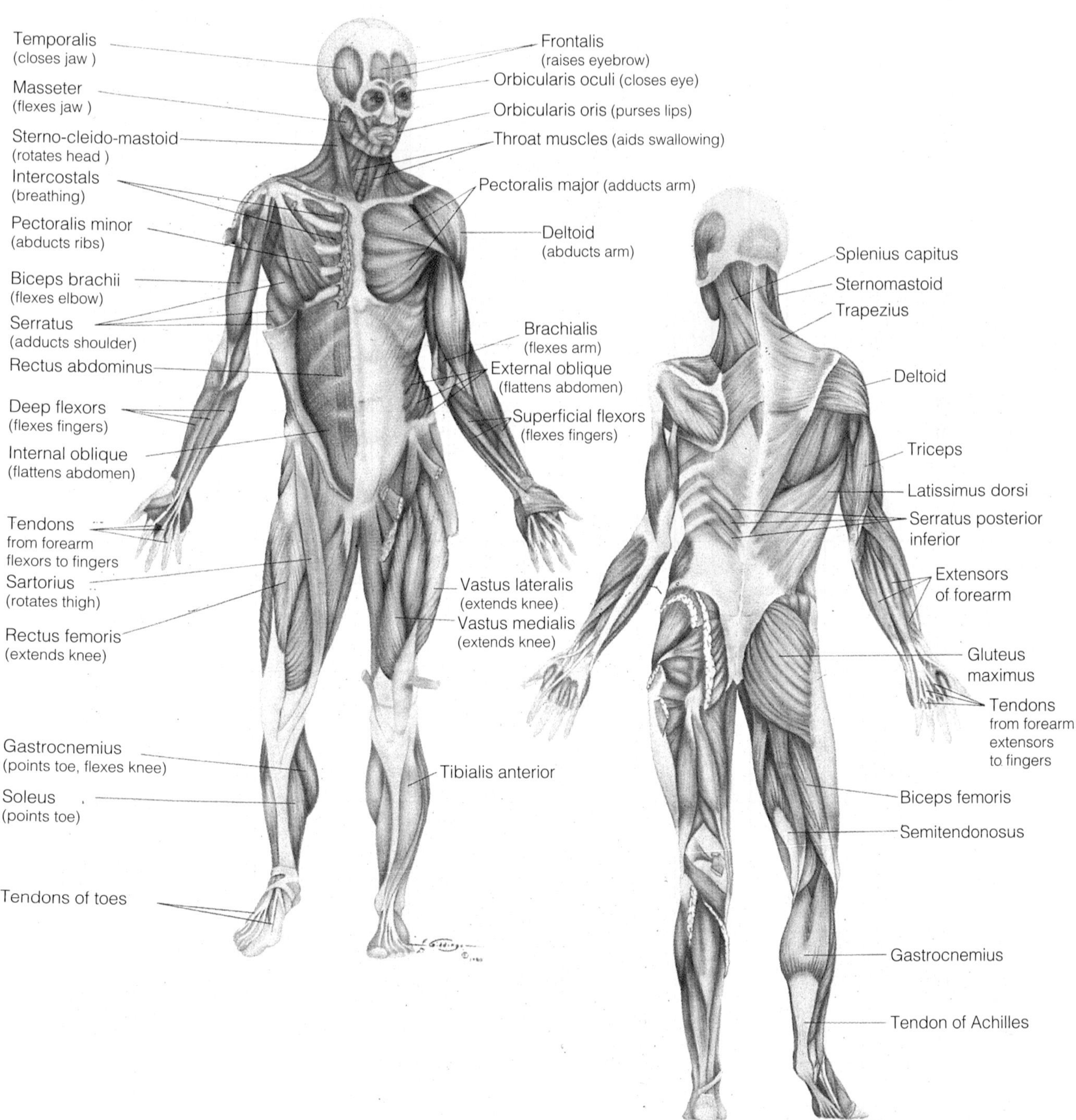

From Basic Physiology and Anatomy by Ellen E. Chaffee and Ivan M. Lytle. Reprinted by permission of F. D. Giddings.

Exercise 36 Back Extension

Action Place your feet under the ankle rollers and the hips over the padded seat. Start with the trunk in a flexed position and the arms crossed over the chest (a). Slowly extend the trunk to a horizontal position (b), hold the extension for 2 to 5 seconds, then slowly flex (lower) the trunk to the original position.

Muscles Developed Erector spinae, gluteus maximus, and quadratus lumborum (lower back)

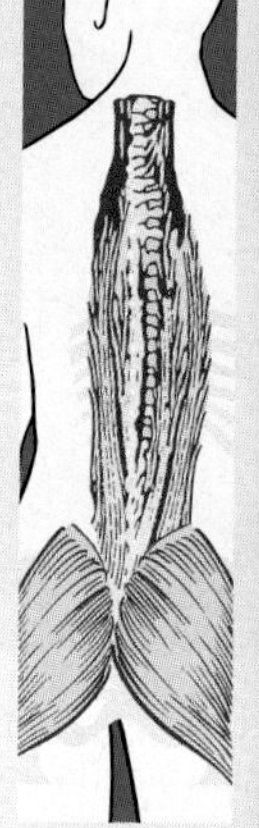
Back

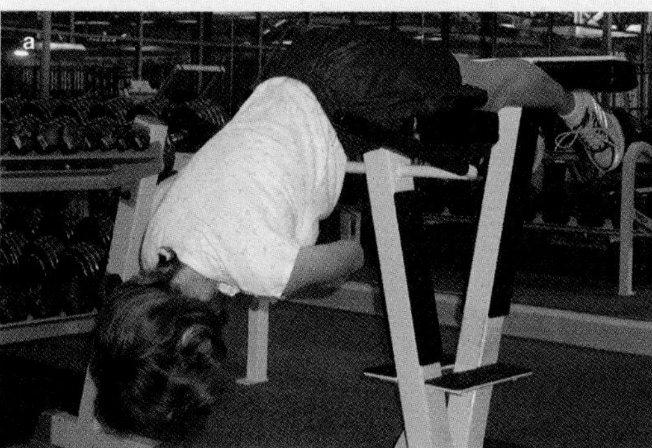

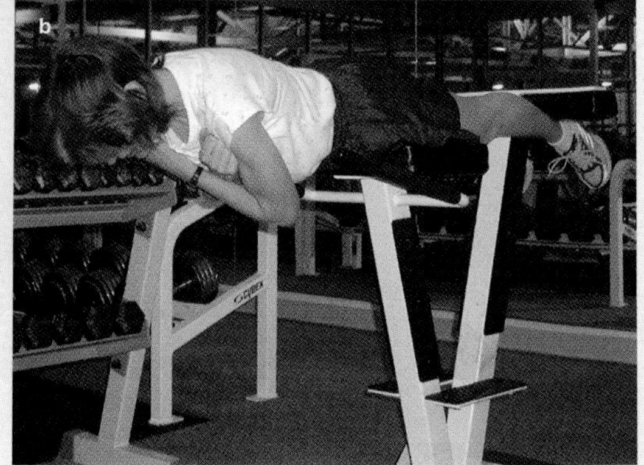

Photos © Fitness & Wellness, Inc.

Exercise 37 Lateral Trunk Flexion

Action Lie sideways on the padded seat with the right foot under the right side of the padded ankle pad (right knee slightly bent) and the left foot stabilized on the vertical bar. Cross the arms over the abdomen or chest and start with the body in a straight line. Raise (flex) your upper body about 30 to 40° and then slowly return to the starting position.

Muscles Developed Erector spinae, rectus abdominus, internal and external abdominal obliques, quadratus lumborum, gluteal muscles

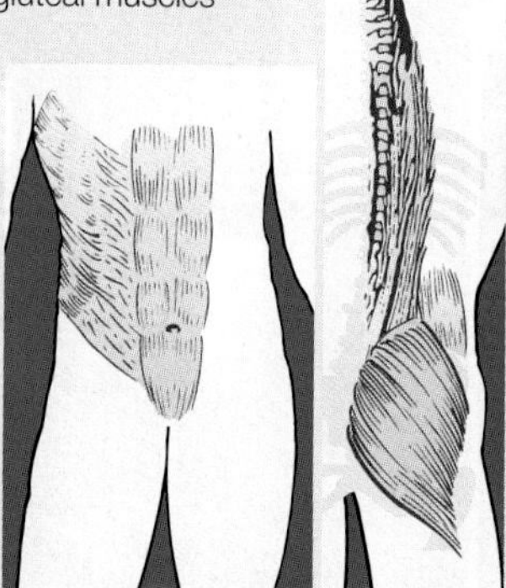
Front

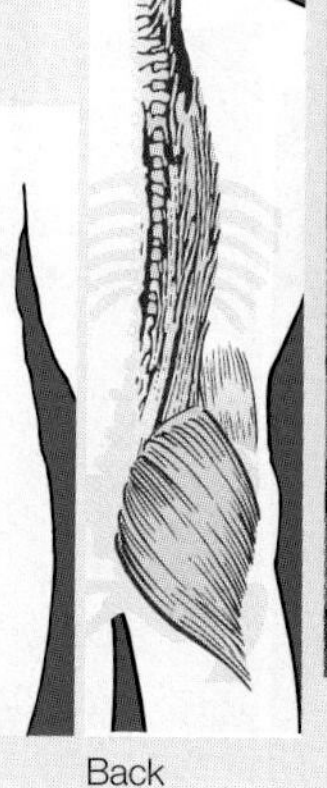
Back

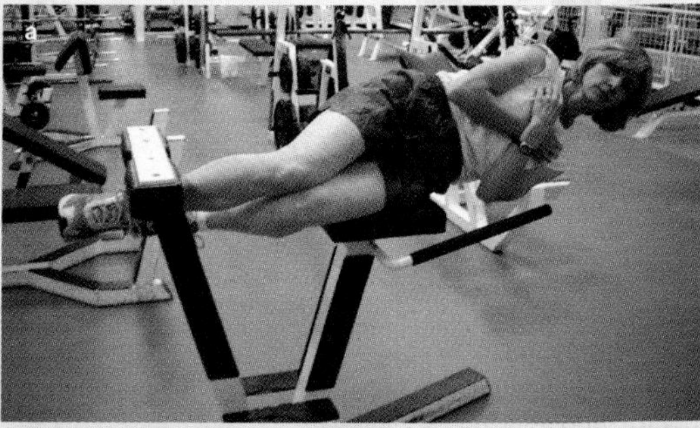

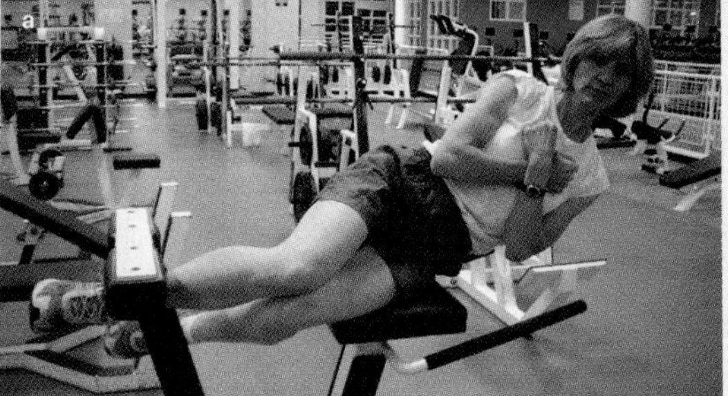

Photos © Fitness & Wellness, Inc.

Stability Ball Exercises

Exercise 38 The Plank

Action Place your knees or feet (increased difficulty) on the ball and raise your body off the floor to a horizontal position. Pull the abdominal muscles in and hold the body in a straight line for 5 to 10 seconds. Repeat the exercise 3 to 5 times.

Muscles Involved Abdominals, erector spinae, lower back, hip flexors, gluteal, quadriceps, hamstrings, chest, shoulder, and triceps

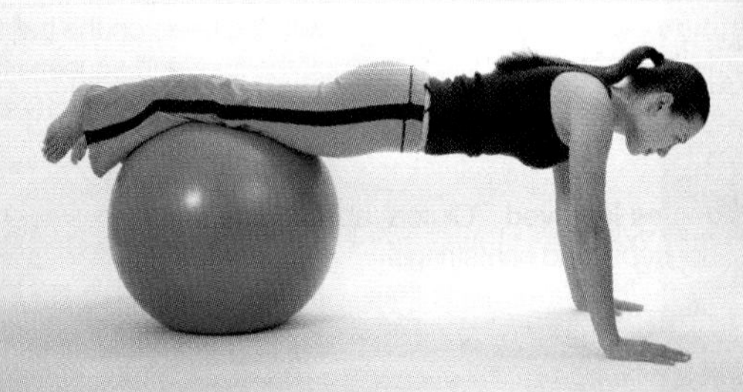

© Fitness & Wellness, Inc.

Exercise 39 Abdominal Crunches

Action On your back and with the feet slightly separated, lie with the ball under your back and shoulder blades. Cross the arms over your chest (a). Press your lower back into the ball and crunch up 20 to 30°. Keep your neck and shoulders in line with your trunk (b). Repeat the exercise 10 to 20 times (you may also do an oblique crunch by rotating the ribcage to the opposite hip at the end of the crunch [c]).

Muscles Involved Rectus abdominus, internal and external abdominal obliques

a

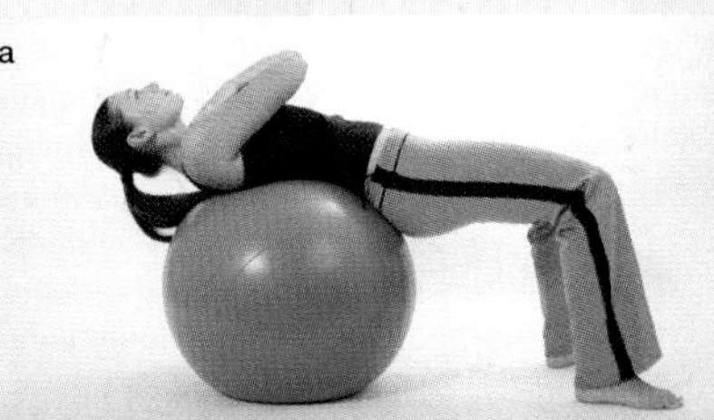

b

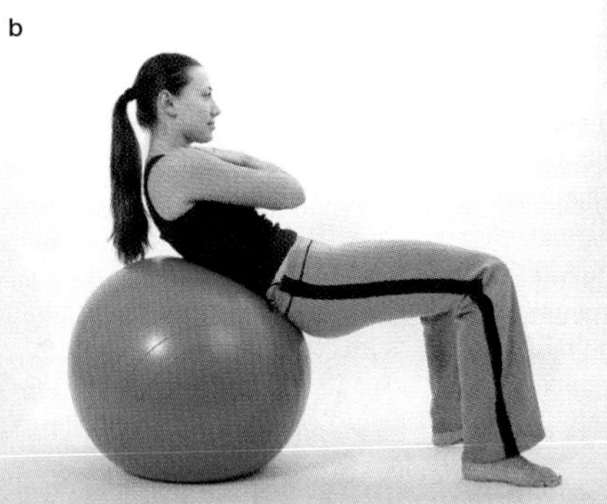

c

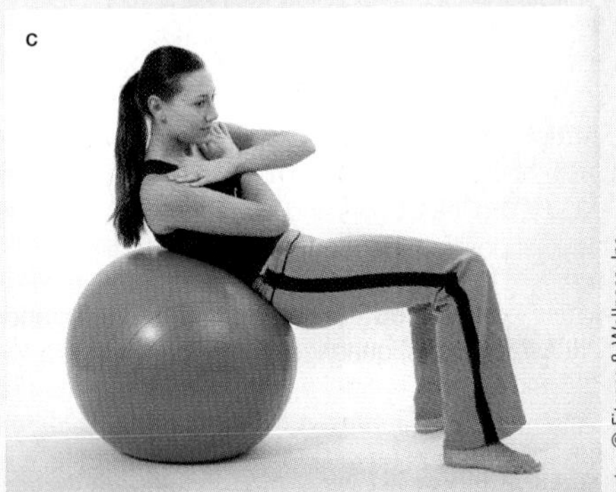

Photos © Fitness & Wellness, Inc.

Exercise 40 Supine Bridge

Action With the feet slightly separated and knees bent, lie with your neck and upper back on the ball; hands placed on the abdomen. Gently squeeze the gluteal muscles while raising your hips off the floor until the upper legs and trunk reach a straight line. Hold this position for 5 to 10 seconds. Repeat the exercise 3 to 5 times.

Muscles Involved Gluteal, abdominals, lower back, hip flexors, quadriceps, and hamstrings

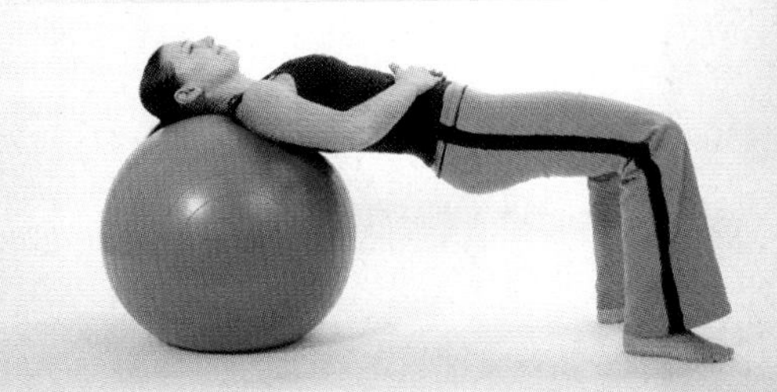

© Fitness & Wellness, Inc.

III. Muscular Strength and Endurance Test

Perform the Muscular Strength and Endurance Test according to the procedure outlined in Figure 7.4, page 215. Record the results, fitness category, and points in the appropriate blanks provided below.

Body weight: ______ lbs.

Lift	Percent of Body Weight (pounds)		Resistance	Repetitions
	Men	Women		
Lat pull-down	.70	.45		
Leg extension	.65	.50		
Bench press	.75	.45		
Bent-leg curl-up or abdominal crunch	NA*	NA*		
Leg curl	.32	.25		
Arm curl	.35	.18		

*Not applicable—no resistance required. Use test described in Figure 7.3, pages 213–214.

IV. Muscular Strength and Endurance Goals

Indicate the muscular strength/endurance category that you would like to achieve by the end of the term: ______

Briefly state your feelings about your current strength level and indicate how you are planning to achieve your strength objective:

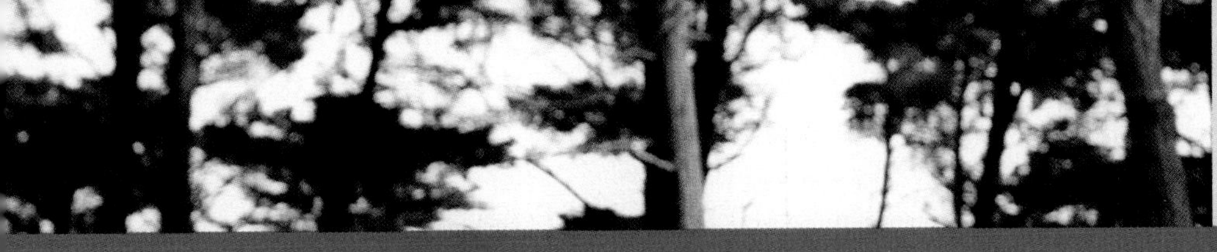

Muscular Flexibility

CHAPTER 8

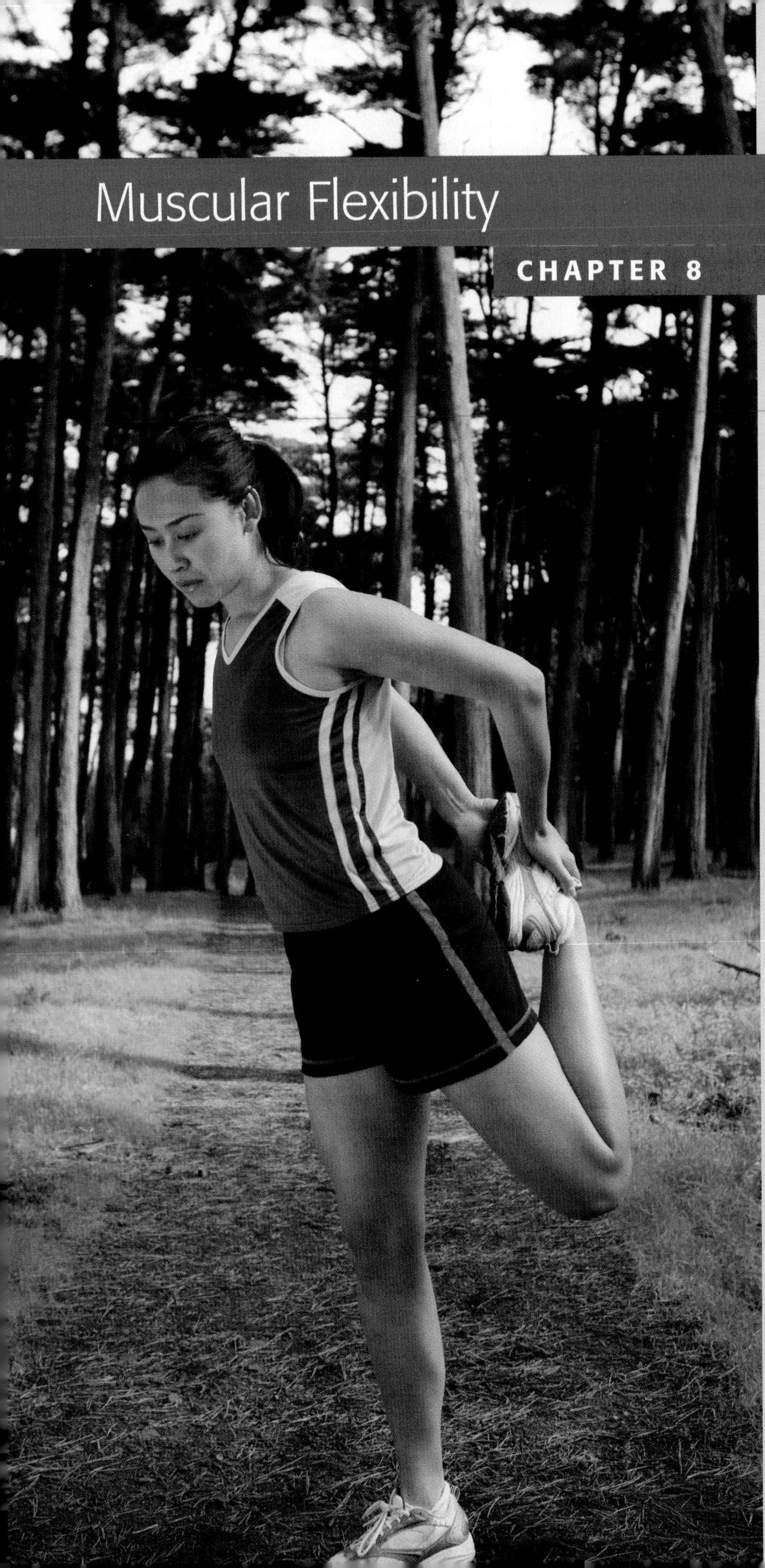

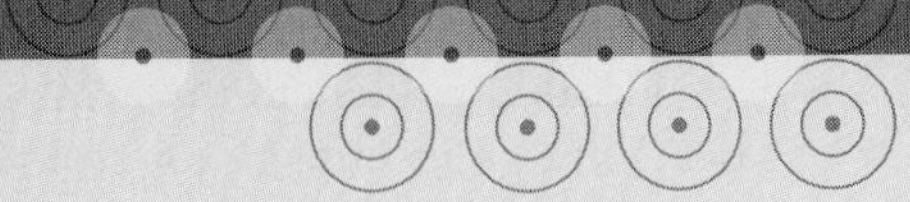

OBJECTIVES

- Explain the importance of muscular flexibility to adequate fitness and preventive health care.
- Identify the factors that affect muscular flexibility.
- Explain the health-fitness benefits of stretching.
- Become familiar with a battery of tests to assess overall body flexibility (Modified Sit-and-Reach Test, Total Body Rotation Test, Shoulder Rotation Test).
- Be able to interpret flexibility test results according to health-fitness and physical-fitness standards.
- Learn the principles that govern development of muscular flexibility.
- List some exercises that may cause injury.
- Become familiar with a program for preventing and rehabilitating low-back pain.

Thomson™ NOW! Go to www.thomsonedu.com/login to:

- Create your personal flexibility profile.
- Check how well you understand the chapter's concepts.

Photo © Drew Kelly/Getty Images

Most people who exercise don't take the time to stretch, and many who do stretch don't stretch properly. When joints are not regularly moved through their normal range of motion, muscles and ligaments shorten in time, and flexibility decreases. Most fitness participants underestimate and overlook the contribution of good muscular flexibility to overall fitness and preventive health care.

Flexibility refers to the achievable range of motion at a joint or group of joints without causing injury. Some muscular/skeletal problems and injuries are related to a lack of flexibility. In daily life, we often have to make rapid or strenuous movements we are not accustomed to making. Abruptly forcing a tight muscle beyond its achievable range of motion may lead to injury.

A decline in flexibility can cause poor posture and subsequent aches and pains that lead to limited and painful joint movement. Inordinate tightness is uncomfortable and debilitating. Approximately 80 percent of all low-back problems in the United States stem from improper alignment of the vertebral column and pelvic girdle, a direct result of inflexible and weak muscles. This backache syndrome costs U.S. industry billions of dollars each year in lost productivity, health services, and worker compensation.

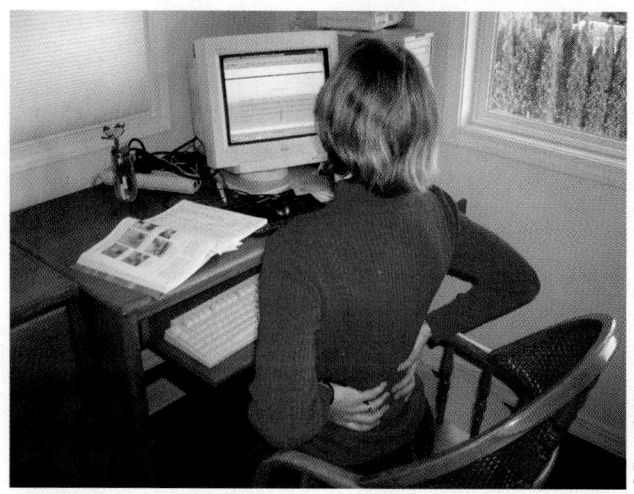

Excessive sitting and lack of physical activity lead to chronic back pain.

Benefits of Good Flexibility

Improving and maintaining good range of motion in the joints enhances the quality of life. Good flexibility promotes healthy muscles and joints. Improving elasticity of muscles and connective tissue around joints enables greater freedom of movement and augments the individual's ability to participate in many types of sports and recreational activities. Adequate flexibility also makes activities of daily living such as turning, lifting, and bending much easier to perform. A person must take care, however, not to overstretch joints. Too much flexibility leads to unstable and loose joints, which may increase injury rate, including joint dislocation and **subluxation.**

Taking part in a regular **stretching** program increases circulation to the muscle(s) being stretched, prevents low-back and other spinal column problems, improves and maintains good postural alignment, promotes proper and graceful body movement, improves personal appearance and self-image, and helps to develop and maintain motor skills throughout life.

Flexibility exercises have been prescribed successfully to treat **dysmenorrhea**[1] (painful menstruation), general neuromuscular tension (stress), and knots (trigger points) in muscles and fascia. Regular stretching helps decrease the aches and pains caused by psychological stress and contributes to a decrease in anxiety, blood pressure, and breathing rate.[2] Stretching also helps relieve muscle cramps encountered at rest or during participation in exercise.

Mild stretching exercises in conjunction with calisthenics are helpful in warm-up routines to prepare for more vigorous aerobic or strength-training exercises, and in cool-down routines following exercise to facilitate the return to a normal resting state. Fatigued muscles tend to contract to a shorter-than-average resting length, and stretching exercises help fatigued muscles reestablish their normal resting length.

Flexibility in Older Adults

Similar to muscular strength, good range of motion is critical in older life (see "Exercise and Aging" in Chapter 9). Because of decreased flexibility, older adults lose mobility and may be unable to perform simple daily tasks such as bending forward or turning. Many older adults cannot turn their head or rotate their trunk to look over their shoulder but, rather, must step around 90° to 180° to see behind them. Adequate flexibility is also important in driving. Individuals who lose range of motion with age are unable to look over their shoulder to switch lanes or to parallel-park, which increases the risk for automobile accidents.

Physical activity and exercise can be hampered severely by lack of good range of motion. Because of the pain during activity, older people who have tight hip flexors (muscles) cannot jog or walk very far. A vicious circle ensues, because the condition usually worsens with further inactivity. Lack of flexibility also may be a cause of falls and subsequent injury in older adults. A simple stretching program can alleviate or prevent this problem and help people return to an exercise program.

Factors Affecting Flexibility

The total range of motion around a joint is highly specific and varies from one joint to another (hip, trunk, shoulder), as well as from one individual to the next. Muscular flexibility relates primarily to genetic factors and to physical activity. Joint structure (shape of the bones), joint cartilage, ligaments, tendons, muscles, skin, tissue injury, and adipose tissue (fat)—all influence range of motion about a joint. Body temperature, age, and gender also affect flexibility.

The range of motion about a given joint depends mostly on the structure of that joint. Greater range of motion, however, can be attained through plastic and elastic elongation. **Plastic elongation** is the permanent lengthening of soft tissue. Even though joint capsules, ligaments, and tendons are basically nonelastic, they can undergo plastic elongation. This permanent lengthening, accompanied by increased range of motion, is best attained through slow-sustained stretching exercises.

Elastic elongation is the temporary lengthening of soft tissue. Muscle tissue has elastic properties and responds to stretching exercises by undergoing elastic or temporary lengthening. Elastic elongation increases extensibility, the ability to stretch the muscles.

Changes in muscle temperature can increase or decrease flexibility by as much as 20 percent. Individuals who warm up properly have better flexibility than people who do not. Cool temperatures have the opposite effect, impeding range of motion. Because of the effects of temperature on muscular flexibility, many people prefer to do their stretching exercises after the aerobic phase of their workout. Aerobic activities raise body temperature, facilitating plastic elongation.

Another factor that influences flexibility is the amount of adipose (fat) tissue in and around joints and muscle tissue. Excess adipose tissue will increase resistance to movement, and the added bulk also hampers joint mobility because of the contact between body surfaces.

On the average, women have better flexibility than men do, and they seem to retain this advantage throughout life. Aging does decrease the extensibility of soft tissue, though, resulting in less flexibility in both sexes.

The most significant contributor to lower flexibility is sedentary living. With less physical activity, muscles lose their elasticity and tendons and ligaments tighten and shorten. Inactivity also tends to be accompanied by an increase in adipose tissue, which further decreases the range of motion around a joint. Finally, injury to muscle tissue and tight skin from excessive scar tissue have negative effects on range of motion.

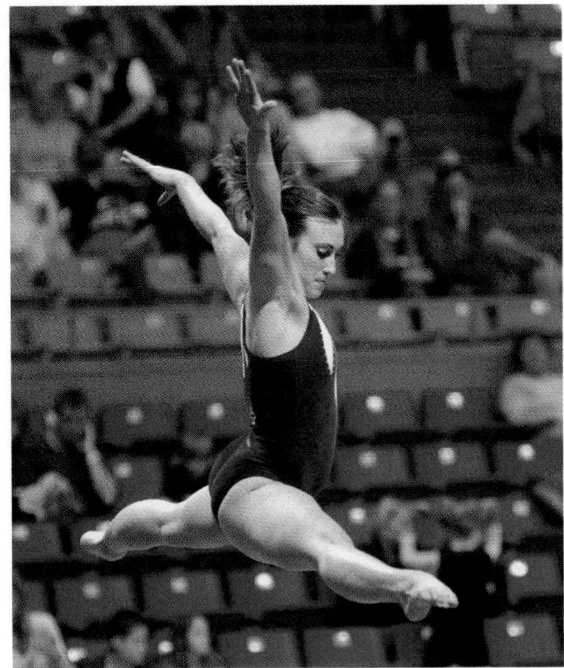

Adequate flexibility helps to develop and maintain sports skill throughout life.

Assessment of Flexibility

Many flexibility tests developed over the years were specific to certain sports or not practical for the general population. Their application in health and fitness programs was limited. For example, the Front-to-Rear Splits Test and the Bridge-Up Test had applications in sports such as gymnastics and several track-and-field events, but they did not represent actions that most people encounter in daily life.

Because of the lack of practical flexibility tests, most health and fitness centers rely strictly on the Sit-and-Reach Test as an indicator of flexibility. This test measures flexibility of the hamstring muscles (back of the thigh) and, to a lesser extent, the lower back muscles.

Flexibility is joint-specific. This means that a lot of flexibility in one joint does not necessarily indicate that other joints are just as flexible. Therefore, the Total Body Rotation Test and the Shoulder Rotation Test—indicators of the ability to perform everyday move-

---

Flexibility The achievable range of motion at a joint or group of joints without causing injury.

Subluxation Partial dislocation of a joint.

Stretching Moving the joints beyond the accustomed range of motion.

Dysmenorrhea Painful menstruation.

Plastic elongation Permanent lengthening of soft tissue.

Elastic elongation Temporary lengthening of soft tissue.

FIGURE 8.1 Procedure for the modified Sit-and-Reach Test.

To perform this test, you will need the Acuflex I* Sit-and-Reach Flexibility Tester, or you may simply place a yardstick on top of a box 12" high.

1. Warm up properly before the first trial.
2. Remove your shoes for the test. Sit on the floor with the hips, back, and head against a wall, the legs fully extended, and the bottom of the feet against the Acuflex I or sit-and-reach box.
3. Place the hands one on top of the other and reach forward as far as possible without letting the head and back come off the wall (the shoulders may be rounded as much as possible, but neither the head nor the back should come off the wall at this time). The technician then can slide the reach indicator on the Acuflex I (or yardstick) along the top of the box until the end of the indicator touches the participant's fingers. The indicator then must be held firmly in place throughout the rest of the test.

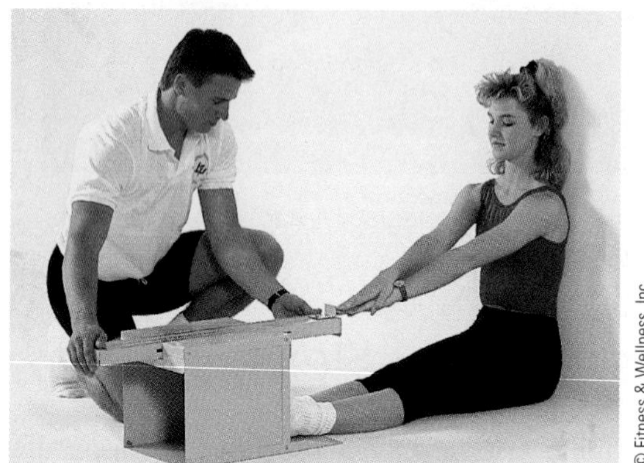

© Fitness & Wellness, Inc.

Determining the starting position for the Modified Sit-and-Reach Test.

4. Now your head and back can come off the wall. Gradually reach forward three times, the third time stretching forward as far as possible on the indicator (or yardstick) and holding the final position for at least 2 seconds. Be sure that during the test you keep the backs of the knees flat against the floor.
5. Record the final number of inches reached to the nearest ½".

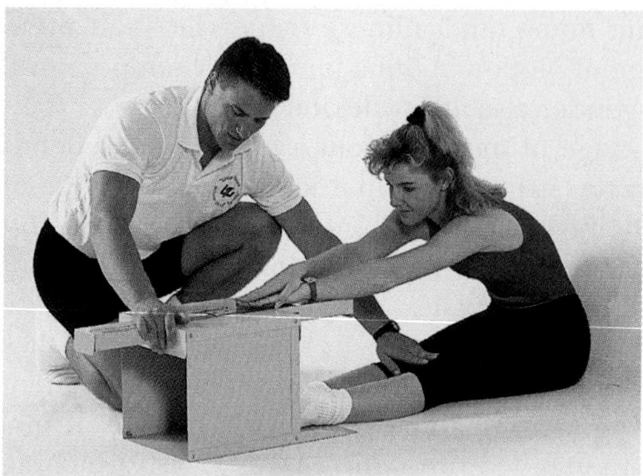

© Fitness & Wellness, Inc.

Modified Sit-and-Reach Test.

You are allowed two trials, and an average of the two scores is used as the final test score. The respective percentile ranks and fitness categories for this test are given in Tables 8.1 and 8.4.

*The Acuflex I Flexibility Tester for the Modified Sit-and-Reach Test can be obtained from Figure Finder Collection, Novel Products, P. O. Box 408, Rockton, IL 61072-0480. Phone: 800-323-5143, Fax 815-624-4866.

ments such as reaching, bending, and turning—are included to determine your flexibility profile.

The Sit-and-Reach Test has been modified from the traditional test to take length of arms and legs into consideration in determining the score (see Figure 8.1). In the original Sit-and-Reach Test, the 15-inch mark of the yardstick used to measure flexibility was always set at the edge of the box where the feet are placed. This does not take into consideration an individual with long arms and/or short legs or one with short arms and/or long legs.[3] All other factors being equal, an individual with longer arms or shorter legs, or both, receives a better rating because of the structural advantage.

The procedures and norms for the flexibility tests are described in Figures 8.1, 8.2, and 8.3 and Tables 8.1, 8.2, and 8.3. The flexibility test results in these three tables are provided in both inches and centimeters (cm). Be sure to use the proper column to read your percentile score based on your test results. For the flexibility profile, you should take all three tests. You will be able to assess your flexibility profile in Lab 8A. Because of the specificity of flexibility, pinpointing an "ideal" level of flexibility is difficult. Nevertheless, flexibility is important to health and independent living, so an assessment will give an indication of your current level of flexibility.

Interpreting Flexibility Test Results

After obtaining your scores and fitness ratings for each test, you can determine the fitness category for each flexibility test using the guidelines given in Table 8.4. You also should look up the number of points assigned for each fitness category in this table. The overall flexibility fitness category is obtained by totaling the number of points from all three tests and using the ratings given in Table 8.5. Record your results in Lab 8A.

Evaluating Body Posture

Good posture enhances personal appearance, self-image, confidence, improves balance and endurance, protects against misalignment-related pains and aches, prevents falls, and enhances your overall sense of well-being.[4] The relationship between different body parts is the essence of posture.

FIGURE 8.2 Procedure for the Total Body Rotation Test.

An Acuflex II* Total Body Rotation Flexibility Tester or a measuring scale with a sliding panel is needed to administer this test. The Acuflex II or scale is placed on the wall at shoulder height and should be adjustable to accommodate individual differences in height. If you need to build your own scale, use two measuring tapes and glue them above and below the sliding panel centered at the 15" mark. Each tape should be at least 30" long. If no sliding panel is available, simply tape the measuring tapes onto a wall oriented in opposite directions as shown below. A line also must be drawn on the floor and centered with the 15" mark.

1. Warm up properly before beginning this test.
2. Stand with one side toward the wall, an arm's length away from the wall, with the feet straight ahead, slightly separated, and the toes touching the center line drawn on the floor. Hold out the arm away from the wall horizontally from the body, making a fist with the hand. The Acuflex II measuring scale (or tapes) should be shoulder height at this time.
3. Rotate the trunk, the extended arm going backward (always maintaining a horizontal plane) and making contact with the panel, gradually sliding it forward as far as possible. If no panel is available, slide the fist alongside the tapes as far as possible. Hold the final position at least 2 seconds. Position the hand with the little finger side forward during the entire sliding movement. **Proper hand position is crucial. Many people attempt to open the hand, or push with extended fingers, or slide the panel with the knuckles—none of which is acceptable.** During the test the knees can be bent slightly, but **the feet cannot be moved or rotated**—they must point forward. The body must be kept as straight (vertical) as possible.
4. Conduct the test on either the right or the left side of the body. Perform two trials on the selected side. Record the farthest point reached, measured to the nearest half inch and held for at least 2 seconds. Use the average of the two trials as the final test score. Refer to Tables 8.2 and 8.4 to determine the percentile rank and flexibility fitness category for this test.

*The Acuflex II Flexibility Tester for the Total Body Rotation Test can be obtained from Figure Finder Collection, Novel Products, P.O. Box 408, Rockton, IL 61072-0408. Phone: 800-323-5143, Fax 815-624-4866.

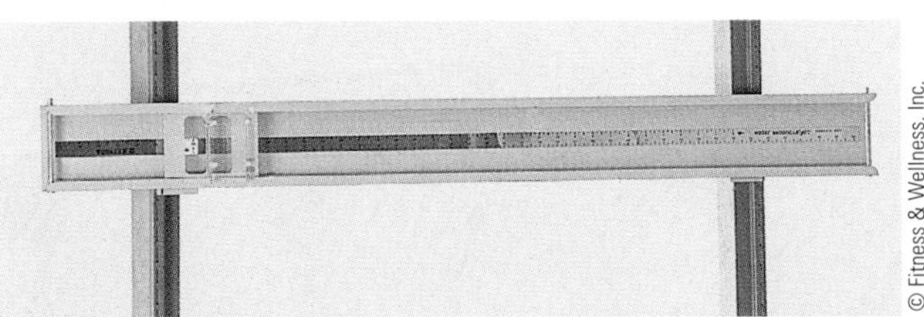

Acuflex II measuring device for the Total Body Rotation Test.

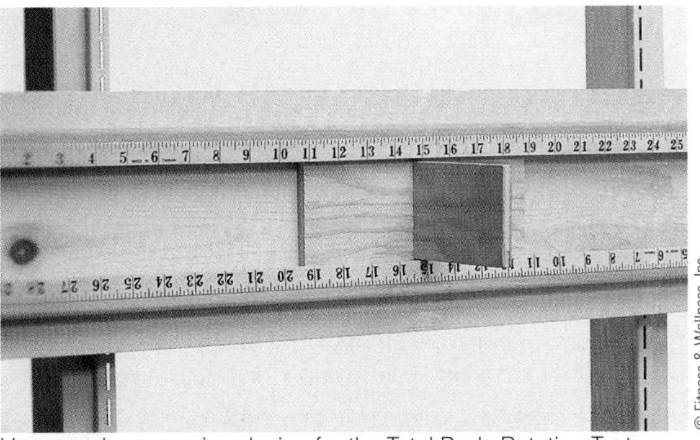

Homemade measuring device for the Total Body Rotation Test.

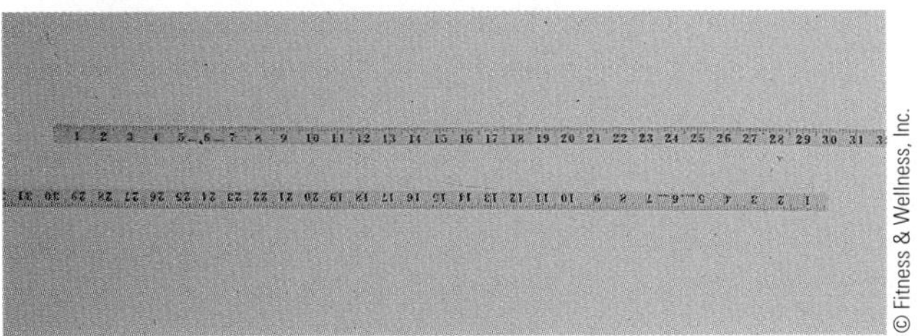

Measuring tapes for the Total Body Rotation Test.

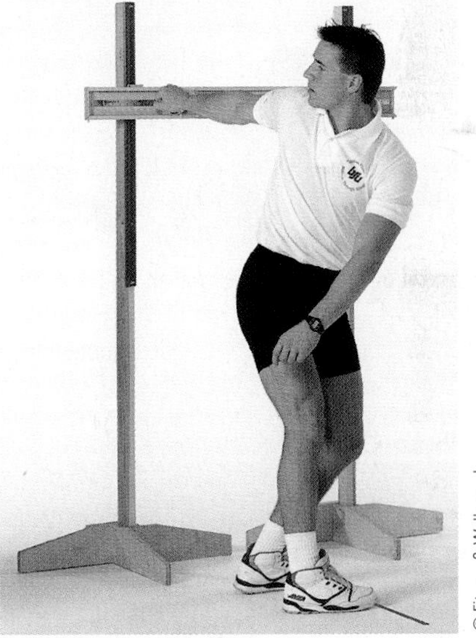

Total Body Rotation Test.

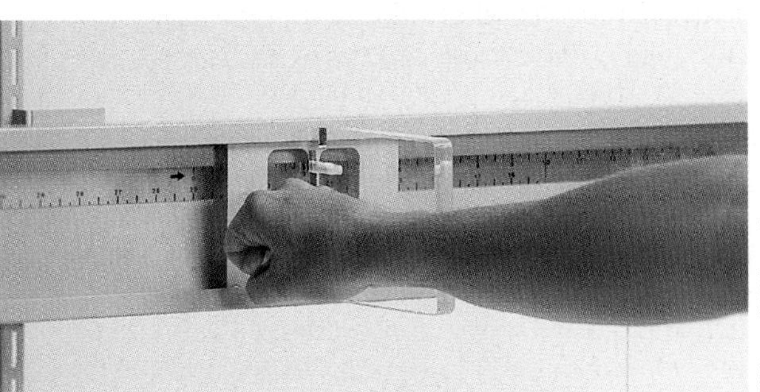

Proper hand position for the Total Body Rotation Test.

FIGURE 8.3 Procedure for the shoulder rotation test.

This test can be done using the Acuflex III* Flexibility Tester, which consists of a shoulder caliper and a measuring device for shoulder rotation. If this equipment is unavailable, you can construct your own device quite easily. The caliper can be built with three regular yardsticks. Nail and glue two of the yardsticks at one end at a 90° angle, and use the third one as the sliding end of the caliper. Construct the rotation device by placing a 60" measuring tape on an aluminum or wood stick, starting at about 6" or 7" from the end of the stick.

1. Warm up before the test.
2. Using the shoulder caliper, measure the biacromial width to the nearest 1/4" (use the top scale on the Acuflex III). Measure biacromial width between the lateral edges of the acromion processes of the shoulders.
3. Place the Acuflex III or homemade device behind the back and use a reverse grip (thumbs out) to hold on to the device. Place the index finger of the right hand next to the zero point of the scale or tape (lower scale on the Acuflex III) and hold it firmly in place throughout the test. Place the left hand on the other end of the measuring device wherever comfortable.
4. Standing straight up and extending both arms to full length, with elbows locked, slowly bring the measuring device over the head until it reaches about forehead level. For subsequent trials, depending on the resistance encountered when rotating the shoulders, move the left grip in ½" to 1" at a time, and repeat the task until you no longer can rotate the shoulders without undue strain or starting to bend the elbows. Always keep the right-hand grip against the zero point of the scale. Measure the last successful trial to the nearest ½". Take this measurement at the inner edge of the left hand on the side of the little finger.
5. Determine the final score for this test by subtracting the biacromial width from the best score (shortest distance) between both hands on the rotation test. For example, if the best score is 35" and the biacromial width is 15", the final score is 20" (35 − 15 = 20). Using Tables 8.3 and 8.4, determine the percentile rank and flexibility fitness category for this test.

*The Acuflex III Flexibility Tester for the Shoulder Rotation Test can be obtained from Figure Finder Collection, Novel Products, Inc., P. O. Box 408, Rockton, IL 61072-0408. Phone: (800) 323-5143, Fax 815-624-4866.

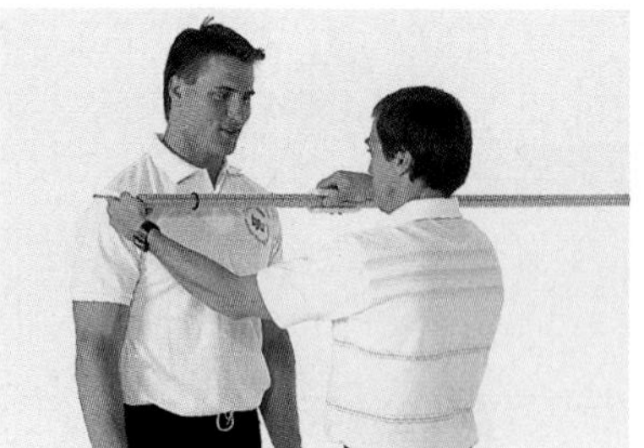
Measuring biacromial width.

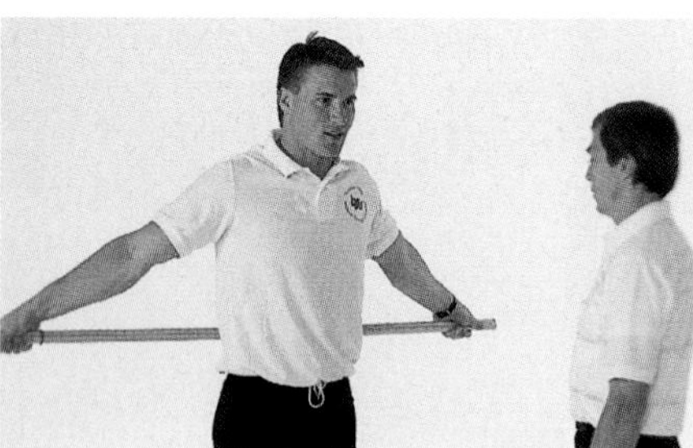
Starting position for the shoulder rotation test (note the reverse grip used for this test).

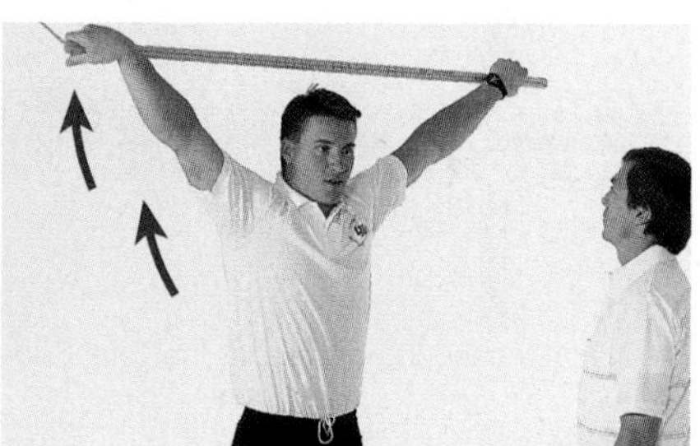
Shoulder rotation test.

TABLE 8.1 Percentile Ranks for the Modified Sit-and-Reach Test

	Age Category—Men							
Percentile	≤18		19–35		36–49		≥50	
Rank	in.	cm	in.	cm	in.	cm	in.	cm
99	20.8	52.8	20.1	51.1	18.9	48.0	16.2	41.1
95	19.6	49.8	18.9	48.0	18.2	46.2	15.8	40.1
90	18.2	46.2	17.2	43.7	16.1	40.9	15.0	38.1
80	17.8	45.2	17.0	43.2	14.6	37.1	13.3	33.8
70	16.0	40.6	15.8	40.1	13.9	35.3	12.3	31.2
60	15.2	38.6	15.0	38.1	13.4	34.0	11.5	29.2
50	14.5	36.8	14.4	36.6	12.6	32.0	10.2	25.9
40	14.0	35.6	13.5	34.3	11.6	29.5	9.7	24.6
30	13.4	34.0	13.0	33.0	10.8	27.4	9.3	23.6
20	11.8	30.0	11.6	29.5	9.9	25.1	8.8	22.4
10	9.5	24.1	9.2	23.4	8.3	21.1	7.8	19.8
05	8.4	21.3	7.9	20.1	7.0	17.8	7.2	18.3
01	7.2	18.3	7.0	17.8	5.1	13.0	4.0	10.2

	Age Category—Women							
Percentile	≤18		19–35		36–49		≥50	
Rank	in.	cm	in.	cm	in.	cm	in.	cm
99	22.6	57.4	21.0	53.3	19.8	50.3	17.2	43.7
95	19.5	49.5	19.3	49.0	19.2	48.8	15.7	39.9
90	18.7	47.5	17.9	45.5	17.4	44.2	15.0	38.1
80	17.8	45.2	16.7	42.4	16.2	41.1	14.2	36.1
70	16.5	41.9	16.2	41.1	15.2	38.6	13.6	34.5
60	16.0	40.6	15.8	40.1	14.5	36.8	12.3	31.2
50	15.2	38.6	14.8	37.6	13.5	34.3	11.1	28.2
40	14.5	36.8	14.5	36.8	12.8	32.5	10.1	25.7
30	13.7	34.8	13.7	34.8	12.2	31.0	9.2	23.4
20	12.6	32.0	12.6	32.0	11.0	27.9	8.3	21.1
10	11.4	29.0	10.1	25.7	9.7	24.6	7.5	19.0
05	9.4	23.9	8.1	20.6	8.5	21.6	3.7	9.4
01	6.5	16.5	2.6	6.6	2.0	5.1	1.5	3.8

High physical fitness standard (rows 99–70) | Health fitness standard (rows 60–01)

FIGURE 8.7 Your back and how to care for it. (continued)

How to Put Your Back to Bed

For proper bed posture, a firm mattress is essential. Bedboards, sold commercially, or devised at home, may be used with soft mattresses. Bedboards, preferably, should be made of 3/4-inch plywood. Faulty sleeping positions intensify swayback and result not only in backache but in numbness, tingling, and pain in arms and legs.

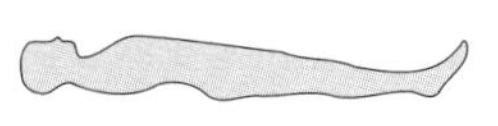

Incorrect:
Lying flat on back makes swayback worse.

Correct:
Lying on side with knees bent effectively flattens the back. Flat pillow may be used to support neck, especially when shoulders are broad.

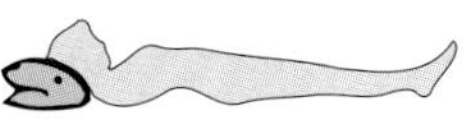

Use of high pillow strains neck, arms, shoulders.

Sleeping on back is restful and correct when knees are properly supported.

Sleeping face down exaggerates swayback, strains neck and shoulders.

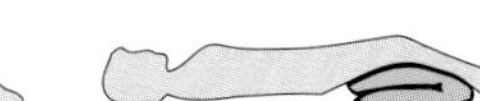

Raise the foot of the mattress eight inches to discourage sleeping on the abdomen.

Bending one hip and knee does not relieve swayback.

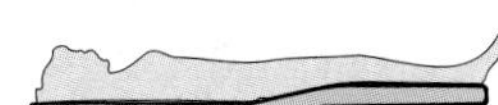

Proper arrangement of pillows for resting or reading in bed.

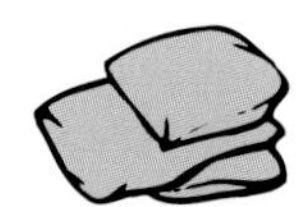

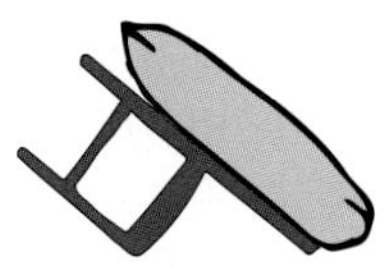

A straight-back chair used behind a pillow makes a serviceable backrest.

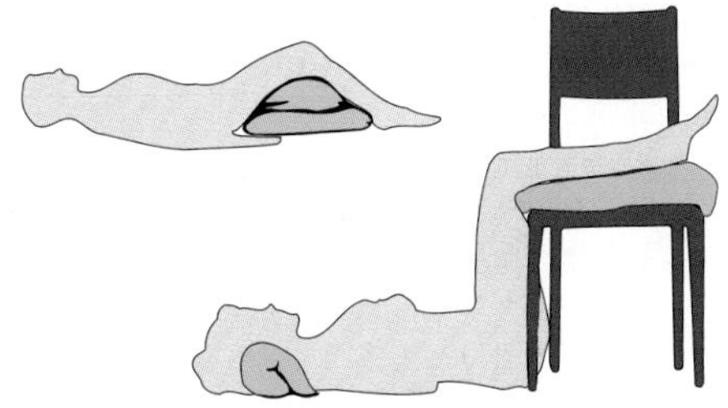

When Doing Nothing, Do it Right

- Rest is the first rule for the tired, painful back. The above positions relieve pain by taking all pressure and weight off the back and legs.
- Note pillows under knees to relieve strain on spine.
- For complete relief and relaxing effect, these positions should be maintained from 5 to 25 minutes.

Exercise Without Getting Out of Bed

Exercises to be performed while lying in bed are aimed not so much at strengthening muscles as at teaching correct positioning. But muscles used correctly become stronger and in time are able to support the body with the least amount of effort.

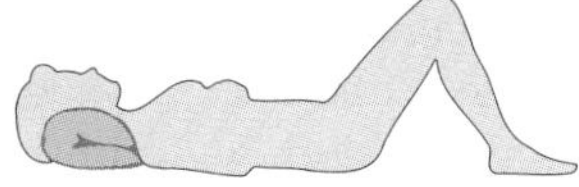

Do all exercises in this position. Legs should not be straightened.

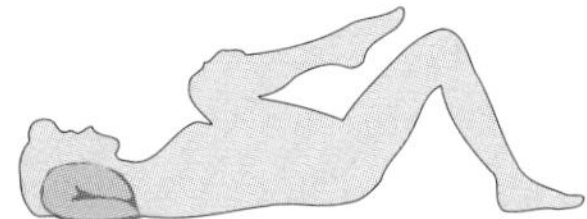

Bring knee up to chest. Lower slowly but do not straighten leg. Relax. Repeat with each leg 10 times.

Exercise Without Attracting Attention

Use these inconspicuous exercises whenever you have a spare moment during the day, both to relax tension and improve the tone of important muscle groups.

1. Rotate shoulders, forward and backward.
2. Turn head slowly side to side.
3. Watch an imaginary plane take off, just below the right shoulder. Stretch neck, follow it slowly as it moves up, around and down, disappearing below the other shoulder. Repeat, starting on left side.
4. Slowly, slowly, touch left ear to left shoulder, right ear to right shoulder. Raise both shoulders to touch ears, drop them as far down as possible.
5. At any pause in the day—waiting for an elevator to arrive, for a specific traffic light to change—pull in abdominal muscles, tighten, hold it for the count of eight without breathing. Relax slowly. Increase the count gradually after the first week, practice breathing normally with the abdomen flat and contracted. Do this sitting, standing, and walking.

Bring both knees slowly up to chest (place your hands on the lower thigh behind the knees). Tighten muscles of abdomen, press back flat against bed. Hold knees to chest 20 seconds, then lower slowly. Relax. Repeat 5 times. This exercise gently stretches the shortened muscles of the lower back, while strengthening abdominal muscles.

Rules to Live By—From Now On

1. Never bend from the waist only; bend the hips and knees.
2. Never lift a heavy object higher than your waist.
3. Always turn and face the object you wish to lift.
4. Avoid carrying unbalanced loads; hold heavy objects close to your body.
5. Never carry anything heavier than you can manage with ease.
6. Never lift or move heavy furniture. Wait for someone to do it who knows the principles of leverage.
7. Avoid sudden movements, sudden "overloading" of muscles. Learn to move deliberately, swinging the legs from the hips.
8. Learn to keep the head in line with the spine, when standing, sitting, lying in bed.
9. Put soft chairs and deep couches on your "don't sit" list. During prolonged sitting, cross your legs to rest your back.
10. Your doctor is the only one who can determine when low-back pain is due to faulty posture and he is the best judge of when you may do general exercises for physical fitness. When you do, omit any exercise that arches or overstrains the lower back: backward bends, or forward bends, touching the toes with the knees straight.
11. Wear shoes with moderate heels, all about the same height. Avoid changing from high to low heels.
12. Put a footrail under the desk and a footrest under the crib.
13. Diaper the baby sitting next to him or her on the bed.
14. Don't stoop and stretch to hang the wash; raise the clothesbasket and lower the washline.
15. Beg or buy a rocking chair. Rocking rests the back by changing the muscle groups used.
16. Train yourself vigorously to use your abdominal muscles to flatten your lower abdomen. In time, this muscle contraction will become habitual, making you the envied possessor of a youthful body profile!
17. Don't strain to open windows or doors.
18. For good posture, concentrate on strengthening "nature's corset"—the abdominal and buttock muscles. The pelvic roll exercise is especially recommended to correct the postural relation between the pelvis and the spine.

Policy and Research. The guidelines suggest that spinal manipulation may help to alleviate discomfort and pain during the first few weeks of an acute episode of low-back pain. Generally, benefits are seen in fewer than 10 treatments. People who have had chronic pain for more than 6 months should avoid spinal manipulation until they have been thoroughly examined by a physician.

Back pain can be reduced greatly through aerobic exercise, muscular flexibility exercise, and muscular strength and endurance training that includes specific exercises to strengthen the spine-stabilizing muscles. Exercise requires effort by the patient, and it may create discomfort initially, but exercise promotes circulation, healing, muscle size, and muscle strength and endurance. Many patients abstain from aggressive physical therapy because they are unwilling to commit the time required for the program.

Aerobic exercise is beneficial because it helps decrease body fat and psychological stress. During an episode of back pain, however, people often avoid activity and cope by getting more rest. Rest is recommended if the pain is associated with a herniated disc, but if your physician rules out a serious problem, exercise is a better choice of treatment. Exercise helps restore physical function, and individuals who start and maintain an aerobic exercise program have back pain less frequently. Individuals who exercise also are less likely to require surgery or other invasive treatments.

In terms of flexibility, regular stretching exercises that help the hip and trunk go through a functional range of motion, rather than increasing the range of motion, are recommended. That is, for proper back care, stretching exercises should not be performed to the extreme range of motion. Individuals with a greater spinal range of motion also have a higher incidence of back injury. Spinal stability, instead of mobility, is desirable for back health.[11]

A strengthening program for a healthy back should be conducted around the endurance threshold—10 to 12 repetitions to near fatigue. Muscular endurance of the muscles that support the spine is more important than absolute strength because these muscles perform their work during the course of an entire day.

Critical Thinking

Consider your own low-back health. Have you ever had episodes of low-back pain? If so, how long did it take you to recover, and what helped you recover from this condition?

Several exercises for preventing and rehabilitating the backache syndrome are given on pages 279–282. These exercises can be done twice or more daily when a person has back pain. Under normal circumstances, doing these exercises three or four times a week is enough to prevent the syndrome. Using some of the additional core exercises listed in Chapter 7 ("Core Strength Training," pages 223–225) will further enhance your low-back management program. Back pain recurs more often in people who rely solely on medication, compared with people who use both medication and exercise therapy to recover.[12]

Lab 8C allows you to develop your own flexibility and low-back conditioning programs. The recommendation calls for isometric contractions of 2 to 20 seconds during each repetition for some of the exercises listed for back health (see Lab 8C) to further increase spinal stability and muscular strength endurance. The length of the hold will depend on your current fitness level and the difficulty of each exercise. For most exercises, you may start with a 2- to 10-second hold. Over the course of several weeks, you can increase the length of the hold from 10 to 20 seconds.

Psychological stress, too, may lead to back pain.[13] Excessive stress causes muscles to contract. In the case of the lower back, frequent tightening of the muscles can throw the back out of alignment and constrict blood vessels that supply oxygen and nutrients to the back. Chronic stress also increases the release of hormones that have been linked to muscle and tendon injuries. Furthermore, people under stress tend to forget proper body mechanics, placing themselves at unnecessary risk for injury. If you are undergoing excessive stress and back pain at the same time, proper stress management (see Chapter 10) should be a part of your comprehensive back-care program.

Assess Your Behavior

Thomson NOW! *Log on to www.thomsonedu.com/login to create a flexibility program and track your progress in incorporating flexibility exercises in your fitness program.*

1. Do you give flexibility exercises the same priority in your fitness program as you do aerobic and strength training?
2. Are stretching exercises a part of your fitness program at least two times per week?
3. Do you include exercises to strengthen and enhance body alignment in your regular strength and flexibility program?

Assess Your Knowledge

Thomson NOW! *Log on to www.thomsonedu.com/login to assess your understanding of this chapter's topics by taking the Student Practice Test and exploring the modules recommended in your Personalized Study Plan.*

1. Muscular flexibility is defined as
   a. the capacity of joints and muscles to work in a synchronized manner.
   b. the achievable range of motion at a joint or group of joints without causing injury.
   c. the capability of muscles to stretch beyond their normal resting length without injury to the muscles.
   d. the capacity of muscles to return to their proper length following the application of a stretching force.
   e. the limitations placed on muscles as the joints move through their normal planes.
2. Good flexibility
   a. promotes healthy muscles and joints.
   b. decreases the risk of injury.
   c. improves posture.
   d. decreases the risk of chronic back pain.
   e. All are correct choices.
3. Plastic elongation means
   a. permanent lengthening of soft tissue.
   b. increased flexibility achieved through dynamic stretching.
   c. temporary elongation of muscles.
   d. the ability of a muscle to achieve a complete degree of stretch.
   e. lengthening of a muscle against resistance.
4. The most significant contributors to loss of flexibility are
   a. sedentary living and lack of physical activity.
   b. weight and power training.
   c. age and injury.
   d. muscular strength and endurance.
   e. excessive body fat and low lean tissue.
5. Which of the following is *not* a mode of stretching?
   a. proprioceptive neuromuscular facilitation
   b. elastic elongation
   c. ballistic stretching
   d. slow-sustained stretching
   e. All are modes of stretching.
6. PNF can help increase
   a. muscular strength.
   b. muscular flexibility.
   c. muscular endurance.
   d. range of motion.
   e. All are correct choices.
7. In any stretching exercises, the degree of stretch should be
   a. through the entire arc of movement.
   b. to about 80 percent of capacity.
   c. to tightness at the end of the range of motion.
   d. applied until the muscle(s) start shaking.
   e. progressively increased until the desired stretch is attained.
8. When you stretch, hold the final stretch for
   a. 1 to 10 seconds.
   b. 15 to 30 seconds.
   c. 30 to 90 seconds.
   d. 1 to 3 minutes.
   e. as long as you are able to sustain the stretch.
9. Low-back pain is associated primarily with
   a. physical inactivity.
   b. faulty posture.
   c. excessive body weight.
   d. improper body mechanics.
   e. All are correct choices.
10. The following exercise helps stretch the lower back and hamstring muscles:
    a. adductor stretch.
    b. cat stretch.
    c. back extension stretch.
    d. single-knee-to-chest stretch.
    e. quad stretch.

Correct answers can be found at the back of the book.

Media Menu

Thomson NOW! *Connections*

- Create your personal flexibility profile.
- Check how well you understand the chapter's concepts.

Internet Connections

Specific Stretching Exercises, with Diagrams

Let Shape Up America show you how to develop an activity program that's right for you. Its online Fitness Center includes valuable information on improvement and assessment of, as well as barriers to, physical fitness.
http://www.shapeup.org

Yoga and Other Stretching Exercises

This site features information on the techniques of yoga, Pilates, and other forms of stretching exercises.
http://www.yoga.com

Stretching to Increase Flexibility

In addition to a comprehensive description of the health benefits of regular stretching, this site features a series of exercises tailored to three levels of fitness levels based on how often you perform stretching exercises.
http://k2.kirtland.cc.mi.us/~balbachl/flex.htm

Notes

1. American College of Obstetricians and Gynecologists, *Guidelines for Exercise During Pregnancy,* 1994.
2. "Stretch Yourself Younger," *Consumer Reports on Health* 11 (August 1999): 6–7.
3. W. W. K. Hoeger and D. R. Hopkins, "A Comparison Between the Sit and Reach and the Modified Sit and Reach in the Measurement of Flexibility in Women," *Research Quarterly for Exercise and Sport* 63 (1992): 191–195; W. W. K. Hoeger, D. R. Hopkins, S. Button, and T. A. Palmer, "Comparing the Sit and Reach with the Modified Sit and Reach in Measuring Flexibility in Adolescents," *Pediatric Exercise Science* 2 (1990): 156–162; D. R. Hopkins and W. W. K. Hoeger, "A Comparison of the Sit and Reach and the Modified Sit and Reach in the Measurement of Flexibility for Males," *Journal of Applied Sports Science Research* 6 (1992): 7–10.
4. "Position Yourself to Stay Well," *Consumer Reports on Health* 18 (February 2006): 8–9.
5. J. Kokkonen and S. Lauritzen, "Isotonic Strength and Endurance Gains Through PNF Stretching," *Medicine and Science in Sports and Exercise* 27 (1995): S22, 127.
6. American College of Sports Medicine, *ACSM's Guidelines for Exercise Testing and Prescription* (Baltimore: Williams & Wilkins, 2006).
7. S. B. Thacker, J. Gilchrist, D. F. Stroup, and C. D. Kimsey, Jr., "The Impact of Stretching on Sports Injury Risk: A Systematic Review of the Literature," *Medicine and Science in Sports and Exercise* 36 (2004): 371–378.
8. D. B. J. Andersson, L. J. Fine, and B. A. Silverstein, "Musculoskeletal Disorders," in *Occupational Health: Recognizing and Preventing Work-Related Disease,* edited by B. S. Levy and D. H. Wegman (Boston: Little, Brown, 1995).
9. M. R. Bracko, "Can We Prevent Back Injuries?" *ACSM's Health & Fitness Journal* 8, no. 4 (2004): 5–11.
10. R. Deyo, "Chiropractic Care for Back Pain: The Physician's Perspective," *HealthNews* 4 (September 10, 1998).
11. See note 9.
12. J. A. Hides, G. A. Jull, and C. A. Richardson, "Long-Term Effects of Specific Stabilizing Exercises for First-Episode Low Back Pain," *Spine* 26 (2001): E243–248.
13. A. Brownstein, "Chronic Back Pain Can Be Beaten," *Bottom Line/Health* 13 (October 1999): 3–4.

Suggested Readings

Alter, M. J. *The Science of Stretching.* Champaign, IL: Human Kinetic Press, 1996.

Alter, M. J. *Sports Stretch.* Champaign, IL: Human Kinetics, 2004.

Anderson, B. *Stretching.* Bolinas, CA: Shelter Publications, 1999.

Bracko, M. R. "Can We Prevent Back Injuries?" *ACSM's Health & Fitness Journal* 8, no. 4 (2004): 5–11.

Hoeger, W. W. K. *The Assessment of Muscular Flexibility: Test Protocols and National Flexibility Norms for the Modified Sit-and-Reach Test, Total Body Rotation Test, and Shoulder Rotation Test.* Rockton, IL: Figure Finder Collection Novel Products, Inc., 2006.

Liemohn, W., and G. Pariser. "Core Strength: Implications for Fitness and Low Back Pain." *ACSM's Health and Fitness Journal* 6, no. 5 (2002): 10–16.

McAtee, R. E., and J. Charland. *Facilitated Stretching.* Champaign, IL: Human Kinetics, 1999.

Flexibility Exercises

Exercise 1 Neck Stretches

Action Slowly and gently tilt the head laterally (a). You may increase the degree of stretch by gently pulling with one hand (b). You may also turn the head about 30° to one side and stretch the neck by raising your head toward the ceiling (see photo c—do not extend your head backward; look straight forward). Now gradually bring the head forward until you feel an adequate stretch in the muscles on the back of the neck (d). Perform the exercises on both the right and left sides. Repeat each exercise several times, and hold the final stretched position for a few seconds.

Areas Stretched Neck flexors and extensors; ligaments of the cervical spine

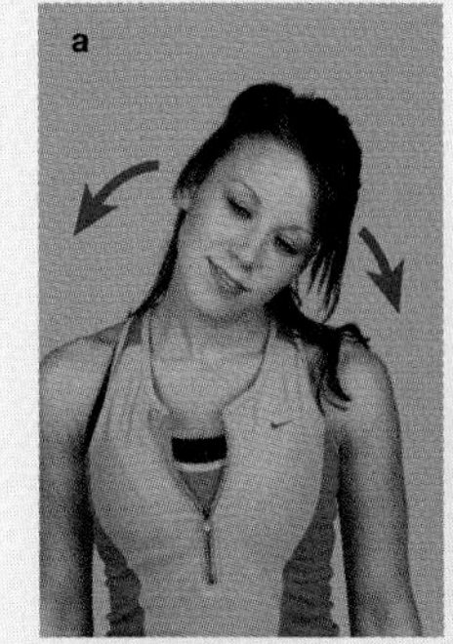

a

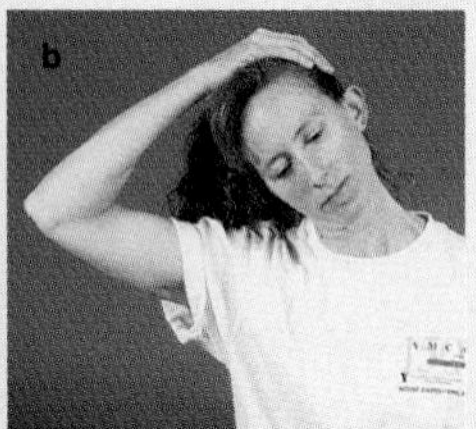

b

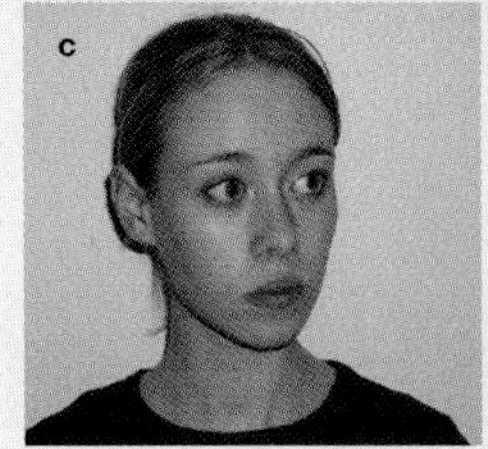

c

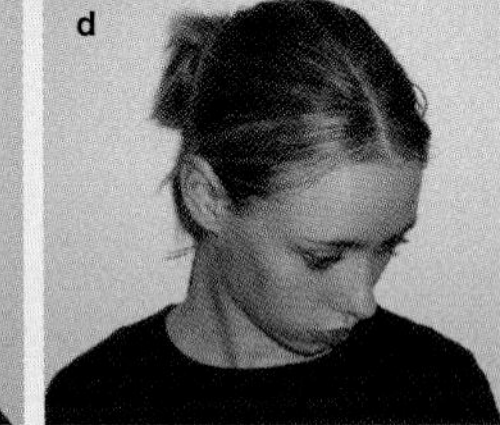

d

Exercise 2 Arm Circles

Action Gently circle your arms all the way around. Conduct the exercise in both directions.

Areas Stretched Shoulder muscles and ligaments

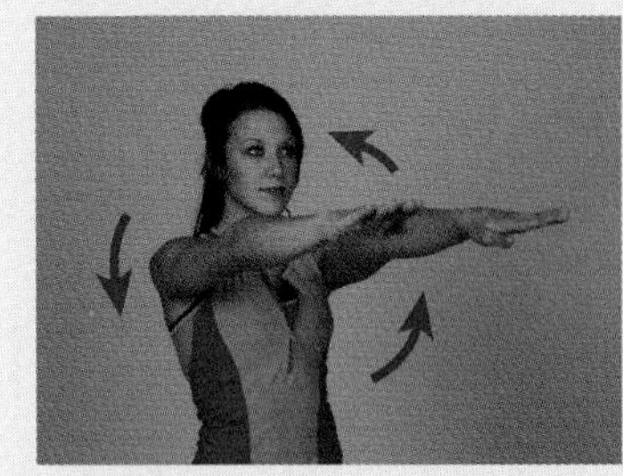

Exercise 3 Side Stretch

Action Stand straight up, feet separated to shoulder-width, and place your hands on your waist. Now move the upper body to one side and hold the final stretch for a few seconds. Repeat on the other side.

Areas Stretched Muscles and ligaments in the pelvic region

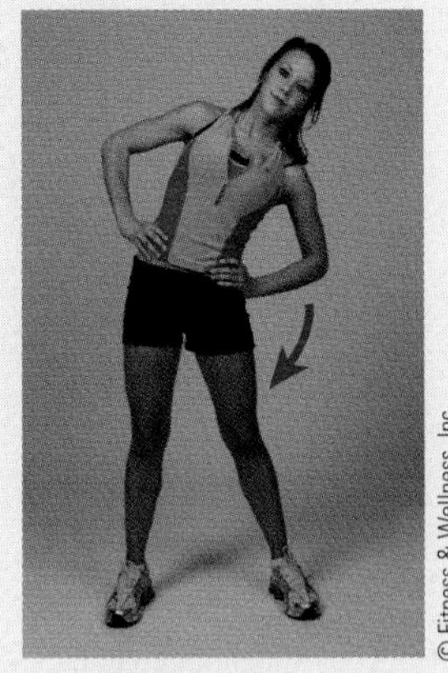

Exercise 4 Body Rotation

Action Place your arms slightly away from the body and rotate the trunk as far as possible, holding the final position for several seconds. Conduct the exercise for both the right and left sides of the body. You also can perform this exercise by standing about 2 feet away from the wall (back toward the wall) and then rotating the trunk, placing the hands against the wall.

Areas Stretched Hip, abdominal, chest, back, neck, and shoulder muscles; hip and spinal ligaments

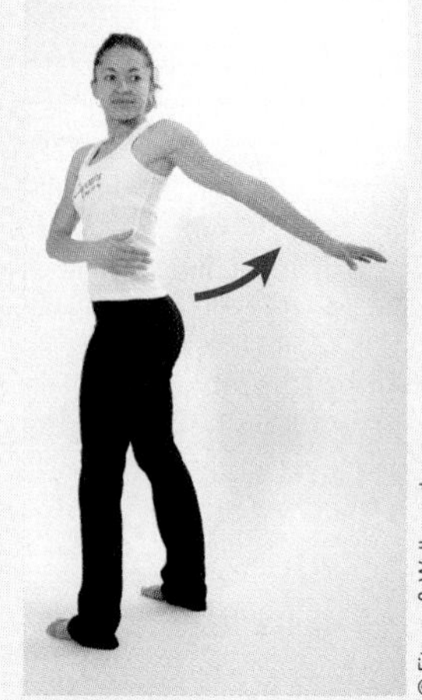

Exercise 5 Chest Stretch

Action Place your hands on the shoulders of your partner, who in turn will push you down by your shoulders. Hold the final position for a few seconds.

Areas Stretched Chest (pectoral) muscles and shoulder ligaments

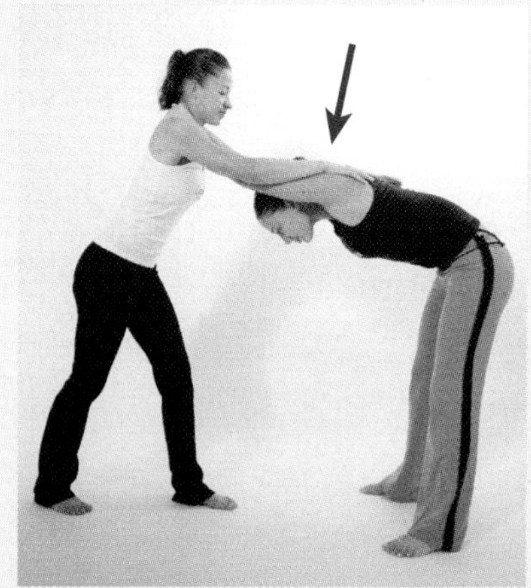

Exercise 6 Shoulder Hyperextension Stretch

Action Have a partner grasp your arms from behind by the wrists and slowly push them upward. Hold the final position for a few seconds.

Areas Stretched Deltoid and pectoral muscles; ligaments of the shoulder joint

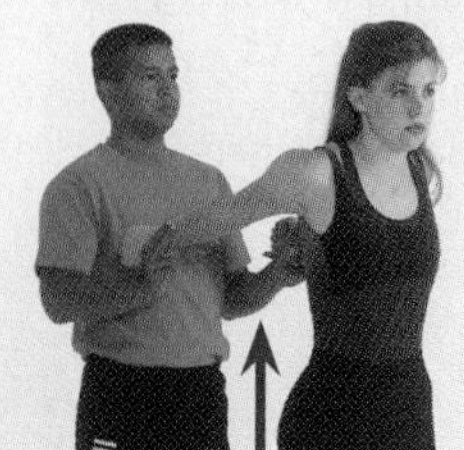

Exercise 7 Shoulder Rotation Stretch

Action With the aid of surgical tubing or an aluminum or wood stick, place the tubing or stick behind your back and grasp the two ends using a reverse (thumbs-out) grip. Slowly bring the tubing or stick over your head, keeping the elbows straight. Repeat several times (bring the hands closer together for additional stretch).

Areas Stretched Deltoid, latissimus dorsi, and pectoral muscles; shoulder ligaments

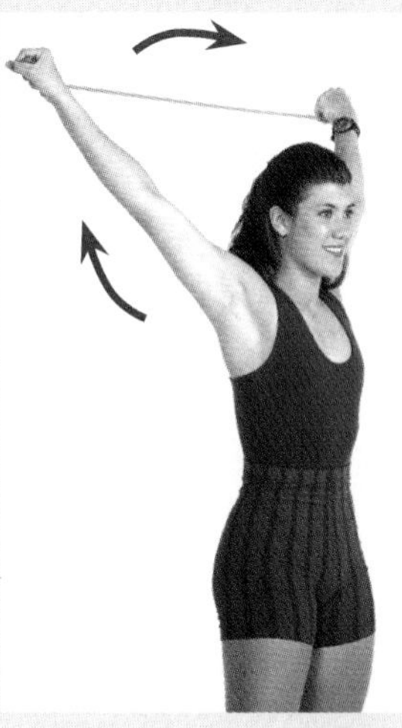

Exercise 8 Quad Stretch

Action Lie on your side and move one foot back by flexing the knee. Grasp the front of the ankle and pull the ankle toward the gluteal region. Hold for several seconds. Repeat with the other leg.

Areas Stretched Quadriceps muscle; knee and ankle ligaments

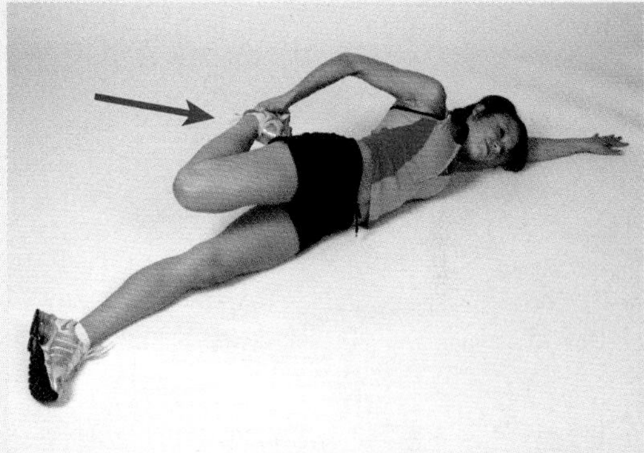

Exercise 9 Heel Cord Stretch

Action Stand against the wall or at the edge of a step and stretch the heel downward, alternating legs. Hold the stretched position for a few seconds.

Areas Stretched Heel cord (Achilles tendon); gastrocnemius and soleus muscles

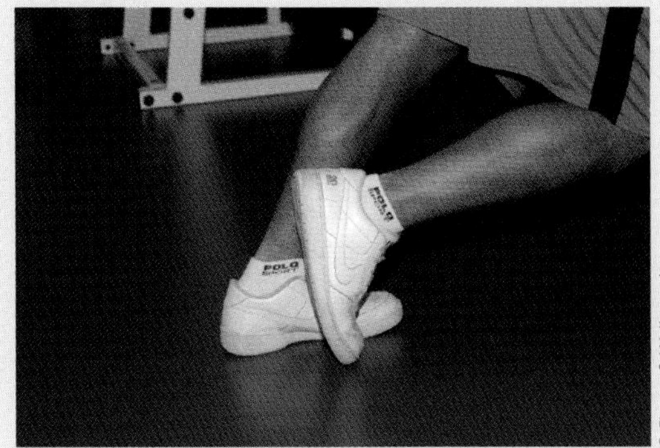

Exercise 10 Adductor Stretch

Action Stand with your feet about twice shoulder-width apart and place your hands slightly above the knees. Flex one knee and slowly go down as far as possible, holding the final position for a few seconds. Repeat with the other leg.

Areas Stretched Hip adductor muscles

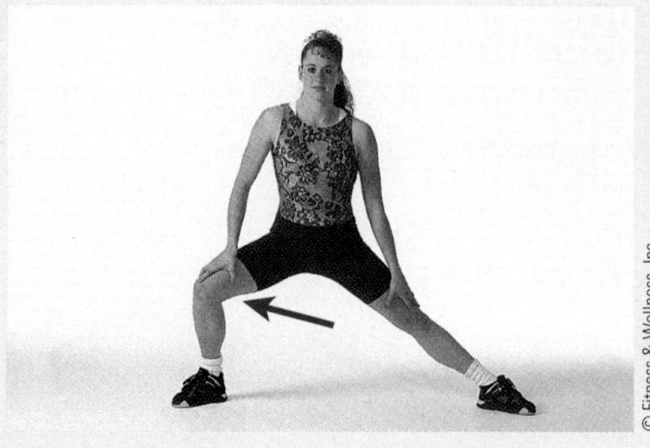

Exercise 11 Sitting Adductor Stretch

Action Sit on the floor and bring your feet in close to you, allowing the soles of the feet to touch each other. Now place your forearms (or elbows) on the inner part of the thigh and push the legs downward, holding the final stretch for several seconds.

Areas Stretched Hip adductor muscles

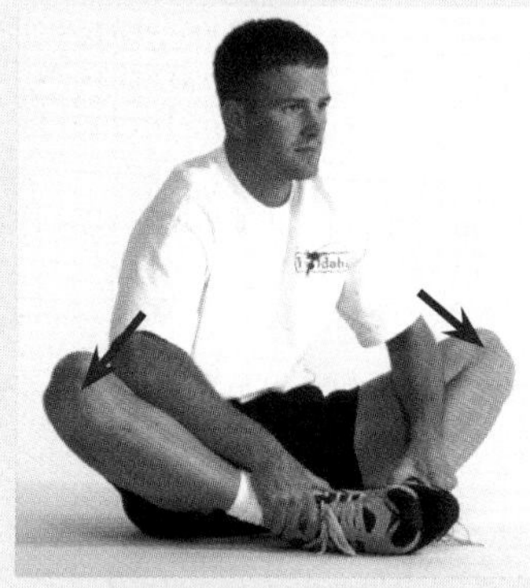

Exercise 12 Sit-and-Reach Stretch

Action Sit on the floor with legs together and gradually reach forward as far as possible. Hold the final position for a few seconds. This exercise also may be performed with the legs separated, reaching to each side as well as to the middle.

Areas Stretched Hamstrings and lower back muscles; lumbar spine ligaments

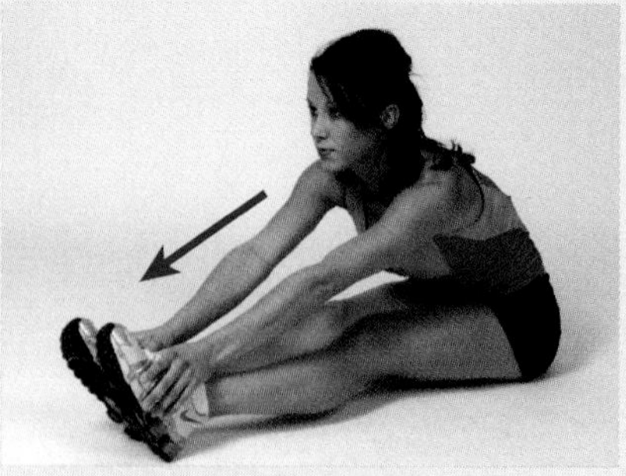

Exercise 20 Back Extension Stretch

Action Lie face down on the floor with the elbows by the chest, forearms on the floor, and the hands beneath the chin. Gently raise the trunk by extending the elbows until you reach an approximate 90° angle at the elbow joint. Be sure the forearms remain in contact with the floor at all times. Do NOT extend the back beyond this point. Hyperextension of the lower back may lead to or aggravate an existing back problem. Hold the stretched position for about 10 seconds.

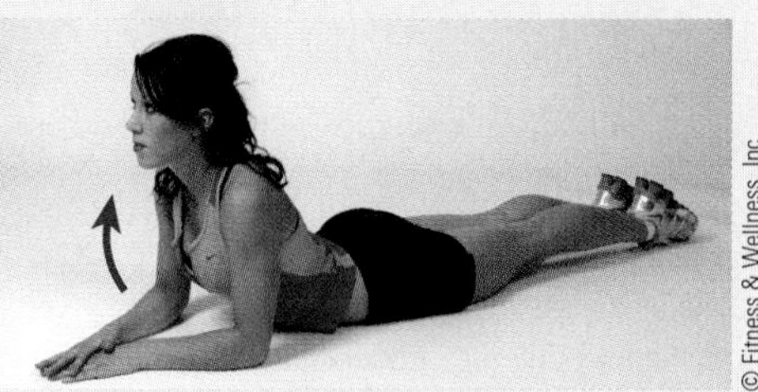

Areas Stretched Abdominal region

Additional Benefits Restore lower back curvature

Exercise 21 Trunk Rotation and Lower Back Stretch

Action Sit on the floor and bend the left leg, placing the right foot on the outside of the left knee. Place the left elbow on the right knee and push against it. At the same time, try to rotate the trunk to the right (clockwise). Hold the final position for a few seconds. Repeat the exercise with the other side.

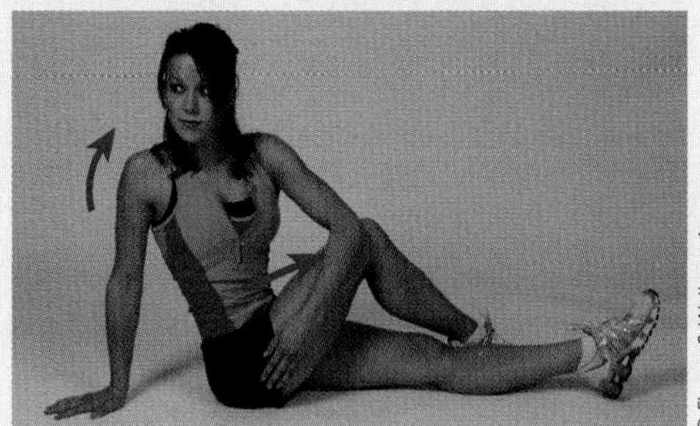

Areas Stretched Lateral side of the hip and thigh; trunk and lower back

Exercise 22 Pelvic Tilt

(See Exercise 12 in Chapter 7, page 235) This is perhaps the most important exercise for the care of the lower back. It should be included as a part of your daily exercise routine and should be performed several times throughout the day when pain in the lower back is present as a result of muscle imbalance.

Exercise 23 The Cat

Action Kneel on the floor and place your hands in front of you (on the floor) about shoulder-width apart. Relax the trunk and lower back (a). Now arch the spine and pull in your abdomen as far as you can and hold this position for a few seconds (b). Repeat the exercise 4–5 times.

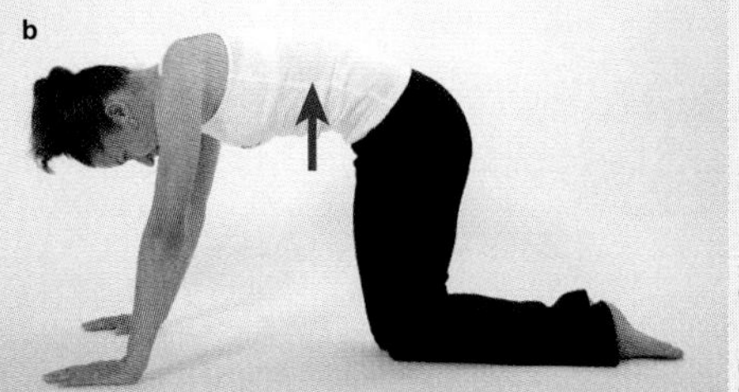

Areas Stretched Low back muscles and ligaments

Areas Strengthened Abdominal and gluteal muscles

Exercise 24 Abdominal Crunch or Abdominal Curl-Up

(See Exercise 4 in Chapter 7, page 232) It is important that you do not stabilize your feet when performing either of these exercises, because doing so decreases the work of the abdominal muscles. Also, remember not to "swing up" but, rather, to curl up as you perform these exercises.

Exercise 25 Reverse Crunch

(See Exercise 11 in Chapter 7, page 235)

Exercise 26 Supine Bridge

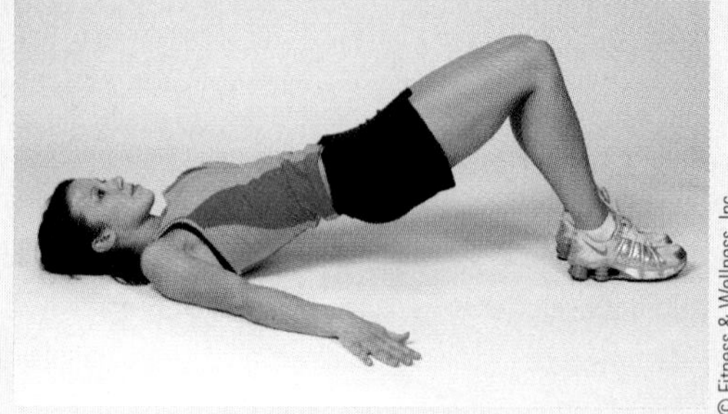

© Fitness & Wellness, Inc.

Action Lie face up on the floor with the knees bent at about 120°. Do a pelvic tilt (Exercise 12 in Chapter 7, page 235) and maintain the pelvic tilt while you raise the hips off the floor until the upper body and upper legs are in a straight line. Hold this position for several seconds.

Areas Strengthened Gluteal and abdominal flexor muscles

Exercise 27 Pelvic Clock

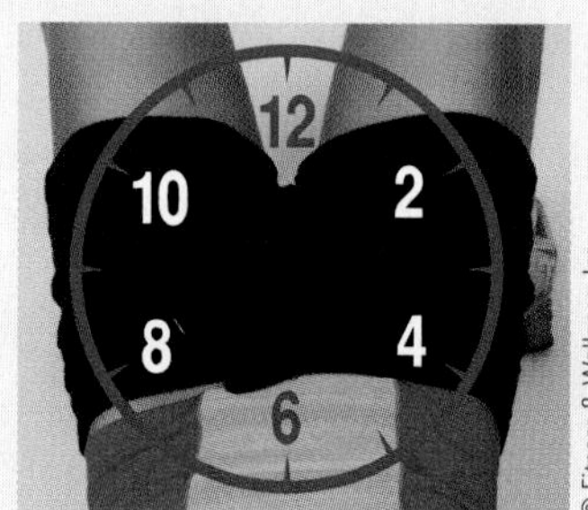

© Fitness & Wellness, Inc.

Action Lie face up on the floor with the knees bent at about 120°. Fully extend the hips as in the supine bridge (Exercise 26). Now progressively rotate the hips in a clockwise manner (2 o'clock, 4 o'clock, 6 o'clock, 8 o'clock, 10 o'clock, and 12 o'clock), holding each position in an isometric contraction for about 1 second. Repeat the exercise counterclockwise.

Areas Strengthened Gluteal, abdominal, and hip flexor muscles

Exercise 28 Lateral Bridge

(See Exercise 13 in Chapter 7, page 235)

Exercise 29 Prone Bridge

(See Exercise 14 in Chapter 7, page 236)

Exercise 30 Leg Press

(See Exercise 16 in Chapter 7, page 237)

Exercise 31 Seated Back

(See Exercise 20 in Chapter 7, page 239)

Exercise 32 Lat Pull-Down

(See Exercise 24 in Chapter 7, page 241)

Exercise 33 Back Extension

(See Exercise 36 in Chapter 7, page 248)

Exercise 34 Lateral Trunk Flexion

(See Exercise 37 in Chapter 7, page 248)

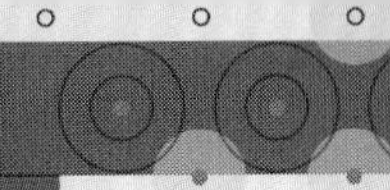

Lab 8B Posture Evaluation

Name: ______ Date: ______ Grade: ______

Instructor: ______ Course: ______ Section: ______

Necessary Lab Equipment

A plumb line, two large mirrors set at about an 85° angle, and a Polaroid camera (the mirrors and the camera are optional—see "Evaluating Body Posture" (pages 260 and 264).

Objective

To determine current body alignment.

Lab Preparation

To conduct the posture analysis, men should wear shorts only and women, shorts and a tank top. Shoes should also be removed for this test.

Lab Assignment

The class should be divided in groups of four students each. The group should carefully study the posture form given in this lab, then proceed to fill out the form for each member according to the instructions given under "Evaluating Body Posture" (pages 260 and 264). If no mirrors and camera are available, three members of the group are to rate the fourth person's posture while he/she first stands with the side of the body and then with the back to the plumb line. A final score is obtained by totaling the points given for each body segment and looking up the posture rating according to the total score found in the table provided below.

Results

Total points: ______

Category: ______

Posture Evaluation Standards

Total Points	Category
≥45	Excellent
40–44	Good
30–39	Average
20–29	Fair
≤19	Poor

Posture Improvement

Indicate how you feel about your posture, identify areas to correct, and specify the steps you can take to make those improvements.

______

______

______

______

______

______

______

______

______

	Good — 5	Fair — 3	Poor — 1	Score
HEAD Left Right	head erect, gravity passes directly through center	head twisted or turned to one side slightly	head twisted or turned to one side markedly	
SHOULDERS Left Right	shoulders level horizontally	one shoulder slightly higher	one shoulder markedly higher	
SPINE Left Right	spine straight	spine slightly curved	spine markedly curved laterally	
HIPS Left Right	hips level horizontally	one hip slightly higher	one hip markedly higher	
KNEES and ANKLES	feet pointed straight ahead, legs vertical	feet pointed out, legs deviating outward at the knee	feet pointed out markedly, legs deviate markedly	
NECK and UPPER BACK	neck erect, head in line with shoulders, rounded upper back	neck slightly forward, chin out, slightly more rounded upper back	neck markedly forward, chin markedly out, markedly rounded upper back	
TRUNK	trunk erect	trunk inclined to rear slightly	trunk inclined to rear markedly	
ABDOMEN	abdomen flat	abdomen protruding	abdomen protruding and sagging	
LOWER BACK	lower back normally curved	lower back slightly hollow	lower back markedly hollow	
LEGS	legs straight	knees slightly hyper-extended	knees markedly hyperextended	
			Total Score	

Adapted from *The New York Physical Fitness Test: A Manual for Teachers of Physical Education*, New York State Education Department (Division of HPER), 1958.

Lab 8C Flexibility Development and Low-Back Conditioning

Name: | Date: | Grade:

Instructor: | Course: | Section:

Necessary Lab Equipment
Minor implements such as a chair, a table, an elastic band (surgical tubing or a wood or aluminum stick), and a stool or steps.

Objective
To develop a flexibility exercise program and a conditioning program for the prevention and rehabilitation of low-back pain.

Lab Preparation
Wear exercise clothing and prepare to participate in a sample stretching exercise session. All of the flexibility and low-back conditioning exercises are illustrated on pages 275–282.

I. Stage of Change for Flexibility Training

Using Figure 2.5 (page 49) and Table 2.3 (page 49), identify your current stage of change for participation in a muscular stretching program:

II. Instruction

Perform all of the recommended flexibility exercises given on pages 275–279. Use a combination of slow-sustained and proprioceptive neuromuscular facilitation stretching techniques. Indicate the technique(s) used for each exercise and, where applicable, the number of repetitions performed and the length of time that the final degree of stretch was held.

Stretching Exercises

Exercise	Stretching Technique	Repetitions	Length of Final Stretch
Lateral head tilt			NA*
Arm circles			NA
Side stretch			
Body rotation			
Chest stretch			
Shoulder hyperextension stretch			
Shoulder rotation stretch			NA
Quad stretch			
Heel cord stretch			
Adductor stretch			
Sitting adductor stretch			
Sit-and-reach stretch			
Triceps stretch			

*Not Applicable

Stretching Schedule (Indicate days, time, and place where you will stretch):

Flexibility-training days: M ___ T ___ W ___ Th ___ F ___ Sa ___ Su ___ Time of day: ___ Place: ___

Low-Back Conditioning Program

Perform all of the recommended exercises for the prevention and rehabilitation of low-back pain given on pages 279–282. Indicate the number of repetitions performed for each exercise.

Flexibility Exercises	Repetitions
Hip flexors stretch	
Single-knee-to-chest stretch	
Double-knee-to-chest stretch	
Upper- and lower-back stretch	
Sit-and-reach stretch	
Gluteal stretch	
Back extension stretch	
Trunk rotation and lower back stretch	

Strength/Endurance Exercises	Repetitions	Seconds Held
Pelvic tilt		
The cat		
Abdominal crunch or abdominal curl-up		
Reverse crunch		
Supine bridge		
Pelvic clock		
Lateral bridge		
Prone bridge		
Leg press		
Seated back		
Lat pull-down		
Back extension		

Proper Body Mechanics

Perform the following tasks using the proper body mechanics given in Figure 8.7 (pages 270–271). Check off each item as you perform the task:

- ☐ Standing (carriage) position
- ☐ Sitting position
- ☐ Bed posture
- ☐ Resting position for tired and painful back
- ☐ Lifting an object

"Rules to Live By — From Now On"

Read the 18 "Rules to Live By—From Now On" given in Figure 8.7 (page 271) and indicate below those rules that you need to work on to improve posture and body mechanics and prevent low-back pain.

Skill Fitness and Fitness Programming

CHAPTER 9

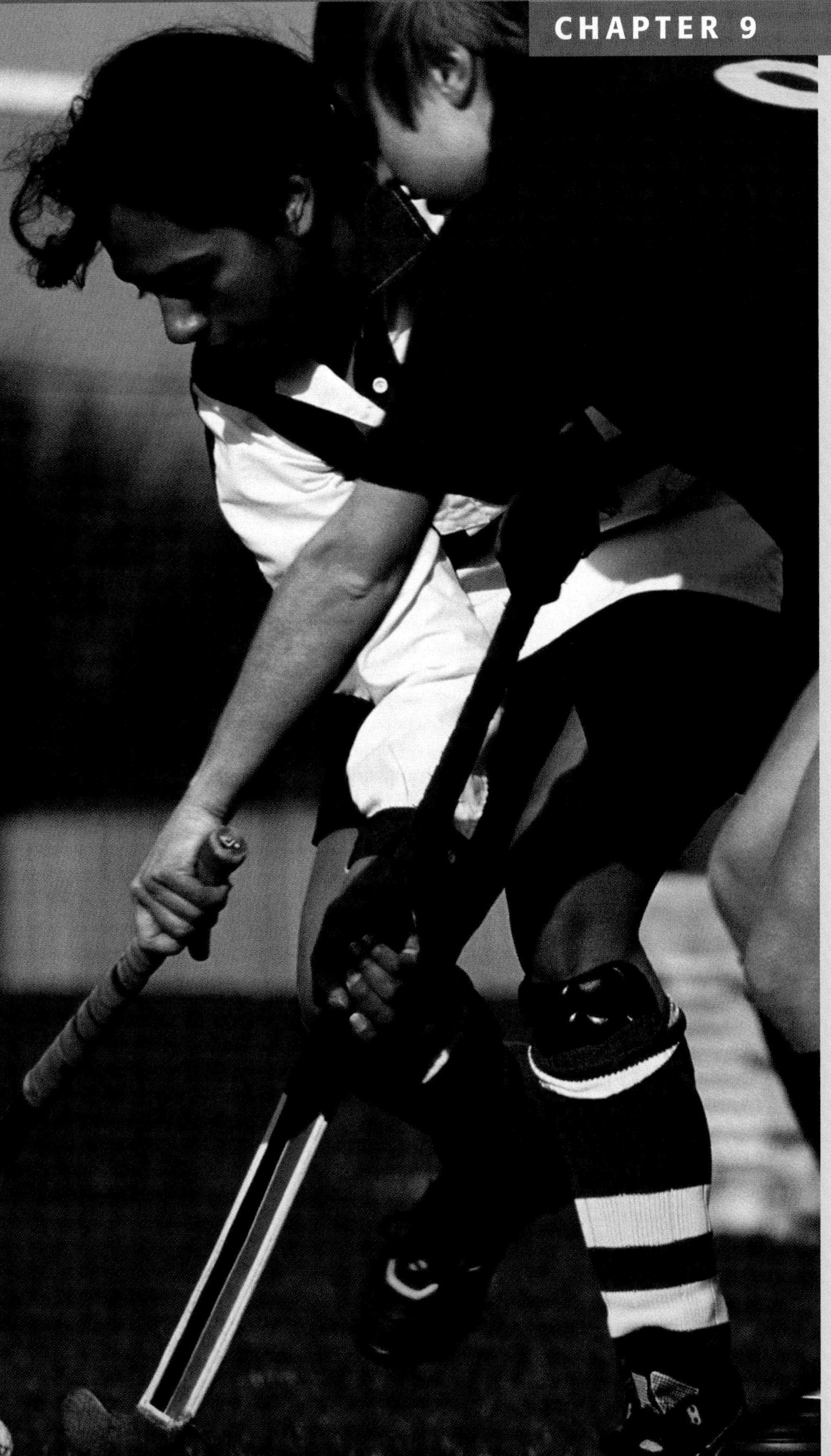

OBJECTIVES

- Learn the benefits of good skill-related fitness.
- Identify and define the six components of skill-related fitness.
- Become familiar with performance tests to assess skill-related fitness.
- Dispel common misconceptions related to physical fitness and wellness.
- Become aware of safety considerations for exercising.
- Learn concepts for preventing and treating injuries.
- Describe the relationship between fitness and aging.
- Be able to write a comprehensive fitness program.

ThomsonNOW! Go to www.thomsonedu.com/login to:

- Evaluate your skill-related fitness levels.
- Check how well you understand the chapter's concepts.

Photo © Adrian Neal/Getty Images

Skill-related fitness is needed for success in athletics and in lifetime sports and activities such as basketball, racquetball, golf, hiking, soccer, and water skiing. Most exercise programs are designed to enhance the health-related components of fitness, but in addition to that, skill-related sports participation also enhances quality of life and helps people cope more effectively in emergency situations.

Outstanding gymnasts, for example, must achieve good skill-related fitness in all components. A significant amount of agility is necessary to perform a double back somersault with a full twist—a skill during which the athlete must simultaneously rotate around one axis and twist around another. Static balance is essential for maintaining a handstand or a scale. Dynamic balance is needed to perform many of the gymnastics routines (such as those on balance beam, parallel bars, and pommel horse).

Coordination is important to successfully integrate multiple skills, each with its own degree of difficulty, into one routine. Power and speed are needed to propel the body into the air, such as when tumbling or vaulting. Quick reaction time is necessary to determine when to end rotation upon a visual clue, such as spotting the floor on a dismount.

The principle of specificity of training applies to skill-related components just as it does to health-related fitness components. The development of agility, balance, coordination, and reaction time is highly task-specific. That is, to develop a certain task or skill, the individual must practice that same task many times. There seems to be very little cross-over learning effect.

For instance, properly practicing a handstand (balance) will lead eventually to successfully performing the skill, but complete mastery of this skill does not ensure that the person will have immediate success when attempting to perform other static-balance positions in gymnastics. In contrast, power and speed may improve with a specific strength-training program or frequent repetition of the specific task to be improved, or both.

The rate of learning in skill-related fitness varies from person to person, mainly because these components seem to be determined to a large extent by genetics. Individuals with good skill-related fitness tend to do better and learn faster when performing a wide variety of skills. Nevertheless, few individuals enjoy complete success in all skill-related components. Furthermore, though skill-related fitness can be enhanced with practice, improvements in reaction time and speed are limited and also seem to be related to genetic endowment.

Although we do not know how much skill-related fitness is desirable, everyone should attempt to develop and maintain a better-than-average level. As pointed out earlier, this type of fitness is crucial for athletes, and it also enables fitness participants to lead a better and happier life. Improving skill-related fitness not only affords an individual more enjoyment and success in lifetime sports (for example, tennis, golf, racquetball, basketball), but it also can help a person cope more effectively in emergency situations. Some of the benefits are as follows:

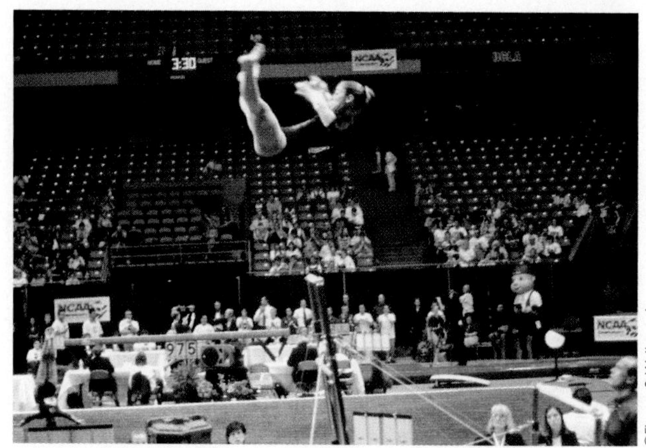

Successful gymnasts demonstrate high levels of skill-fitness.

1. Good reaction time, balance, coordination, and/or agility can help you avoid a fall or break a fall and thereby minimize injury.
2. The ability to generate maximum force in a short time (power) may be crucial to ameliorate injury or even preserve life if you ever have to lift a heavy object that has fallen on another person or even on yourself.
3. In our society, where the average lifespan continues to expand, maintaining speed can be especially important for elderly people. Many of these individuals and, for that matter, many unfit/overweight young people no longer have the speed they need to cross an intersection safely before the light changes or run for help if someone else needs assistance.

Regular participation in a health-related fitness program can heighten performance of skill-related components. For example, significantly overweight people do not have good agility or speed. Because participating in aerobic and strength-training programs helps take off body fat, an overweight individual who loses weight through such an exercise program can improve agility and speed. A sound flexibility program decreases resistance to motion about body joints, which may increase agility, balance, and overall coordination. Improvements in strength definitely help develop power. People who have good skill-related fitness usually participate in lifetime sports and games, which in turn helps develop and/or maintain health-related fitness.

Critical Thinking

If you are interested in health fitness, should you participate in skill-fitness activities? Explain the pros and cons of participating in skill-fitness activities. Should you participate in skill-fitness activities to get fit, or should you get fit to participate in skill-fitness activities?

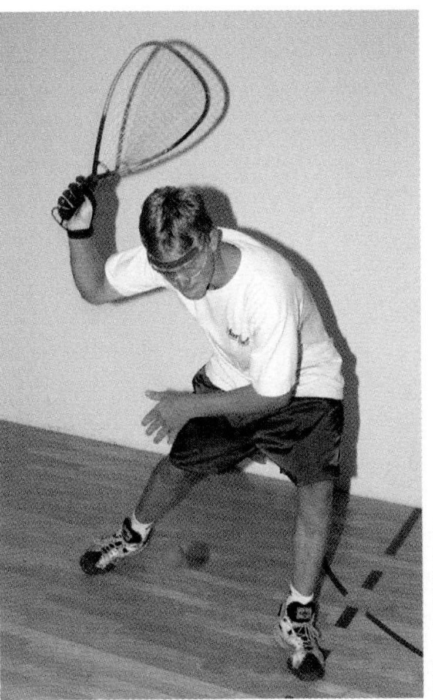

Good racquetball players have excellent agility and reaction time.

©Fitness & Wellness, Inc.

Performance Tests for Skill-Related Fitness

The following six performance tests will assess the various components of skill-related fitness. Results of the performance tests, expressed in percentile ranks, are given in Table 9.1 (men) and Table 9.2 (women) on page 295. Fitness categories for skill-fitness components are established according to percentile rankings only. These rankings fall into categories that are similar to those given for muscular strength and endurance and for flexibility (see Table 9.3 on page 295). You can record the results of your skill-related fitness tests in Lab 9A.

Agility

Agility is the ability to quickly and efficiently change body position and direction. Agility is important in sports such as basketball, soccer, and racquetball, in which the participant must change direction rapidly and also maintain proper body control.

Agility Test SEMO Agility Test[1]

Objective To measure general body agility

Procedure The free-throw area of a basketball court or any other smooth area 12 by 19 feet with adequate running space around it can be used for this test. Four plastic cones or similar objects are placed on each corner of the free-throw lane, as shown in Figure 9.1.

Start on the outside of the free-throw lane at point A, with your back to the free-throw line. When given the "go" command, side step from A to B (do not make crossover steps), backpedal from B to D, sprint forward from D to A, again backpedal from A to C, sprint forward from C to B, and sidestep from B to the finish line at A.

During the test, always go outside each corner cone. A stopwatch is started at the "go" command and stopped when you cross the finish line. Take a practice trial and then use the best of two trials as the final test score. Record the time to the nearest tenth of a second.

FIGURE 9.1 Graphic description of the SEMO Test for agility.

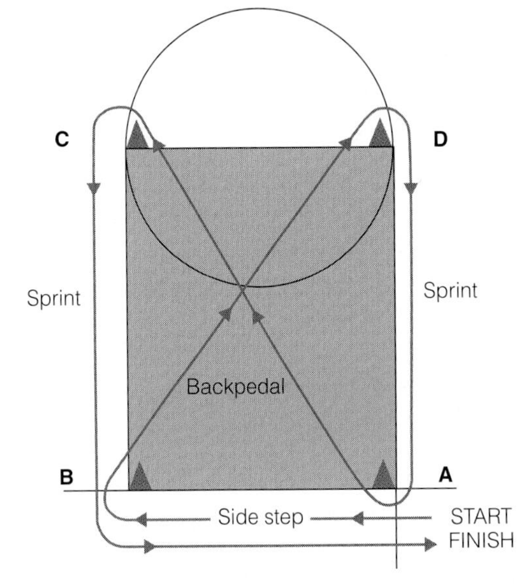

Balance

The ability to maintain the body in proper equilibrium, balance, is vital in activities such as gymnastics, diving, ice skating, skiing and even football and wrestling, in which the athlete attempts to upset the opponent's equilibrium.

Balance Test One-Foot Stand Test (preferred foot, without shoes)

Objective To measure the static balance of the participant

Procedure A flat, smooth floor, not carpeted, is used for this test. Remove your shoes and socks and

Skill-related fitness Fitness components important for success in skillful activities and athletic events; encompasses agility, balance, coordination, power, reaction time, and speed.

One-Foot Stand Test for Balance.

©Fitness & Wellness, Inc.

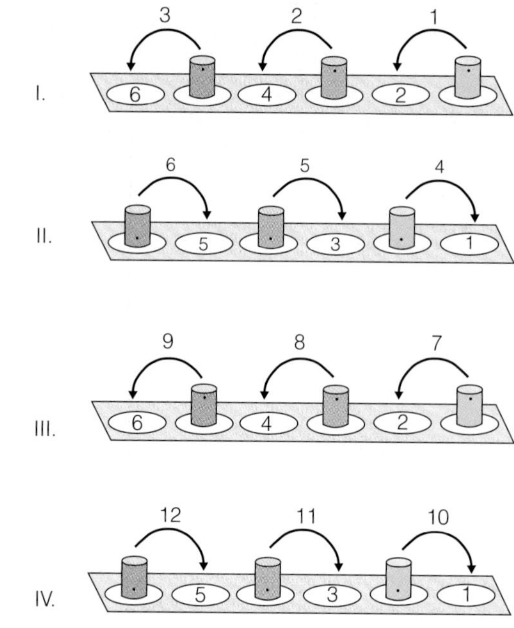

FIGURE 9.2 Graphic illustration of "Soda Pop" Test.

stand on your preferred foot, placing the other foot on the inside of the supporting knee, and the hands on the sides of the hips. When the "go" command is given, raise your heel off the floor and balance yourself as long as possible without moving the ball of the foot from its initial position.

The test is terminated when any of the following conditions occur:

1. The supporting foot moves (shuffles)
2. The raised heel touches the floor
3. The hands are moved from the hips
4. A minute has elapsed

The test is scored by recording the number of seconds that the testee maintains balance on the selected foot, starting with the "go" command. After a practice trial, use the best of two trials as the final performance score. Record the time to the nearest tenth of a second.

Coordination

Coordination is the integration of the nervous and the muscular systems to produce correct, graceful, and harmonious body movements. This component is important in a wide variety of motor activities such as golf, baseball, karate, soccer, and racquetball in which hand-eye and/or foot-eye movements, or both, must be integrated.

Coordination Test Soda Pop Test

Objective To assess overall motor/muscular control and movement time

Procedure

Administrator: Homemade equipment is necessary to perform this test. Draw a straight line lengthwise through the center of a piece of cardboard approximately 32 inches long by 5 inches wide. Draw six marks exactly 5 inches away from each other on this line (draw the first mark about $2\frac{1}{2}$ inches from the edge of the cardboard). Using a compass, draw six circles, each $3\frac{1}{4}$ inches in diameter (that is, having a radius 1 centimeter larger than a can of soda pop), which must be centered on the six marks along the line. See Figure 9.2.

For the purpose of this test, each circle is assigned a number starting with 1 for the first circle on the right of the test taker and ending with 6 for the last circle on the left. The cardboard, three unopened (full) cans of soda pop, a table, a chair, and a stopwatch are needed to perform the test.

Place the cardboard on a table and have the person sit in front of it with the center of the cardboard bisecting the body. Use the preferred hand for this test. If this is the right hand, place the three cans of soda pop on the cardboard in the following manner: can one centered in circle 1 (farthest to the right), can two in circle 3, and can three in circle 5.

Participant: To start the test, place the right hand, with the thumb up, on can one with the elbow joint bent at about 100°–120°. When the tester gives the signal and the stopwatch is started, turn the cans of soda pop upside down, placing can one inside circle 2, followed by can two inside circle 4, and then can three inside circle 6. Immediately return all three cans, starting with can one, then can two, and can three, turning them right side up to their original placement. On this "return trip," grasp the cans with the hand in a thumb-down position.

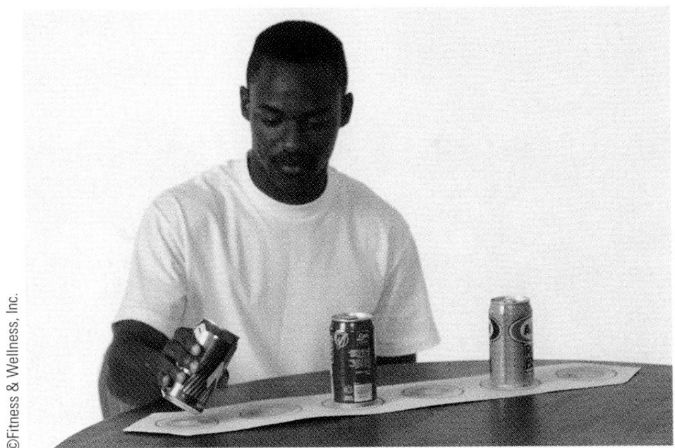

"Soda Pop" Test for coordination.

FIGURE 9.3 Correct placement of feet for start of standing long jump.

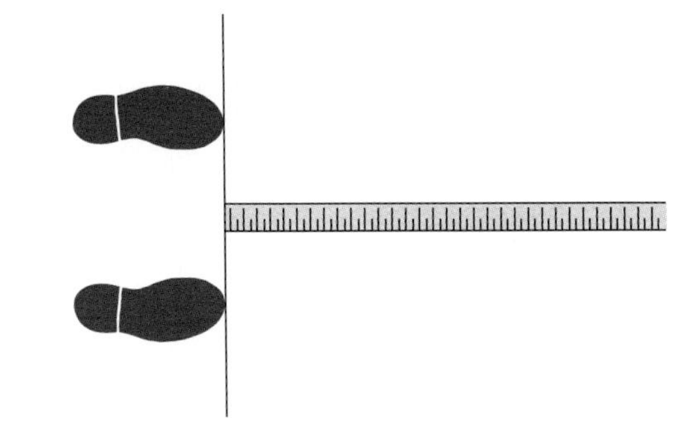

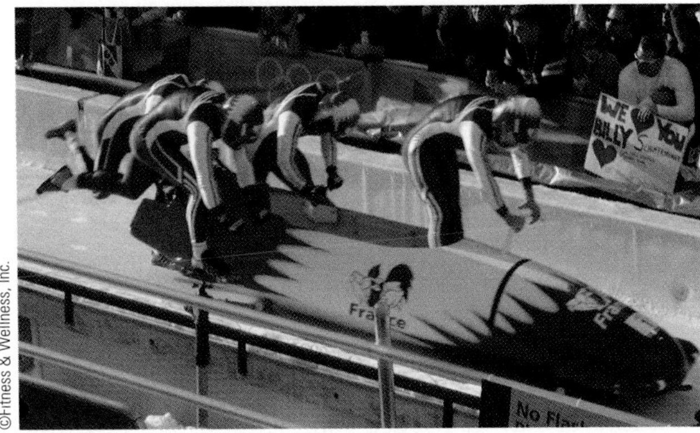

Fast starts in bob sleigh require exceptional leg power.

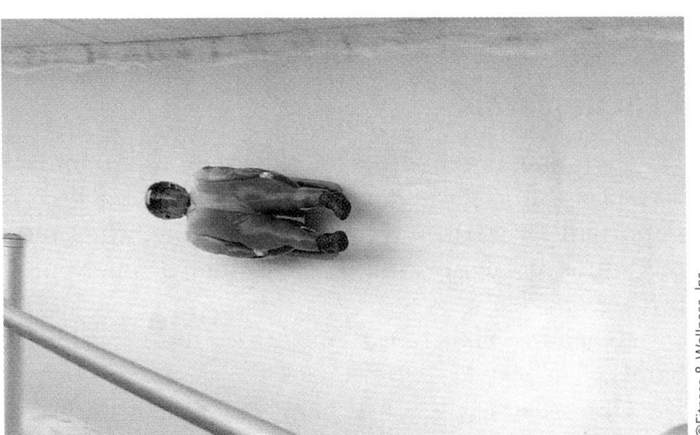

Luge athletes exhibit excellent reaction time and coordination.

The entire procedure is done twice, without stopping, and is counted as one trial. Two "trips" down and up are required to complete one trial. The watch is stopped when the last can of soda pop is returned to its original position, following the second trip back. The preferred hand (in this case, the right hand) is used throughout the entire task, and the objective of the test is to perform the task as fast as possible, making sure the cans are always placed within each circle.

If the person misses a circle at any time during the test (that is, if a can is placed on a line or outside a circle), the trial must be repeated from the start. A graphic illustration of this test is provided in Figure 9.2.

If using the left hand, the participant follows the same procedure, except the cans are placed starting from the left, with can one in circle 6, can two in circle 4, and can three in circle 2. The procedure is initiated by turning can one upside down onto circle 5, can two onto circle 3, and so on.

Prior to initiating the test, two practice trials are allowed. Two test trials then are administered, and the best time, recorded to the nearest tenth of a second, is used as the test score. If the person has a mistrial (misses a circle), the test is repeated until two consecutive successful trials are accomplished.

Power

Power is defined as the ability to produce maximum force in the shortest time. The two components of power are speed and force (strength). An effective combination of these two components allows a person to produce explosive movements such as in jumping, putting the shot, and spiking/throwing/hitting a ball.

Power is necessary to perform many activities of daily living that require strength and speed such as climbing stairs, lifting objects, preventing falls, or hurrying to catch a bus. Power is also beneficial in sports such as soccer, tennis, softball, golf, and volleyball.

Power Test Standing Long Jump Test[2]

Objective To measure leg power

Procedure

Administrator: Draw a takeoff line on the floor and place a 10-foot tape measure perpendicular to this line. Have the participant stand with feet several inches apart, centered on the tape measure, and toes just behind the takeoff line (see Figure 9.3).

Participant: Prior to the jump, swing your arms backward and bend your knees. Perform the jump by extending your knees and swinging your arms forward at the same time.

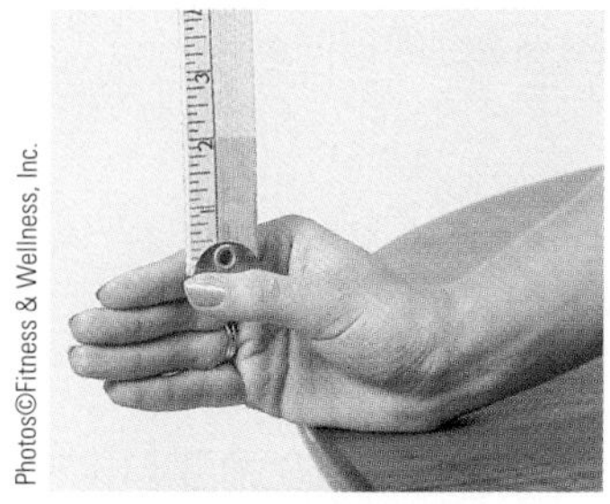
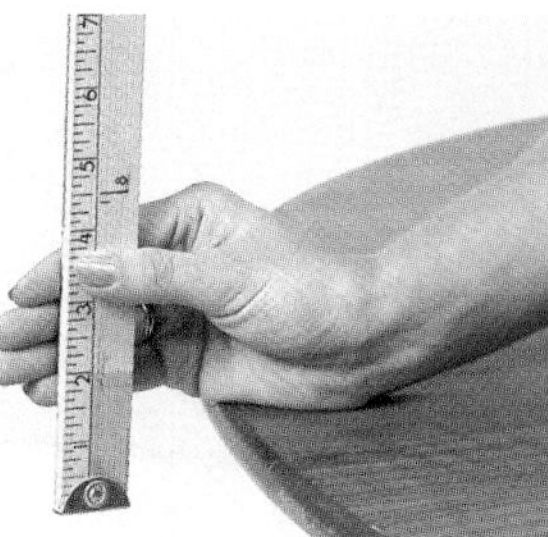

Photos©Fitness & Wellness, Inc.

"Yardstick" Reaction Time Test.

The distance is recorded from the takeoff line to the heel or other body part that touches the floor nearest the takeoff line. Three trials are allowed, and the best trial, measured to the nearest inch, becomes the final test score.

Reaction Time

Reaction time is defined as the time required to initiate a response to a given stimulus. Good reaction time is important for starts in track and swimming, when playing tennis at the net, and in sports such as ping pong, boxing, and karate.

Reaction Time Test Yardstick Test (preferred hand)

Objective To measure hand reaction time in response to a visual stimulus

Procedure

Administrator: For this test you will need a regular yardstick with a shaded "concentration zone" marked on the first 2 inches of the stick (see the photo above). Administer the test with the participant sitting in a chair adjacent to a table and the preferred forearm and hand resting on the table.

Participant: Hold the tips of the thumb and fingers in a "ready-to-pinch" position, about 1 inch apart and 3 inches beyond the edge of the table, with the upper edges of the thumb and index finger parallel to the floor. With the person administering the test holding the yardstick near the upper end and the zero point of the stick even with the upper edge of your thumb and index finger (the administrator may steady the middle of the stick with the other hand), look at the "concentration zone" and react by catching the stick when it is dropped. Do not look at the administrator's hand or move your hand up or down while trying to catch the stick.

Twelve trials make up the test, each preceded by the preparatory command "ready." The administrator makes a random 1- to 3-second count between the "ready" command and each drop of the stick. Each trial is scored to the nearest half-inch, read just above the upper edge of the thumb. Three practice trials are given before the actual test to be sure the subject understands the procedure. The three lowest and the three highest scores are discarded, and the average of the middle six is used as the final test score. The testing area should be as free from distractions as possible.

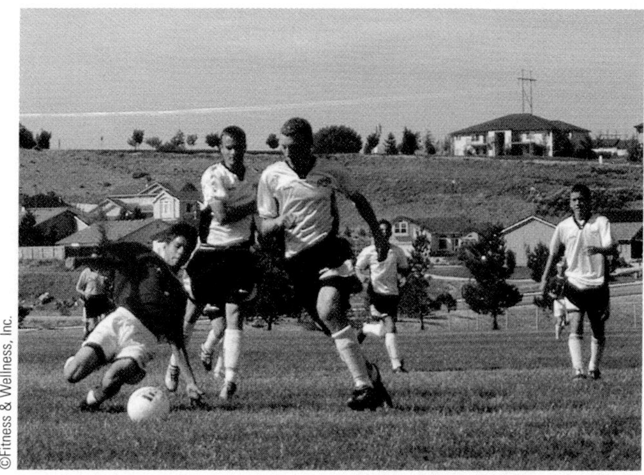

©Fitness & Wellness, Inc.

Speed is essential in the sport of soccer.

Speed

Speed is the ability to rapidly propel the body or a part of the body from one point to another. Examples of activities that require good speed for success are soccer, basketball, sprints in track, and stealing a base in baseball. In everyday life, speed can be important in a wide variety of emergency situations.

Speed Test 50-Yard Dash[3]

Objective To measure speed

Procedure Two participants take their positions behind the starting line. The starter raises one arm and asks, "Are you ready?" and the gives the command "go" while swinging the raised arm downward as a signal for the timer (or timers) at the finish line to start the stopwatch (or stopwatches).

The score is the time that elapses between the starting signal and the moment the participant crosses the finish line, recorded to the nearest tenth of a second.

Interpreting Test Results

Look up your score for each test in Table 9.1 or 9.2, then use Table 9.3 to see your level of fitness in that particular skill.

Team Sports

Choosing activities that you enjoy will greatly enhance your adherence to exercise. People tend to repeat things they enjoy doing. Enjoyment by itself is a reward. In this regard, combining individual activities (such as jogging, swimming, cycling) can deepen your commitment to fitness.

TABLE 9.1 Percentile Ranks and Fitness Category for Skill-Related Fitness Components—Men

	Agility*	Balance*	Coordination*	Power*	Reaction Time*	Speed**
99	9.5	59.8	5.8	9'10"	3.5	5.4
95	10.3	46.9	7.5	8'5"	4.2	5.9
90	10.6	41.1	7.7	8'2"	4.5	6.0
80	11.1	24.9	8.5	7'10"	4.9	6.3
70	11.5	15.4	8.9	7'7"	5.3	6.4
60	11.7	12.0	9.3	7'5"	5.5	6.5
50	11.9	9.2	9.6	7'2"	5.8	6.6
40	12.1	7.3	9.9	7'0"	6.1	6.8
30	12.4	5.8	10.2	6'8"	6.5	7.0
20	12.9	4.3	10.7	6'4"	6.7	7.1
10	13.7	3.1	11.3	5'10"	7.2	7.5
5	14.0	2.6	11.8	5'3"	7.4	7.9

* Norms developed at Boise State University, Department of Kinesiology.
** From *AAHPERD Youth Fitness: Test Manual.* 1976.

TABLE 9.2 Percentile Ranks and Fitness Category for Skill-Related Fitness Components—Women

	Agility*	Balance*	Coordination*	Power*	Reaction Time*	Speed**
99	11.1	59.9	7.5	7'6"	3.3	6.4
95	12.0	39.1	8.0	6'9"	4.5	6.8
90	12.2	25.8	8.2	6'6"	4.7	7.0
80	12.5	16.7	8.6	6'2"	5.1	7.3
70	12.9	11.9	9.0	5'11"	5.3	7.5
60	13.2	9.8	9.2	5'9"	5.9	7.6
50	13.4	7.6	9.5	5'5"	6.1	7.9
40	13.9	6.2	9.6	5'3"	6.4	8.0
30	14.2	5.0	9.9	5'0"	6.7	8.2
20	14.8	4.2	10.3	4'9"	7.2	8.5
10	15.5	2.9	10.7	4'4"	7.8	9.0
5	16.2	1.8	11.2	4'1"	8.4	9.5

* Norms developed at Boise State University, Department of Kinesiology.
** From *AAHPERD Youth Fitness: Test Manual.* 1976.

TABLE 9.3 Skill-Fitness Categories

Percentile Rank	Fitness Category
≥81	Excellent
61–80	Good
41–60	Average
21–40	Fair
≤20	Poor

TABLE 9.4 Contribution of Selected Activities to Skill-Related Components

Activity	Ability	Balance	Coordination	Power	Reaction Time	Speed
Alpine skiing	4	5	4	2	3	2
Archery	1	2	4	2	3	1
Badminton	4	3	4	2	4	3
Baseball	3	2	4	4	5	4
Basketball	4	3	4	3	4	3
Bowling	2	2	4	1	1	1
Cross-country skiing	3	4	3	2	2	1
Football	4	4	4	4	4	3
Golf	1	2	5	3	1	3
Gymnastics	5	5	5	4	3	3
Ice skating	5	5	5	3	3	3
In-line skating	4	4	4	3	2	4
Judo/Karate	5	5	5	4	5	4
Racquetball	5	4	4	4	5	4
Soccer	5	3	5	5	3	4
Table tennis	5	3	5	3	5	3
Tennis	4	3	5	3	5	3
Volleyball	4	3	5	4	5	3
Water skiing	3	4	3	2	2	1
Wrestling	5	5	5	4	5	4

1 = Low, 2 = Fair, 3 = Average, 4 = Good, 5= Excellent.

People with good skill-related fitness usually participate in lifetime sports and games, which in turn helps develop health-related fitness. Individuals who enjoyed basketball or soccer in their youth tend to stick to those activities later in life. The availability of teams and community leagues may be all that is needed to stop contemplating and start participating. The social element of team sports provides added incentive to participate. Team sports offer an opportunity to interact with people who share a common interest. Being a member of a team creates responsibility—another incentive to exercise because you are expected to be there. Furthermore, team sports foster lifetime friendships, strengthening the social and emotional dimensions of wellness.

For those who were not able to participate in youth sports, it's never too late to start (see the discussion of behavior modification and motivation in Chapter 2). Don't be afraid to select a new activity, even if that means learning new skills. The fitness and social rewards will be ample.

Similar to the fitness benefits of the aerobic activities discussed in Chapter 6 (see Table 6.10, page 191), the contributions of skill-related activities also vary among activities and individuals. The extent to which an activity helps develop each skill-related component varies by the effort the individual makes and, most important, by proper execution of the skill (knowledgeable coaching is highly recommended to achieve good technique) and the individual's potential based on genetic endowment. A summary of potential contributions to skill-related fitness for selected activities is provided in Table 9.4.

Critical Thinking

Participation in sports is a good predictor of adherence to exercise later in life. What previous experiences have you had with participation in sports? Were these experiences positive? What effect do they have on your current physical activity patterns?

Specific Exercise Considerations

In addition to the exercise-related issues already discussed in this book, many other concerns require clarification or are somewhat controversial. Let's examine some of these issues.

1. Does aerobic exercise make a person immune to heart and blood vessel disease?

Although aerobically fit individuals as a whole have a lower incidence of cardiovascular disease, a regular aerobic exercise program by itself does not offer an absolute guarantee against cardiovascular disease. The best way to minimize the risk for cardiovascular disease is to manage the risk factors. Many factors, including a genetic predisposition, can increase the risk. In any case, experts believe that a regular aerobic exercise program will delay the onset of cardiovascular problems and also will improve the chances of surviving a heart attack.

Even moderate increases in aerobic fitness significantly lower the incidence of premature cardiovascular deaths. Data from the research study on death rates by physical fitness groups (illustrated in Figure 1.9, page 12) indicate that the decrease in cardiovascular mortality is greatest between the unfit and the moderately fit groups. A further decrease in cardiovascular mortality is observed between the moderately fit and the highly fit groups, although the difference is not as pronounced as that between the unfit and moderately fit groups.

2. How much aerobic exercise is required to decrease the risk for cardiovascular disease?

Even though research has not yet indicated the exact amount of aerobic exercise required to lower the risk for cardiovascular disease, Dr. Ralph Paffenbarger and his co-researchers showed that expending 2,000 calories per week as a result of physical activity yielded the lowest risk for cardiovascular disease among a group of almost 17,000 Harvard alumni.[4] Expanding 2,000 calories per week represents about 300 calories per daily exercise session.

3. Do people get a "physical high" during aerobic exercise?

During vigorous exercise, **endorphins** are released from the pituitary gland in the brain. Endorphins can create feelings of euphoria and natural well-being. Higher levels of endorphins often result from aerobic endurance activities and may remain elevated for as long as 30 to 60 minutes after exercise. Many experts believe these higher levels explain the physical high that some people get during and after prolonged exercise.

Endorphin levels also have been shown to increase during pregnancy and childbirth. Endorphins act as painkillers. The higher levels could explain a woman's greater tolerance for the pain and discomfort of natural childbirth and her pleasant feelings shortly after the baby's birth. Several reports have indicated that well-conditioned women have shorter and easier labor. These women may attain higher endorphin levels during delivery, making childbirth less traumatic than it is for untrained women.

4. Can people with asthma exercise?

Asthma, a condition that causes difficult breathing, is characterized by coughing, wheezing, and shortness of breath induced by narrowing of the airway passages because of contraction (bronchospasm) of the airway muscles, swelling of the mucous membrane, and excessive secretion of mucus. In a few people, asthma can be triggered by exercise itself, particularly in cool and dry environments. This condition is referred to as *exercise-induced asthma* (EIA).

People with asthma need to obtain proper medication from a physician prior to initiating an exercise program. A regular program is best, because random exercise bouts are more likely to trigger asthma attacks. In the initial stages of exercise, an intermittent program (with frequent rest periods during the exercise session) is recommended. Gradual warm-up and cool-down are essential to reduce the risk of an acute attack. Furthermore, exercising in warm and humid conditions (such as swimming) is better because it helps to moisten the airways and thereby minimizes the asthmatic response. For land-based activities (such as walking and aerobics), drinking water before, during, and after exercise helps to keep the airways moist, decreasing the risk of an attack. During the winter months, wearing an exercise mask is recommended to increase the warmth and humidity of inhaled air. People with asthma should not exercise alone and always should carry their medication with them during workouts.

5. What types of activities are recommended for people with arthritis?

Individuals who have arthritis should participate in a combined stretching, aerobic, and strength-training program. The participant should do mild stretching prior to aerobic exercise to relax tight muscles. A regular flexibility program following aerobic exercise is encouraged to help maintain good joint mobility. During the aerobic portion of the exercise program, individuals with arthritis should avoid high-impact ac-

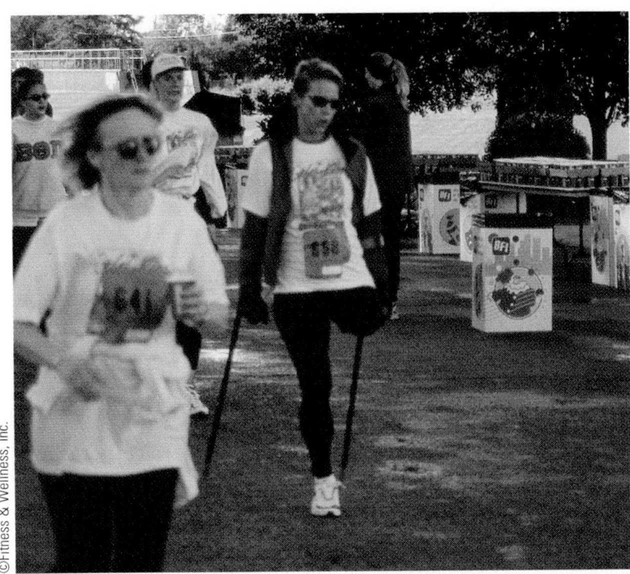

Physically challenged people can participate in and derive health and fitness benefits from a high-intensity exercise program.

tivities because these may cause greater trauma to arthritic joints. Low-impact activities such as swimming, water aerobics, and cycling are recommended. A complete strength-training program also is recommended, with special emphasis on exercises that will support the affected joint(s). As with any other program, individuals with arthritis should start with low-intensity or resistance exercises and build up gradually to a higher fitness level.

6. What precautions should diabetics take with respect to exercise?

According to the Centers for Disease Control and Prevention, there were more than 20 million reported diabetics in the United States in 2006, and more than 1 million new cases are diagnosed each year. At the current rate, one in three children born in the United States will develop the disease.

There are two types of diabetes:

type 1, or insulin-dependent diabetes (IDDM)
type 2, or non–insulin-dependent diabetes (NIDDM).

In type 1, found primarily in young people, the pancreas produces little or no insulin. With type 2, the pancreas may not produce enough insulin or the cells become insulin-resistant, thereby keeping glucose from entering the cell. Type 2 accounts for more than 90 percent of all cases of diabetes, and it occurs mainly in overweight people. (A more thorough discussion of the types of diabetes is given in Chapter 11, pages 376–378.)

If you have diabetes, consult your physician before you start exercising. You may not be able to begin until the diabetes is under control. Never exercise alone, and always wear a bracelet that identifies your condition. If you take insulin, the amount and timing of each dose may have to be regulated with your physician. If you inject insulin, do so over a muscle that won't be exercised, then wait an hour before exercising. For type 1 diabetics, it is recommended that you ingest 15 to 30 grams of carbohydrates during each 30 minutes of intense exercise and follow it with a carbohydrate snack after exercise.

Both types of diabetes improve with exercise, although the results are more notable in patients with type 2 diabetes. Exercise usually lowers blood sugar and helps the body use food more effectively. The extent to which the blood glucose level can be controlled in overweight type 2 diabetics seems to be related directly to how long and how hard a person exercises. Normal or near-normal blood glucose levels can be achieved through a proper exercise program.

As with any fitness program, the exercise must be done regularly to be effective against diabetes. The benefits of a single exercise bout on blood glucose are highest between 12 and 24 hours following exercise. These benefits are completely lost within 72 hours after exercise. Thus, regular participation is crucial to derive ongoing benefits. In terms of fitness, all diabetic patients can achieve higher fitness levels, including reductions in weight, blood pressure, and total cholesterol and triglycerides.

According to the ACSM, patients with type 2 diabetes should adhere to the following guidelines to make their exercise program safe and derive the most benefit:[5]

- Expend a minimum of 1,000 calories per week through your exercise program.
- Exercise at a low-to-moderate intensity (40 to 70 percent of HRR). Start your program with 10 to 15 minutes per session, on at least 3 nonconsecutive days, but preferably exercise 5 days per week. Gradually increase the time you exercise to 30 minutes until you achieve your goal of at least 1,000 calories weekly. Diabetic individuals with a weight problem should build up daily physical activity to 60 minutes per session.
- Choose an activity that you enjoy doing, and stay with it. As you select your activity, be aware of your condition. For example, if you have lost sensation in your feet, swimming or stationary cycling is better than walking or jogging to minimize the risk for injury.
- Check your blood glucose levels before and after exercise. If you are on insulin or diabetes medication, monitor your blood glucose regularly and

Endorphins Morphine-like substances released from the pituitary gland (in the brain) during prolonged aerobic exercise; thought to induce feelings of euphoria and natural well-being.

check it at least twice within 30 minutes of starting exercise.
- Schedule your exercise 1 to 3 hours after a meal, and avoid exercise when your insulin is peaking.
- Be ready to treat low blood sugar with a fast-acting source of sugar, such as juice, raisins, or other source recommended by your doctor.
- If you feel that a reaction is about to occur, discontinue exercise immediately. Check your blood glucose level and treat the condition as needed.
- When you exercise outdoors, always do so with someone who knows what to do in a diabetes-related emergency.

In addition, strength training twice per week, using 8 to 10 exercises with a minimum of one set of 10 to 15 repetitions to near fatigue, is recommended for individuals with diabetes. A complete description of strength-training programs is provided in Chapter 7.

7. Is exercise safe during pregnancy?

Exercise is beneficial during pregnancy. According to the American College of Obstetricians and Gynecologists (ACOG), in the absence of contraindications, healthy pregnant women are encouraged to participate in regular, moderate-intensity physical activities to continue to derive health benefits during pregnancy.[6] Pregnant women, however, should consult with their respective physicians to ensure that they have no contraindications to exercise during pregnancy.

As a general rule, healthy pregnant women can also accumulate 30 minutes of moderate-intensity physical activity on most, if not all, days of the week. Physical activity strengthens the body and helps prepare for the challenges of labor and childbirth.

The average labor and delivery lasts 10–12 hours. In most cases, labor and delivery are highly intense, with repeated muscular contractions interspersed with short rest periods. Proper conditioning will better prepare the body for childbirth. Moderate exercise during pregnancy also helps to prevent back pain and excessive weight gain, and it speeds recovery following childbirth.

The most common recommendations for exercise during pregnancy for healthy pregnant women with no additional risk factors are as follows:

- Don't start a new or more rigorous exercise program without proper medical clearance.
- Accumulate 30 minutes of moderate-intensity physical activities on most days of the week.
- Instead of using heart rate to monitor intensity, exercise at an intensity level between "fairly light" and "somewhat hard," using the Rate of Perceived Exertion (RPE) scale in Figure 6.7 (see page 186).
- Gradually switch from weight-bearing and high-impact activities, such as jogging and aerobics, to nonweight-bearing/lower-impact activities, such as walking, stationary cycling, swimming, and water aerobics. The latter activities minimize the risk of injury and may allow exercise to continue throughout pregnancy.
- Avoid exercising at an altitude above 6,000 feet (1,800 meters), as well as scuba diving because either may compromise the availability of oxygen to the fetus.
- Women who are accustomed to strenuous exercise may continue in the early stages of pregnancy but should gradually decrease the amount, intensity, and exercise mode as pregnancy advances (most healthy pregnant women, however, slow down during the first few weeks of pregnancy until morning sickness and fatigue subside).
- Pay attention to the body's signals of discomfort and distress, and never exercise to exhaustion. When fatigued, slow down or take a day off. Do not stop exercising altogether unless you experience any of the contraindications for exercise listed in the box on the next page.
- To prevent fetal injury, avoid activities that involve potential contact, loss of balance, or cause even mild trauma to the abdomen. Examples of these activities are basketball, soccer, volleyball, Nordic or water skiing, ice skating, road cycling, horseback riding, and motorcycle riding.
- During pregnancy, don't exercise for weight loss purposes.

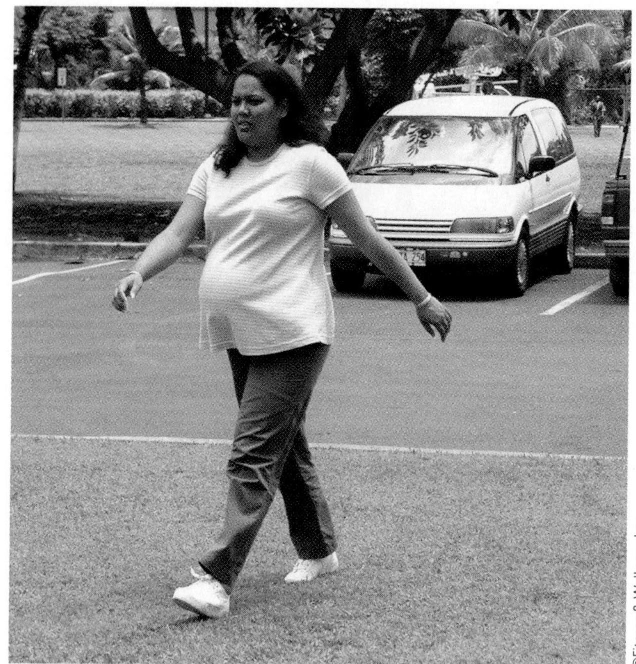

Mild-to-moderate intensity exercise is recommended throughout pregnancy.

CONTRAINDICATIONS TO EXERCISE DURING PREGNANCY

Stop exercise and seek medical advice if you experience any of the following symptoms:

- Unusual pain or discomfort, especially in the chest or abdominal area
- Cramping, primarily in the pelvic or lower back areas
- Muscle weakness, excessive fatigue, or shortness of breath
- Abnormally high heart rate or a pounding (palpitations) heart rate
- Decreased fetal movement
- Insufficient weight gain
- Amniotic fluid leakage
- Nausea, dizziness, or headaches
- Persistent uterine contractions
- Vaginal bleeding or rupture of the membranes
- Swelling of ankles, calves, hands, or face

- Get proper nourishment (pregnancy requires between 150 and 300 extra calories per day), and eat a small snack or drink some juice 20 to 30 minutes prior to exercise.
- Prevent dehydration by drinking a cup of fluids 20 to 30 minutes before exercise, and drink 1 cup of liquid every 15 to 20 minutes during exercise.
- During the first 3 months in particular, don't exercise in the heat. Wear clothing that allows for proper dissipation of heat. A body temperature above 102.6°F (39.2°C) can harm the fetus.
- After the first trimester, avoid exercises that require lying on the back. This position can block blood flow to the uterus and the baby.
- Perform stretching exercises gently because hormonal changes during pregnancy increase the laxity of muscles and connective tissue. Although these changes facilitate delivery, they also make women more susceptible to injuries during exercise.

8. Does exercise help relieve dysmenorrhea?

Although exercise has not been shown to either cure or aggravate **dysmenorrhea,** it has been shown to relieve menstrual cramps because it improves circulation to the uterus. Less severe menstrual cramps also could be caused by higher levels of endorphins produced during prolonged physical activity, which may counteract pain. Particularly, stretching exercises of the muscles in the pelvic region seem to reduce and prevent painful menstruation that is not the result of disease.[7]

9. Does participation in exercise hinder menstruation?

In some instances, highly trained athletes develop **amenorrhea** during training and competition. This condition is seen most often in extremely lean women who also engage in sports that require strenuous physical effort over a sustained time. It is by no means irreversible. At present, we do not know whether the condition is caused by physical or emotional stress related to high-intensity training, excessively low body fat, or other factors.

Although, on the average, women have a lower physical capacity during menstruation, medical surveys at the Olympic Games have shown that women have broken Olympic and world records at all stages of the menstrual cycle. Menstruation should not keep a woman from exercising, and it will not necessarily have a negative impact on performance.

10. Does exercise offset the detrimental effects of cigarette smoking?

Physical exercise often motivates a person to stop smoking, but it does not offset any ill effects of smoking. Smoking greatly decreases the ability of the blood to transport oxygen to working muscles.

Oxygen is carried in the circulatory system by hemoglobin, the iron-containing pigment of the red blood cells. Carbon monoxide, a byproduct of cigarette smoke, has 210 to 250 times greater affinity for hemoglobin over oxygen. Consequently, carbon monoxide combines much faster with hemoglobin, decreasing the oxygen-carrying capacity of the blood.

Chronic smoking also increases airway resistance, requiring the respiratory muscles to work much harder and consume more oxygen just to ventilate a given amount of air. If a person quits smoking, exercise does help increase the functional capacity of the pulmonary system.

A regular exercise program seems to be a powerful incentive to quit smoking. A random survey of 1,250 runners conducted at the 6.2-mile Peachtree Road Race in Atlanta provided impressive results. The survey indicated that, of the men and women who smoked cigarettes when they started running, 81 percent and 75 percent, respectively, had quit before the date of the race.

11. How long should a person wait after a meal before exercising strenuously?

The length of time to wait before exercising after a meal depends on the amount of food eaten. On the average, after a regular meal, you should wait about 2 hours before participating in strenuous physical activity. But a walk or some other light physical activity is fine following a meal. If anything, it helps burn extra calories and may help the body metabolize fats more efficiently.

Dysmenorrhea Painful menstruation.

Amenorrhea Cessation of regular menstrual flow.

FIGURE 9.4 What to look for in a good pair of shoes.

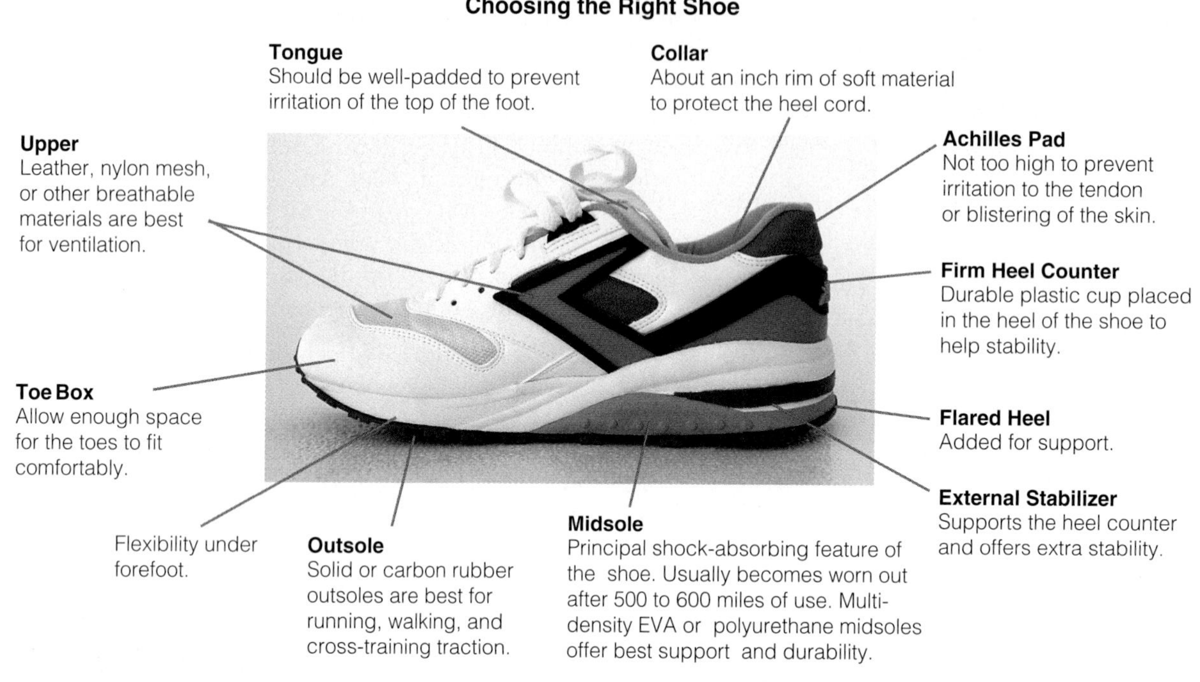

12. What type of clothing should I wear when I exercise?

The type of clothing you wear during exercise is important. In general, clothing should fit comfortably and allow free movement of the various body parts. Select clothing according to air temperature, humidity, and exercise intensity. Avoid nylon and rubberized materials and tight clothes that interfere with the cooling mechanism of the human body or obstruct normal blood flow. Choose fabrics made of polypropylene, Capilene, Thermax, or any synthetic that draws (wicks) moisture away from the skin, enhancing evaporation and cooling of the body. It's also important to consider your exercise intensity, because the harder you exercise, the more heat your body produces.

When exercising in the heat, avoid the hottest time of the day between 11:00 AM and 5:00 PM. Surfaces such as asphalt, concrete, and artificial turf absorb heat, which then radiates to the body. Therefore, these surfaces are not recommended. (Also see the discussion about heat and humidity in Question 14, page 301.)

Only a minimal amount of clothing is necessary during exercise in the heat, to allow for maximal evaporation. Clothing should be lightweight, light-colored, loose-fitting, airy, and absorbent. Examples of commercially available products that can be used during exercise in the heat are Asic's Perma Plus, Cool-max, and Nike's Dri-F.I.T. Double-layer acrylic socks are more absorbent than cotton and help to prevent blistering and chafing of the feet. A straw-type hat can be worn to protect the eyes and head from the sun. (Clothing for exercise in the cold is discussed in Question 16, page 302.)

A good pair of shoes is vital to prevent injuries to lower limbs. Shoes manufactured specifically for your choice of activity are a must (see Figure 9.4). When selecting proper footwear, you should consider body type, tendency toward pronation (rotating the foot outward) or supination (rotating the foot inward), and exercise surfaces. Shoes should have good stability, motion control, and comfortable fit. Purchase shoes in the middle of the day when your feet have expanded and might be one-half size larger. For increased breathability, choose shoes with nylon or mesh uppers.

Generally, salespeople at reputable athletic shoe stores are knowledgeable and can help you select a good shoe that fits your needs. After 300 to 500 miles or 6 months, examine your shoes and obtain a new pair if they are worn out. Old shoes are frequently responsible for injuries to the lower limbs.

13. What time of the day is best for exercise?

You can do intense exercise almost any time of the day, with the exception of about 2 hours following a heavy meal or the mid-day and early afternoon hours on hot, humid days. Moderate exercise seems to be beneficial shortly after a meal, because exercise enhances the **thermogenic response.** A walk shortly after a meal burns more calories than a walk several hours after a meal.

Many people enjoy exercising early in the morning because it gives them a boost to start the day. People who exercise in the morning also seem to stick with it more than others, because the chances of putting off the exercise session for other reasons are minimized. Some prefer the lunch hour for weight-control reasons. By exercising at noon, they do not eat as big a lunch, which helps keep down the daily caloric intake. Highly stressed people seem to like the evening hours because of the relaxing effects of exercise.

14. Why is exercising in hot and humid conditions unsafe?

When a person exercises, only 30 to 40 percent of the energy the body produces is used for mechanical work or movement. The rest of the energy (60 to 70 percent) is converted into heat. If this heat cannot be dissipated properly because the weather is too hot or the relative humidity is too high, body temperature increases and, in extreme cases, it can result in death.

The specific heat of body tissue (the heat required to raise the temperature of the body by 1° C) is .38 calories per pound of body weight (.38 cal/lb). This indicates that if no body heat is dissipated, a 150-pound person has to burn only 57 calories (150 × .38) to increase total body temperature by 1° C. If this person were to conduct an exercise session requiring 300 calories (e.g., running about 3 miles) without any dissipation of heat, the inner body temperature would increase by 5.3° C (300 ÷ 57), which is the equivalent of going from 98.6° F to 108.1° F.

This example illustrates clearly the need for caution when exercising in hot or humid weather. If the relative humidity is too high, body heat cannot be lost through evaporation because the atmosphere already is saturated with water vapor. In one instance, a football casualty occurred when the temperature was only 64° F, but the relative humidity was 100 percent. People must be cautious when air temperature is above 90° F and the relative humidity is above 60 percent.

The American College of Sports Medicine recommends avoiding strenuous physical activity when the readings of a wet-bulb globe thermometer exceed 82.4° F. With this type of thermometer, the wet bulb is cooled by evaporation, and on dry days it shows a lower temperature than the regular (dry) thermometer. On humid days, the cooling effect is less because of less evaporation; hence, the difference between the wet and dry readings is not as great.

Following are descriptions of, and first-aid measures for, the three major signs of heat illness:

- **Heat cramps.** Symptoms include cramps, spasms, and muscle twitching in the legs, arms, and abdomen. To relieve heat cramps, stop exercising, get out of the heat, massage the painful area, stretch slowly, and drink plenty of fluids (water, fruit drinks, or electrolyte beverages).
- **Heat exhaustion.** Symptoms include fainting; dizziness; profuse sweating; cold, clammy skin; weakness; headache; and a rapid, weak pulse. If you incur any of these symptoms, stop and find a cool place to rest. If conscious, drink cool water. Do not give water to an unconscious person. Loosen or remove clothing and rub your body with a cool, wet towel or apply ice packs. Place yourself in a supine position with the legs elevated 8 to 12 inches. If you are not fully recovered in 30 minutes, seek immediate medical attention.
- **Heat stroke.** Symptoms include serious disorientation; warm, dry skin; no sweating; rapid, full pulse; vomiting; diarrhea; unconsciousness; and high body temperature. As the body temperature climbs, unexplained anxiety sets in. When the body temperature reaches 104° F to 105° F, the individual may feel a cold sensation in the trunk of the body, goosebumps, nausea, throbbing in the temples, and numbness in the extremities. Most people become incoherent after this stage.

  When body temperature reaches 105° F to 107° F, disorientation, loss of fine-motor control, and muscular weakness set in. If the temperature exceeds 106° F, serious neurologic injury and death may be imminent.

  Heat stroke requires immediate emergency medical attention. Request help and get out of the sun and into a cool, humidity-controlled environ-

SYMPTOMS OF HEAT ILLNESS

If any of these symptoms occur, stop physical activity, get out of the sun, and start drinking fluids.

- Decreased perspiration
- Cramping
- Weakness
- Flushed skin
- Throbbing head
- Nausea/vomiting
- Diarrhea
- Numbness in the extremities
- Blurred vision
- Unsteadiness
- Disorientation
- Incoherency

Thermogenic response Amount of energy required to digest food.

Heat cramps Muscle spasms caused by heat-induced changes in electrolyte balance in muscle cells.

Heat exhaustion Heat-related fatigue.

Heat stroke Emergency situation resulting from the body being subjected to high atmospheric temperatures.

ment. While you are waiting to be taken to the hospital emergency room, you should be placed in a semi-seated position and your body should be sprayed with cool water and rubbed with cool towels. If possible, cold packs should be placed in areas that receive an abundant blood supply, such as the head, neck, armpits, and groin. Fluids should not be given if you are unconscious. In any case of heat-related illness, if the person refuses water, vomits, or starts to lose consciousness, an ambulance should be summoned immediately. Proper initial treatment of heat stroke is vital.

15. What should a person do to replace fluids lost during prolonged aerobic exercise?

The main objective of fluid replacement during prolonged aerobic exercise is to maintain the blood volume so circulation and sweating can continue at normal levels. Adequate water replacement is the most important factor in preventing heat disorders. Drinking about 6 to 8 ounces of cool water every 15 to 20 minutes during exercise is recommended to prevent dehydration. Cold fluids seem to be absorbed more rapidly from the stomach.

Other relevant points are the following:

- Drinking commercially prepared sports drinks is recommended when exercise will be strenuous and carried out for more than an hour. For exercise lasting less than an hour, water is just as effective in replacing lost fluid. The sports drinks you select may be based on your personal preference. Try different drinks at 6 to 8 percent glucose concentration to see which drink you tolerate best and suits your tastes as well.
- Commercial fluid-replacement solutions (such as Powerade® and Gatorade®) contain about 6 to 8 percent glucose, which seems to be optimal for fluid absorption and performance. Sugar does not become available to the muscles until about 30 minutes after consumption of a glucose solution.
- Drinks high in fructose or with a glucose concentration above 8 percent are not recommended because they slow water absorption during exercise in the heat.
- Most sodas (both cola and non-cola) contain between 10 and 12 percent glucose, which is too high for proper rehydration during exercise in the heat.
- Do not overhydrate with just water during a very long or ultra-long distance event, as such can lead to hyponatremia (also see "Hyponatremia" in Chapter 3, page 92) or low sodium concentration in the blood. When water loss through sweat during prolonged exercise is replaced by water alone, blood sodium is diluted to the point where it creates serious health problems, including seizures and coma in severe cases.

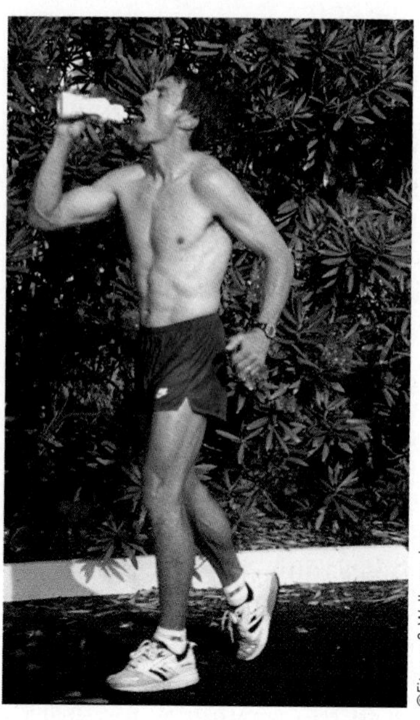

Fluid and carbohydrate replacement is essential when exercising in the heat or for a prolonged period.

16. What precautions must a person take when exercising in the cold?

When exercising in the cold, the two factors to consider are frostbite and **hypothermia.** In contrast to hot and humid conditions, cold weather usually does not threaten health because clothing can be selected for heat conservation, and exercise itself increases the production of body heat.

Most people actually overdress for exercise in the cold. Because exercise increases body temperature, a moderate workout on a cold day makes a person feel that the temperature is 20 to 30 degrees warmer than it actually is. Overdressing for exercise can make the clothes damp from excessive perspiration. The risk for hypothermia increases when a person is wet or after exercise stops when the person is not moving around sufficiently to increase (or maintain) body heat.

Initial warning signs of hypothermia include shivering, losing coordination, and having difficulty speaking. With a continued drop in body temperature, shivering stops, the muscles weaken and stiffen, and the person feels elated or intoxicated and eventually loses consciousness. To prevent hypothermia, use common sense, dress properly, and be aware of environmental conditions.

The popular belief that exercising in cold temperatures (32° F and lower) freezes the lungs is false, because the air is warmed properly in the air passages before it reaches the lungs. Cold is not what poses a threat; wind velocity is what increases the chill factor most.

For example, exercising at a temperature of 25° F with adequate clothing is not too cold to exercise, but if the wind is blowing at 25 miles per hour, the chill factor lowers the actual temperature to 15° F. This effect is even worse if a person is wet and exhausted. When the weather is windy, the individual should exercise (jog or cycle) against the wind on the way out and with the wind upon returning.

Even though the lungs are under no risk when you exercise in the cold, your face, head, hands, and feet should be protected because they are subject to frostbite. Watch for signs of frostbite: numbness and discoloration. In cold temperatures, as much as half of the body's heat can be lost through an unprotected head and neck. A wool or synthetic cap, hood, or hat will help to hold in body heat. Mittens are better than gloves, because they keep the fingers together so the surface area from which to lose heat is less. Inner linings of synthetic material to wick moisture away from the skin are recommended. Avoid cotton next to the skin, because once cotton gets wet whether from perspiration, rain, or snow it loses its insulating properties.

Wearing several layers of lightweight clothing is preferable to wearing one single, thick layer because warm air is trapped between layers of clothes, enabling greater heat conservation. As body temperature increases, you can remove layers as necessary.

The first layer of clothes should wick moisture away from the skin. Polypropylene, Capilene, and Thermax are recommended materials. Next, a layer of wool, dacron, or polyester fleece insulates well even when wet. Lycra tights or sweatpants help protect the legs. The outer layer should be waterproof, wind-resistant, and breathable. A synthetic material such as Gore-Tex is best, so moisture can still escape from the body. A ski mask or face mask helps protect the face. In extremely cold conditions, exposed skin, such as the nose, cheeks, and around the eyes, can be insulated with petroleum jelly.

For lengthy or long-distance workouts (cross-country skiing or long runs), take a small backpack to carry the clothing you removed. You also can carry extra warm and dry clothes in case you stop exercising away from shelter. If you remain outdoors following exercise, added clothing and continuous body movement are essential to maintain body temperature and avoid hypothermia.

17. Can I exercise when I have a cold or the flu?

The most important consideration is to use common sense and pay attention to your symptoms. Usually, you may continue to exercise if your symptoms include a runny nose, sneezing, or a scratchy throat. But, if your symptoms include fever, muscle ache, vomiting, diarrhea, or a hacking cough, you should avoid exercise. After an illness, be sure to ease back gradually into your program. Do not attempt to return at the same intensity and duration that you were used to prior to your illness.

Exercise-Related Injuries

To enjoy and maintain physical fitness, preventing injury during a conditioning program is essential. Exercise-related injuries, nonetheless, are common in individuals who participate in exercise programs. Surveys indicate that more than half of all new participants incur injuries during the first 6 months of the conditioning program.

The four most common causes of injuries are

1. high-impact activities,
2. rapid conditioning programs (doing too much too quickly),
3. improper shoes or training surfaces, and
4. anatomical predisposition (that is, body propensity).

High-impact activities and a significant increase in quantity, intensity, or duration of activities are by far the most common causes of injuries. The body requires time to adapt to more intense activities. Most of these injuries can be prevented through a more gradual and correct conditioning (low-impact) program.

Proper shoes for specific activities are essential. Shoes should be replaced when they show a lot of wear and tear. Softer training surfaces, such as grass and dirt, produce less trauma than asphalt and concrete.

Because few people have perfect body alignment, injuries associated with overtraining may occur eventually. In case of injury, proper treatment can avert a lengthy recovery process. A summary of common exercise-related injuries and how to manage them follows.

Acute Sports Injuries

The best treatment always has been prevention. If an activity causes unusual discomfort or chronic irritation, you need to treat the cause by decreasing the intensity, switching activities, substituting equipment, or upgrading clothing (such as buying properly fitting shoes).

In cases of acute injury, the standard treatment is rest, cold application, compression or splinting (or both), and elevation of the affected body part. This is commonly referred to as **RICE:**

R = rest
I = ice (cold) application
C = compression
E = elevation

Hypothermia A breakdown in the body's ability to generate heat; a drop in body temperature below 95° F.

RICE An acronym used to describe the standard treatment procedure for acute sports injuries: Rest, Ice (cold application), Compression, and Elevation.

TABLE 9.5 Reference Guide for Exercise-Related Problems

Injury	Signs/Symptoms	Treatment*
Bruise (contusion)	Pain, swelling, discoloration	Cold application, compression, rest
Dislocations/Fracture	Pain, swelling, deformity	Splinting, cold application, seek medical attention
Heat cramp	Cramps, spasms, and muscle twitching in the legs, arms, and abdomen	Stop activity, get out of the heat, stretch, massage the painful area, drink plenty of fluids
Heat exhaustion	Fainting, profuse sweating, cold/clammy skin, weak/rapid pulse, weakness, headache	Stop activity, rest in a cool place, loosen clothing, rub body with cool/wet towel, drink plenty of fluids, stay out of heat for 2–3 days
Heat stroke	Hot/dry skin, no sweating, serious disorientation, rapid/full pulse, vomiting, diarrhea, unconsciousness, high body temperature	**Seek immediate medical attention,** request help and get out of the sun, bathe in cold water/spray with cold water/rub body with cold towels, drink plenty of cold fluids
Joint sprains	Pain, tenderness, swelling, loss of use, discoloration	Cold application, compression, elevation, rest; heat after 36 to 48 hours (if no further swelling)
Muscle cramps	Pain, spasm	Stretch muscle(s), use mild exercises for involved area
Muscle soreness and stiffness	Tenderness, pain	Mild stretching, low-intensity exercise, warm bath
Muscle strains	Pain, tenderness, swelling, loss of use	Cold application, compression, elevation, rest; heat after 36 to 48 hours (if no further swelling)
Shin splints	Pain, tenderness	Cold application prior to and following any physical activity, rest; heat (if no activity is carried out)
Side stitch	Pain on the side of the abdomen below the rib cage	Decrease level of physical activity or stop altogether, gradually increase level of fitness
Tendinitis	Pain, tenderness, loss of use	Rest, cold application, heat after 48 hours

* Cold should be applied three to five times a day for 15 minutes. Heat can be applied three times a day for 15 to 20 minutes.

Cold should be applied three to five times a day for 15 minutes at a time during the first 36 to 48 hours, by submerging the injured area in cold water, using an ice bag, or applying ice massage to the affected part. An elastic bandage or wrap can be used for compression. Elevating the body part decreases blood flow (and therefore swelling) in that body part.

The purpose of these treatment modalities is to minimize swelling in the area, which hastens recovery time. After the first 36 to 48 hours, heat can be used if the injury shows no further swelling or inflammation. If you have doubts as to the nature or seriousness of the injury (such as suspected fracture), seek a medical evaluation.

Obvious deformities (exhibited by fractures, dislocations, or partial dislocations, as examples) call for splinting, cold application with an ice bag, and medical attention. Do not try to reset any of these conditions by yourself, because you could further damage muscles, ligaments, and nerves. Treatment of these injuries always should be left to specialized medical personnel. A quick reference guide for the signs or symptoms and treatment of exercise-related problems is provided in Table 9.5.

Muscle Soreness and Stiffness

Individuals who begin an exercise program or participate after a long layoff from exercise often develop muscle soreness and stiffness. The acute soreness that sets in the first few hours after exercise is thought to be related to general fatigue of the exercised muscles.

Delayed muscle soreness that appears several hours after exercise (usually about 12 hours later) and lasts 2 to 4 days may be related to actual tiny tears in muscle tissue, muscle spasms that increase fluid retention (stimulating the pain nerve endings), and overstretching or tearing of connective tissue in and around muscles and joints.

Mild stretching before and adequate stretching after exercise help to prevent soreness and stiffness. Gradually progressing into an exercise program is important, too. A person should not attempt to do too much too quickly. To relieve pain, mild stretching, low-intensity exercise to stimulate blood flow, and a warm bath might help.

Exercise Intolerance

When starting an exercise program, participants should stay within the safe limits. The best method to determine whether you are exercising too strenuously is to check your heart rate and make sure it does not exceed the limits of your target zone. Exercising above this target zone may not be safe for unconditioned or high-risk individuals. You do not have to exercise beyond your target zone to gain the desired cardiorespiratory benefits.

Several physical signs will tell you when you are exceeding your functional limitations, that is, experiencing **exercise intolerance.** Signs of intolerance include rapid or irregular heart rate, difficult breathing, nausea, vomiting, lightheadedness, headache, dizziness, unusually flushed or pale skin, extreme weakness, lack of energy, shakiness, sore muscles, cramps, and tightness in the chest. Learn to listen to your body. If you notice any of these symptoms, seek medical attention before continuing your exercise program.

Recovery heart rate is another indicator of overexertion. To a certain extent, recovery heart rate is related to fitness level. The higher your cardiorespiratory fitness level, the faster your heart rate will decrease following exercise. As a rule, heart rate should be below 120 beats per minute 5 minutes into recovery. If your heart rate is above 120, you most likely have overexerted yourself or possibly could have some other cardiac abnormality. If you lower the intensity or duration of exercise, or both, and you still have a fast heart rate 5 minutes into recovery, you should consult your physician.

Side Stitch

Side stitch can develop in the early stages of participation in exercise. It occurs primarily in unconditioned beginners and in trained individuals when they exercise at higher intensities than usual. As one's physical condition improves, this condition tends to disappear unless training is intensified.

The exact cause is unknown. Some experts suggest that it could relate to a lack of blood flow to the respiratory muscles during strenuous physical exertion. Some people encounter side stitch during downhill running. If you get side stitch during exercise, slow down. If it persists, stop altogether. Lying down on your back and gently bringing both knees to the chest and holding that position for 30 to 60 seconds also helps.

Some people get side stitch if they drink juice or eat anything shortly before exercise. Drinking only water 1 to 2 hours prior to exercise sometimes prevents side stitch. Other individuals have problems with commercially available sports drinks during high-intensity exercise. Unless carbohydrate replacement is crucial to complete an event (such as a marathon or a triathlon), drink cool water for fluid replacement or try a different carbohydrate solution.

Shin Splints

Shin splints, one of the most common injuries to the lower limbs, usually results from one or more of the following: (a) lack of proper and gradual conditioning, (b) doing physical activities on hard surfaces (wooden floors, hard tracks, cement, or asphalt), (c) fallen arches, (d) chronic overuse, (e) muscle fatigue, (f) faulty posture, (g) improper shoes, or (h) participating in weight-bearing activities when excessively overweight.

To manage shin splints:

1. Remove or reduce the cause (exercise on softer surfaces, wear better shoes or arch supports, or completely stop exercise until the shin splints heal);
2. Do stretching exercises before and after physical activity;
3. Use ice massage for 10 to 20 minutes before and after exercise;
4. Apply active heat (whirlpool and hot baths) for 15 minutes, two to three times a day; or
5. Use supportive taping during physical activity (a qualified athletic trainer can teach you the proper taping technique).

Muscle Cramps

Muscle cramps are caused by the body's depletion of essential electrolytes or a breakdown in the coordination between opposing muscle groups. If you have a muscle cramp, you should first attempt to stretch the muscles involved. In the case of the calf muscle, for example, pull your toes up toward the knees. After stretching the muscle, rub it down gently, and, finally, do some mild exercises requiring the use of that muscle.

In pregnant and lactating women, muscle cramps often are related to a lack of calcium. If women get cramps during these times, calcium supplements usually relieve the problem. Tight clothing also can cause cramps by decreasing blood flow to active muscle tissue.

Exercise and Aging

For the first time in U.S. history, the elderly constitute the fastest-growing segment of the population. The number of Americans ages 65 and older has increased from 3.1 million in 1900 (4.1 percent of the population) to about 36 million (12 percent) in 2003. By the year 2030, more than 72 million people, or 20 percent of the U.S. population, are expected to be older than age 65.

The main objective of fitness programs for older adults should be to help them improve their functional status and contribute to healthy aging. This implies the ability to maintain independent living status and to

---

Exercise intolerance Inability to function during exercise because of excessive fatigue or extreme feelings of discomfort.

Side stitch A sharp pain in the side of the abdomen.

Shin splints Injury to the lower leg characterized by pain and irritation in the shin region of the leg.

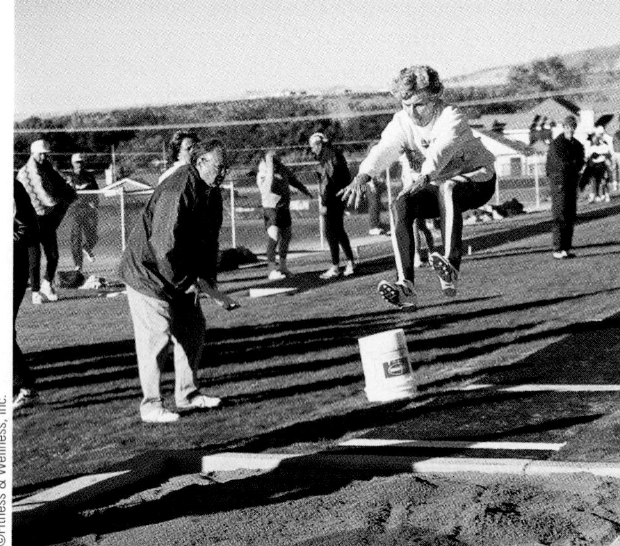

A high level of physical fitness can be maintained throughout the life span.

TABLE 9.6 Effects of Physical Activity and Inactivity on Older Men

	Exercisers	Non-exercisers
Age (yrs)	68.0	69.8
Weight (lbs)	160.3	186.3
Resting heart rate (bpm)	55.8	66.0
Maximal heart rate (bpm)	157.0	146.0
Heart rate reserve* (bpm)	101.2	80.0
Blood pressure (mm Hg)	120/78	150/90
Maximal oxygen uptake (ml/kg/min)	38.6	20.3

* Heart rate reserve = maximal heart rate − resting heart rate.
Data from F. W. Kash, J. L. Boyer, S. P. Van Camp, L. S. Verity, and J. P. Wallace, "The Effect of Physical Activity on Aerobic Power in Older Men (A Longitudinal Study)," *The Physician and Sports Medicine* 18, no. 4 (1990): 73–83.

avoid disability. Older adults are encouraged to participate in programs that will help develop cardiorespiratory endurance, muscular strength and endurance, muscular flexibility, agility, balance, and motor coordination.

Physical Training in the Older Adult

Regular participation in physical activity provides both physical and psychological benefits to older adults.[8] Cardiorespiratory endurance training helps to increase functional capacity, decrease the risk for disease, improve health status, and increase life expectancy. Strength training decreases the rate at which strength and muscle mass are lost. Among the psychological benefits are preserved cognitive function, reduced symptoms and behaviors related to depression, and improved self-confidence and self-esteem.

The trainability of older men and women alike and the effectiveness of physical activity in enhancing health have been demonstrated in research. Older adults who increase their physical activity experience significant changes in cardiorespiratory endurance, strength, and flexibility. The extent of the changes depends on their initial fitness level and the types of activities they select for their training (walking, cycling, strength training, and so on).

Improvements in maximal oxygen uptake in older adults are similar to those of younger people, although older people seem to require a longer training period to achieve these changes. Declines in maximal oxygen uptake average about 1 percent per year between ages 25 and 75.[9] A slower rate of decline is seen in people who maintain a lifetime aerobic exercise program.

Results of research on the effects of aging on the cardiorespiratory system of male exercisers versus nonexercisers showed that the maximal oxygen uptake of regular exercisers was almost twice that of the nonexercisers (see Table 9.6).[10] The study revealed a decline in maximal oxygen uptake between ages 50 and 68 of only 13 percent in the active group, compared to 41 percent in the inactive group. These changes indicate that about one-third of the loss in maximal oxygen uptake results from aging and two-thirds of the loss comes from inactivity. Blood pressure, heart rate, and body weight also were remarkably better in the exercising group. Furthermore, aerobic training seems to decrease high blood pressure in the older patients at the same rate as in young hypertensive people.[11]

In terms of aging, muscle strength declines by 10 to 20 percent between ages 20 and 50, but between ages 50 and 70, it drops by another 25 to 30 percent. Through strength training, frail adults in their 80s or 90s can double or triple their strength in just a few months. The amount of muscle hypertrophy achieved, however, decreases with age. Strength gains close to 200 percent have been found in previously inactive adults older than age 90.[12] In fact, research has shown that regular strength training improves balance, gait, speed, **functional independence,** morale, depression symptoms, and energy intake.[13]

Although muscle flexibility drops by about 5 percent per decade of life, 10 minutes of stretching every other day can prevent most of this loss as a person ages.[14] Improved flexibility also enhances mobility skills.[15] The latter promotes independence because it helps older adults successfully perform activities of daily living.

In terms of body composition, inactive adults continue to gain body fat after age 60 despite their tendency toward lower body weight. The increase in body fat is most likely related to a decrease in physical activity, lean body mass, and basal metabolic rate, along with increased caloric intake above that required to maintain daily energy requirements.[16]

Older adults who wish to initiate or continue an exercise program are strongly encouraged to have a complete medical exam, including a stress electrocardiogram test (see Chapter 11). Recommended activities for older adults include calisthenics, walking, jogging, swimming, cycling, and water aerobics.

Older people should avoid isometric and very high-intensity weight-training exercises (see Chapter 7). Activities that require all-out effort or require participants to hold their breath tend to lessen blood flow to the heart, cause a significant increase in blood pressure, and increase the load placed on the heart. Older adults should participate in activities that require continuous and rhythmic muscular activity (about 40 to 60 percent of HRR). These activities do not cause large increases in blood pressure or overload the heart.

Preparing for Sports Participation

To enhance your participation in sports, it is better to get fit before playing sports rather than playing sports to get fit.[17] A good pre-season training program will help make the season more enjoyable and prevent exercise-related injuries.

Properly conditioned individuals can participate safely in sports and enjoy the activities to their fullest with few or no limitations. Unfortunately, sport injuries often are the result of poor fitness and lack of sport-specific conditioning. Many injuries occur when fatigue sets in following overexertion by unconditioned individuals.

Base Fitness Conditioning

Pre-activity screening that includes a health history (see "Clearance for Exercise Participation," page 29) and/or a medical evaluation appropriate to your sport selection is recommended. Once cleared for exercise, start by building a base of general athletic fitness that includes the four health-related fitness components: cardiorespiratory fitness, muscular strength and endurance, flexibility, and recommended body composition. The base fitness conditioning program should last a minimum of 6 weeks.

As explained in Chapter 6, for cardiorespiratory fitness select an activity that you enjoy (such as walking, jogging, cycling, **step aerobics,** cross-country skiing, stair climbing, endurance games) and train three to five times per week at a minimum of 20 minutes of continuous activity per session. Exercise in the moderate- to high-intensity zones for adequate conditioning. You should feel as though you are training "somewhat hard" to "hard" at these intensity levels.

Strength (resistance) training helps maintain and increase muscular strength and endurance. Following the guidelines provided in Chapter 7, select 10 to 12 exercises that involve the major muscle groups and train two or three times per week on nonconsecutive days. Select a resistance (weight) that allows you to do 3 to 20 repetitions (based on your fitness goals—see Chapter 7) to near fatigue. That is, the resistance will be heavy enough so that when you perform one set of an exercise, you will not be able to do more than the predetermined number of repetitions at that weight. Begin your program slowly and perform between one and three sets of each exercise. Recommended exercises include the bench press, lat pull-down, leg press, leg curl, triceps extension, arm curl, rowing torso, heel raise, abdominal crunch, and back extension.

Flexibility is important in sports participation to enhance the range of motion in the joints. Using the guidelines from Chapter 8, schedule flexibility training two or three days per week. Perform each stretching exercise four times, and hold each stretch for 15 to 30 seconds. Examples of stretching exercises include the side body stretch, body rotation, chest stretch, shoulder stretch, sit-and-reach stretch, adductor stretch, quad stretch, heel cord stretch, and knee-to-chest stretch.

In terms of body composition, excess body fat hinders sports performance and increases the risk for injuries. Depending on the nature of the activity, fitness goals for body composition range from 12 to 20 percent body fat for men and 17 to 25 percent for most women.

Sport-Specific Conditioning

Once you have achieved the general fitness base, continue with the program but make adjustments to add sport-specific training. This training should match the sport's requirements for aerobic/anaerobic capabilities, muscular strength and endurance, and range of motion.

During the sport-specific training, about half of your aerobic/anaerobic training should involve the same muscles you used during your sport. Ideally, allocate 4 weeks of sport-specific training before you start participating in the sport. Then continue the sport-specific training on a more limited basis throughout the season. Depending on the nature of the sport (aerobic versus anaerobic), once the season starts, sports participation itself can take the place of some or all of your aerobic workouts.

Functional independence Ability to carry out activities of daily living without assistance from other individuals.

Step aerobics A form of exercise that combines stepping up and down from a bench accompanied by arm movements.

The next step is to look at the demands of the sport. For example, soccer, bicycle racing, cross-country skiing, and snowshoeing are aerobic activities, whereas basketball, racquetball, alpine skiing, snowboarding, and ice hockey are stop-and-go sports that require a combination of aerobic and anaerobic activity. Consequently, aerobic training may be appropriate for cross-country skiing, but it will do little to prepare your muscles for the high-intensity requirements of combined aerobic and anaerobic sports.

Interval training, performed twice per week, is added to the program at this time. The intervals consist of a 1:3 work-to-rest ratio. This means you'll work at a fairly high intensity for, say, 15 seconds, and then spend 45 seconds on low-intensity recovery. Be sure to keep moving during the recovery phase. Perform four or five intervals at first, then gradually progress to 10 intervals. As your fitness improves, lengthen the high-intensity proportion of the intervals progressively to 1 minute and use a 1:2 work-to-rest ratio in which you work at high intensity for 1 minute and then at low intensity for 2 minutes.

For aerobic sports, interval training once a week also improves performance. These intervals, however, can be done on a 3-minute to 3-minute work-to-rest ratio. You also can do a 5- to 10-minute work interval followed by 1 to 2 minutes of recovery, but the intensity of these longer intervals should not be as high, and only three to five intervals are recommended. The interval-training workouts are not performed in addition to the regular aerobic workouts but, instead, take the place of one of these workouts.

Consider sport-specific strength requirements as well. Look at the primary muscles used in your sport, and make sure your choice of exercises works those muscles. Try to perform your strength training through a range of motion similar to that used in your sport. Aerobic/anaerobic sports require greater strength. During the season, the recommendation is three sets of 8 to 12 repetitions to near fatigue, two or three times per week. For aerobic endurance sports, the recommendation is a minimum of one set of 8 to 12 repetitions to near fatigue, once or twice per week during the season.

Stop-and-go sports (basketball, racquetball, soccer) require greater strength than pure endurance sports (triathlon, long-distance running, cross-country skiing). For example, recreational participants during the sport-specific training phase for stop-and-go sports perform three sets of 8 to 12 repetitions to near fatigue, two to three times per week. Competitive athletes and those desiring greater strength gains typically conduct three to five sets of 4 to 12 repetitions to near fatigue three times per week.

For some winter sports, such as alpine skiing and snowboarding, gravity supplies most of the propulsion and the body acts more as a shock absorber. Muscles in the hips, knees, and trunk are used to control the forces on the body and equipment. Multi-joint exercises, such as the leg press, squats, and lunges, are suggested for these activities.

Before the season starts, make sure your equipment is in proper working condition. For example, alpine skiers' bindings should be cleaned and adjusted properly so they will release as needed. This is one of the most important things you can do to help prevent knee injuries. A good pair of bindings is cheaper than knee surgery.

The first few times you participate in the sport of your choice, go easy, practice technique, and do not continue once you are fatigued. Gradually increase the length and intensity of your workouts. Consider taking a lesson to have someone watch your technique and help correct flaws early in the season. Even Olympic athletes have coaches watching them. Proper conditioning allows for a more enjoyable and healthier season.

Overtraining

In any fitness conditioning program, rest is important. Although the term **overtraining** is associated most frequently with athletic performance, it applies just as well to fitness participants. We all know that hard work improves fitness and performance. Hard training without adequate recovery, however, breaks down the body and leads to loss of fitness.

Physiological improvements in fitness and conditioning programs occur during the rest periods following training. As a rule, a hard day of training must be followed by a day of light training. Equally, a few weeks of increased training **volume** are to be followed by a few days of light recovery work. During these recovery periods, body systems strengthen and compensate for the training load, leading to a higher level of fitness. If proper recovery is not built into the training routine, overtraining occurs. Decreased performance, staleness, and injury are frequently seen with overtraining. Thus, to obtain optimal results, training regimens are altered during different phases of the year.

Periodization

Periodization is a training approach that uses a systematic variation in intensity and volume to enhance fitness and performance. This model was designed around the premises that the body becomes stronger as a result of training, but if similar workouts are constantly repeated, the body tires and enters a state of staleness and fatigue.

Periodization is used most frequently for athletic conditioning. Because athletes cannot maintain peak fitness during an entire season, most athletes seeking peak performance use a periodized training approach.

Behavior Modification Planning

COMMON SIGNS AND SYMPTOMS OF OVERTRAINING

- Decreased fitness
- Decreased sports performance
- Increased fatigue
- Loss of concentration
- Staleness and burnout
- Loss of competitive drive
- Increased resting and exercise heart rate
- Decreased appetite
- Loss of body weight
- Altered sleep patterns
- Decreased sex drive
- Generalized body aches and pains
- Increased susceptibility to illness and injury
- Mood disturbances
- Depression

Try It

If following several weeks or months of hard training you experience some of the above symptoms, you need to substantially decrease training volume and intensity for a week or two. This recovery phase will allow the body to recover, strengthen, and prepare for the next training phase. In your Behavior Change Tracker or your Online Journals, modify your training program to allow a light week of training following each 5 to 8 weeks of hard exercise training.

Studies have documented that greater improvements in fitness are achieved by using a variety of training loads. Using the same program and attempting to increase volume and intensity over a prolonged time will be manifested in overtraining.

The periodization training system involves three cycles:

1. macrocycles
2. mesocycles
3. microcycles

These cycles vary in length depending on the requirements of the sport. Typically, the overall training period (season or year) is referred to as a *macrocycle*. For athletes who need to peak twice a year, such as cross-country and track runners, two macrocycles can be developed within the year.

Macrocycles are divided into smaller weekly or monthly training phases known as *mesocycles*. A typical season, for example, is divided into the following mesocycles: base fitness conditioning (off-season), pre-season or sport-specific conditioning, competition, peak performance, and transition (active recovery from sport-specific training and competition).

In turn, mesocycles are divided into smaller weekly or daily *microcycles*. During microcycles, training follows the general objective of the mesocycle, but the workouts are altered to avoid boredom and fatigue.

The concept behind periodizing can be used in both aerobic and anaerobic sports. In the case of a long-distance runner, for instance, training can start with a general strength-conditioning program and cardiorespiratory endurance **cross-training** (jogging, cycling, swimming) during the off-season. In pre-season, the volume of strength training is decreased and the total weekly running mileage, at moderate intensities, is progressively increased. During the competitive season, the athlete maintains a limited strength-training program but now increases the intensity of the runs while decreasing the total weekly mileage. During the peaking phase, volume (miles) of training is reduced even further while the intensity is maintained at a high level. At the end of the season, a short transition period of 2 to 4 weeks, involving low- to moderate-intensity activities other than running and lifting weights, is recommended.

Periodization is frequently used for development of muscular strength, progressively cycling through the various components (hypertrophy, strength, and power) of strength training. Research indicates that varying the volume and intensity over time is more effective for long term progression than either single- or multiple-set programs with no variations. Training volume and intensity are typically increased only for large muscle/multi-joint lifts (for example bench press, squats, and lat pull-downs). Single-joint lifts (triceps extension, biceps curls, hamstrings curls) usually remain in the range of three sets of 8 to 12 repetitions.

A sample sequence—one macrocycle—of periodized training is provided in Table 9.7. The program starts with high volume and low intensity. During subsequent mesocycles (divided among the objectives of hypertrophy, strength, and power), the volume is decreased and the intensity (resistance) increases. Follow-

Interval training A system of exercise in which a short period of intense effort is followed by a specified recovery period according to a prescribed ratio; for instance, a 1:3 work-to-recovery ratio.

Overtraining An emotional, behavioral, and physical condition marked by increased fatigue, decreased performance, persistent muscle soreness, mood disturbances, and feelings of "staleness" or "burnout" as a result of excessive physical training.

Volume (of training) The total amount of training performed in a given work period (day, week, month, or season).

Periodization A training approach that divides the season into three cycles (macrocycles, mesocycles, and microcycles) using a systematic variation in intensity and volume of training to enhance fitness and performance.

Cross-training A combination of aerobic activities that contribute to overall fitness.

TABLE 9.7 Periodization Program for Strength

	One Macrocycle			
	Mesocycle 1*	Mesocycle 2*	Mesocycle 3*	Mesocycle 4*
	Hypertrophy	Strength & Hypertrophy	Strength & Power	Peak Performance
Sets per exercise	3–5	3–5	3–5	1–3
Repetitions	8–12	6–9	1–5	1–3
Intensity (resistance)	Low	Moderate	High	Very High
Volume	High	Moderate	Low	Very Low
Weeks (microcycles)	6–8	4–6	3–5	1–2

* Each mesocycle is followed by several days of light training.

ing each mesocycle, the recommendation is up to seven days of very light training. This brief resting period allows the body to fully recuperate, preventing overtraining and risk for injury. Other models of periodization are available, but the example provided is the most commonly used.

For aerobic endurance sports, one to three sets of 8 to 12 repetitions to near-fatigue performed once or twice per week is recommended. Although strength training does not enhance maximal oxygen uptake (VO_{2max}), and while strength requirements are not as high with endurance sports, data indicate that strength training does help the individual sustain submaximal exercise for longer periods of time.

In recent years, altering or cycling workouts has become popular among fitness participants. Research indicates that periodization is not limited to athletes but has been used successfully by fitness enthusiasts who are preparing for a special event such a 10K run, a triathlon, a bike race, or those who are simply aiming for higher fitness. Altering training is also recommended for people who progressed nicely in the initial weeks of a fitness program but now feel "stale" and "stagnant." Studies indicate that even among general fitness participants, systematically altering volume and intensity of training is most effective for progress in long-term fitness. Because training phases change continually during a macrocycle, periodization breaks the staleness and the monotony of repeated workouts.

For the non-athlete, a periodization program does not have to account for every detail of the sport. You can periodize workouts by altering mesocycles every 2 to 8 weeks. You can use different exercises, change the number of sets and repetitions, vary the speed of the repetitions, alter recovery time between sets, and even cross-train.

Periodization is not for everyone. People who are starting an exercise program, who enjoy a set routine, or who are satisfied with their fitness routine and fitness level do not need to periodize. For new participants, the goal is to start and adhere to exercise long enough to adopt the exercise behavior.

Personal Fitness Programming: An Example

Now that you understand the principles of fitness assessment and exercise prescription given in Chapters 6 through 8 and this chapter, you can review this program to cross-check and improve the design of your own fitness program. Let's look at an example.

Mary is 20 years old and 5 feet 6 inches tall. She participated in organized sports on and off throughout high school. During the last 2 years, however, she has participated only minimally in physical activity. She was not taught the principles for exercise prescription and has not participated in regular exercise to improve and maintain the various health-related components of fitness.

Mary became interested in fitness and contemplated signing up for a fitness and wellness course. As she was preparing her class schedule for the semester, she noted a "Lifetime Fitness and Wellness" course. In registering for the course, Mary anticipated some type of structured aerobic exercise. She knew that good fitness was important to health and weight management, but she didn't quite know how to plan and implement a program.

Once the new course started, she and her classmates received the "Stages of Change Questionnaire." Mary learned that she was in the Preparation stage for cardiorespiratory endurance, the Precontemplation stage for muscular strength and endurance, the Maintenance stage for flexibility, and the Preparation stage for body composition (see the discussion of the transtheoretical model in Chapter 2, pages 42–44). Various fitness assessments determined that her cardiorespiratory endurance level was fair, her muscular strength and endurance were poor, her flexibility was good, and her percent body fat was 25 percent (Moderate category).

Critical Thinking

In your own experience with personal fitness programs throughout the years, what factors have motivated you and helped you to stay with a program the most? What factors have kept you from being physically active, and what can you do to change these factors?

Cardiorespiratory Endurance

At the beginning of the semester, the instructor informed the students that the course would require self-monitored participation in activities outside the regularly scheduled class hours. Thus, Mary was in the Preparation stage for cardiorespiratory endurance. She knew she would be starting exercise in the next couple of weeks.

While in this Preparation stage, Mary chose three processes of change to help her implement her program (see Chapter 2, Table 2.1, page 45). She thought she could adopt an aerobic exercise program (Positive Outlook process of change) and set a realistic goal to reach the "Good" category for cardiorespiratory endurance by the end of the semester (Goal Setting). By staying in this course, she committed to go through with exercise (Commitment). She prepared a 12-week Personalized Cardiorespiratory Exercise Prescription (see Figure 9.5), wrote down her goal, signed the prescription (now a contract), and shared the program with her instructor and roommates.

As her exercise modalities, Mary selected walking/jogging and aerobics. Initially she walked/jogged twice a week and did aerobics once a week. By the tenth week of the program, she was jogging three times per week and participating in aerobics twice a week. She also selected Self-monitoring, Self-reevaluation, and Countering as techniques of change (see Chapter 2, Table 2.2, page 48). Using the exercise log in Figure 6.10 (Chapter 6, page 196) and the online exercise log (Figure 9.6), she monitored her exercise program. At the end of 6 weeks, she scheduled a follow-up cardiorespiratory assessment test (Self-reevaluation process of change), and she replaced her evening television hour with aerobics (Countering).

Mary also decided to increase her daily physical activity. She chose to walk 10 minutes to and from school, take the stairs instead of elevators whenever possible, and add 5-minute walks every hour during study time. On Saturdays, she cleaned her apartment and went to a school-sponsored dance at night. On Sundays, she opted to walk to and from church and took a 30-minute leisurely walk after the dinner meal. Mary now was fully in the Action stage of change for cardiorespiratory endurance.

Muscular Strength and Endurance

After Mary had started her fitness and wellness course, she wasn't yet convinced that she wanted to strength-train. Still, she contemplated strength training because a small part of her grade depended on it. When she read the information on the importance of lean body mass in regulating basal metabolic rate and weight maintenance (the Consciousness-Raising process of change), she thought that perhaps it would be good to add strength training to her program. She also was contemplating the long-term consequences of loss of lean body mass, its effect on her personal appearance, and the potential for decreased independence and quality of life (Emotional Arousal process of change).

Mary visited with her course instructor for additional guidance. Following this meeting, Mary committed herself to strength-train. While yet in the Preparation stage, she outlined a 10-week periodized training program (see Figure 9.7) and opted to aim for the "Good" strength category by the end of the program.

Because this was the first time Mary had lifted weights, the course instructor introduced Mary to two other students who were lifting already (Helping Relationships process of change). She also monitored her program with the form provided in Chapter 7, Figure 7.7, on page 230. Mary promised herself a movie and dinner out if she completed the first 5 weeks of strength training, and a new blouse if she made it through 10 weeks (Rewards process and technique for change).

Muscular Flexibility

Good flexibility was not a problem for Mary because she regularly stretched 15 to 30 minutes while watching the evening news on television. She had developed this habit the last 2 years of high school to maintain flexibility as a member of the dance-drill team (Environment Control process of change—as a team member, she needed good flexibility).

Because Mary had been stretching regularly for more than 3 years, she was in the Maintenance stage for flexibility. The flexibility fitness tests revealed that she had good flexibility. These results allowed her to pursue her stretching program because she thought she would be excellent for this fitness component (Self-Evaluation process of change).

To gain greater improvements in flexibility, Mary chose slow-sustained stretching and proprioceptive neuromuscular facilitation (PNF). She would need help to carry out the PNF technique. She spoke to one of her lifting classmates, and together they decided to allocate 20 minutes at the end of strength training to stretching (Helping Relationships process of change) and they chose the sequence of exercises presented in Chapter 8, Lab 8C, pages 287–288 (Consciousness-Raising and Goal Setting).

FIGURE 9.5 Sample online cardiorespiratory exercise prescription.

Personalized Cardiorespiratory Exercise Prescription

Fitness & Wellness Series
Thomson Wadsworth

Thomson NOW!

Mary Johnson September 1, 2007
Maximal heart rate: 200 bpm Resting heart rate: 76 bpm
Present cardiorespiratory fitness level: Fair Age: 20

The following is your personal program for cardiorespiratory fitness development and maintenance. If you have been exercising regularly and you are in the average or good category, you may start at week 5. If you are in the excellent category, you can start at week 10.

Week	Time (min.)	Frequency (per week)	Training Intensity (beats per minute)	Pulse (10 sec. count)
1	15	3	126–138	21–23 beats
2	15	4	126–138	21–23 beats
3	20	4	126–138	21–23 beats
4	20	5	126–138	21–23 beats
5	20	4	138–150	23–25 beats
6	20	5	138–150	23–25 beats
7	30	4	138–150	23–25 beats
8	30	5	138–150	23–25 beats
9	30	4	150–181	25–30 beats
10	30	5	150–181	25–30 beats
11	30–40	5	150–181	25–30 beats
12	30–40	5-6	150–181	25–30 beats

You may participate in any combination of activities that are aerobic and continuous in nature such as walking, jogging, swimming, cross-country skiing, aerobic exercise, rope skipping, cycling, aerobic dancing, racquetball, stair climbing, stationary running or cycling, etc. As long as the heart rate reaches the desired rate, and it stays at that level for the period of time indicated, the cardiorespiratory system will improve.

Following the 12-week program, in order to maintain your fitness level, you should exercise to reach between 150 and 181 bpm for about 30 minutes, a minimum of three times per week on nonconsecutive days. When you exercise, allow about 5 minutes for a gradual warm-up period and another 5 for gradual cool-down. Also, when you check your exercise heart rate, only count your pulse for 10 seconds (start counting with 0) and then refer to the above 10-second pulse count. You may also multipy by 6 to obtain your rate in beats per minute.

Good cardiorespiratory fitness will greatly contribute to the enhancement and maintenance of good health. It is especially important in the prevention of cardiovascular disease. We encourage you to be persistent in your exercise program and to participate regularly.

Training days: ✓ M ✓ T __ W __ Th ✓ F ✓ S __ S Training time: 7:00 am

Signature: Mary Johnson Goal: Good Date: 9/01/07

FIGURE 9.6 Sample exercise record using the online exercise log option at ThomsonNOW.

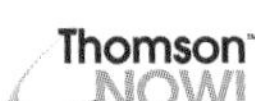

Exercise Log

Fitness & Wellness Series
Thomson Wadsworth

Mary Johnson

Date	Exercise	Body Weight (lbs)	Heart Rate (bpm)	Duration (min)	Distance (miles)	Calories Burned
09/01/2007	Walking (4.5 mph)	140.0	138	15	1.00	95
09/03/2007	Aerobics/Moderate	140.0	144	20		182
09/05/2007	Walking (4.5 mph)	141.0	138	15	1.00	95
09/06/2007	Dance/Moderate	141.0	100	60		254
09/07/2007	Walking (4.5 mph)	140.0	132	30	2.00	189
09/08/2007	Jogging (11 min/mile)	140.0	138	15	1.25	147
09/10/2007	Aerobics/Moderate	140.0	138	20		182
09/11/2007	Jogging (11 min/mile)	139.0	138	15	1.25	146
09/12/2007	Jogging (11 min/mile)	139.0	134	15	1.25	146
09/13/2007	Dance/Moderate	140.0	96	75		315
09/14/2007	Walking (4.5 mph)	139.0	126	30	2.50	188
09/15/2007	Jogging (11 min/mile)	139.0	134	20	2.00	195
09/16/2007	Strength Training	138.0	96	30		207
09/17/2007	Step-Aerobics	139.0	138	30		292
09/18/2007	Jogging (11 min/mile)	138.0	138	20	2.00	193
09/19/2007	Jogging (11 min/mile)	138.0	138	20	2.00	193
	Strength Training	138.0	96	30		207
09/20/2007	Dance/Moderate	138.0	90	30		124
09/21/2007	Walking (4.5 mph)	138.0	126	30	2.50	186
09/22/2007	Jogging (11 min/mile)	137.0	136	20	2.00	192
09/23/2007	Step-Aerobics	138.0	138	30		290
	Strength Training	138.0	96	40		276
09/24/2007	Jogging (8.5 min/mile)	138.0	144	20	2.50	248
09/25/2007	Step-Aerobics	137.0	136	20		192
09/26/2007	Strength Training	137.0	92	40		274
	Jogging (8.5 min/mile)	137.0	140	20	2.50	247
09/27/2007	Dance/Moderate	136.0	94	90		367
09/28/2007	Walking (4.5 mph)	136.0	120	30	2.50	184
Totals				13 hr 50 min	28.25	5806
Average per exercise session Number of exercise sessions: 28		138.5	124	30	1.88	207
Average per day exercised Number of days exercised: 25				33		232

Distance summary

Total miles run: 16.8
Total miles walked: 11.5

FIGURE 9.7 Sample starting muscular strength and endurance periodization program.

	Learning Lifting Technique	Muscular Strength	Muscular Endurance	Muscular Strength
Sets per exercise	1–2	2	2	3
Repetitions	10	12	18–20	8–12 (RM)
Intensity (resistance)	Very low	Moderate	Low	High
Volume	Low	Moderate	Moderate	High
Sessions per week	2	2	2	3
Weeks	2	3	2	3

Selected exercises: Bench press, leg press, leg curl, lat pull-down, rowing torso, rotary torso, seated back, and abdominal crunch.

Training days: ☐ M ☑ T ☐ W ☐ Th ☐ F ☑ S ☐ S Training time: 3:00 pm

Signature: Mary Johnson Goal: Average Date: 9-10-07

Body Composition

One of the motivational factors to enroll in a fitness course was Mary's desire to learn how to better manage her weight. She had gained a few pounds since entering college. To prevent further weight gain, she thought it was time to learn sound principles for weight management (Behavior Analysis process of change). She was in the Preparation stage of change because she was planning to start a diet and exercise program but wasn't sure how to get it done. All Mary needed was a little Consciousness-Raising to get her into the Action stage.

With the knowledge she had now gained, Mary planned her program. At 25 percent body fat and 140 pounds, she decided to aim for 23 percent body fat so she would be in the "Good" category for body composition (Goal Setting). This meant she would have to lose about 4 pounds (see Chapter 4, Lab 4B, page 127).

Mary's daily estimated energy requirement was about 2,027 calories (see Table 5.3, page 149). Mary also figured out that she was expending an additional 400 calories per day through her newly adopted exercise program and increased level of daily physical activity. Thus, her total daily energy intake would be around 2,427 calories (2,027 + 400).

To lose weight, Mary could decrease her caloric intake by 700 calories per day (body weight × 5; see Chapter 5, Lab 5A, page 159), yielding a target daily intake of 1,727 calories. By decreasing the intake by 700 daily calories daily, Mary should achieve her target weight in about 20 days (4 pounds of fat × 3,500 calories per pound of fat ÷ 700 fewer calories per day = 20 days). Mary picked the 1,800 calorie diet and eliminated one daily serving of grains (80 calories) to avoid exceeding her target 1,727 daily calorie intake.

The processes of change that will help Mary in the Action stage for weight management are Goal Setting, Countering (exercising instead of watching television), Monitoring, Environment Control, and Rewards. To monitor her daily caloric intake, Mary uses the 1,800-calorie diet plan in Chapter 5, Lab 5B (page 163). To further exert control over her environment, she gave away all of her junk food. She determined that she would not eat out while on the diet, and she bought only low-to-moderate fat/complex carbohydrate foods during the 3 weeks. As her reward, she achieved her target body weight of 136 pounds.

Leisure-Time Physical Activity

Accepted that individuals exhibit notable differences, the average person in developed countries has about 3½ hours of "free" or leisure time daily. In our current automated society, most of this time is spent in sedentary living. People would be better off doing some physical activities based on personal interests. Motivational factors include health, aesthetics, weight control, competition and challenge, fun, social interaction, mental arousal, relaxation, and stress management.

Frequently, leisure-time physical activity does not include exercise performed during a regular exercise program. It consists of activities such as walking, hiking, gardening, yard work, occupational work and chores, and moderate sports such as tennis, table tennis, badminton, golf, or croquet.

Every small increase in daily physical activity contributes to better health and wellness. Small increases in physical activity have a large impact in decreasing early risks for disease and premature death. Therefore, a new, concerted effort must be made to spend leisure time in activities that will promote the expenditure of energy, provide a break from daily tasks, and contribute to health-related fitness.

You Can Get It Done

Once they understand the proper exercise, nutrition, and behavior modification guidelines, people find that implementing a fitness lifestyle program is not as difficult as they thought. With adequate preparation and a personal behavioral analysis, you are now ready to design, implement, evaluate, and adhere to a lifetime fitness program that can enhance your functional capacity and zest for life.

Using the concepts provided thus far in this book and the exercise prescription principles that you have learned, you should now update your personal fitness program in Lab 9B. You also have an opportunity to revise your current stage of change, fitness category for each health-related component of physical fitness, and number of daily steps taken. You have the tools—the rest is up to you!

Assess Your Behavior

Log on to www.thomsonedu.com/login to create or update your personal log to include all your fitness activities.

1. Do you participate in recreational sports as a means to further improve your fitness and add enjoyment to training?
2. Have you been able to meet your cardiorespiratory endurance, muscular strength, muscular flexibility, and recommended body composition goals?
3. Are you able to incorporate a variety of activities into your fitness program, and do you vary exercise intensity and duration from time to time in your training?

Assess Your Knowledge

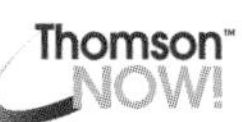

Log on to www.thomsonedu.com/login to assess your understanding of this chapter's topics by taking the Student Practice Test and exploring the modules recommended in your Personalized Study Plan.

1. Which of the following is *not* a skill-related fitness component?
   a. agility
   b. speed
   c. power
   d. strength
   e. balance
2. The ability to quickly and efficiently change body position and direction is known as
   a. agility.
   b. coordination.
   c. speed.
   d. reaction time.
   e. mobility.
3. The two components of power are
   a. strength and endurance.
   b. speed and force.
   c. speed and endurance.
   d. strength and force.
   e. endurance and force.
4. Diabetics should
   a. not exercise alone.
   b. wear a bracelet that identifies their condition.
   c. exercise at a low-to-moderate intensity.
   d. check blood glucose levels before and after exercise.
   e. follow all four guidelines above.
5. During pregnancy a woman should
   a. accumulate 30 minutes of moderate-intensity activity on most days of the week.
   b. exercise between "fairly light" and "somewhat hard."
   c. avoid exercising at an altitude above 6,000 feet.
   d. All of the above choices are correct.
   e. None of the choices is correct.

6. During exercise in the heat, drinking about a cup of cool water every __________ minutes seems to be ideal to prevent dehydration.
   a. 5
   b. 15 to 20
   c. 30
   d. 30 to 45
   e. 60
7. One of the most common causes of activity-related injuries is
   a. high impact.
   b. low level of fitness.
   c. exercising without stretching.
   d. improper warm-up.
   e. All choices cause about an equal number of injuries.
8. Improvements in maximal oxygen uptake in older adults (as compared with younger adults) as a result of cardiorespiratory endurance training are
   a. lower.
   b. higher.
   c. difficult to determine.
   d. non-existent.
   e. similar.
9. To participate in sports, it is recommended that you have
   a. base fitness and sport-specific conditioning.
   b. at least a good rating on skill fitness.
   c. good-to-excellent agility.
   d. basic speed.
   e. all of the above.
10. Periodization is a training approach that
   a. uses a systematic variation in intensity and volume.
   b. helps enhance fitness and performance.
   c. is commonly used by athletes.
   d. helps prevent staleness and overtraining.
   e. All are correct choices.

Correct answers can be found at the back of the book.

Media Menu

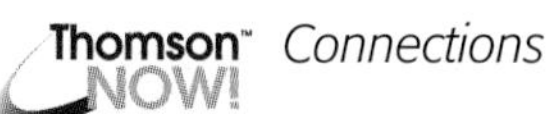

Connections

- Evaluate your skill-related fitness levels.
- Check how well you understand the chapter's concepts.

Internet Connections

Fitness Jumpsite

A comprehensive search engine guides you to information on nutrition, weight management, fitness equipment, and healthy lifestyles.
http://www.primusweb.com/fitnesspartner

President's Council on Physical Fitness and Sports

This site features fitness basics, workout plans, and exercise principles.
http://www.hoptechno.com/book11.htm

Notes

1. R. F. Kirby, "A Simple Test of Agility," *Coach and Athlete* (June 1971): 30–31
2. American Alliance for Health, Physical Education, Recreation and Dance (AAHPERD), *Youth Fitness: Test Manual* (Reston, VA: AAHPERD, 1976).
3. See note 2, AAHPERD.
4. R. S. Paffenbarger, Jr., R. T. Hyde, A. L. Wing, and C. H. Steinmetz, "A Natural History of Athleticism and Cardiovascular Health," *Journal of the American Medical Association* 252 (1984): 491–495.
5. American College of Sports Medicine, "Position Stand: Exercise and Type 2 Diabetes," *Medicine and Science in Sports and Exercise* 32 (2000): 1345–1360.
6. American College of Obstetricians and Gynecologists, "Exercise During Pregnancy and the Postpartum Period," ACOG Committee Opinion No. 267, *International Journal of Gynecology and Obstetrics* 77 (2002): 79–81.
7. University of California at Berkeley, *The Wellness Guide to Lifelong Fitness* (New York: Random House, 1993): 198.
8. American College of Sports Medicine, "Position Stand: Exercise and Physical Activity for Older Adults," *Medicine and Science in Sports and Exercise* 30 (1998): 992–1008.
9. R. J. Shephard, "Exercise and Aging: Extending Independence in Older Adults," *Geriatrics* 48 (1993): 61–64.
10. F. W. Kash, J. L. Boyer, S. P. Van Camp, L. S. Verity, and J. P. Wallace, "The Effect of Physical Activity on Aerobic Power in Older Men (A Longitudinal Study)," *Physician and Sports Medicine* 18, no. 4 (1990): 73–83.

11. J. Hagberg, S. Blair, A. Ehsani, N. Gordon, N. Kaplan, C. Tipton, and E. Zambraski, "Position Stand: Physical Activity, Physical Fitness, and Hypertension," *Medicine and Science in Sports and Exercise* 25 (1993): i–x.
12. W. S. Evans, "Exercise, Nutrition and Aging," *Journal of Nutrition* 122 (1992): 796–801.
13. See note 8.
14. The Editors, "Exercise for the Ages," *Consumer Reports on Health* (Yonkers, NY: July, 1996).
15. J. M. Walker, D. Sue, N. Miles-Elkousy, G. Ford, and H. Trevelyan, "Active Mobility of the Extremities in Older Subjects," *Physical Therapy* 64 (1994): 919–923.
16. S. B. Roberts et al., "What Are the Dietary Needs of Adults?" *International Journal of Obesity* 16 (1992): 969–976.
17. J. M. Moore and W. W. K. Hoeger, "Game On! Preparing Your Clients for Recreational Sports," *ACSM's Health & Fitness Journal* 9 no. 3 (2005): 14–19.

Suggested Readings

American College of Obstetricians and Gynecologists. "Exercise During Pregnancy and the Postpartum Period." ACOG Committee Opinion No. 267. *International Journal of Gynecology and Obstetrics* 77 (2002): 79–81.

Coleman, E. *Eating for Endurance.* Palo Alto, CA: Bull Publishing, 2003.

Pfeiffer, R. P., and B. C. Mangus. *Concepts of Athletic Training.* Boston: Jones and Bartlett, 2005.

Prentice, W., and D. D. Arnheim. *Arnheim's Principles of Athletic Training.* Boston: McGraw-Hill, 2003.

Unruh, N., S. Unruh, and E. Scantling. "Heat Can Kill: Guidelines to Prevent Heat Illness in Athletics and Physical Education." *Journal of Physical Education, Recreation & Dance* 73 no. 6 (2002): 36–38.

VIII. Body Composition and Fitness Benefits

List all of the activities in which you participate regularly and rate the respective contribution to body composition and other fitness components. Use the following rating scale: 1 = low, 2 = fair, 3 = average, 4 = good, and 5 = excellent.

Activity	Body Composition	Cardiorespiratory	Musc. Strength	Musc. Flexibility	Agility	Balance	Coordination	Power	Reaction Time	Speed
Example: Jogging	*5*	*5*	*2*	*1*	*2*	*2*	*1*	*2*	*1*	*2*

IX. Contract

I hereby commit to carry out the above described fitness plan and complete my goals by ____________.

Upon completion of all my fitness goals I will present my results to ____________ and will reward myself with ____________.

____________ ____________

My signature Date

____________ ____________

Witness signature Date

Stress Management

CHAPTER 10

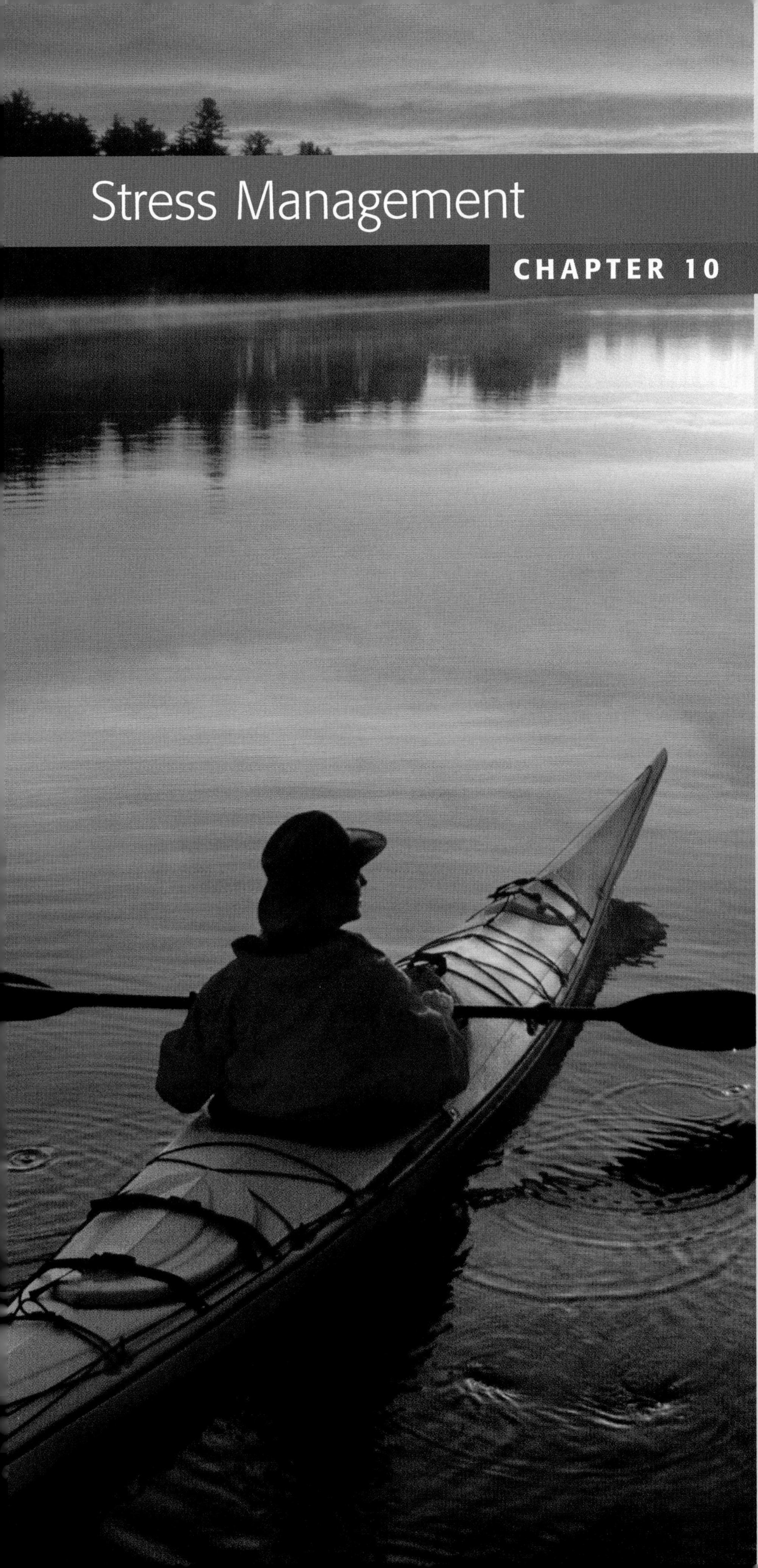

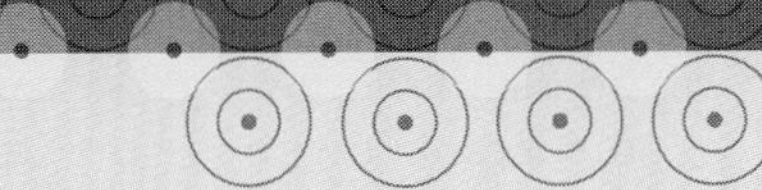

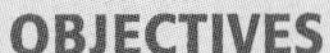

OBJECTIVES

- Define stress, eustress, and distress.
- Explain the role of stress in maintaining health and optimal performance.
- Identify the major sources of stress in life.
- Define the two major types of behavior patterns.
- Learn to lower your vulnerability to stress.
- Develop time management skills.
- Define the role of physical exercise in reducing stress.
- Describe and learn to use various stress management techniques.

Thomson NOW! Go to www.thomsonedu.com/login to:

- Identify the stressors in your life and develop a change plan to deal more effectively with them.
- Check how well you understand the chapter's concepts.

A growing body of evidence indicates that virtually every illness known to modern humanity—from arthritis to migraine headaches, from the common cold to cancer—is influenced for good or bad by our emotions. To a profound extent, emotions affect our susceptibility to disease and our **immunity.** The way we react to what comes along in life can determine in great measure how we will react to the disease-causing organisms that we face. The feelings we have and the way we express them can either boost our immune system or weaken it.

Emotional health is a key part of total wellness. Most emotionally healthy people take care of themselves physically—they eat well, exercise, and get enough rest. They work to develop supportive personal relationships. In contrast, many people who are emotionally unhealthy are self-destructive. For example, they may abuse alcohol and other drugs or may overwork and not have balance in their lives. Emotional health is so important that it affects what we do, who we meet, who we marry, how we look, how we feel, the course of our lives, and even how long we live.

The Mind/Body Connection

Emotions cause physiological responses that can influence health. Certain parts of the brain are associated with specific emotions and specific hormone patterns. The release of certain hormones is associated with various emotional responses, and those hormones affect health. These responses may contribute to development of disease. Emotions have to be expressed somewhere, somehow. If they are suppressed repeatedly, and/or if a person feels conflict about controlling them, they often reveal themselves through physical symptoms. These physiological responses may weaken the immune system over time.

The Brain

The brain is the most important part of the nervous system. For the body to survive, the brain must be maintained. All other organs sacrifice to keep the brain alive and functioning when the entire body is under severe stress.

The brain directs nerve impulses that are carried throughout the body. It controls voluntary processes, such as the direction, strength, and coordination of muscle movements; the processes involved in smelling, touching, and seeing; and involuntary functions over which you have no conscious control. Among the latter are many automatic, vital functions in the body, such as breathing, heart rate, digestion, control of the bowels and bladder, blood pressure, and release of hormones.

The brain is the cognitive center of the body, the place where ideas are generated, memory is stored, and emotions are experienced. The brain has a powerful influence over the body via the link between the emotions and the immune system. That link is extremely complex.

The emotions that the brain produces are a mixture of feelings and physical responses. Every time the brain manufactures an emotion, physical reactions accompany it. The brain's natural chemicals form literal communication links that connect the brain, its thought processes, and the cells of the body, including those of the immune system.

The Immune System

The immune system patrols and guards the body against attackers. This system consists of about a trillion cells called **lymphocytes** (the cells responsible for waging war against disease or infection) and about a hundred million trillion molecules called **antibodies.** The brain and the immune system are closely linked in a connection that allows the mind to influence both susceptibility and resistance to disease. A number of immune system cells—including those in the thymus gland, spleen, bone marrow, and lymph nodes—are laced with nerve cells.

Cells of the immune system are therefore equipped to respond to chemical signals from the central nervous system. For example, the surface of the lymphocytes contains receptors for a variety of central nervous system chemical messengers, such as catecholamines, prostaglandins, serotonin, endorphins, sex hormones, the thyroid hormone, and the growth hormone. Certain white blood cells also possess the ability to receive messages from the brain.

Because of these receptors on the lymphocytes, physical and psychological stress alters the immune system. Stress causes the body to release several powerful neurohormones that bind with the receptors on the lymphocytes and suppress immune function.

Stress

Living in today's world is nearly impossible without encountering **stress.** In an unpredictable world that changes with every new day, most people find that working under pressure has become the rule rather than the exception. As a result, stress has become one of the most common problems we face and undermines our ability to stay well. Current estimates indicate that the annual cost of stress and stress-related diseases in the United States exceeds $100 billion, a direct result of health-care costs, lost productivity, and absenteeism. Many medical and stress researchers believe that "stress should carry a health warning" as well.

The good news is that stress can be self-controlled. Unfortunately, most people have accepted stress as a normal part of daily life and, even though everyone has

FIGURE 10.1 Relationship between stress and health and performance.

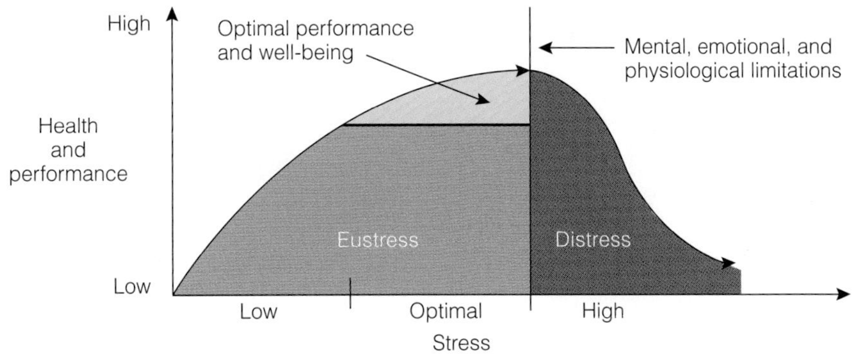

to face it, few seem to understand it or know how to cope with it effectively. It is difficult to succeed and have fun in life without "runs, hits, and errors." In fact, stress should not be avoided entirely, because a certain amount is necessary for optimum health, performance, and well-being.

Just what is stress? Dr. Hans Selye, one of the foremost authorities on stress, defined it as "the nonspecific response of the human organism to any demand that is placed upon it."[1] "Nonspecific" indicates that the body reacts in a similar fashion, regardless of the nature of the event that leads to the stress response. In simpler terms, stress is the body's mental, emotional, and physiological response to any situation that is new, threatening, frightening, or exciting.

The body's response to stress has been the same ever since humans first walked the earth. Stress prepares the organism to react to the stress-causing event, also called the **stressor.** The problem arises in the way in which we react to stress. Many people thrive under stress; others under similar circumstances are unable to handle it. An individual's reaction to a stress-causing agent determines whether that stress is positive or negative.

Dr. Selye defined the ways in which we react to stress as either eustress or distress. In both cases, the nonspecific response is almost the same. In the case of **eustress,** health and performance continue to improve even as stress increases. On the other hand, **distress** refers to the unpleasant or harmful stress under which health and performance begin to deteriorate. The relationship between stress and performance is illustrated in Figure 10.1.

Stress is a fact of modern life, and every person does need an optimal level of stress that is most conducive to adequate health and performance. When stress levels reach mental, emotional, and physiological limits, however, stress becomes distress and the person no longer functions effectively.

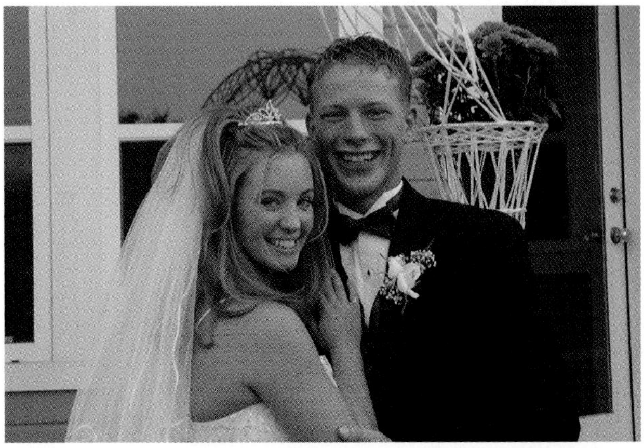

Marriage is an example of positive stress, also known as eustress.

Chronic distress raises the risk for many health disorders—among them, coronary heart disease, hypertension, eating disorders, ulcers, diabetes, asthma, depression, migraine headaches, sleep disorders, and chronic fatigue—and may even play a role in the development of certain types of cancers.[2] Recognizing this

Immunity The function that guards the body from invaders, both internal and external.

Lymphocytes Immune system cells responsible for waging war against disease or infection.

Antibodies Substances produced by the white blood cells in response to an invading agent.

Stress The mental, emotional, and physiological response of the body to any situation that is new, threatening, frightening, or exciting.

Stressor Stress-causing event.

Eustress Positive stress: Health and performance continue to improve, even as stress increases.

Distress Negative stress: Unpleasant or harmful stress under which health and performance begin to deteriorate.

FIGURE 10.2 General adaptation syndrome: The body's response to stress can end in exhaustion, illness, or recovery.

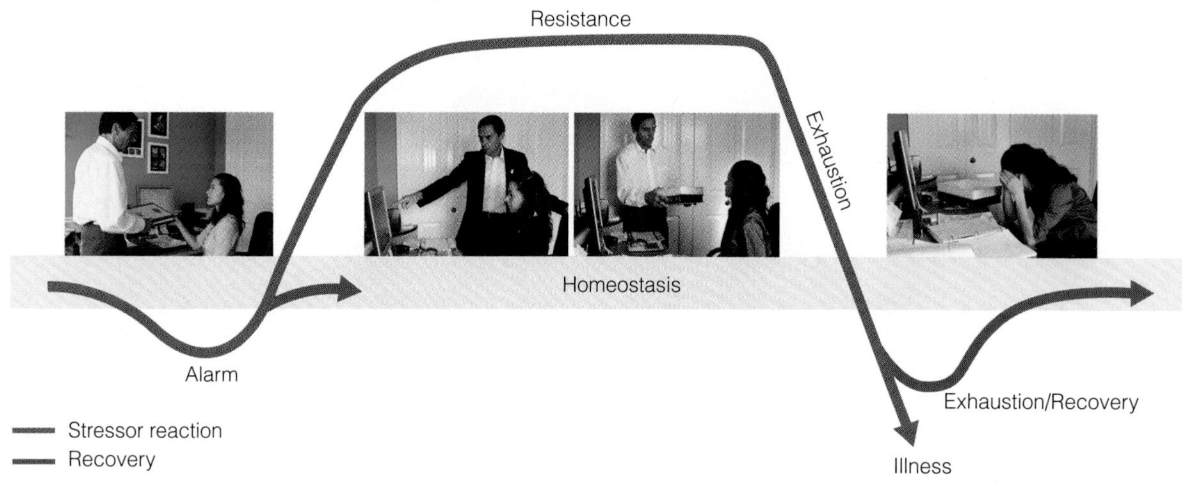

and overcoming the problem quickly and efficiently are crucial in maintaining emotional and physiological stability.

Critical Thinking

Can you identify sources of eustress and distress in your personal life during this past year? Explain your emotional and physical response to each stressor and how the two differ.

Stress Adaptation

The body continually strives to maintain a constant internal environment. This state of physiological balance, known as **homeostasis,** allows the body to function as effectively as possible. When a stressor triggers a nonspecific response, homeostasis is disrupted. This reaction to stressors, best explained by Dr. Selye through the **general adaptation syndrome (GAS),** is composed of three stages: alarm reaction, resistance, and exhaustion/recovery.

Alarm Reaction

The alarm reaction is the immediate response to a stressor (whether positive or negative). During the alarm reaction, the body evokes an instant physiological reaction that mobilizes internal systems and processes to minimize the threat to homeostasis (see also "Coping with Stress" on page 335). If the stressor subsides, the body recovers and returns to homeostasis.

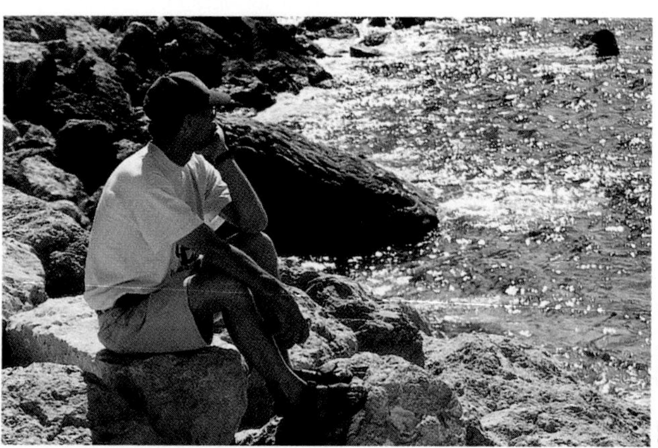

Taking time out during stressful life events is critical for good health and wellness.

Resistance

If the stressor persists, the body calls upon its limited reserves to build up its resistance as it strives to maintain homeostasis. For a short while, the body copes effectively and meets the challenge of the stressor until it can be overcome (see Figure 10.2).

Exhaustion/Recovery

If stress becomes chronic and intolerable, the body spends its limited reserves and loses its ability to cope, entering the exhaustion/recovery stage. During this stage, the body functions at a diminished capacity while it recovers from stress. In due time, following an "adequate" recovery period (which varies greatly), the body recuperates and is able to return to homeostasis. If chronic stress persists during the exhaustion stage, however, immune function is compromised, which can damage body systems and lead to disease.

An example of the stress response through the general adaptation syndrome can be illustrated by college test performance. As you prepare to take an exam, you experience an initial alarm reaction. If you understand the material, study for the exam, and do well (eustress), the body recovers and stress is dissipated. If, however, you are not adequately prepared and fail the exam, you trigger the resistance stage. You are now concerned about your grade, and you remain in the resistance stage until the next exam. If you prepare and do well, the body recovers. But, if you fail once again and can no longer bring up the grade, exhaustion sets in and physical and emotional breakdowns may occur. Exhaustion may be further aggravated if you are struggling in other courses as well.

The exhaustion stage is often manifested by athletes and the most ardent fitness participants. Staleness is usually a manifestation of overtraining. Peak performance can be sustained for only about 2 to 3 weeks at a time. Any attempts to continue intense training after peaking leads to exhaustion, diminished fitness, and mental and physical problems associated with overtraining (see "Overtraining," Chapter 9, page 308). Thus, athletes and some fitness participants also need an active recovery phase following the attainment of peak fitness.

Perceptions and Health

The habitual manner in which people explain the things that happen to them is their **explanatory style.** It is a way of thinking when all other factors are equal and when there are no clear-cut right and wrong answers. The contrasting explanatory styles are pessimism and optimism. People with a pessimistic explanatory style interpret events negatively; people with an optimistic explanatory style interpret events in a positive light—every cloud has a silver lining.

A pessimistic explanatory style can delay healing time and worsen the course of illness in several major diseases. For example, it can affect the circulatory system and general outlook for people with coronary heart disease. Blood flow actually changes as thoughts, feelings, and attitudes change. People with a pessimistic explanatory style have a higher risk of developing heart disease.

Studies of explanatory style verify that a negative explanatory style also compromises immunity. Blood samples taken from people with a negative explanatory style revealed suppressed immune function, a low ratio of helper/suppressor T-cells, and fewer lymphocytes.

In contrast, an optimistic style tends to increase the strength of the immune system. An optimistic explanatory style and the positive attitude it fosters can also enhance the ability to resist infections, allergies, autoimmunities, and even cancer. A change in explanatory style can lead to a remarkable change in the course of disease. An optimistic explanatory style and the positive emotions it embraces—such as love, acceptance, and forgiveness—stimulate the body's healing systems.

Self-Esteem

Self-esteem is a way of viewing and assessing yourself. Positive self-esteem is a sense of feeling good about one's capabilities, goals, accomplishments, place in the world, and relationship to others. People with high self-esteem respect themselves. Self-esteem is a powerful determinant of health behavior and, therefore, of health status. Healthy self-esteem is one of the best things a person can develop for overall health, both mental and physical. A good, strong sense of self can boost the immune system, protect against disease, and aid in healing.

Whether people get sick—and how long they stay that way—may depend in part on the strength of their self-esteem. For example, low self-esteem worsens chronic pain. The higher the self-esteem, the more rapid the recovery. If we have strong self-esteem, the outlook is good. If our self-esteem is poor, however, our health can decline in direct proportion, as our attitude and negative perceptions worsen.

Belief in oneself is one of the most powerful weapons people have to protect health and live longer, more satisfying lives. It has a dramatic and positive impact on wellness, and we can work to harness it to our advantage.

A Fighting Spirit

A **fighting spirit** involves the healthy expression of emotions, whether they are negative or positive. At the other extreme is hopelessness, a surrender to despair. Fighting spirit can play a major role in recovery from disease. People with a fighting spirit accept their disease diagnosis, adopt an optimistic attitude filled with faith, seek information about how to help themselves, and are determined to fight the disease. A fighting spirit makes a person take charge.

Homeostasis A natural state of equilibrium; the body attempts to maintain this equilibrium by constantly reacting to external forces that attempt to disrupt this fine balance.

General adaptation syndrome (GAS) A theoretical model that explains the body's adaptation to sustained stress which includes three stages: Alarm reaction, resistance, and exhaustion/recovery.

Explanatory style The way people perceive the events in their lives, from an optimistic or a pessimistic perspective.

Self-esteem A sense of positive self-regard and self-respect.

Fighting spirit Determination; the open expression of emotions, whether negative or positive.

A fighting spirit may be the underlying factor in what is called **spontaneous remission** from incurable illness. More and more physicians believe that the phenomenon is real and that the patient is the key in spontaneous remission. They believe the patient's attitude, especially the presence of a fighting spirit, is responsible for victory over disease. Fighters are not stronger or more capable than others—they simply do not give up as easily. They enjoy better health and live longer, even when physicians and laboratory tests say they should not. Fighters are intrinsically different from people who give up, and their health status reflects those differences.

Sources of Stress

Several instruments have been developed to assess sources of stress in life. The most practical instrument is the **Life Experiences Survey,** presented in Lab 10A, which identifies the life changes within the last 12 months that may have an impact on your physical and psychological well-being.

The Life Experiences Survey is divided into two sections. Section 1, to be completed by all respondents, contains a list of 47 life events plus three blank spaces for other events experienced but not listed in the survey. Section 2 contains an additional 10 questions designed for students only (students should fill out both sections). Common stressors in the lives of college students are depicted in Figure 10.3.

The survey requires the testee to rate the extent to which his or her life events had a positive or negative impact on his or her life at the time these events occurred. The ratings are on a 7-point scale. A rating of –3 indicates an extremely undesirable impact. A rating of zero (0) suggests neither a positive nor a negative impact **(neustress).** A rating of +3 indicates an extremely desirable impact.

FIGURE 10.3 Stressors in the lives of college students.

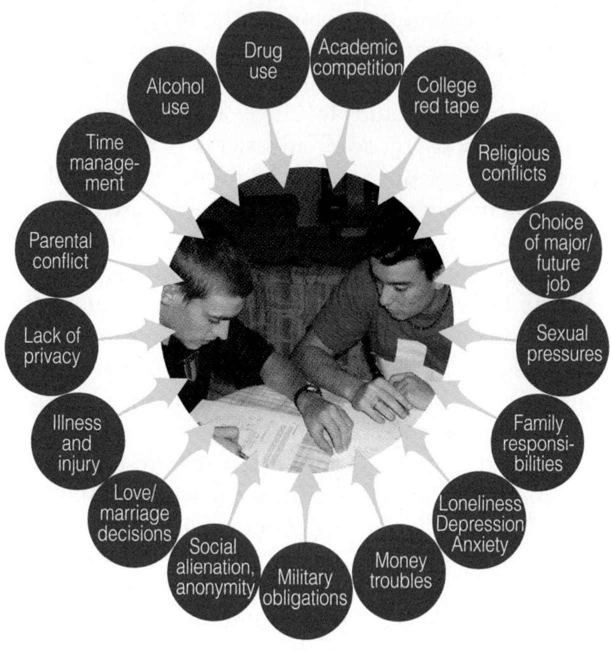

Adapted from W. W. K. Hoeger, L. W. Turner, and B. Q. Hafen. *Wellness Guidelines for a Healthy Lifestyle.* Wadsworth/Thomson Learning, 2007.

Critical Thinking

Technological advances provide many benefits to our lives. What positive and negative effects do these advances have upon your daily living activities, and what impact are they having on your stress level?

After the person evaluates his or her life events, the negative and the positive points are totaled separately. Both scores are expressed as positive numbers (for example, positive ratings of 2, 1, 3, and 3 = 9 points positive score; negative ratings of –3, –2, –2, –1, and –2 = 10 points negative score). A final "total life change" score can be obtained by adding the positive score and the negative score together as positive numbers (total life change score: 9 + 10 = 19 points).

Because negative and positive changes alike can produce nonspecific responses, the total life change score is a good indicator of total life stress. Most research in this area, however, suggests that the negative change score is a better predictor of potential physical and psychological illness than the total change score. More research is necessary to establish the role of total change and the role of the ratio of positive to negative stress.

Behavior Patterns

Common life events are not the only source of stress in life. All too often, individuals bring on stress as a result of their behavior patterns. The two main types of behavior patterns, Type A and Type B, are based on several observable characteristics.

Several attempts have been made to develop an objective scale to identify Type A individuals properly, but these questionnaires are not as valid and reliable as researchers would like them to be. Consequently, the main assessment tool to determine behavioral type is still the **structured interview,** during which a person is asked to reply to several questions that describe Type A and Type B behavior patterns. The interviewer notes not only the responses to the questions but also the in-

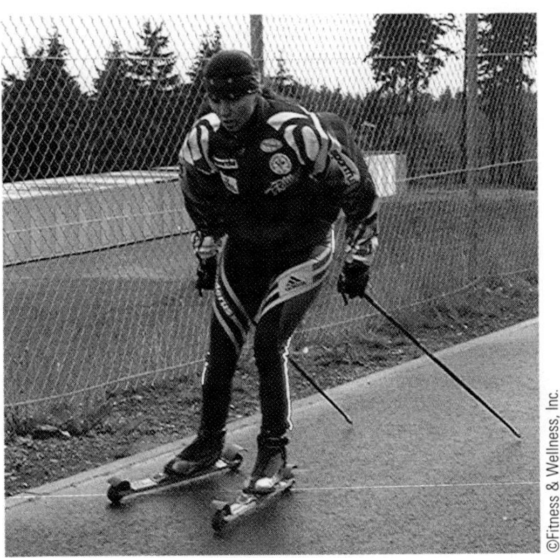

Physical activity: An excellent tool to control stress.

to as **endorphins** are thought to be released from the pituitary gland in the brain. These substances not only act as painkillers but also seem to induce the soothing, calming effect often associated with aerobic exercise.

Another way by which exercise helps lower stress is to deliberately divert stress to various body systems. Dr. Hans Selye explains in his book *Stress Without Distress* that, when one specific task becomes difficult, a change in activity can be as good or better than rest itself.[5] For example, if a person is having trouble with a task and does not seem to be getting anywhere, jogging or swimming for a while is better than sitting around and getting frustrated. In this way the mental strain is diverted to the working muscles, and one system helps the other to relax.

Other psychologists indicate that, when muscular tension is removed from the emotional strain, the emotional strain disappears. In many cases, the change of activity suddenly clears the mind and helps put the pieces together.

Researchers have found that physical exercise gives people a psychological boost because exercise does all the following:

- Lessens feelings of anxiety, depression, frustration, aggression, anger, and hostility.
- Alleviates insomnia.
- Provides an opportunity to meet social needs and develop new friendships.
- Allows the person to share common interests and problems.
- Develops discipline.
- Provides the opportunity to do something enjoyable and constructive that will lead to better health and total well-being.

Beyond the short-term benefits of exercise in lessening stress, a regular aerobic exercise program actually strengthens the cardiovascular system itself. Because the cardiovascular system seems to be affected seriously by stress, a stronger system should be able to cope more effectively. For instance, good cardiorespiratory endurance has been shown to lower resting heart rate and blood pressure. Because both heart rate and blood pressure rise in stressful situations, initiating the stress response at a lower baseline will counteract some of the negative effects of stress. Cardiorespiratory-fit individuals can cope more effectively and are less affected by the stresses of daily living.

Relaxation Techniques

Although benefits are reaped immediately after engaging in any of the several relaxation techniques, several months of regular practice may be necessary for total mastery. The relaxation exercises that follow should not be considered cure-alls. If these exercises do not prove to be effective, more specialized textbooks and professional help are called for. (Some symptoms may not be caused by stress but may be related to a medical disorder.)

Biofeedback

Clinical application of **biofeedback** has been used for many years to treat various medical disorders. Besides its successful application in managing stress, it is commonly used to treat medical disorders such as essential hypertension, asthma, heart rhythm and rate disturbances, cardiac neurosis, eczematous dermatitis, fecal incontinence, insomnia, and stuttering. Biofeedback as a treatment modality has been defined as a technique in which a person learns to influence physiological responses that are not typically under voluntary control or responses that normally are regulated but regulation has broken down as a result of injury, trauma, or illness.

In simpler terms, biofeedback is the interaction with the interior self. This interaction enables a person to learn the relationship between the mind and the biological response. The person actually can "feel" how thought processes influence biological responses (such as heart rate, blood pressure, body temperature, and muscle tension) and how biological responses influence the thought process.

As an illustration of this process, consider the association between a strange noise in the middle of a

---

Fight or flight Physiological response of the body to stress that prepares the individual to take action by stimulating the body's vital defense systems.

Endorphins Morphine-like substances released from the pituitary gland in the brain during prolonged aerobic exercise, thought to induce feelings of euphoria and natural well-being.

Biofeedback A stress management technique in which a person learns to influence physiological responses that are not typically under voluntary control or responses that typically are regulated but for which regulation has broken down as a result of injury, trauma, or illness.

dark, quiet night and the heart rate response. At first the heart rate shoots up because of the stress the unknown noise induces. The individual may even feel the heart palpitating in the chest and, while still uncertain about the noise, attempts not to panic to prevent an even faster heart rate. Upon realizing that all is well, the person can take control and influence the heart rate to come down. The mind, now calm, is able to exert almost complete control over the biological response.

Complex electronic instruments are required to conduct biofeedback. The process itself entails a three-stage, closed-loop feedback system:

1. A biological response to a stressor is detected and amplified.
2. The response is processed.
3. Results of the response are fed back to the individual immediately.

The person uses this new input and attempts to change the physiological response voluntarily—this attempt, in turn, is detected, amplified, and processed. The results then are fed back to the person. The process continues with the intent of teaching the person to reliably influence the physiological response for the better (see Figure 10.5). The most common methods used to measure physiological responses are monitoring the heart rate, finger temperature, and blood pressure; electromyograms; and electroencephalograms. The goal of biofeedback training is to transfer the experiences learned in the laboratory to everyday living.

Although biofeedback has significant applications in treating various medical disorders, including stress, it requires adequately trained personnel and, in many cases, costly equipment. Therefore, several alternative methods that yield similar results are frequently substituted for biofeedback. For example, research has shown that exercise and progressive muscle relaxation, used successfully in stress management, seem to be just as effective as biofeedback in treating essential hypertension.

FIGURE 10.5 Biofeedback mechanism.

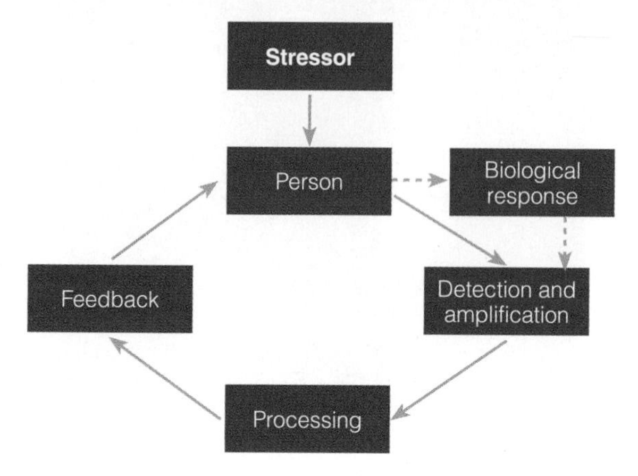

Progressive Muscle Relaxation

Progressive muscle relaxation enables individuals to relearn the sensation of deep relaxation. The technique involves progressively contracting and relaxing muscle groups throughout the body. Because chronic stress leads to high levels of muscular tension, acute awareness of how progressively tightening and relaxing the muscles feels can release the tension in the muscles and teach the body to relax at will.

Feeling the tension during the exercises also helps the person to be more alert to signs of distress, because this tension is similar to that experienced in stressful situations. In everyday life, these feelings then can cue the person to do relaxation exercises.

Relaxation exercises should be done in a quiet, warm, well-ventilated room. The recommended exercises and the duration of the routine vary from one person to the next. Most important is that the individual pay attention to the sensation he or she feels each time the muscles are tensed and relaxed.

The exercises should encompass all muscle groups of the body. Following is an example of a sequence of progressive muscle relaxation exercises. The instructions for these exercises can be read to the person, memorized, or tape-recorded. At least 20 minutes should be set aside to complete the entire sequence. Doing the exercises any faster will defeat their purpose. Ideally, the sequence should be done twice a day.

The individual performing the exercises stretches out comfortably on the floor, face up, with a pillow under the knees, and assumes a passive attitude, allowing the body to relax as much as possible. Each muscle group is to be contracted in sequence, taking care to avoid any strain. Muscles should be tightened to only about 70 percent of the total possible tension to avoid cramping or some type of injury to the muscle itself.

To produce the relaxation effects, the person must pay attention to the sensation of tensing up and relaxing. The person holds each contraction about 5 seconds and then allows the muscles to go totally limp. The person should take enough time to contract and relax each muscle group before going on to the next. An example of a complete progressive muscle relaxation sequence is as follows:

1. Point your feet, curling the toes downward. Study the tension in the arches and the top of the feet. Hold, continue to note the tension, then relax. Repeat once.
2. Flex the feet upward toward the face and note the tension in your feet and calves. Hold and relax. Repeat once.

Behavior Modification Planning

CHARACTERISTICS OF GOOD STRESS MANAGERS

Good stress managers

- are physically active, eat a healthy diet, and get adequate rest every day.
- believe they have control over events in their life (have an internal locus of control, see page 40).
- understand their own feelings and accept their limitations.
- recognize, anticipate, monitor, and regulate stressors within their capabilities.
- control emotional and physical responses when distressed.
- use appropriate stress management techniques when confronted with stressors.
- recognize warning signs and symptoms of excessive stress.
- schedule daily time to unwind, relax, and evaluate the day's activities.
- control stress when called upon to perform.
- enjoy life despite occasional disappointments and frustrations.
- look success and failure squarely in the face and keep moving along a predetermined course.
- move ahead with optimism and energy and do not spend time and talent worrying about failure.
- learn from previous mistakes and use them as building blocks to prevent similar setbacks in the future.
- give of themselves freely to others.
- have a deep meaning in life.

Try It

Change for many people is threatening, but often required. Pick three of the above strategies and apply them in your life. After several days, determine the usefulness of these strategies to your physical, mental, social, and emotional well-being.

3. Push your heels down against the floor as if burying them in the sand. Hold and note the tension at the back of the thigh. Relax. Repeat once.
4. Contract the right thigh by straightening the leg, gently raising the leg off the floor. Hold and study the tension. Relax. Repeat with the left leg. Hold and relax. Repeat each leg.
5. Tense the buttocks by raising your hips ever so slightly off the floor. Hold and note the tension. Relax. Repeat once.
6. Contract the abdominal muscles. Hold them tight and note the tension. Relax. Repeat once.
7. Suck in your stomach. Try to make it reach your spine. Flatten your lower back to the floor. Hold and feel the tension in the stomach and lower back. Relax. Repeat once.

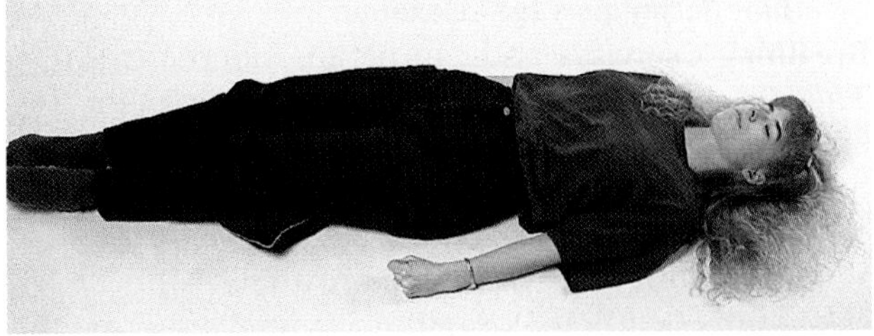

Practicing progressive muscle relaxation on a regular basis helps reduce stress.

8. Take a deep breath and hold it, then exhale. Repeat. Note your breathing becoming slower and more relaxed.
9. Place your arms at the sides of your body and clench both fists. Hold, study the tension, and relax. Repeat.
10. Flex the elbow by bringing both hands to the shoulders. Hold tight and study the tension in the biceps. Relax. Repeat.
11. Place your arms flat on the floor, palms up, and push the forearms hard against the floor. Note the tension on the triceps. Hold, and relax. Repeat.
12. Shrug your shoulders, raising them as high as possible. Hold and note the tension. Relax. Repeat.
13. Gently push your head backward. Note the tension in the back of the neck. Hold, relax. Repeat.
14. Gently bring the head against the chest, push forward, hold, and note the tension in the neck. Relax. Repeat.
15. Press your tongue toward the roof of your mouth. Hold, study the tension, and relax. Repeat.
16. Press your teeth together. Hold, and study the tension. Relax. Repeat.
17. Close your eyes tightly. Hold them closed and note the tension. Relax, leaving your eyes closed. Do this one more time.
18. Wrinkle your forehead and note the tension. Hold and relax. Repeat.

When time is a factor during the daily routine and an individual is not able to go through the entire sequence, he or she may do only the exercises specific to the area that feels most tense. Performing a partial sequence is better than not doing the exercises at all. Completing the entire sequence, of course, yields the best results.

Progressive muscle relaxation A stress management technique that involves sequential contraction and relaxation of muscle groups throughout the body.

Breathing Techniques for Relaxation

Breathing exercises also can be an antidote to stress. These exercises have been used for centuries in the Orient and India to improve mental, physical, and emotional stamina. In breathing exercises, the person concentrates on "breathing away" the tension and inhaling a large amount of air with each breath. Breathing exercises can be learned in only a few minutes and require considerably less time than the progressive muscle relaxation exercises.

As with any other relaxation technique, these exercises should be done in a quiet, pleasant, well-ventilated room. Any of the three examples of breathing exercises presented here will help relieve tension induced by stress.

1. Deep breathing. Lie with your back flat against the floor and place a pillow under your knees. Feet are slightly separated, with toes pointing outward. (The exercise also may be done while sitting up in a chair or standing straight up.) Place one hand on your abdomen and the other hand on your chest.

Slowly breathe in and out so the hand on your abdomen rises when you inhale and falls as you exhale. The hand on the chest should not move much at all. Repeat the exercise about ten times. Next, scan your body for tension and compare your present tension with the tension you felt at the beginning of the exercise. Repeat the entire process once or twice.

2. Sighing. Using the abdominal breathing technique, breathe in through your nose to a specific count (e.g., 4, 5, or 6). Now exhale through pursed lips to double the intake count (e.g., 8, 10, or 12). Repeat the exercise eight to ten times whenever you feel tense.

3. Complete natural breathing. Sit in an upright position or stand straight up. Breathing through your nose, gradually fill your lungs from the bottom up. Hold your breath for several seconds. Now exhale slowly by allowing your chest and abdomen to relax completely. Repeat the exercise eight to ten times.

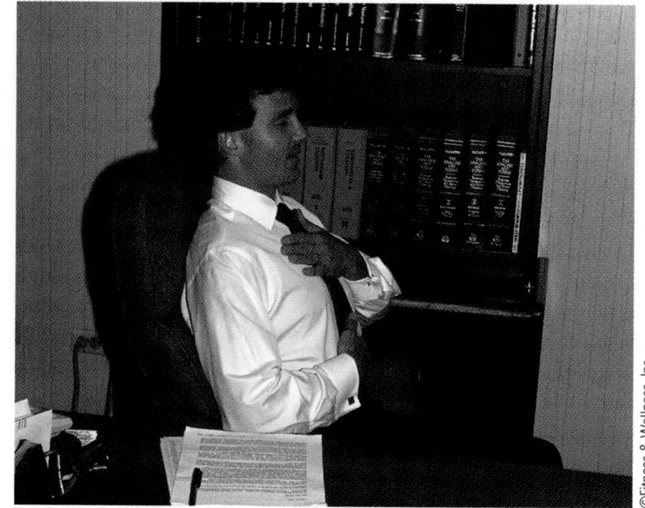

Breathing exercises help dissipate stress.

Critical Thinking

List the three most common stressors that you face as a college student. What techniques have you used to manage these situations, and in what way have they helped you cope?

Visual Imagery

Visual or mental **imagery** has been used as a healing technique for centuries in various cultures around the world. In Western medicine, the practice of imagery is relatively new and not widely accepted among health-care professionals.

Research is now being done to study the effects of imagery on the treatment of conditions such as cancer, hypertension, asthma, chronic pain, and obesity. Imagery induces a state of relaxation that rids the body of the stress that leads to illness. It improves circulation and increases the delivery of healing antibodies and white blood cells to the site of illness.[6] Imagery also helps to boost self-confidence, regain control and power over the body, and lower feelings of hopelessness, fear, and depression.

Visual imagery involves the creation of relaxing visual images and scenes in times of stress to elicit body and mind relaxation. Imagery works by offsetting the stressor with the visualization of relaxing scenes such as a sunny beach, a beautiful meadow, a quiet mountaintop, or some other peaceful setting. If you are ill, you can also visualize your white blood cells attacking an infection or a tumor. Imagery is also used in conjunction with breathing exercises, meditation, and yoga.

As with other stress management techniques, imagery should be performed in a quiet and comfortable environment. You can either sit or lie down for the exercise. If you lie down, use a soft surface and place a pillow under your knees. Be sure that your clothes are loose and that you are as comfortable as you can be.

To start the exercise, close your eyes and take a few breaths using one of the breathing techniques previously described. You then can proceed to visualize one of your favorite scenes in nature. Place yourself into the scene and visualize yourself moving about and experiencing nature to its fullest. Enjoy the people, the animals, the colors, the sounds, the smells, and even the temperature in your scene. After 10 to 20 minutes of visualization, open your eyes and compare the tension in your body

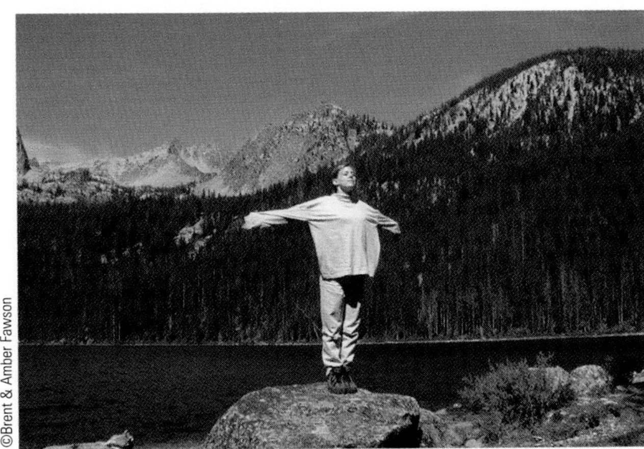

©Brent & Amber Fawson

Visual imagery of beautiful and relaxing scenes helps attenuate the stress response.

and mind at this point with how you felt prior to the exercise. You can repeat this exercise as often as you deem necessary when you are feeling tension or stress.

You may not always be able to find a quiet/comfortable setting in which to sit or lie down for 10 to 20 minutes. If you think imagery works for you, however, you can perform this technique while standing or sitting in an active setting. If you are able, close your eyes and disregard your surroundings for a short moment and visualize one of your favorite scenes. Once you feel that you have regained some control over the stressor, open your eyes and continue with your assigned tasks.

Autogenic Training

Autogenic training is a form of self-suggestion in which people place themselves in an autohypnotic state by repeating and concentrating on feelings of heaviness and warmth in the extremities. This technique was developed by Johannes Schultz, a German psychiatrist who noted that hypnotized individuals developed sensations of warmth and heaviness in the limbs and torso. The sensation of warmth is caused by dilation of blood vessels, which increases blood flow to the limbs. Muscular relaxation produces the feeling of heaviness.

In this technique the person lies down or sits in a comfortable position, eyes closed, and concentrates progressively on six fundamental stages and says (or thinks) the following:

1. Heaviness
   My right (left) arm is heavy.
   Both arms are heavy.
   My right (left) leg is heavy.
   Both legs are heavy.
   My arms and legs are heavy.
2. Warmth
   My right (left) arm is warm.
   Both arms are warm.
   My right (left) leg is warm.
   Both legs are warm.
   My arms and legs are warm.
3. Heart
   My heartbeat is calm and regular. (Repeat four or five times.)
4. Respiration
   My body breathes itself. (Repeat four or five times.)
5. Abdomen
   My abdomen is warm. (Repeat four or five times.)
6. Forehead
   My forehead is cool. (Repeat four or five times.)

The autogenic training technique is more difficult to master than any of those mentioned previously. The person should not move too fast through the entire exercise, because this actually may interfere with learning and relaxation. Each stage must be mastered before proceeding to the next.

Meditation

Meditation is a mental exercise that can bring about psychological and physical benefits. Regular meditation has been shown to decrease blood pressure, stress, anger, anxiety, fear, negative feelings, chronic pain, and increase activity in the brain's left frontal region—an area associated with positive emotions.[7] The objective of meditation is to gain control over one's attention by clearing the mind and blocking out the stressor(s) responsible for the higher tension.

This technique can be learned rather quickly, but first-time users often drop out before reaping benefits because they feel intimidated, confused, bored, or frustrated. In such cases, a group setting is best to get started. Many colleges, community programs, health clubs, and hospitals offer classes.

Initially the person who is learning to meditate should choose a room that is comfortable, quiet, and free of all disturbances (including telephones). After learning the technique, the person will be able to med-

---

Breathing exercises A stress management technique wherein the individual concentrates on "breathing away" the tension and inhaling fresh air to the entire body.

Imagery Mental visualization of relaxing images and scenes to induce body relaxation in times of stress or as an aid in the treatment of certain medical conditions such as cancer, hypertension, asthma, chronic pain, and obesity.

Autogenic training A stress management technique using a form of self-suggestion, wherein an individual is able to place himself or herself in an autohypnotic state by repeating and concentrating on feelings of heaviness and warmth in the extremities.

Meditation A stress management technique used to gain control over one's attention by clearing the mind and blocking out the stressor(s) responsible for the increased tension.

itate just about anywhere. A time block of approximately 10 to 15 minutes is adequate to start, but as you become more comfortable with meditation you can lengthen the time to 30 minutes or longer. To use meditation effectively, meditate daily—as just once or twice per week may not provide noticeable benefits.

Of the several forms of meditation, the following routine is recommended to get started.

1. Sit in a chair in an upright position with the hands resting either in your lap or on the arms of the chair. Close your eyes and focus on your breathing. Allow your body to relax as much as possible. Do not try to consciously relax, because trying means work. Rather, assume a passive attitude and concentrate on your breathing.
2. Allow the body to breathe regularly, at its own rhythm, and repeat in your mind the word "one" every time you inhale, and the word "two" every time you exhale. Paying attention to these two words keeps distressing thoughts from entering into your mind.
3. Continue to breathe in this way about 15 minutes. Because the objective of meditation is to bring about a hypometabolic state leading to body relaxation, do not use an alarm clock to remind you that the 15 minutes have expired. The alarm will only trigger your stress response again, defeating the purpose of the exercise. Opening your eyes once in a while to keep track of the time is fine, but do not rush or anticipate the end of the session. This time has been set aside for meditation, and you need to relax, take your time, and enjoy the exercise.

Yoga

Yoga is an excellent stress-coping technique. It is a school of thought in the Hindu religion that seeks to help the individual attain a higher level of spirituality and peace of mind. Although its philosophical roots can be considered spiritual, yoga is based on principles of self-care.

Practitioners of yoga adhere to a specific code of ethics and a system of mental and physical exercises that promote control of the mind and the body. In Western countries, many people are familiar mainly with the exercise portion of yoga. This system of exercises (called postures or asanas) can be used as a relaxation technique for stress management. The exercises include a combination of postures, diaphragmatic breathing, muscle relaxation, and meditation that help buffer the biological effects of stress.

Western interest in yoga exercises developed gradually over the last century, particularly since the 1970s. The practice of yoga exercises helps align the musculoskeletal system and increases muscular flexibility, muscular strength and endurance, and balance.[8] People pursue yoga exercises to help dispel stress by raising self-esteem, clearing the mind, slowing respiration, promoting neuromuscular relaxation, and increasing body awareness. In addition, the exercises help relieve back pain and control involuntary body functions like heart rate, blood pressure, oxygen consumption, and metabolic rate. Yoga also is used in many hospital-based programs for cardiac patients to help manage stress and decrease blood pressure.

In addition, yoga exercises have been used to help treat chemical dependency, insomnia, and prevent injury. Research on patients with coronary heart disease who practiced yoga (among other lifestyle changes) has shown that it slows down or even reverses atherosclerosis. These patients were compared with others who did not use yoga as one of the lifestyle changes.[9]

Of the many different styles of yoga, more than 60 are presently taught in the United States. Classes vary according to their emphasis. Some styles of yoga are athletic, others are passive in nature.

The most popular variety of yoga in the Western world is **hatha yoga,** which incorporates a series of static-stretching postures performed in specific sequences ("asanas") that help induce the relaxation response. The postures are held for several seconds while participants concentrate on breathing patterns, meditation, and body awareness.

Most yoga classes now are variations of hatha yoga and many of the typical stretches used in flexibility exercises today have been adapted from hatha yoga. Examples include

1. *integral yoga* and *viny yoga,* which focus on gentle/static stretches,
2. *iyengar yoga,* which promotes muscular strength and endurance,
3. *yogalates,* which incorporates Pilates exercises to increase muscular strength, and
4. *power yoga* or *yogarobics,* which is a high-energy form that links many postures together in a dance-like routine to promote cardiorespiratory fitness.

As with flexibility exercises, the stretches in hatha yoga should not be performed to the point of discomfort. Instructors should not push participants beyond their physical limitations. Similar to other stress management techniques, yoga exercises are best performed in a quiet place for 15 to 60 minutes per session. Many yoga participants like to perform the exercises daily.

To appreciate yoga exercises, a person has to experience them. The discussion here serves only as an introduction. Although yoga exercises can be practiced with the instruction of a book or video, most participants take classes. Many of the postures are difficult and complex, and few individuals can master the entire sequence in the first few weeks.

Individuals who are interested in yoga exercises should initially pursue under qualified instruction.

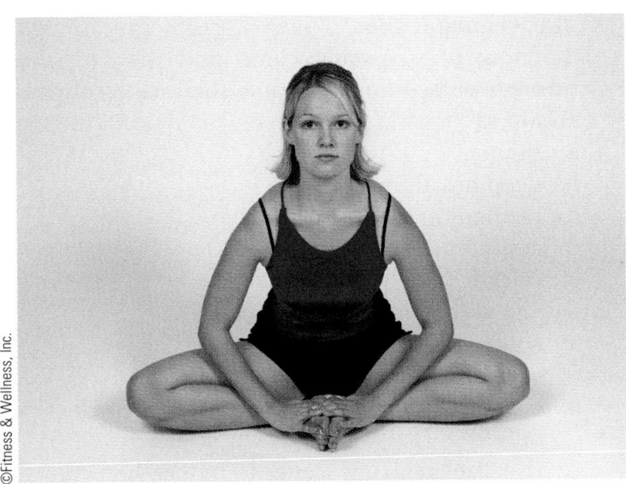

©Fitness & Wellness, Inc.

Yoga exercises help induce the relaxation response.

Many universities offer yoga courses, and you also can check the phone book for a listing of yoga instructors or classes. Yoga courses are offered at many health clubs and recreation centers. Because instructors and yoga styles vary, you may want to sit in on a class before enrolling. The most important thing is to look for an instructor whose views on wellness parallel your own. Instructors are not subject to any national certification standards. If you are new to yoga, you are encouraged to compare a couple of instructors before you select a class.

Which Technique Is Best?

Each person reacts to stress differently. Therefore, the best coping strategy depends mostly on the individual. Which technique is used does not really matter, as long as it works. An individual may want to experiment with several or all of them to find out which works best. A combination of two or more is best for many people.

All of the coping strategies discussed here help to block out stressors and promote mental and physical relaxation by diverting the attention to a different, nonthreatening action. Some of the techniques are easier to learn and may take less time per session. As a part of your class experience, you may participate in a stress management session (see Lab 10E). Regardless of which technique you select, the time spent doing stress management exercises (several times a day, as needed) is well worth the effort when stress becomes a significant problem in life.

Keep in mind that most individuals need to learn to relax and take time for themselves. Stress is not what makes people ill; it's the way they react to the stress-causing agent. Individuals who learn to be diligent and start taking control of themselves find that they can enjoy a better, happier, and healthier life.

Yoga A school of thought in the Hindu religion that seeks to help the individual attain a higher level of spirituality and peace of mind.

Hatha yoga A form of yoga that incorporates specific sequences of static-stretching postures to help induce the relaxation response.

Assess Your Behavior

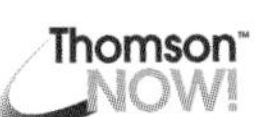

Log on to www.thomsonedu.com/login and take the stress inventory to identify the main stressors in your life and to create a plan for dealing more effectively with those stressors.

1. Are you able to channel your emotions and feelings to exert a positive effect on your mind, health, and wellness?
2. Do you use time management strategies on a regular basis?
3. Do you use stress management techniques, and do they allow you to be in control over the daily stresses of life?

Assess Your Knowledge

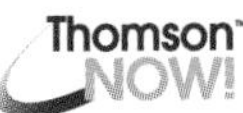

Log on to www.thomsonedu.com/login to assess your understanding of this chapter's topics by taking the Student Practice Test and exploring the modules recommended in your Personalized Study Plan.

1. Positive stress is also referred to as
   a. eustress.
   b. posstress.
   c. functional stress.
   d. distress.
   e. physiostress.
2. Which of the following is *not* a stage of the general adaptation syndrome?
   a. alarm reaction
   b. resistance
   c. compliance
   d. exhaustion/recovery
   e. All are stages of the general adaptation syndrome.

3. The behavior pattern of highly stressed individuals who do not seem to be at higher risk for disease is known as Type
   a. A.
   b. B.
   c. C.
   d. X.
   e. Z.

4. Effective time managers
   a. delegate.
   b. learn to say "no."
   c. protect from boredom.
   d. set aside "overtimes."
   e. do all of the above.

5. Hormonal changes that occur during a stress response
   a. decrease heart rate.
   b. sap the body's strength.
   c. diminish blood flow to the muscles.
   d. induce relaxation.
   e. increase blood pressure.

6. Exercise decreases stress levels by
   a. deliberately diverting stress to various body systems.
   b. metabolizing excess catecholamines.
   c. diminishing muscular tension.
   d. stimulating alpha-wave activity in the brain.
   e. doing all of the above.

7. Biofeedback is
   a. the interaction with the interior self.
   b. the biological response to stress.
   c. the nonspecific response to a stress-causing agent.
   d. used to identify biological factors that cause stress.
   e. most readily achieved while in a state of self-hypnosis.

8. The technique where a person breathes in through the nose to a specific count and then exhales through pursed lips to double the intake count is known as
   a. sighing.
   b. deep breathing.
   c. meditation.
   d. autonomic ventilation.
   e. release management.

9. During autogenic training, a person
   a. contracts each muscle to about 70 percent of capacity.
   b. concentrates on feelings of warmth and heaviness.
   c. visualizes relaxing scenes to induce body relaxation.
   d. learns to reliably influence physiological responses.
   e. notes the positive and negative impact of frequent stressors on various body systems.

10. Yoga exercises have been successfully used to
   a. stimulate ventilation.
   b. increase metabolism during stress.
   c. slow down atherosclerosis.
   d. decrease body awareness.
   e. accomplish all of the above.

Correct answers can be found at the back of the book.

Media Menu

Thomson™ NOW! *Connections*

- Identify the stressors in your life and develop a change plan to deal more effectively with them.
- Check how well you understand the chapter's concepts.

Internet Connections

Stress: Who Has Time For It?

This is a visually appealing site that describes the symptoms of stress and how to manage your daily stress.
http://www.familydoctor.org/handouts/278.html

Workplace Stress

This site, sponsored by the American Institute of Stress, provides research-based, practical information on occupational stress and its effect on health.
http://www.stress.org/job.htm

Mind Tools

This site covers a variety of topics on stress management, including recognizing stress, exercise, time management, self-hypnosis, meditation, breathing exercises, coping mechanisms, and more. The site also features a free comprehensive personal self-assessment with questions pertaining to work and home stressors, physical and behavioral signs and symptoms, as well as personal coping skills and resources.
http://www.mindtools.com/smpage.html

Notes

1. H. Selye, *Stress Without Distress* (New York: Signet, 1974).
2. E. Gullete et al., "Effects of Mental Stress on Myocardial Ischemia during Daily Life," *Journal of the American Medical Association* 277 (1997): 1521–1525. C. A. Lengacher et al., "Psychoneuroimmunology and Immune System Link for Stress, Depression, Health Behaviors, and Breast Cancer," *Alternative Health Practitioner* 4 (1998): 95–108.
3. R. J. Kriegel and M. H. Kriegel, *The C Zone: Peak Performance Under Stress* (Garden City, NY: Anchor Press/ Doubleday, 1985).
4. Lengacher; J. Moses et al., "The Effects of Exercise Training on Mental Well-Being in the Normal Population: A Controlled Trial," *Journal of Psychosomatic Research* 33 (1989): 47–61; C. Shang, "Emerging Paradigms in Mind-Body Medicine," *Journal of Complementary and Alternative Medicine* 7 (2001): 83–91.
5. See note 1, Selye.
6. M. Samuels, "Use Your Mind to Heal Your Body," *Bottom Line/Health* 19 (February 2005): 13–14.
7. S. Bodian, "Meditate Your Way to Much Better Health," *Bottom Line/Health* 18 (June 2004): 11–13.
8. D. Mueller, "Yoga Therapy," *ACSM's Health & Fitness Journal* 6 (2002): 18–24.
9. S. C. Manchanda et al., "Retardation of Coronary Atherosclerosis with Yoga Lifestyle Intervention," *Journal of the Association of Physicians of India* 48 (2000): 687–694.

Suggested Readings

Girdano, D. A., D. E. Dusek, and G. S. Everly. *Controlling Stress and Tension.* San Francisco: Benjamin Cummings, 2005.

Greenberg, J. S. *Comprehensive Stress Management.* New York: McGraw-Hill/Primis Custom Publishing, 2002.

Olpin, M., and M. Hesson. *Stress Management for Life.* Belmont, CA: Wadsworth/ Thomson Learning, 2007.

Schwartz, M. S., and F. Andrasik. *Biofeedback: A Practitioner's Guide.* New York: Guilford Press, 2004.

Selye, H. *The Stress of Life.* New York: McGraw-Hill, 1978.

Smith, J. S. *Stress Management: A Comprehensive Handbook of Techniques and Strategies.* New York: Springer, 2002.

Lab 10A Life Experiences Survey

Name:		Date:		Grade:	
Instructor:		Course:		Section:	

Necessary Lab Equipment
None required.

Objective
To determine stressful life experiences within the last 12 months that may affect your physical and psychological well-being and your Type A personality rating.

I. Life Experiences Survey

Introduction

The Life Experiences Survey contains a list of events that sometimes bring about change in the lives of those who experience them and that necessitate social readjustment. Please check events that you have experienced in the past 12 months. Be sure all checkmarks are directly across from the items to which they correspond (check only those that apply). For each item checked, please indicate the type and extent of impact the event had on your life at the time the event occurred. A rating of −3 would indicate an extremely negative impact. A rating of 0 suggests no impact either positive or negative. A rating of +3 would indicate an extremely positive impact.

Section 1

Event							
1. Marriage	−3	−2	−1	0	+1	+2	+3
2. Detention in jail or comparable institution	−3	−2	−1	0	+1	+2	+3
3. Death of spouse	−3	−2	−1	0	+1	+2	+3
4. Major change in sleeping habits (much more or much less sleep)	−3	−2	−1	0	+1	+2	+3
5. Death of close family member:							
a. mother	−3	−2	−1	0	+1	+2	+3
b. father	−3	−2	−1	0	+1	+2	+3
c. brother	−3	−2	−1	0	+1	+2	+3
d. sister	−3	−2	−1	0	+1	+2	+3
e. grandmother	−3	−2	−1	0	+1	+2	+3
f. grandfather	−3	−2	−1	0	+1	+2	+3
g. other (specify)	−3	−2	−1	0	+1	+2	+3
6. Major change in eating habits (much more or much less food intake)	−3	−2	−1	0	+1	+2	+3
7. Foreclosure on mortgage or loan	−3	−2	−1	0	+1	+2	+3
8. Death of close friend	−3	−2	−1	0	+1	+2	+3
9. Outstanding personal achievement	−3	−2	−1	0	+1	+2	+3
10. Minor law violations (traffic tickets, disturbing the peace, etc.)	−3	−2	−1	0	+1	+2	+3
11. Male: Wife/girlfriend's pregnancy	−3	−2	−1	0	+1	+2	+3
12. Female: Pregnancy	−3	−2	−1	0	+1	+2	+3
13. Changed work situation (different work responsibility, major change in working conditions or working hours, etc.)	−3	−2	−1	0	+1	+2	+3
14. New job	−3	−2	−1	0	+1	+2	+3
15. Serious illness or injury of close family member:							
a. father	−3	−2	−1	0	+1	+2	+3
b. mother	−3	−2	−1	0	+1	+2	+3
c. sister	−3	−2	−1	0	+1	+2	+3

Continued

From Sarason, I. G., et al., "Assessing the Impact of Life Changes: Development of the Life Experiences Survey," *Journal of Consulting and Clinical Psychology* 46 (1978): 932–946.

Item							
d. brother	−3	−2	−1	0	+1	+2	+3
e. grandfather	−3	−2	−1	0	+1	+2	+3
f. grandmother	−3	−2	−1	0	+1	+2	+3
g. spouse	−3	−2	−1	0	+1	+2	+3
h. other (specify)	−3	−2	−1	0	+1	+2	+3
16. Sexual difficulties	−3	−2	−1	0	+1	+2	+3
17. Trouble with employer (in danger of losing job or of being suspended or demoted, etc.)	−3	−2	−1	0	+1	+2	+3
18. Trouble with in-laws	−3	−2	−1	0	+1	+2	+3
19. Major change in financial status (a lot better off or a lot worse off)	−3	−2	−1	0	+1	+2	+3
20. Major change in closeness of family members (increased or decreased closeness)	−3	−2	−1	0	+1	+2	+3
21. Gaining a new family member (through birth, adoption, family member moving in, etc.)	−3	−2	−1	0	+1	+2	+3
22. Change of residence	−3	−2	−1	0	+1	+2	+3
23. Marital separation from mate (due to conflict)	−3	−2	−1	0	+1	+2	+3
24. Major change in church activities (increased or decreased attendance)	−3	−2	−1	0	+1	+2	+3
25. Marital reconciliation with mate	−3	−2	−1	0	+1	+2	+3
26. Major change in number of arguments with spouse (a lot more or a lot less arguments)	−3	−2	−1	0	+1	+2	+3
27. Married male: Change in wife's work outside the home (beginning work, ceasing work, changing to a new job, etc.)	−3	−2	−1	0	+1	+2	+3
28. Married female: Change in husband's work (loss of job, beginning new job, retirement, etc.)	−3	−2	−1	0	+1	+2	+3
29. Major change in usual type and/or amount of recreation	−3	−2	−1	0	+1	+2	+3
30. Borrowing more than $10,000 (buying home, business, etc.)	−3	−2	−1	0	+1	+2	+3
31. Borrowing less than $10,000 (buying car or TV, getting school loan, etc.)	−3	−2	−1	0	+1	+2	+3
32. Being fired from job	−3	−2	−1	0	+1	+2	+3
33. Male: Wife/girlfriend having abortion	−3	−2	−1	0	+1	+2	+3
34. Female: Having abortion	−3	−2	−1	0	+1	+2	+3
35. Major personal illness or injury	−3	−2	−1	0	+1	+2	+3
36. Major change in social activities (participation in parties, movies, visiting, etc.)	−3	−2	−1	0	+1	+2	+3
37. Major change in living conditions of family (building new home or remodeling, deterioration of home or neighborhood, etc.)	−3	−2	−1	0	+1	+2	+3
38. Divorce	−3	−2	−1	0	+1	+2	+3
39. Serious injury or illness of close friend	−3	−2	−1	0	+1	+2	+3
40. Retirement from work	−3	−2	−1	0	+1	+2	+3
41. Son or daughter leaving home (because of marriage, college, etc.)	−3	−2	−1	0	+1	+2	+3
42. End of formal schooling	−3	−2	−1	0	+1	+2	+3
43. Separation from spouse (because of work, travel, etc.)	−3	−2	−1	0	+1	+2	+3
44. Engagement	−3	−2	−1	0	+1	+2	+3
45. Breaking up with boyfriend/girlfriend	−3	−2	−1	0	+1	+2	+3
46. Leaving home for the first time	−3	−2	−1	0	+1	+2	+3
47. Reconciliation with boyfriend/girlfriend	−3	−2	−1	0	+1	+2	+3
48. Others______________________	−3	−2	−1	0	+1	+2	+3
49. ______________________	−3	−2	−1	0	+1	+2	+3
50. ______________________	−3	−2	−1	0	+1	+2	+3

A Healthy Lifestyle

CHAPTER 11

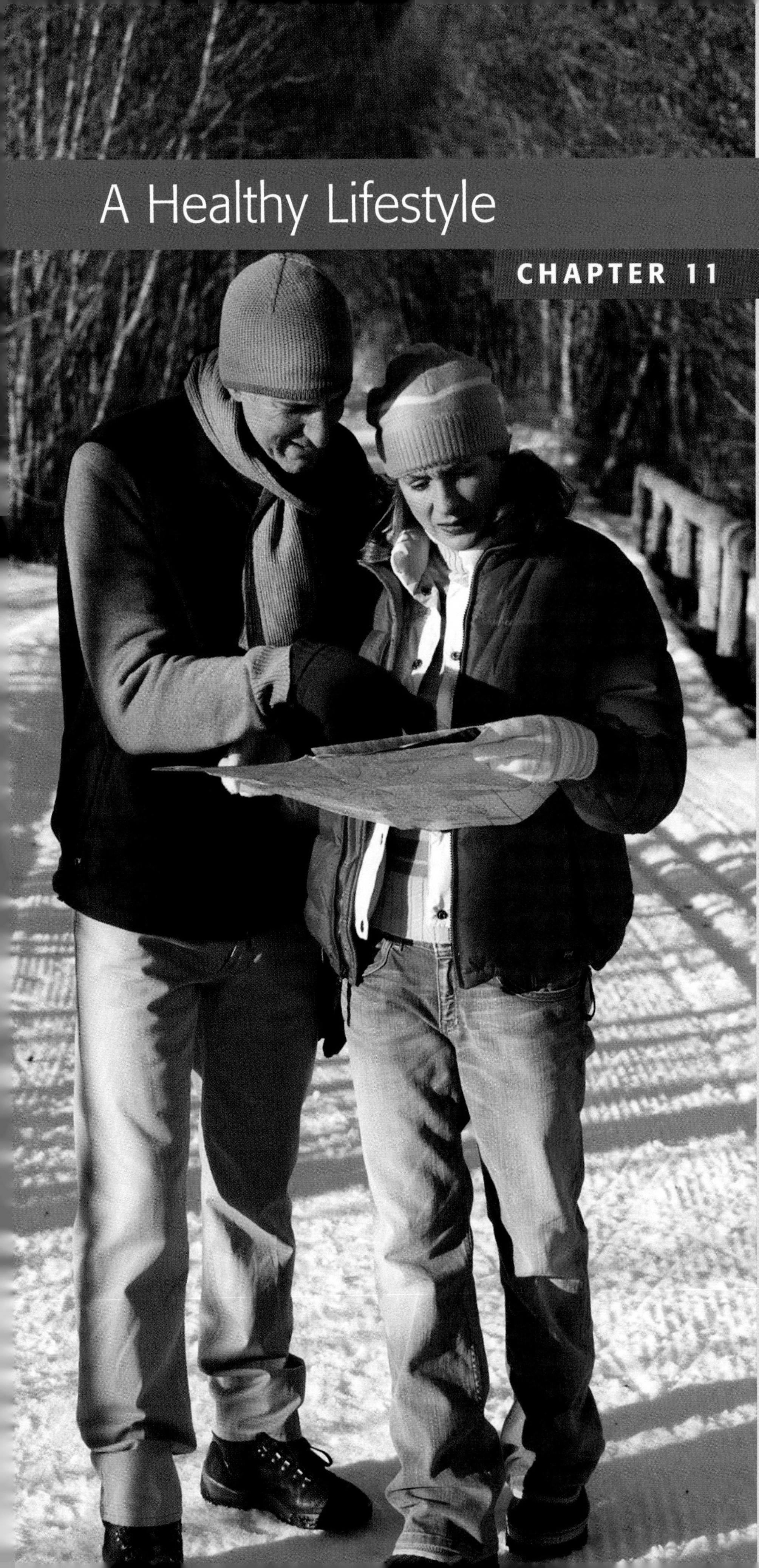

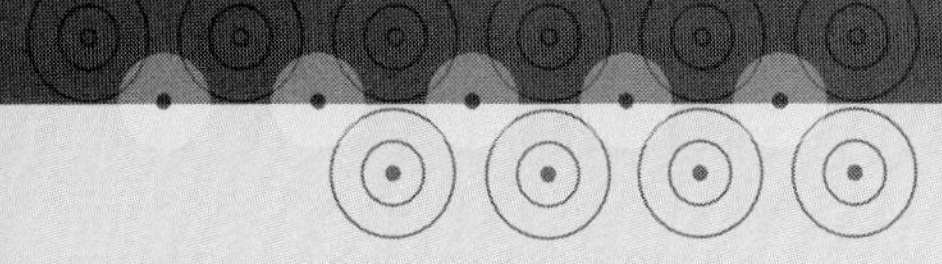

OBJECTIVES

- State the importance of implementing a healthy lifestyle program.
- Identify the major risk factors for coronary heart disease.
- Cite the cancer-prevention guidelines.
- Explain the relationship between spirituality and wellness.
- Learn the health consequences of chemical abuse and irresponsible sex.
- Differentiate physiological age from chronological age.
- Give some guidelines for preventing consumer fraud.
- Enumerate factors to consider when selecting a health/fitness club.
- Explain how to select appropriate exercise equipment.
- Record your own health/fitness accomplishments and chart a wellness program for the future.
- Estimate your life expectancy and determine your real physiological age.

Thomson™ NOW! Go to www.thomsonedu.com/login to:

- Determine your risk for heart disease.
- Check how well you understand the chapter's concepts.

Most people recognize that participating in fitness programs improves their quality of life. Improving physical fitness alone, however, is not sufficient to lower the risk for disease and ensure better health. For example, individuals who run 3 miles (about 5 km) a day, lift weights regularly, participate in stretching exercises, and watch their body weight can easily be classified as having good or excellent health-related fitness. If these same people, however, have high blood pressure, smoke, suffer constant stress, drink alcohol excessively, consume too much saturated and trans fat, and have an excessive caloric intake, they are not fit. All of these behaviors increase **risk factors** for chronic diseases and undermine physiologic fitness (see Chapter 1, page 8).

Good health is no longer viewed as simply the absence of illness. The notion of good health has evolved notably in the last three decades and continues to change as scientists understand lifestyle factors that bring on illness and affect wellness. Once we realized that improving the health-related components of fitness by themselves would not ensure good health, a wellness concept developed in the 1980s.

Wellness has been defined as the constant and deliberate effort to stay healthy and achieve the highest potential for well-being. Wellness covers a variety of activities aimed at helping individuals recognize lifestyle components that are detrimental to their health. Wellness living requires implementing positive programs to change behavior to improve health and quality of life, prolong life, and achieve total well-being.

FIGURE 11.1 Dimensions of wellness.

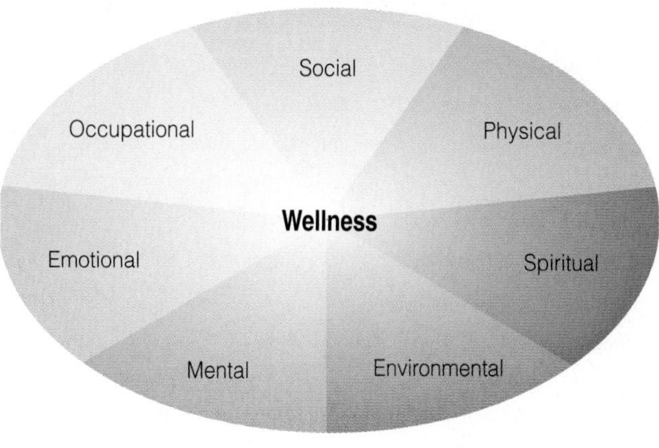

The Seven Dimensions of Wellness

To enjoy a wellness lifestyle, a person has to practice behaviors that will lead to positive outcomes in the seven dimensions of wellness: physical, emotional, mental, social, environmental, occupational, and spiritual (see Figure 11.1). These dimensions are interrelated; each dimension frequently affects the others. For example, a person who is emotionally "down" often has no desire to exercise, study, socialize with friends, or attend church, and, therefore, may be more susceptible to illness and disease.

High-level wellness goes beyond optimal fitness and the absence of disease. Wellness incorporates factors such as adequate fitness, proper nutrition, stress management, disease prevention, spirituality, smoking cessation, personal safety, substance abuse control, regular physical examinations, health education, and environmental support. For a wellness way of life, individuals must be physically fit and avoid risk factors that cause disease.

Consequently, your biggest challenge in the 21st century is to learn how to take control of your personal health habits by engaging in positive lifestyle activities. To help you achieve this goal, researchers have pointed out 12 lifestyle habits that can significantly increase health and longevity:

1. Be physically active (including exercise).
2. Do not use tobacco.
3. Eat a healthy diet.
4. Avoid snacking between meals.
5. Maintain recommended body weight.
6. Sleep 7 to 8 hours each night.
7. Decrease stress levels.
8. Drink alcohol moderately or not at all.
9. Surround yourself with healthy relationships.
10. Be informed about the environment and avoid environmental risk factors.
11. Increase education (more-educated people live longer).
12. Take personal safety measures.

Spiritual Well-Being

The definition of **spirituality** by the National Interfaith Coalition on Aging encompasses Christians and non-Christians alike. It assumes that all people are spiritual in nature. Spiritual health provides a unifying power that integrates the dimensions of wellness (see Figure 11.2). Basic characteristics of spiritual people include a sense of meaning and direction in life, a relationship to a higher being, freedom, prayer, faith, love, closeness to others, peace, joy, fulfillment, and altruism.

Although not everyone claims an affiliation with a certain religion or denomination, most surveys indicate that 95 percent of the U.S. population believes in God or a universal spirit functioning as God. People, furthermore, believe to varying extents that (a) a relationship with God is meaningful; (b) God can grant help, guidance, and assistance in daily living; and (c) mortal existence has a purpose. If we accept any or all of these

FIGURE 11.2 Components of spiritual well-being.

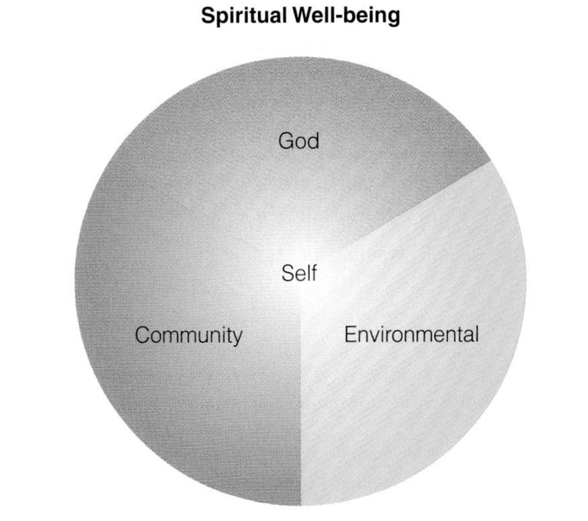

FIGURE 11.3 Underlying causes of death in United States, year 2000.

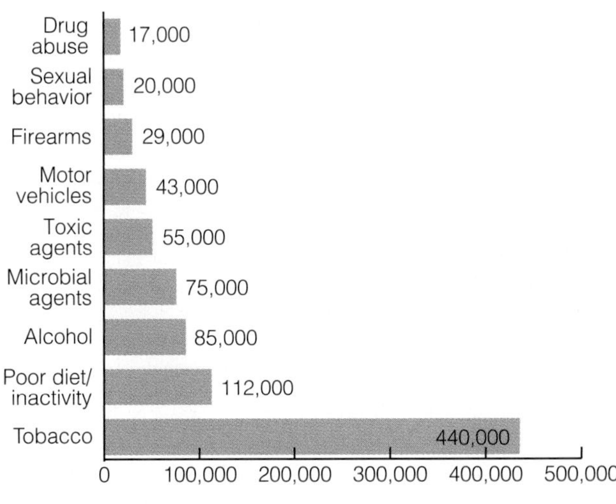

Source: Centers for Disease Control and Prevention. Atlanta, GA, 2003.

statements, attaining spirituality will have a definite effect on our happiness and well-being.

The reasons that religious affiliation enhances wellness are difficult to determine. Possible reasons include the promotion of healthy lifestyle behaviors, social support, assistance in times of crisis and need, and counseling to overcome one's weaknesses.

Prayer is a signpost of our spirituality, at the core of most spiritual experiences. It is communication with a higher power. Prayers are offered for a multiplicity of reasons, including guidance, wisdom, thanksgiving, strength, protection, and health. More than 200 studies have been conducted on the effects of prayer on health. About two-thirds of these studies have linked prayer to positive health outcomes, as long as these prayers are offered with sincerity, humility, love, empathy, and compassion. Some studies have shown faster healing time and fewer complications in patients who didn't even know they were being prayed for, compared with patients that were not prayed for.[1]

Altruism, a key attribute of spiritual people, seems to enhance health and longevity. Researchers believe that doing good to others is good for oneself, especially for the immune system. In a study of more than 2,700 people in Michigan, the investigators found that people who did regular volunteer work lived longer.[2] People who did not perform regular (at least once a week) volunteer work had a 250 percent higher risk for mortality during the course of the study.

Wellness requires a balance among the dimensions of physical, mental, social, emotional, occupational, environmental, and spiritual well-being. The relationship between spirituality and wellness, therefore, is meaningful in our quest for a better quality of life. As with other parameters of wellness, optimum spirituality requires developing the spiritual nature to its fullest potential.

Leading Causes of Death

Over the years, lack of wellness leads to a loss of health, vitality, and zest for life. Fortunately, most of the leading causes of premature illness and death are self-controlled, and you, the individual, can do more for your health and well-being than the entire medical establishment.

Of all deaths in the United States, approximately 60 percent are caused by cardiovascular disease and cancer.[3] Close to 80 percent of these deaths could be prevented by following a healthy lifestyle. The third and fourth leading causes of death, chronic lower respiratory disease and accidents, also are preventable, primarily by abstaining from tobacco and other drugs, wearing seat belts, and using common sense.

The underlying causes of death in the United States (see Figure 11.3) indicate that 8 of the 9 causes are related to lifestyle and lack of common sense. Of

Risk factors Lifestyle and genetic variables that may lead to disease.

Wellness The constant and deliberate effort to stay healthy and to achieve the highest potential for well-being.

Spirituality A sense of meaning and direction in life, a relationship to a higher being, freedom, prayer, faith, love, closeness to others, peace, joy, fulfillment, and altruism.

Prayer Sincere and humble communication with a higher power.

Altruism True concern for and action on behalf of others (opposite of egoism); a sincere desire to serve others above one's personal needs.

TABLE 11.1 Estimated Prevalence and Yearly Number of Deaths from Cardiovascular Disease, 2003

	Prevalence	Deaths
All forms of cardiovascular diseases*	71,300,000	910,600
Coronary heart disease	13,200,000	**
Heart attack	6,500,000	479,300
Stroke	5,500,000	157,800
High blood pressure	65,000,000	52,600***

*Includes people with one or more forms of cardiovascular disease.
**Number of deaths included under heart attack.
***Mortality figures appear to be low because many heart attack and stroke deaths are caused by high blood pressure.
Source: American Heart Association, *Heart Disease and Stroke Statistics—2004 Update* (Dallas: AHA, 2003).

WARNING SIGNALS OF A HEART ATTACK

Any of the following symptoms may occur during a heart attack. If you experience any of these and they last longer than a few minutes, call 911 and seek immediate medical attention. Failure to do so may result in death.

- Discomfort, pressure, fullness, squeezing, or pain in the middle of the chest that persists for several minutes. It may go away and return later.
- Pain that radiates to the shoulders, neck, or arms.
- Chest discomfort with lightheadedness, shortness of breath, nausea, sweating, or fainting.

the approximately 2.4 million yearly deaths in the United States, the "big three"—tobacco use, poor diet and inactivity, and alcohol abuse—are responsible for about 632,000 deaths each year.

Diseases of the Cardiovascular System

The most prevalent degenerative conditions in the United States are **cardiovascular diseases.** Almost 35 percent of all deaths in the United States are attributed to heart and blood vessel disease.[4] The American Heart Association estimated the cost of cardiovascular disease in the United States at more than $368 billion in 2004.

Cardiovascular diseases include afflictions such as coronary heart disease (CHD), heart attacks, peripheral vascular disease, congenital heart disease, rheumatic heart disease, atherosclerosis, strokes, high blood pressure, and congestive heart failure. Table 11.1 provides the estimated prevalence and annual number of deaths caused by the major types of cardiovascular disease.

One in five adults has some form of cardiovascular disease. More than 60 percent of the people who die from heart disease die suddenly and unexpectedly—with no previous symptoms of the disease. About 1.2 million people have a first-time or recurrent heart attack each year, and nearly 500,000 of them die as a result. Approximately 80 percent of deaths from CHD in people under age 65 occur during the first heart attack. More than half of these deaths occur within an hour of the onset of symptoms, before the person reaches the hospital.[5] Almost half of these deaths occur outside of the hospital, most likely because people fail to recognize early warning symptoms of a heart attack. It follows that the risk of death is higher in the least-educated segment of the population.

FIGURE 11.4 Incidence of cardiovascular disease in the United States for selected years: 1900–2000.

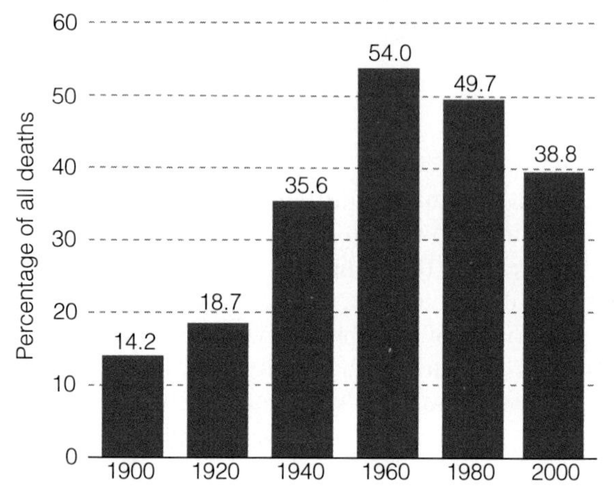

Source: Centers for Disease Control

Although heart and blood vessel disease is still the number-one health problem in the United States, the incidence has declined by almost 28 percent since 1960 (see Figure 11.4). The main reason for this dramatic decrease is health education. More people are now aware of the risk factors for cardiovascular disease and are changing their lifestyle to lower their potential risk for these diseases. In Lab 11A, you will have the opportunity to evaluate lifestyle habits that help decrease your risk for cardiovascular disease.

Coronary Heart Disease

The heart and the coronary arteries are illustrated in Figure 11.5. The major form of cardiovascular disease is **coronary heart disease (CHD),** in which the arteries that supply the heart muscle with oxygen and nutrients are narrowed by fatty deposits, such as cholesterol and triglycerides. Narrowing of the coronary arteries diminishes the blood supply to the heart muscle, which can precipitate a heart attack. CHD is the single leading cause of death in the United States, accounting for 20

FIGURE 11.5 The heart and its blood vessels (coronary arteries).

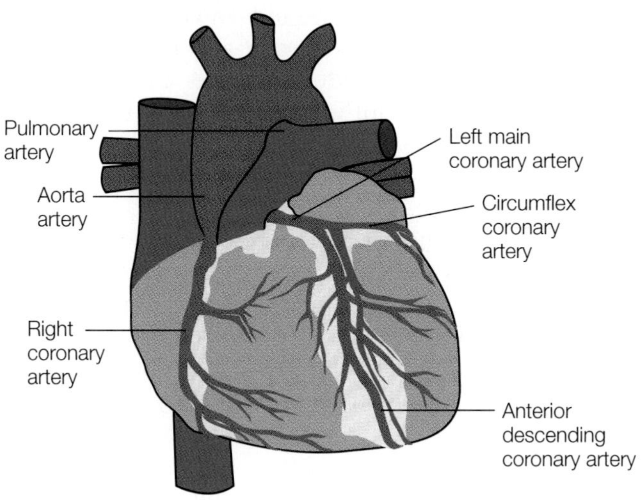

FIGURE 11.6 Relationship between fitness levels and cardiovascular mortality.

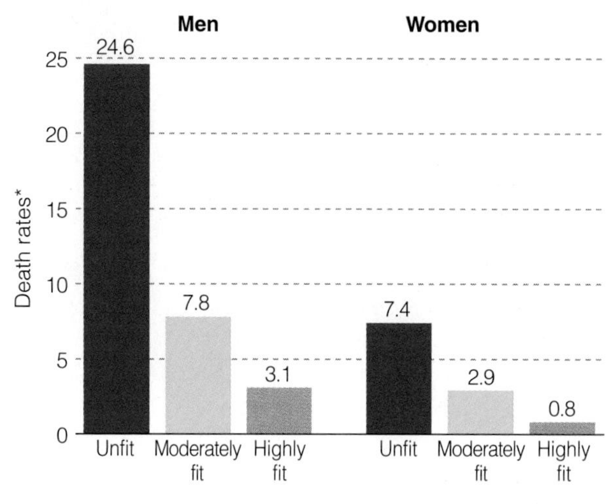

*Age-adjusted death rates per 10,000 person-years of follow-up, 1978–1985. From S. N. Blair, H. W. Kohl, III, R. S. Paffenbarger, Jr., D. B. Clark, D. H. Cooper, and L. W. Gibbons, "Physical Fitness and All-Cause Mortality: A Prospective Study of Healthy Men and Women," *Journal of the American Medical Association* 262 (1989): 2395–2401. Reprinted with permission.

percent of all deaths and approximately half of all cardiovascular deaths.[6]

The leading contributors to the development of CHD are

- Physical inactivity
- High blood pressure
- High body mass index (BMI 30 or higher)
- Low HDL cholesterol
- Elevated LDL cholesterol
- Elevated triglycerides
- Elevated homocysteine
- Inflammation
- Diabetes
- Abnormal electrocardiograms (ECG)
- Tobacco use
- Stress
- Personal and family history of cardiovascular disease
- Gender
- Age

Although genetic inheritance plays a role in CHD, the most important determinant is personal lifestyle. Several of the major risk factors for CHD are preventable and reversible. All of the preceding risk factors are discussed in the following pages.

Physical Inactivity

Improving cardiorespiratory endurance through aerobic exercise has perhaps the greatest impact in reducing the overall risk for cardiovascular disease. In this age of mechanized societies, we cannot afford *not* to exercise. Research on the benefits of aerobic exercise in reducing cardiovascular disease is too impressive to be ignored.

Guidelines for implementing an aerobic exercise program are discussed thoroughly in Chapters 6 and 9. Following these guidelines will promote cardiorespiratory fitness, enhance health, and extend the lifespan. Even moderate amounts of aerobic exercise can reduce cardiovascular risk considerably. As shown in Figure 11.6, work conducted at the Aerobics Research Institute in Dallas showed a much higher incidence of cardiovascular deaths in unfit people, compared to moderately fit and highly fit people.[7]

A regular aerobic exercise program helps control most of the major risk factors that lead to heart and blood vessel disease. Aerobic exercise will do all of the following:

- Increase cardiorespiratory endurance.
- Decrease and control blood pressure.
- Reduce body fat.
- Lower blood lipids (cholesterol and triglycerides).
- Improve HDL cholesterol (see "Abnormal Cholesterol Profile" on pages 366–368).
- Help control or decrease the risk for diabetes.
- Decrease low-grade inflammation in the body.
- Increase and maintain good heart function, sometimes improving certain ECG abnormalities.
- Motivate toward quitting smoking.

Cardiovascular diseases The array of conditions that affect the heart and the blood vessels.

Coronary heart disease (CHD) Condition in which the arteries that supply the heart muscle with oxygen and nutrients are narrowed by fatty deposits, such as cholesterol and triglycerides.

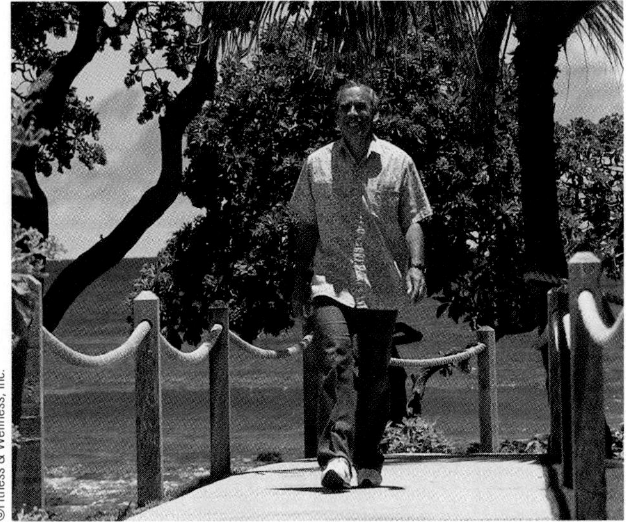

Regular physical activity helps control most of the major risk factors that lead to cardiovascular disease.

- Alleviate stress.
- Counteract a personal history of heart disease.

High Blood Pressure (Hypertension)

Blood pressure should be checked regularly. The pressure is measured in milliliters of mercury (mm Hg), usually expressed in two numbers. The higher (first) number reflects the **systolic pressure,** which is exerted during the forceful contraction of the heart. The lower (second) value, **diastolic pressure,** is taken during the heart's relaxation phase, when no blood is being ejected. Ideal blood pressure is 120/80 or below. All blood pressures above 140/90 are considered **hypertension.**

High blood pressure can be controlled with various medications, along with the lifestyle changes described below for people with mild hypertension. Because people respond differently to these medications, a physician may try different medications to find one that produces the best results with the fewest side effects.

The recommended treatment for people with mild hypertension consists of regular aerobic exercise, weight control, a low-salt/low-fat and high-potassium/high-calcium diet, lower alcohol and caffeine intake, smoking cessation, and stress management. People with high blood pressure should follow their physician's advice and continue to take any prescribed medication.

Comprehensive reviews of the effects of aerobic exercise on blood pressure found that, in general, an individual can expect exercise-induced reductions of approximately 4 to 5 mm Hg in resting systolic blood pressure and 3 to 4 mm Hg in resting diastolic blood pressure.[8] Although these reductions do not seem large, a decrease of about 5 mm Hg in resting diastolic blood pressure has been associated with a 40 percent decrease in the risk for stroke and a 15 percent reduction in the risk for coronary heart disease.[9]

Even in the absence of any decrease in resting blood pressure, hypertensive individuals who exercise have a lower risk of all-cause mortality than do hypertensive/sedentary individuals.[10] The research also shows that exercise, not weight loss, is the major contributor to the lower blood pressure of exercisers. If aerobic exercise is discontinued, the individual does not maintain these changes.

Another extensive review of research studies on the effects of at least 4 weeks of strength training on resting blood pressure yielded similar results.[11] Both systolic and diastolic blood pressures decreased by an average of 3 mm Hg. Participants in these studies, however, were primarily individuals with normal blood pressure. Of greater significance, strength training did not cause an increase in resting blood pressure. More research remains to be done on hypertensive subjects.

Excessive Body Fat

As defined in Chapter 4, body composition delineates the fat and non-fat components of the human body. If a person has too much fat weight, he or she is overweight or obese. Obesity (BMI of 30 or higher) is recognized by the American Heart Association as a major risk factor for coronary heart disease.

Maintaining recommended body weight (fat percent) is essential in any cardiovascular risk-reduction program. For individuals with excessive body fat, even a modest weight reduction of 5 to 10 percent can reduce high blood pressure and total cholesterol levels. The causes of obesity are complex, including the combination of an individual's genetics, behavior, and lifestyle factors. Guidelines for a comprehensive weight management program are given in Chapter 5.

Abnormal Cholesterol Profile

The term **blood lipids** generally refers to cholesterol and triglycerides. Because these substances cannot float around freely in the water-based medium of the blood, they are packaged and transported by complex molecules called **lipoproteins.**

If you never have had a blood lipid test, you are strongly encouraged to do so. The blood test identifies levels of total **cholesterol,** high-density lipoprotein cholesterol (HDL cholesterol), low-density lipoprotein cholesterol (LDL cholesterol), and triglycerides. A significant elevation in blood lipids has been linked to heart and blood vessel disease.

A poor blood lipid profile is thought to be the most important predisposing factor in developing CHD, accounting for almost half of all cases. The general recommendation by the National Cholesterol Education Program (NCEP) is to keep total cholesterol levels below 200 milligrams per deciliter (mg/dl) of blood (see Table 11.2). The risk for heart attack in-

TABLE 11.2 Standards for Blood Lipids

	Amount	Rating
Total Cholesterol	<200 mg/dl	Desirable
	200–239 mg/dl	Borderline high
	≥240 mg/dl	High risk
LDL Cholesterol	<100 mg/dl	Optimal
	100–129 mg/dl	Near or above optimal
	130–159 mg/dl	Borderline high
	160–189 mg/dl	High
	≥190 mg/dl	Very high
HDL Cholesterol	<40 mg/dl	Low (high risk)
	≥60 mg/dl	High (low risk)
Triglycerides	<150 mg/dl	Desirable
	150–199 mg/dl	Borderline-high
	200–499 mg/dl	High
	≥500 mg/dl	Very high

Source: Cholesterol data from National Cholesterol Education Program; triglyceride data from National Heart, Lung and Blood Institute.

creases 2 percent for every 1 percent increase in total cholesterol.[12]

Cholesterol levels between 200 and 239 mg/dl are borderline high, and levels of 240 mg/dl and above indicate high risk for disease. Approximately 51 percent, or 104.7 million American adults, have total cholesterol values of 200 mg/dl or higher, and 18.3 percent (37 million adults) have values at or above 240 mg/dl.[13]

As important as it is, total cholesterol is no longer the best predictor for cardiovascular risk. More significant is the way in which cholesterol is carried in the bloodstream. Cholesterol is transported primarily in the form of **high-density lipoprotein (HDL)** cholesterol and **low-density lipoprotein (LDL)** cholesterol.

In a process known as "reverse cholesterol transport," HDL, the "good cholesterol," acts as a scavenger, removing cholesterol from the body and preventing plaque from forming in the arteries. The functioning parts of HDL are the protein molecules found in the coating of the molecules. When HDL comes in contact with cholesterol-filled cells, these protein molecules attach to the cells and take their cholesterol.

The "bad cholesterol," LDL, tends to release cholesterol, which then may penetrate into the arteries and speed up the process of **atherosclerosis.** The NCEP guidelines provided in Table 11.2 state that an LDL cholesterol value below 100 mg/dl is optimal.

LDL cholesterol particles are of two types: large or type A, and small or type B. Small particles are thought to pass through the inner lining of the coronary arteries more readily, increasing the risk for a heart attack. Predominance of small particles can mean a threefold to fivefold increase in the risk for CHD. If an individual is at risk for heart disease, the blood lipid analysis should include LDL particle size.

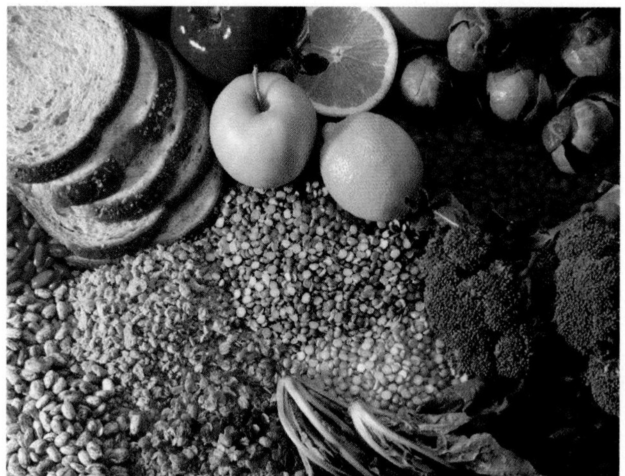

Low-fat/high-fiber foods are necessary to control blood lipids.

A genetic variation of LDL cholesterol known as Lp(a) is noteworthy because a high level of these particles leads to earlier development of atherosclerosis. Certain substances in the arterial wall are thought to interact with Lp(a), leading to premature formation of plaque. Only medications help decrease Lp(a), and drug options should be discussed with a physician.

The more HDL cholesterol (particularly the subcategory HDL_2), the better. HDL cholesterol, the "good" cholesterol, offers some protection against heart disease. In fact, a low level of HDL cholesterol is one of the best predictors of CHD; it has the strongest relationship to CHD at all levels of total cholesterol, including levels below 200 mg/dl.

Research suggests that, for every 1 mg/dl increase in HDL cholesterol, the risk for CHD drops up to 3 per-

---

Blood pressure A measure of the force exerted against the walls of the vessels by the blood flowing through them.

Systolic blood pressure Pressure exerted by the blood against the walls of the arteries during the forceful contraction (systole) of the heart.

Diastolic blood pressure Pressure exerted by the blood against the walls of the arteries during the relaxation phase (diastole) of the heart.

Hypertension Chronically elevated blood pressure.

Blood lipids (fats) Cholesterol and triglycerides.

Lipoproteins Complex molecules that transport cholesterol in the bloodstream.

Cholesterol A waxy substance, technically a steroid alcohol, found only in animal fats and oil; used in making cell membranes, as a building block for some hormones, in the fatty sheath around nerve fibers, and in other necessary substances.

High-density lipoprotein (HDL) Cholesterol-transporting molecules in the blood; the "good" cholesterol.

Low-density lipoprotein (LDL) Cholesterol-transporting molecules in the blood; the "bad" cholesterol.

Atherosclerosis Fatty/cholesterol deposits in the walls of the arteries leading to the formation of plaque.

cent in men and 5 percent in women.[14] The recommended HDL cholesterol values to minimize the risk for CHD are a minimum of 40. HDL cholesterol levels above 60 mg/dl help to reduce the risk for CHD.

For the most part, HDL cholesterol is determined genetically, and women in general have higher levels than men. Because the female sex hormone estrogen tends to raise HDL, premenopausal women have a much lower incidence of heart disease. African-American children and adult African-American men have higher values than Caucasians. HDL cholesterol also decreases with age.

Increasing HDL Cholesterol Increasing HDL cholesterol improves the cholesterol profile and lessens the risk for CHD. Habitual aerobic exercise, weight loss, high-dose niacin, and quitting smoking all help raise HDL cholesterol levels. Drug therapy (see pages 370–371) may also promote higher HDL cholesterol levels.

HDL cholesterol is clearly related to participation in a regular aerobic exercise program (exercising at high intensity, or above 6 METs, for at least 20 minutes three times per week—see Chapter 6). Individual responses to aerobic exercise differ, but, generally, the more one exercises, the higher is the HDL cholesterol level.

Even when more LDL cholesterol is present than the cells can use, cholesterol seems not to cause a problem until it is oxidized by **free radicals** (see discussion on antioxidants, Chapter 3, pages 84–87). After cholesterol is oxidized, white blood cells invade the arterial wall, take up the cholesterol, and clog the arteries.

The antioxidant effect of vitamins C and E may provide other benefits, too. Data suggest that a single unstable free radical can damage LDL particles, accelerating the atherosclerotic process. Vitamin C seems to deactivate free radicals and slow the oxidation of LDL cholesterol. Vitamin E apparently protects LDL from oxidation and thereby helps prevent heart disease, but studies suggest that this vitamin does not seem to be helpful in reversing damage once it has taken place.

Although the average adult in the United States consumes between 400 and 600 mg of cholesterol daily, the body actually manufactures more than that. Saturated and trans fats raise cholesterol levels more than anything else in the diet. These fats produce approximately 1,000 mg of cholesterol per day. Because of individual differences, some people can have a higher-than-normal intake of saturated and trans fats and still maintain normal cholesterol levels. Others who have a lower intake of these fats can have abnormally high cholesterol levels.

Saturated fats are found mostly in meats and dairy products and seldom in foods of plant origin. Poultry and fish contain less saturated fat than beef does but still should be eaten in moderation (about 3 to 6 ounces per day—see Chapter 3). Unsaturated fats are mainly of plant origin and cannot be converted to cholesterol.

Trans Fats Foods that contain trans fatty acids, hydrogenated fat, or partially hydrogenated vegetable oil should be avoided. Studies indicate that these foods elevate LDL cholesterol as much as saturated fats do. Trans fats also increase triglycerides and lower HDL cholesterol. These changes contribute not only to heart disease, but also to gallstone formation. Trans fats are found primarily in processed foods.

Hydrogen frequently is added to monounsaturated and polyunsaturated fats to increase shelf life and to solidify them so they are more spreadable. Hydrogenation can change the position of hydrogen atoms along the carbon chain, transforming the fat into a trans fatty acid. Margarine and spreads, chips, commercially produced crackers and cookies, and fast foods often contain trans fatty acids. Small amounts of trans fats are also found naturally in some meats, dairy products, and other animal-based foods.

In June of 2006, the American Heart Association (AHA) became the first major health organization to issue dietary guidelines for trans fat intake. In the 2006 revision of its *Diet and Lifestyle Recommendations,* the AHA limits trans fat intake to less than 1 percent of the total daily caloric intake.[15] This amount represents about 1.5 grams of trans fats a day for a 1,500 calorie diet, 2 grams for 2,000 calories, and 3 grams for 3,000 calories. Because the FDA now requires that all food labels list the trans fat content, you can keep better track of your daily trans fat intake by paying attention to food labels. Additional information on trans fats is found under the "Trans Fatty Acids" section in Chapter 3 (see pages 67–68).

The U. S. Food and Drug Administration (FDA) allows food manufacturers to label any product that has less than half a gram of trans fat per serving as zero. Be aware that if you eat three or four servings of a particular food containing near half a gram of trans fat, you may be getting your maximum daily allowance (1 gram per 1,000 calories of daily caloric intake). Thus, you are encouraged to look at the list of ingredients and search for the words "partially hydrogenated" as an indicator of hidden trans fats.

The labels "partially hydrogenated" and "trans fatty acids" indicate that the product carries a health risk just as high as that of saturated fat. Now that trans fats are listed on food labels, companies are trying to reformulate their products to reduce or eliminate these fats. Some products that once had a high trans fat content now may have none. As a consumer, you are encouraged to check food labels often to obtain current information. Table 11.3 lists the average trans fat content of some foods. These values may vary between brands according to food formulation and ingredients and may change in the near future as man-

TABLE 11.3 Average Trans Fat Content of Selected Foods*

Food Item	Amount	Grams
Fats/Oils		
Margarine, stick	1 tbsp	2.0
Margarine, tub	1 tbsp	0.5
Butter	1 tbsp	0.3
Shortening	1 tbsp	4.0
Mayonnaise	1 tbsp	0.0
Snacks		
Oreo cookies	3	2.5
Chips Ahoy Chocolate Chip Cookies	3	1.5
Ritz crackers	5	1.5
Flavorite Honey Maid Grahams	8 sections	1.5
Fig Newtons	2	1.0
Potato chips	2 oz	3.0
Cake, pound	1 slice (3 oz)	4.5
Candy bar	1	3.0
Fast Foods		
Dunkin' Donuts Apple Fritter	1	2.5
Krispy Kreme Apple Fritter	1	7.0
Krispy Kreme Doughnut, glazed	1	4.0
McDonald's Biscuit	1	5.0
McDonald's Cinnamon Roll	1	4.5
McDonald's Baked Apple Pie	1	4.0
McDonald's Chicken McNuggets	10 pieces	2.5
Burger King French Toast Sticks	5 pieces	4.5
Burger King Chicken Tenders	5 pieces	2.5
Burger King Fish Sandwich	1	1.5
KFC Extra Crispy Breast	6 oz	4.5
KFC Breast, original recipe	6 oz	2.5
French fries	1 med (4 oz)	5.0
Taco Bell Taco	1	0.5
Taco Bell Taco Supreme	1	1.0
Taco Bell Burrito	1	2.0
Taco Bell Burrito Supreme, beef	1	2.0

Note: Trans fat intake should be limited to no more than 1 percent of total daily caloric intake or the equivalent of 1 gram per 1,000 calories of energy intake.

*Trans fat content in food items may decrease significantly in the near future as food manufacturers look to lower the amount in their products because of FDA regulations that require trans fats to be listed on food labels. Trans fat content also varies between different brands based on food formulation and ingredients. Check food labels regularly to obtain current information.

ufacturers alter food formulations to decrease or eliminate trans fat content.

Critical Thinking

What do think is your own risk for diseases of the cardiovascular system? Is this something you need to concern yourself with at this point in your life? Why or why not?

Lowering LDL Cholesterol If LDL cholesterol is higher than ideal, it can be lowered by participating in a regular aerobic exercise program, manipulating the diet, losing body fat, and taking medication. As part of the dietary regimen to lower LDL cholesterol significantly, total daily fiber intake must be in the range of 25 to 38 grams per day (see Chapter 3).

Fiber intake of most people in the United States averages less than 15 grams per day. Fiber, in particular the soluble type, has been shown to lower cholesterol. Soluble fiber dissolves in water and forms a gel-like substance that encloses food particles. This property helps bind and excrete fats from the body. Soluble fibers also bind intestinal bile acids that could be recycled into additional cholesterol. Soluble fibers are found primarily in oats, fruits, barley, legumes, and psyllium.

Psyllium is a grain that is added to some multigrain breakfast cereals. As little as 3 daily grams (a generous tablespoon) of psyllium can lower LDL cholesterol by 20 percent. Commercially available fiber supplements that contain psyllium (such as Metamucil) can be used to increase soluble fiber intake. Three tablespoons daily will add about 10 grams of soluble fiber to the diet.

The incidence of heart disease is very low in populations where daily fiber intake exceeds 30 grams per day. Further, a Harvard University Medical School study of 43,000 middle-aged men who were followed for more than 6 years showed that increasing fiber intake to 30 daily grams resulted in a 41 percent reduction in heart attacks.[16]

In terms of dietary fat, consumption can be in the range of 30 percent of total daily caloric intake as long as most of the fat is unsaturated fat and the average cholesterol consumption is lower than 300 mg per day (preferably less than 200 mg). Research on the effects of a "typical" 30-percent-fat diet (including saturated fat) has shown that it has little or no effect in lowering cholesterol, and that CHD actually continues to progress in people who have the disease. Thus, some practitioners recommend a 10 percent or less fat-calorie diet combined with a regular aerobic exercise program for people trying to lower their cholesterol.

A daily 10 percent total-fat diet requires the person to limit fat intake to an absolute minimum. Some health-care professionals contend that a diet like this is difficult to follow indefinitely. People with high cholesterol levels, however, may not have to follow that diet indefinitely but should adopt the 10 percent-fat diet while attempting to lower cholesterol. Thereafter, eating a 20 to 30 percent-fat diet may be adequate to maintain recommended cholesterol levels as long as most of the intake is from unsaturated fats. (National data indicate that current fat consumption in the United States averages 34 percent of total calories—see Table 3.5, page 72.)

Free radicals Oxygen compounds produced in normal metabolism.

Behavior Modification Planning

DIETARY GUIDELINES TO LOWER LDL CHOLESTEROL

- Consume between 25 and 38 grams of fiber daily, including a minimum of 10 grams of soluble fiber (good sources are oats, fruits, barley, legumes, and psyllium).
- Increase consumption of vegetables, fruits, whole grains, and beans.
- Do not consume more than 200 mg of dietary cholesterol a day.
- Consume red meats (3 ounces per serving) fewer than 3 times per week and no organ meats (such as liver and kidneys).
- Do not eat commercially baked foods.
- Avoid foods that contain trans fatty acids, hydrogenated fat, or partially hydrogenated vegetable oil.
- Increase intake of omega-3 fatty acids (see Chapter 3) by eating two to three omega-3–rich fish meals per week.
- Consume 25 grams of soy protein a day.
- Drink low-fat milk (1 percent or less fat, preferably) and use low-fat dairy products.
- Do not use coconut oil, palm oil, or cocoa butter.
- Limit egg consumption to fewer than three eggs per week (this is for people with high cholesterol only; others may consume eggs in moderation).
- Use margarines and salad dressings that contain stanol ester instead of butter and regular margarine.
- Bake, broil, grill, poach, or steam food instead of frying.
- Refrigerate cooked meat before adding to other dishes. Remove fat hardened in the refrigerator before mixing the meat with other foods.

Try It

Dietary guidelines for health and wellness were thoroughly discussed in Chapter 3, Nutrition for Wellness. Record in your Online Journal or class notebook how your dietary habits have changed since studying these guidelines. How well do they now follow the above recommendations for lowering LDL cholesterol?

A drawback of very low-fat diets (less than 25 percent fat) is that they tend to lower HDL ("good") cholesterol and increase triglycerides. If HDL cholesterol is already low, monounsaturated and polyunsaturated fats should be added to the diet. Olive, canola, corn, and soybean oils and nuts are examples of food items that are high in monounsaturated fats and polyunsaturated fats. Appendix A, Nutritive Value of Selected Foods, can be used to determine food items that are high in monounsaturated and polyunsaturated fats (also see Figure 3.9, page 79).

The NCEP guidelines for people who are trying to decrease cholesterol allow for a diet with up to 35 percent of calories from fat, as long as less than 7 percent is derived from saturated fats, up to 10 percent from polyunsaturated fats, and up to 20 percent from monounsaturated fats. Carbohydrate intake would be in the range of 50 to 60 percent of calories and protein 15 percent of calories.[17]

Margarines and salad dressings that contain stanol ester, a plant-derived compound that interferes with cholesterol absorption in the intestine, are now also on the market. Over the course of several weeks, daily intake of about 3 grams of margarine or 6 tablespoons of salad dressing containing stanol ester lowers LDL cholesterol by 14 percent.

Dietary guidelines to lower LDL cholesterol levels are provided in the box at the left. Dietary manipulation by itself, however, is not as effective in lowering LDL cholesterol as a combination of diet plus aerobic exercise.

If, after 6 months on a low-cholesterol, low-fat diet, cholesterol remains unacceptably high, the NCEP guidelines recommend that people consider drug therapy. An unacceptable level is an LDL cholesterol above 190 mg/dl for people with fewer than two risk factors and no signs of heart disease. For people with more than two risk factors and with a history of heart disease, LDL cholesterol above 160 mg/dl is unacceptable.

Cholesterol-lowering drugs, most notably the statins group, can lower cholesterol by 25 to 60 percent in 2 to 3 months—see "Medications" below.

Elevated Triglycerides **Triglycerides,** also known as free fatty acids, make up most of the fat in our diet and most of the fat that circulates in the blood. In combination with cholesterol, triglycerides speed up formation of plaque in the arteries. Triglycerides are carried in the bloodstream primarily by very low-density lipoproteins (VLDLs) and **chylomicrons.**

Although they are found in poultry skin, lunch meats, and shellfish, these fatty acids are manufactured mainly in the liver from refined sugars, starches, and alcohol. High intake of alcohol and sugars (honey and fruit juices included) significantly raises triglyceride levels. To lower triglycerides, the person should avoid pastries, candies, soft drinks, fruit juices, white bread, pasta, and alcohol. In addition, cutting down on overall fat consumption, quitting smoking, reducing weight (if overweight), and doing aerobic exercise are helpful. The desirable blood triglyceride level is less than 150 mg/dl (see Table 11.2).

Medications There are now very effective medications to treat elevated cholesterol and triglycerides. Most notably among these are the statins group (Lipitor, Mevacor, Pravachol, Lescol, and Zocor), which can lower cholesterol by up to 60 percent in 2 to 3 months. Statins slow down cholesterol production, decrease absorption of cholesterol in the intestines, and increase the liver's ability to remove blood cholesterol. They also decrease triglycerides and produce a small increase in HDL levels.

In general, lowering LDL cholesterol without medication is better because drugs often produce undesirable side effects, such as muscle or joint pain or altered liver enzyme levels. People with heart disease, however, frequently must take cholesterol-lowering medication. It is best if medication is combined with lifestyle changes to augment the cholesterol-lowering effect. For example, when Zocor was taken alone over 3 months, LDL cholesterol decreased by 30 percent; but when a Mediterranean diet was adopted in combination with Zocor therapy, LDL cholesterol decreased by 41 percent.[18]

Other drugs effective in reducing LDL cholesterol are bile acid sequestrans, which bind cholesterol found in bile acids. Cholesterol subsequently is excreted in the stools. These drugs are often used in combination with statin drugs.

High doses of nicotinic acid or niacin (a B vitamin) also help lower LDL cholesterol and triglycerides, and they help increase HDL cholesterol. A fourth group of drugs, known as fibrates, is used primarily to lower triglycerides.

Elevated Homocysteine

Clinical data indicating that many heart attack victims have normal cholesterol levels have led researchers to look for other risk factors that may contribute to atherosclerosis. Although it is not a blood lipid, a high concentration of **homocysteine** in the blood is thought to enhance the formation of plaque and subsequent blockage of the arteries.[19]

The body uses homocysteine to help build proteins and carry out cellular metabolism. Homocysteine is formed during an intermediate step in the creation of another amino acid. This process requires folate and vitamins B_6 and B_{12}. Typically, homocysteine is metabolized rapidly and, therefore, it does not accumulate in the blood or damage the arteries.

A large number of people have high blood levels of homocysteine. This might be attributable to either a genetic inability to metabolize homocysteine or a deficiency in the vitamins required for its conversion. Homocysteine typically is measured in micromoles per liter (μmol/l). Guidelines to interpret homocysteine levels are provided in Table 11.4. A 10-year follow-up study of people with high homocysteine levels showed that those individuals with a level above 14.25 μmol/l had almost twice the risk of stroke compared with individuals whose level was below 9.25 μmol/l.[20]

Accumulation of homocysteine is theorized to be toxic because it may do some or all of the following:

1. Cause damage to the inner lining of the arteries (the initial step in the process of atherosclerosis).
2. Stimulate the proliferation of cells that contribute to plaque formation.
3. Encourage clotting, which may completely obstruct an artery.

TABLE 11.4 Homocysteine Guidelines

Level	Rating
<9.0 μmol/l	Desirable
9–12 μmol/l	Mild elevation
13–15 μmol/l	Elevated
>15 μmol/l	Extreme elevation

Adapted from K. S. McCully, "What You Must Know Now About Homocysteine," *Bottom Line /Health* 18 (January 2004): 7–9.

Keeping homocysteine from accumulating in the blood seems to be as simple as eating the recommended daily servings of vegetables, fruits, grains, and some meat and legumes. Increasing evidence that folate can prevent heart attacks has led to the recommendation that people consume 400 mcg per day of folate. Five daily servings of fruits and vegetables can provide sufficient levels of folate and vitamin B_6 to clear homocysteine from the blood. Unfortunately, estimates indicate that more than 80 percent of Americans do not get 400 daily mcg of folate.[21] People who consume the recommended five servings of fruits and vegetables daily most likely do not need a vitamin B complex supplement.

Vitamin B_{12} is found primarily in animal flesh and animal products. Vitamin B_{12} deficiency is rarely a problem because 1 cup of milk or an egg provides the daily requirement. The body also recycles most of this vitamin and, therefore, it takes years to develop a deficiency.

Inflammation

In addition to homocysteine, scientists are looking at inflammation as a major risk factor for heart attacks. Low-grade inflammation can occur in a variety of places throughout the body. For years it has been known that inflammation plays a role in CHD and that inflammation hidden deep in the body is a common trigger of heart attacks, even when cholesterol levels are normal or low and arterial plaque is minimal.

To evaluate ongoing inflammation in the body, physicians have turned to **C-reactive protein (CRP),** a

---

Triglycerides Fats formed by glycerol and three fatty acids; also known as free fatty acids.

Chylomicrons Molecules that transport triglycerides in the blood.

Homocysteine Intermediate amino acid in the interconversion of two other amino acids: methionine and cysteine. High levels increase the risk for heart disease and stroke.

C-reactive protein (CRP) A protein whose blood levels increase with inflammation, at times hidden deep in the body; elevation of this protein is an indicator of potential cardiovascular events.

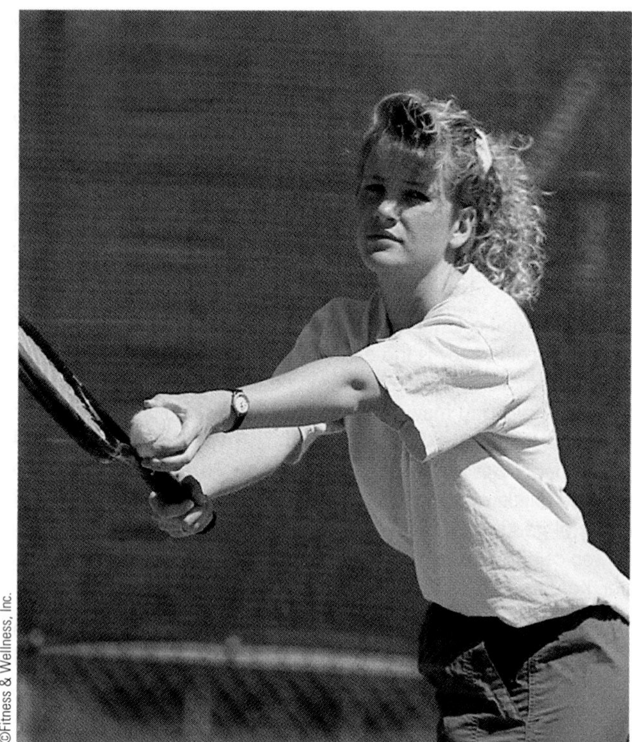
©Fitness & Wellness, Inc.

Physical activity is an excellent tool to control stress.

Behavior Modification Planning

2006 AMERICAN HEART ASSOCIATION DIET AND LIFESTYLE RECOMMENDATIONS FOR CARDIOVASCULAR DISEASE REDUCTION

- Balance caloric intake and physical activity to achieve or maintain a healthy body weight.
- Consume a diet rich in vegetables and fruits.
- Consume whole-grain, high-fiber foods.
- Consume fish, especially oily fish, at least twice a week.
- Limit your intake of saturated fat to less than 7 percent and trans fat to less than 1 percent of total daily caloric intake.
- Limit cholesterol intake to less than 300 mg per day.
- Minimize your intake of beverages and foods with added sugars.
- Choose and prepare foods with little or no salt.
- If you consume alcohol, do so in moderation.
- When you eat food that is prepared outside of the home, follow the above recommendations.
- Avoid use of and exposure to tobacco products.

Try It

In your Online Journal or class notebook, record which of the above recommendations you fall short on and propose at least one thing you could do to improve.

A six-step plan to help people stop smoking is contained in the box on the previous page. The most important factor in quitting cigarette smoking is a sincere desire to do so. More than 95 percent of successful ex-smokers have been able to quit on their own, either by quitting cold turkey or by using self-help kits available from organizations such as the American Cancer Society, the American Heart Association, and the American Lung Association. Only 3 percent of ex-smokers quit as a result of formal cessation programs.

Stress

Stress has become a part of life. People have to deal daily with goals, deadlines, responsibilities, pressures. What creates the health hazard is not the **stressor** itself, but, rather, the individual's response to it.

The human body responds to stress by producing more catecholamines to prepare the body for what is called **fight or flight.** If the person actually fights or flees, the catecholamines are metabolized and the body is able to return to a normal state. If, however, a person is under constant stress and is unable to take physical action (as in the death of a close relative or friend, loss of a job, trouble at work, financial insecurity), the catecholamines remain elevated in the bloodstream.

People who are not able to relax are placing a constant low-level strain on their cardiovascular system that could manifest itself as heart disease. In addition, when a person is in a stressful situation, the coronary arteries that feed the heart muscle constrict, reducing the oxygen supply to the heart. If the blood vessels are largely blocked by atherosclerosis, abnormal heart rhythms or even a heart attack could follow.

Individuals who are under a lot of stress and do not cope well with stress need to take measures to counteract the effects of stress in their lives. They must identify the sources of stress and learn how to cope with them. People need to take control of themselves, examine and act upon the things that are most important in their lives, and ignore less meaningful details.

One of the best ways to relieve stress is physical activity—in essence, mimicking the "fight" or the "flight." If you are subjected to stress regularly, try to schedule exercise soon thereafter. Exercise also steps up muscular activity, which contributes to muscular relaxation.

Many executives in large cities are choosing the evening hours for their physical activity programs, stopping after work at the health or fitness club. In doing this, they are able to burn up the excess tension accumulated during the day and enjoy the evening. This has proven to be one of the best stress management techniques.

Personal and Family History

Individuals who have a family history of, or have already experienced cardiovascular problems are at higher risk than those who never have had a problem. People with this sort of history are strongly encouraged to keep the other risk factors as low as possible. Because most risk factors are reversible, the risk for future problems will decrease significantly.

Critical Thinking

Do you have any relatives with cardiovascular disease? If so, what steps are you taking to prevent a cardiovascular event in your life, and can you do anything to help others in your family do the same?

Age and Gender

Age becomes a risk factor for men over age 45 and women over age 55. The higher incidence of heart disease may stem in part from lifestyle changes (less physical activity, poor nutrition, obesity, and so on) as people get older. Earlier in life, men are at greater risk for cardiovascular disease than women are. Following menopause, women's risk increases. Based on final mortality statistics for 2003, more women (483,800) than men (426,800) died from cardiovascular disease.[28]

Cancer

Cell growth is controlled by **deoxyribonucleic acid (DNA)** and **ribonucleic acid (RNA).** When nuclei lose their ability to regulate and control cell growth, cell division is disrupted and mutant cells may develop. Some of these cells may grow uncontrollably and abnormally, forming a mass of tissue called a tumor, which can be either **benign** or **malignant.** Although benign tumors can interfere with normal bodily functions, they rarely cause death. About 23 percent of all deaths in the United States are attributable to **cancer.** More than 1.3 million new cases are reported each year, and more than half a million people die every year from cancer.

Cancer is not a singular term, as more than 100 types of cancer can develop in the body. The commonality is that cancer cells grow for no reason and multiply, destroying normal tissue. If the spread of cells is not controlled, death ensues. A normal cell can duplicate as many as 100 times during its lifetime, and the DNA molecule normally is duplicated perfectly during cell division. In the few cases when the DNA molecule is not replicated exactly, specialized enzymes make repairs quickly. Occasionally, however, cells with defective DNA keep dividing and ultimately form a small tumor. As more mutations occur, the altered cells continue to divide and can become malignant. A decade or more can pass between carcinogenic exposure or mutations and the time cancer is diagnosed.

A critical turning point in the development of cancer is when a tumor reaches about one million cells. At this stage it is referred to as **carcinoma in situ.** It is at an early stage and is encapsulated—that is, it has not spread. If undetected, the tumor may go for months and years without any significant growth.

While encapsulated, a tumor does not pose a serious threat to human health. To continue growing, however, the tumor requires more oxygen and nutrients. In time, a few of the cancer cells start producing chemicals that enhance **angiogenesis.** In a process called **metastasis,** cells break away from a malignant tumor and migrate through the new blood vessels to other parts of the body, where they can cause new cancer.

Although the immune system and the **blood turbulence** destroy most cancer cells, only one abnormal cell lodging elsewhere can start a new cancer. These cells also will grow and multiply uncontrollably, destroying normal tissue.

Once cancer cells metastasize, treatment becomes more difficult. Therapy can kill most cancer cells, but a few cells may become resistant to treatment. These cells then can grow into a new tumor that will not respond to the same treatment.

Like cardiovascular disease, cancer is largely preventable. As much as 80 percent of all human cancer is related to lifestyle or environmental factors (including diet, tobacco use, excessive use of alcohol, sexual and reproductive activity, and exposure to environmental hazards).

Significantly, more than 9.8 million Americans with a history of cancer were alive in 2005. Currently, 6 of 10 people diagnosed with cancer are expected to be alive 5 years from the initial diagnosis.

Stress The mental, emotional, and physiological response of the body to any situation that is new, threatening, frightening, or exciting.

Stressor Stress-causing event.

Fight or flight Physiological response of the body to stress that prepares the individual to take action by stimulating the vital defense systems.

Deoxyribonucleic acid (DNA) Genetic substance of which genes are made; molecule that bears cell's genetic code.

Ribonucleic acid (RNA) Genetic material involved in the formation of cell proteins.

Benign Noncancerous.

Malignant Cancerous.

Cancer Group of diseases characterized by uncontrolled growth and spread of abnormal cells into malignant tumors.

Carcinoma in situ Encapsulated malignant tumor that has not spread.

Angiogenesis Capillary (blood vessel) formation into a tumor.

Metastasis The movement of bacteria or body cells from one part of the body to another.

Blood turbulence Agitated or tumultuous flow of the blood through the vascular system.

The biggest factor in fighting cancer today is health education. People need to be informed about the risk factors for cancer and the guidelines for early detection. The most effective way to protect against cancer is to change negative lifestyle habits and behaviors. Following are some guidelines for preventing cancer.

Dietary Changes

The American Cancer Society estimates that one-third of all cancers in the United States are related to nutrition. A healthy diet, therefore, is crucial to decrease the risk for cancer. The diet should be predominately vegetarian, high in fiber, and low in fat (particularly from animal sources). **Cruciferous vegetables,** tea, soy products, calcium, and omega-3 fats are encouraged. Protein intake should be kept within the recommended nutrient guidelines. If alcohol is used, it should be consumed in moderation. Obesity should be avoided.

Fruits and Vegetables

Green and dark yellow vegetables, cruciferous vegetables (cauliflower, broccoli, cabbage, Brussels sprouts, and kohlrabi), and beans (legumes) seem to protect against cancer. Folate, found naturally in dark green leafy vegetables, dried beans, and orange juice, may reduce the risk of colon and cervical cancers. Brightly colored fruits and vegetables also contain **carotenoids** and vitamin C. Lycopene, one of the many carotenoids (a phytonutrient—see discussion on the following page), has been linked to lower risk of cancers of the prostate, colon, and cervix. Lycopene is especially abundant in cooked tomato products.

Antioxidants

Researchers believe the antioxidant effect of vitamins and the mineral selenium help protect the body from oxygen free radicals. As discussed in Chapter 3 (under "Antioxidants," pages 84–87), during normal metabolism most of the oxygen in the human body is converted into stable forms of carbon dioxide and water. A small amount, however, ends up in an unstable form known as oxygen *free radicals,* which are thought to attack and damage the cell membrane and DNA, leading to the formation of cancers. Antioxidants are thought to absorb free radicals before they can cause damage and also interrupt the sequence of reactions once damage has begun.

Phytonutrients

A promising horizon in cancer prevention is the discovery of **phytonutrients.** These compounds, found in abundance in fruits and vegetables, seem to prevent cancer by blocking the formation of cancerous tumors and disrupting the process at almost every step of the way. Experts recommend that to obtain the highest possible protection, these foods should be consumed several times during the day (instead of in one meal) to maintain phytonutrients at effective levels throughout the day. Blood phytonutrient levels drop within 3 hours of produce consumption.

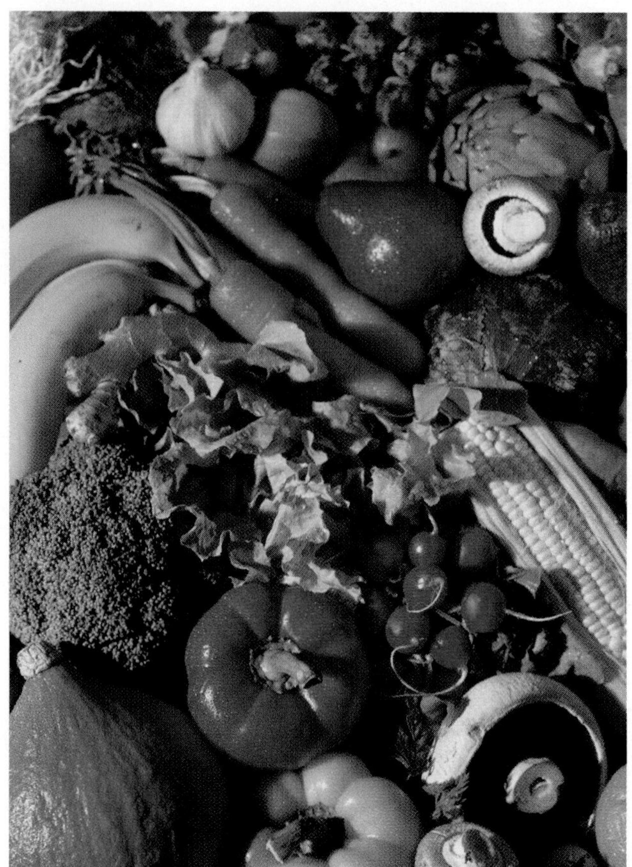

Phytonutrients, found in abundance in fruits and vegetables, seem to have a powerful effect in decreasing cancer risk.

Fiber

Although one recent study failed to show an association, many studies have linked low intake of fiber to increased risk for colon cancer. Fiber binds to bile acids in the intestine for excretion from the body in the stools. The interaction of bile acids with intestinal bacteria releases carcinogenic byproducts. Production of bile acid increases with higher fat content in the small intestine (created, of course, by higher fat content in the diet).

Daily consumption of fiber—at least 25 grams for women and 38 grams for men—is recommended. Grains are high in fiber and also contain vitamins and minerals (folate, selenium, and calcium), which seem to decrease the risk for colon cancer.

Selenium also protects against prostate cancer and, possibly, lung cancer. Calcium may also protect against colon cancer by preventing rapid growth of cells in the colon, especially in people with colon polyps.

Polyphenols in Tea

Polyphenols (a group of phytonutrients) are potent cancer-fighting antioxidants found in fresh fruits and vegetables and many grains. A prime source is tea. Green, black, and red tea all seem to provide protection. Evidence also points to certain components in tea that can block the spread of cancers to other parts of the body. Polyphenols are known to block the formation of **nitrosamines** and quell the activation of **carcinogens.** Polyphenols are also thought to fight cancer by shutting off the formation of cancer cells, turning up the body's natural detoxification defenses and thereby suppressing progression of the disease.

Green tea and black tea have similar amounts of polyphenols. Green tea seems to be especially helpful in preventing gastrointestinal cancers, including those of the stomach, small intestines, pancreas, and colon. Consumption of green tea also has been linked to a lower incidence of lung, esophageal, and estrogen-related cancers, including most breast cancers.

Research on tea-drinking habits in China showed that people who regularly drank green tea had about half the risk for chronic gastritis and stomach cancer.[29] The risk further decreased as the years of green tea drinking increased.

In Japan, where people drink green tea regularly but smoke twice as much as do people in the United States, the incidence of lung cancer is half that of the United States. The antioxidant effect of one of the polyphenols in green tea—epigallocatechin gallate, or EGCG—is at least 25 times more effective than vitamin E and 100 times more effective than vitamin C at protecting cells and the DNA from damage believed to cause cancer, heart disease, and other diseases associated with free radicals.[30] EGCG is also twice as strong as the red wine antioxidant resveratrol in helping prevent heart disease.

The recommendation in a cancer-prevention diet is two or more cups of green tea daily. Herbal teas do not provide the same benefits as regular tea.

Vitamin C

Foods high in vitamin C may deter some cancers. Salt-cured, smoked, and nitrite-cured foods have been associated with cancers of the esophagus and stomach. Processed meats should be consumed sparingly and always with orange juice or other vitamin C-rich foods. Vitamin C seems to discourage the formation of nitrosamines. These potentially cancer-causing compounds are formed when nitrites and nitrates, which are used to prevent the growth of harmful bacteria in processed meats, combine with other chemicals in the stomach.

Spices

Although still in the early stages, research is uncovering cancer-fighting phytonutrients in many traditional spices. These phytonutrients alter damaging carcinogenic pathways, provide antioxidant effects, promote cancer-fighting enzymes, decrease inflammation, stimulate the immune system, and suppress the development of tumors.[31] Ginger, oregano, curry, pepper, cloves, fennel, rosemary, and turmeric are all encouraged for use in cooking and at the table.

Fat Intake

High fat intake promotes excessive weight and cancer. Fat intake should be primarily monounsaturated and omega-3 fats (found in many types of fish and flaxseeds), which seem to offer protection against colorectal, pancreatic, breast, oral, esophageal, and stomach cancers. Omega-3 fats block the synthesis of prostaglandins, bodily compounds that promote the growth of tumors.

Protein

Salt-cured, smoked, and nitrite-cured foods have been associated with cancers of the esophagus, stomach, colon, and rectum. Processed meats (hot dogs, ham, bacon, sausage, and lunch meats) should be consumed sparingly and always with orange juice or other vitamin C-rich foods, as vitamin C seems to discourage the formation of nitrosamines (see "Vitamin C" above).

Nutritional guidelines also discourage excessive intake of protein. The daily protein intake for some people is almost twice the amount the human body needs. Too much animal protein seems to decrease blood enzymes that prevent precancerous cells from developing into tumors. According to the National Cancer Institute, eating substantial amounts of red meat may increase the risk of colorectal, pancreatic, breast, prostate, and renal cancer.

Cooking protein at high temperature should be avoided or done only occasionally. The data suggest that grilling, broiling, or frying meat, poultry, or fish at high temperatures to "medium-well" or "well-done" leads to the formation of carcinogenic substances known as het-

---

Cruciferous vegetables Plants that produce cross-shaped leaves (cauliflower, broccoli, cabbage, Brussels sprouts, and kohlrabi); these vegetables seem to protect against cancer.

Carotenoids Pigment substances in plants, some of which are precursors to vitamin A. Over 600 carotenoids are found in nature, and about 50 of them are precursors to vitamin A (the most potent one is beta-carotene).

Phytonutrients Compounds, found in fruits and vegetables, that block the formation of cancerous tumors and disrupt the process of cancer.

Nitrosamines Potentially cancer-causing compounds formed when nitrites and nitrates, which are used to prevent the growth of harmful bacteria in processed meats, combine with other chemicals in the stomach.

Carcinogens Substances that contribute to the formation of cancers.

Behavior Modification Planning

TIPS FOR A HEALTHY CANCER-FIGHTING DIET

Increase intake of phytonutrients, fiber, cruciferous vegetables, and more antioxidants by

- Eating a predominantly vegetarian diet
- Eating more fruits and vegetables every day (six to eight servings per day maximize anticancer benefits)
- Increasing the consumption of broccoli, cauliflower, kale, turnips, cabbage, kohlrabi, Brussels sprouts, hot chili peppers, red and green peppers, carrots, sweet potatoes, winter squash, spinach, garlic, onions, strawberries, tomatoes, pineapple, and citrus fruits in your regular diet
- Eating vegetables raw or quickly cooked by steaming or stir-frying
- Substituting tea, fruit, and vegetable juices for coffee and soda
- Eating whole-grain breads
- Including calcium in the diet (or from a supplement)
- Including soy products in the diet
- Using whole-wheat flour instead of refined white flour in baking
- Using brown (unpolished) rice instead of white (polished) rice

Decrease daily fat intake to 20 percent of total caloric intake by

- Limiting consumption of beef, poultry, or fish to no more than 3 to 6 ounces (about the size of a deck of cards) once or twice a week
- Trimming all visible fat from meat and removing skin from poultry prior to cooking
- Decreasing the amount of fat and oils used in cooking
- Substituting low-fat for high-fat dairy products
- Using salad dressings sparingly
- Using only half to three-quarters the amount of fat required in baking recipes
- Limiting fat intake to mostly monounsaturated (olive oil, canola oil, nuts, and seeds) and omega-3 fats (fish, flaxseed, and flaxseed oil)
- Eating fish once or twice a week
- Including flaxseed oil in the diet

Try It

Make a copy of this "Cancer-Fighting Diet" chart and each week incorporate into your lifestyle two additional dietary behaviors from the above list.

erocyclic amines (HCAs) and polycyclic aromatic hydrocarbons (PAHs). Individuals who cook their meat at high temperatures to "medium-well" or "well-done" have a much higher risk for colorectal and stomach cancers.

Microwaving meat for a couple of minutes before barbecuing decreases the risk, as long as the fluid released by the meat is discarded. Most of the potential carcinogens collect in this solution. Removing the skin before serving and cooking at lower heat to "medium" rather than "well done" also seem to lower the risk. An electric contact grill (such as a George Foreman grill) is preferable when cooking meats because cooking temperatures are easily controlled.

Soy Protein

Soy protein also seems to decrease the formation of carcinogens during cooking of meats. Soy foods may help because soy contains chemicals that prevent cancer. Although further research is merited, isoflavones (phytonutrients) found in soy are structurally similar to estrogen and may prevent breast, prostate, lung, and colon cancers. These isoflavones are frequently referred to as "phytoestrogens" or "plant estrogens." Isoflavones also block angiogenesis. Presently, it is not known if the health benefits of soy are derived from isoflavones by themselves or in combination with other nutrients found in soy.

One drawback of soy was found in animal studies in which animals with tumors were given large amounts of soy, in which the estrogen-like activity of soy isoflavones actually led to the growth of estrogen-dependent tumors. Experts, therefore, caution women with breast cancer or a history of this disease to limit soy intake because it may stimulate cancer cells by closely imitating the actions of estrogen.

No specific recommendations are presently available as to the amount of daily soy protein intake for cancer prevention. Based on the traditional diets of people (including children) in China and Japan who regularly consume soy foods, there doesn't appear to be an unsafe natural level of consumption. Soy protein powder supplementation, however, may elevate soy protein intake to an unnatural (and perhaps unsafe) level.

Alcohol Consumption

Alcohol should be consumed in moderation, because too much alcohol raises the risk for developing certain cancers. In combination with tobacco use, consuming alcohol increases the risk for cancers of the mouth, larynx, throat, esophagus, and liver significantly. The combined action of heavy alcohol and tobacco use can increase odds of developing cancer of the oral cavity fifteenfold. Approximately 17,000 deaths from cancer yearly are attributed to excessive use of alcohol, often in combination with smoking or smokeless tobacco.

Body Weight

Maintaining recommended body weight is also encouraged. Based on estimates, excess weight accounts for 14 percent of deaths from cancer in men and 20 percent in women. Furthermore, obese men and women have an increased risk of more than 50 percent of dying from any form of cancer.[32] Obesity has been associated with cancers of the colon, rectum, breast, prostate, endometrium, and kidney.

Tobacco Use

Cigarette smoking by itself is a major health hazard. If we include all related deaths, smoking is responsible for more than 440,000 unnecessary deaths in the United States each year. The World Health Organization estimates that smoking causes 5 million deaths worldwide annually. The average life expectancy for a chronic smoker is about 15 years shorter than for a nonsmoker.[33]

Of all cancers, at least 30 percent are tied to smoking, and 87 percent of lung cancers are tied to smoking. The biggest carcinogenic exposure in the workplace is cigarette smoke. Use of smokeless tobacco also can lead to nicotine addiction and dependence, as well as increased risk for cancers of the mouth, larynx, throat, and esophagus.

Excessive Sun Exposure

Too much exposure to ultraviolet radiation (both UVB and UVA rays) is a major contributor to skin cancer. The most common sites of skin cancer are those areas exposed to the sun most often (face, neck, and back of the hands).

The three types of skin cancer are

1. Basal cell carcinoma
2. Squamous cell carcinoma
3. Malignant melanoma

Nearly 90 percent of the almost 1 million cases of basal cell or squamous cell skin cancers reported yearly in the United States could have been prevented by protecting the skin from the sun's rays. **Melanoma** is the most deadly, causing approximately 7,600 deaths in 2003. One in every six Americans will eventually develop some type of skin cancer.

Nothing is healthy about a "healthy tan." Tanning of the skin is the body's natural reaction to permanent and irreversible damage from too much exposure to the sun. Even small doses of sunlight add up to a greater risk for skin cancer and premature aging. Although the tan fades at the end of the summer season,

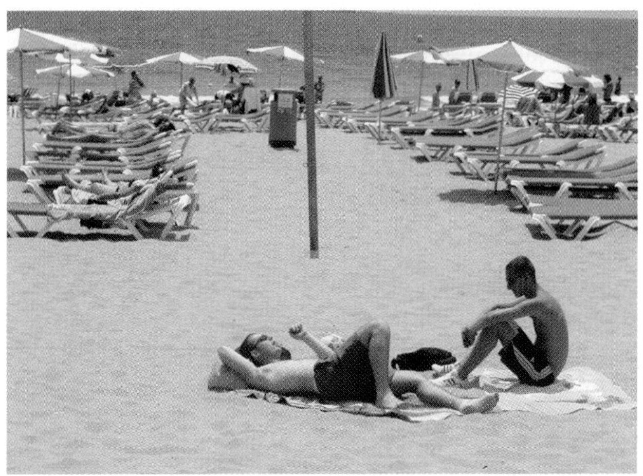

Tanning leads to premature aging of the skin and poses a risk for skin cancer from overexposure to ultraviolet rays.

the underlying skin damage does not disappear. Ultraviolet rays are strongest when the sun is high in the sky. You should avoid sun exposure between 10:00 AM and 4:00 PM. Take the shadow test: If your shadow is shorter than you, the UV rays are at their strongest.

The sting of sunburn comes from **ultraviolet B (UVB) rays,** which also are thought to be the main cause of premature wrinkling and skin aging, roughened/leathery/sagging skin, and skin cancer. Unfortunately, the damage may not become evident until up to 20 years later. By comparison, skin that has not been overexposed to the sun remains smooth and unblemished and shows less evidence of aging over time.

Sun lamps and tanning parlors provide mainly ultraviolet A (UVA) rays. Once thought to be safe, they are now known to be damaging and have been linked to melanoma, the most serious form of skin cancer. As little as 15 to 30 minutes of exposure to UVA can be as dangerous as a day spent in the sun. Similar to regular exposure to the sun, exposure to short-term recreational tanning at a salon causes DNA alterations that can lead to skin cancer.

Sunscreen lotion should be applied about 30 minutes before lengthy exposure to the sun because the skin takes that long to absorb the protective ingredients. A **sun protection factor (SPF)** of at least 15 is recommended. SPF 15 means that the skin takes 15 times longer to burn than it does with no lotion. If you ordinarily get a mild sunburn after 20 minutes of noonday sun, an SPF 15 allows you to remain in the sun about 300 minutes before burning. The higher the number, the stronger the pro-

---

Melanoma The most virulent, rapidly spreading form of skin cancer.

Ultraviolet B (UVB) rays Portion of sunlight that causes sunburn and encourages skin cancers.

Sun protection factor (SPF) Degree of protection offered by ingredients in sunscreen lotion; at least SPF 15 is recommended.

tection. When swimming or sweating, you should reapply waterproof sunscreens more often, because all sunscreens lose strength when they are diluted.

Estrogen, Radiation, and Potential Occupational Hazards

The intake of estrogen has been linked to endometrial cancer in some studies, but other evidence contradicts those findings. Although exposure to radiation increases the risk for cancer, the benefits of X-rays may outweigh the risks involved, particularly because most medical facilities use the lowest dose possible to keep the risk to a minimum. Occupational hazards such as asbestos fibers, nickel and uranium dusts, chromium compounds, vinyl chloride, and bischloromethyl ether increase the risk for cancer. Cigarette smoking magnifies the risk from occupational hazards.

FIGURE 11.8 Association between physical fitness and cancer mortality.

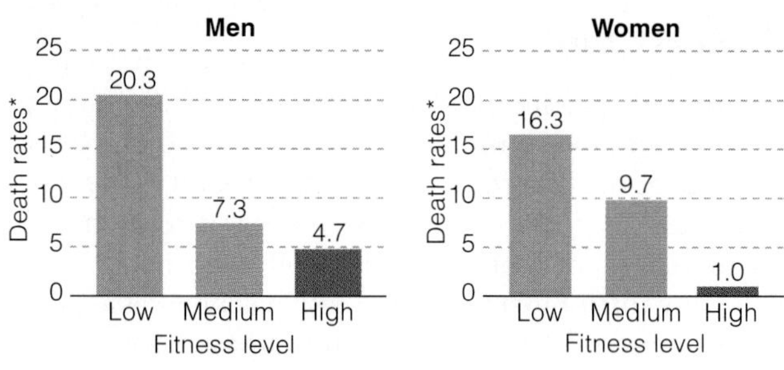

*Age-adjusted per 10,000 person-years at follow-up.

Source: S. N. Blair, H. W. Kohl III, R. S. Paffenbarger, Jr., D. G. Clark, K. H. Cooper, and L. W. Gibbons, "Physical Fitness and All-Cause Mortality: A Prospective Study of Healthy Men and Women," *Journal of the American Medical Association* 262 (1989): 2395–2401.

Physical Activity

An active lifestyle has been shown to have a protective effect against cancer. Although the mechanism is not clear, physical fitness and cancer mortality in men and women may have a graded and consistent inverse relationship (see Figure 11.8). A daily 30-minute, moderate-intensity exercise program lowers the risk for colon cancer and may lower the risk for cancers of the breast and reproductive system. Data indicate that regular exercise lowers the risk for breast cancer in women by up to 30 percent, and women who are active throughout life cut their risk of endometrial cancer by about 40 percent. Those who started exercise in adulthood cut their risk by about 25 percent.[34]

Among women diagnosed with breast cancer, women who walk 2 to 3 miles per hour one to three times per week are 20 percent less likely to die of the disease. Those who walk three to five times per week cut their risk in half.[35] Researchers believe that the decreasing levels of circulating ovarian hormones through physical activity decreases breast cancer risk.

Other data suggest that in men 65 or older, exercising vigorously at least three times per week decreases the risk of advanced or fatal prostate cancer by 70 percent.[36] In addition, growing evidence suggests that the body's autoimmune system may play a role in preventing cancer, and that moderate exercise improves the autoimmune system.

Early Detection

Fortunately, many cancers can be controlled or cured through early detection. The real problem comes when cancerous cells spread, because they become more difficult to destroy. Therefore, effective prevention, or at least early detection, is crucial. Herein lies the importance of periodic screening. Once a month, women should practice breast self-examination (BSE) and men, testicular self-examination (TSE). Men should pick a regular day each month (for example, the first day of each month) to do a TSE, and women should perform a BSE 2 or 3 days after the menstrual period is over.

Other Factors

The influence of many of the other much-publicized factors contributing to cancer is not as significant as those just pointed out. Intentional food additives, saccharin, processing agents, pesticides, and packaging materials currently used in the United States and other developed countries seem to have minimal consequences. High levels of tension and stress and poor coping skills may affect the autoimmune system negatively and thus render the body less effective in dealing with the various cancers. In the workplace, the biggest carcinogenic factor is exposure to cigarette smoke.

Genetics plays a role in susceptibility in about 10 percent of all cancers. Most of the effect is seen in the early childhood years. Some cancers reflect a combination of genetic and environmental liability; genetics may add to the environmental risk of certain types of cancers. "Environment," however, means more than pollution and smoke. It incorporates diet, lifestyle-related events, viruses, and physical agents such as X-rays and exposure to the sun.

Critical Thinking

Have you ever had or do you now have any family members with cancer? Can you identify any lifestyle or environmental factors as possible contributors to the disease? If not, are you concerned about your genetic predisposition, and are you making any lifestyle changes to decrease such risk?

Behavior Modification Planning

LIFESTYLE FACTORS THAT DECREASE CANCER RISK

Factor	Function
Physical activity	Controls body weight, may influence hormone levels, strengthens the immune system.
Fiber	Contains anti-cancer substances, increases stool movement, blunts insulin secretion.
Fruits and vegetables	Contain phytonutrients and vitamins that thwart cancer.
Recommended weight	Helps control hormones that promote cancer.
Healthy grilling	Prevents formation of heterocyclic amines (HCAs) and polycyclic aromatic hydrocarbons (PAHs), both carcinogenic substances.
Tea	Contains polyphenols, which neutralize free radicals, including epigallocatechin gallate (EGCG), which protects cells and the DNA from damage believed to cause cancer.
Spices	Provide phytonutrients and strengthen the immune system.
Vitamin D	Disrupts abnormal cell growth.
Monounsaturated fat	May contribute to cancer cell destruction.

Try It

The above are factors that you can use at once to decrease overall cancer risk. Note in your Online Journal or class notebook ways you can incorporate all of these factors into your everyday lifestyle.

Warning Signals of Cancer

Everyone should become familiar with the following seven warning signals for cancer and bring them to a physician's attention if any are present:

1. Change in bowel or bladder habits.
2. Sore that does not heal.
3. Unusual bleeding or discharge.
4. Thickening or lump in breast or elsewhere.
5. Indigestion or difficulty in swallowing.
6. Obvious change in wart or mole.
7. Nagging cough or hoarseness.

The recommendations for early detection of cancer in asymptomatic people by the American Cancer Society, outlined in Table 11.6, should be heeded in regular physical examinations as part of a cancer-prevention program. In Lab 11A you will be able to determine how well you are doing in terms of your risk management for cardiovascular disease and for cancer prevention and also respond to a questionnaire developed by the American Medical Association to alert people to symptoms that may indicate a serious health problem. Although in most cases nothing serious will be found, any of the symptoms calls for a physician's attention as soon as possible.

Scientific evidence and testing procedures for prevention and early detection of cancer do change. Studies continue to provide new information. The intent of cancer-prevention programs is to educate and guide individuals toward a lifestyle that will help prevent cancer and enable early detection of malignancy.

Treatment of cancer should always be left to specialized physicians and cancer clinics. Current treatment modalities include surgery, radiation, radioactive substances, chemotherapy, hormones, and immunotherapy.

Chronic Lower Respiratory Disease

Chronic lower respiratory disease (CLRD) is a general term that encompasses chronic obstructive pulmonary disease, emphysema, and chronic bronchitis (all diseases of the respiratory system). The incidence of CLRD increases proportionately with smoking cigarettes (and other forms of smoked tobacco) and exposure to certain types of industrial pollution. In the case of emphysema, genetic factors also may play a role.

Accidents

Even though most people do not consider accidents to be a health problem, accidents are the fourth leading cause of death in the United States, affecting the total well-being of millions of Americans each year. Accident prevention and personal safety are part of a health-enhancement program aimed at achieving a higher quality of life. Proper nutrition, exercise, abstinence from cigarette smoking, and stress management are of little

---

Chronic lower respiratory disease (CLRD) A general term that includes chronic obstructive pulmonary disease, emphysema, and chronic bronchitis (all diseases that limit air flow).

the near future. It is the end result of **human immunodeficiency virus (HIV),** which spreads among individuals who engage in risky behavior such as having unprotected sex or sharing hypodermic needles. When a person becomes infected with HIV, the virus multiplies, then attacks and destroys white blood cells. These cells are part of the immune system, whose function is to fight off infections and diseases in the body.

As the number of white blood cells killed increases, the body's immune system breaks down gradually or may be destroyed totally. Without a functioning immune system, a person becomes susceptible to **opportunistic infections** or cancers that are not ordinarily seen in healthy people.

HIV is a progressive disease. At first, people who contract the virus may not know they are infected. An incubation period of weeks, months, or years may pass during which no symptoms appear. The virus can live in the body 10 years or longer before any symptoms emerge.

As the infection progresses to the point at which certain diseases develop, the person is said to have AIDS. HIV itself doesn't kill. Nor do people die from AIDS. AIDS is the final stage of HIV infection. Death results from a weakened immune system that is unable to fight off opportunistic diseases. On the average, 9 to 10 years elapse after infection before the individual develops the symptoms that fit the case definition of AIDS.

No one has to become infected with HIV. At present, once infected with the virus, a person will never become uninfected. The only answer is to protect oneself against this infection. No one should be so ignorant as to believe that it can never happen to him or her!

HIV is transmitted by the exchange of cellular body fluids—blood, semen, vaginal secretions, and maternal milk. These fluids may be exchanged during sexual intercourse, by using hypodermic needles used previously by infected individuals, between a pregnant woman and her developing fetus, during childbirth, less frequently during breast feeding, and rarely from a blood transfusion or an organ transplant.

AIDS is an "equal opportunity epidemic." People do not get HIV because of who they are but, rather, because of what they *do.* HIV and AIDS threaten anyone, anywhere: men, women, children, teenagers, young people, older adults, whites, African Americans, Hispanic Americans, homosexuals, heterosexuals, bisexuals, druggies, Americans, Africans, Asians, Europeans. Nobody is immune to HIV.

You cannot tell if people are infected with HIV or have AIDS simply by looking at them or taking their word. Not you, not a nurse, not even a doctor can tell without getting the results of an HIV antibody test. Therefore, every time you engage in risky behavior, you run the risk of contracting HIV. The two most basic risky behaviors are (a) having unprotected vaginal, anal, or oral sex with an HIV-infected person, and (b) sharing hypodermic needles or other drug paraphernalia with someone who is infected.

About 1.1 million people in the United States are infected with HIV. About 25 percent of them are unaware of the infection. One in every 300 Americans is infected, and about 26 percent of the newly reported cases are women. Through the end of 2004, a cumulative total of 944,305 AIDS cases had been diagnosed in the United States, and 529,113 people had died from the diseases caused by HIV. About 70 percent of the people who died are in the 25- to 44-year-old age group. Of the reported AIDS cases, 756,399 were in males.

Although more than half of all AIDS cases in the United States initially occurred in homosexual or bisexual men, HIV infection now is spreading at a faster rate in heterosexuals. Many heterosexuals have unprotected sex because they don't believe it can happen to their segment of the population. HIV is an epidemic that does not discriminate by sexual orientation. Worldwide, up to 80 percent of the AIDS cases have been reported in heterosexuals.

As with any other serious illness, AIDS patients deserve respect, understanding, and support. Rejection and discrimination are traits of immature, hateful, and ignorant people. Education, knowledge, and responsible behaviors are the best ways to minimize fear and discrimination.

Critical Thinking

Many individuals who have sexually transmitted infections withhold this information from potential sexual partners. Do you think it should be considered a criminal action for an individual to knowingly transmit an STI to someone else?

Guidelines for Preventing STIs

The good news is that you can do things to prevent the spread of STIs and take precautions to keep yourself from becoming a victim. The facts are in: The best prevention technique is a mutually monogamous sexual relationship—sex with only one person who has sexual relations only with you. That one behavior will remove you almost completely from any risk for developing an STI.

Unfortunately, in today's society, trust is an elusive concept. You may be led to believe you are in a monogamous relationship when your partner actually (a) may be cheating on you and gets infected, (b) has a one-night stand with someone who is infected, (c) got the virus several years ago before the present relationship and still doesn't know about the infection, (d) may choose not to tell you about the infection, or (e) is shooting up drugs and becomes infected. In any of these cases, HIV can be passed on to you.

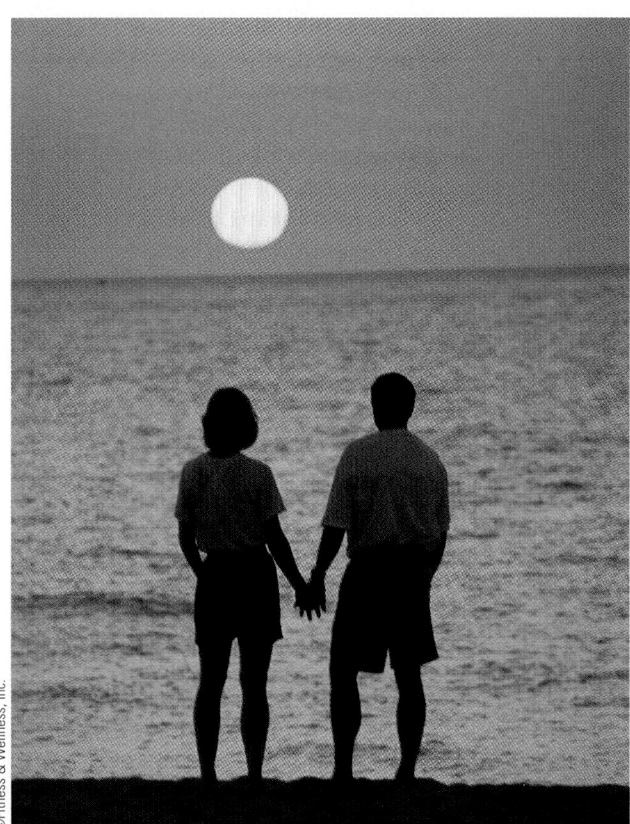

©Fitness & Wellness, Inc.

A monogamous sexual relationship almost completely removes people from the risk of HIV infection and the danger of contracting other sexually transmitted infections.

Because your future and your life are at stake, and because you may never know if your partner is infected, you should give serious and careful consideration to postponing sex until you believe you have found a lifetime monogamous relationship. In doing so, you will not have to live with the fear of catching HIV or other STIs or deal with an unplanned pregnancy.

As strange as this may seem to some, many people postpone sexual activity until they are married. This is the best guarantee against HIV. Married life will provide plenty of time for fulfilling and rewarding sex.

If you choose to delay sex, do not let peers pressure you into having sex. Some people would have you believe you are not a "real" man or woman if you don't have sex. Manhood and womanhood are not proven during sexual intercourse but, instead, through mature, responsible, and healthy choices.

Other people lead you to believe that love cannot be present without sex. Sex in the early stages of a relationship is not the product of love but, rather, simply the fulfillment of a physical, and often selfish, drive. A loving relationship develops over a long time as mutual respect for each other grows.

Teenagers are especially susceptible to peer pressure leading to premature sexual intercourse. As a result, more than a million teens become pregnant each year, with a 43 percent pregnancy rate for all girls at least once as a teenager. Too many young people wish they had postponed sex and silently admire those who do. Sex lasts only a few minutes. The consequences of irresponsible sex may last a lifetime—and in some cases, they are fatal.

Some people brag about their sexual conquests and mock people who choose to wait. Many of these conquests are just fantasies expounded in an attempt to gain popularity with peers.

Sexual promiscuity never leads to a trusting, loving, and lasting relationship. Mature people respect others' choices. If someone does not respect your choice to wait, he or she certainly does not deserve your friendship or, for that matter, anything else.

There is no greater sex than that between two loving and responsible individuals who mutually trust and admire each other. Contrary to many beliefs, these relationships are possible. They are built upon unselfish attitudes and behaviors.

As you look around, you will find people who have these values. Seek them out and build your friendships and future around people who respect you for who you are and what you believe. You don't have to compromise your choices or values. In the end, you will reap the greater rewards of a fulfilling and lasting relationship, free of AIDS and other STIs.

Also, be prepared so you will know your course of action before you get into an intimate situation. Look for common interests and work together toward them. Express your feelings openly: "I'm not ready for sex; I just want to have fun and kissing is fine with me." If your friend does not accept your answer and is not willing to stop the advances, be prepared with a strong response. Statements like "Please stop" or "Don't!" are for the most part ineffective. Use a firm statement such as, "No, I'm not willing to do it" or "I've already thought about this and I'm not going to have sex." If this still doesn't work, label the behavior rape: "This is rape, and I'm going to call the police."

What about those who do not have—or do not desire—a monogamous relationship? Risky behaviors that significantly increase the chances of contracting an STI, including HIV infection, are the following:

1. Multiple or anonymous sexual partners, such as a pickup or prostitute.
2. Anal sex with or without a condom.
3. Vaginal or oral sex with someone who shoots drugs or participates in anal sex.
4. Sex with someone you know has several sex partners.

Human immunodeficiency virus (HIV) Virus that leads to acquired immunodeficiency syndrome (AIDS).

Opportunistic infections Diseases that arise in the absence of a healthy immune system that would fight them off in healthy people.

5. Unprotected sex (without a condom) with an infected person.
6. Sexual contact of any kind with anyone who has symptoms of AIDS or who is a member of a group at high risk for AIDS.
7. Sharing toothbrushes, razors, or other implements that could become contaminated with blood from anyone who is, or might be, infected with HIV.

Avoiding risky behaviors that destroy quality of life and life itself is a critical component of a healthy lifestyle. Learning the facts so you can make responsible choices can protect you and those around you from unpleasant, and perhaps even fatal, consequences. Keys to averting both physical and psychological damage include using alcohol moderately (or not at all), refraining from substance abuse, and avoiding sexually transmitted infections.

An Educated Fitness/Wellness Consumer

The rapid growth of the fitness and wellness industry during the last three decades has spurred the promotion of fraudulent products that deceive consumers into "miraculous," quick, and easy ways to achieve total well-being. **Quackery** and **fraud** have been defined as the conscious promotion of unproven claims for profit.

Today's market is saturated with "special" foods, diets, supplements, pills, cures, equipment, books, and videos that promise quick, dramatic results. Advertisements for these products often are based on testimonials, unproven claims, secret research, half-truths, and quick-fix statements that the uneducated consumer wants to hear. In the meantime, the organization or enterprise making the claims reaps a large profit from the consumers' willingness to pay for astonishing and spectacular solutions to problems caused by their unhealthy lifestyle.

Television, magazine, and newspaper advertisements are not necessarily reliable. For instance, one piece of equipment sold through television and newspaper advertisements promised to "bust the gut" through 5 minutes of daily exercise that appeared to target the abdominal muscle group. This piece of equipment consisted of a metal spring attached to the feet on one end and held in the hands on the other end. According to distributors, the equipment was "selling like hotcakes," and companies could barely keep up with consumer demand.

Three problems became apparent to the educated consumer. First, there is no such thing as spot-reducing; therefore, the claims could not be true. Second, 5 minutes of daily exercise burn hardly any calories and, therefore, have no effect on weight loss. Third, the intended abdominal (gut) muscles were not really involved during the exercise. The exercise engaged mostly the gluteal and lower-back muscles. This piece of equipment now can be found at garage sales for about a tenth of its original cost!

Although people in the United States tend to be firm believers in the benefits of physical activity and positive lifestyle habits as a means to promote better health, most do not reap these benefits because they simply do not know how to put into practice a sound fitness and wellness program that will give them the results they want. Unfortunately, many uneducated wellness consumers are targets of deception by organizations making fraudulent claims for their products.

If you have questions or concerns about a health product, you may write to the National Council Against Health Fraud (NCAHF), 119 Foster Street, Peabody, MA 01960. The purpose of this organization is to provide the consumer with responsible, reliable, evidence-driven health information. NCAHF also monitors deceitful advertising, investigates complaints, and offers public information regarding fraudulent health claims. You may report any type of quackery to its Web site at http://www.ncahf.org/. The site contains an updated list of reliable and unreliable health Web sites for the consumer.

Even though deceit is all around us, we can protect ourselves from consumer fraud. The first step, of course, is education. You have to be an informed consumer of the product you intend to purchase. If you do not have or cannot find the answers, seek the advice of a reputable professional. Ask someone who understands the product but does not stand to profit from the transaction. As examples, a physical educator or an exercise physiologist can advise you regarding exercise equipment; a registered dietitian can provide information on nutrition and weight-control programs; a physician can offer advice on nutritive supplements. Also, be alert to those who bill themselves as "experts." Look for qualifications, degrees, professional experience, certifications, and reputation.

Another clue to possible fraud is that if it sounds too good to be true, it probably is. Phrases like quick-fix, miraculous, special, secret, mail-order only, money-back guarantee, and testimonials often are heard in advertisements of fraudulent promotions. When claims are made, ask where the claims are published. Newspapers, magazines, and trade books are apt to be unreliable sources of information, whereas refereed scientific journals are the most reliable. When a researcher submits information for publication in a refereed journal, at least two qualified and reputable professionals in the field conduct blind reviews of the manuscript. A blind review means the author does not know who will review the manuscript and the reviewers do not know who submitted the manuscript. Acceptance for publication is based on this input and relevant changes.

RELIABLE SOURCES OF HEALTH, FITNESS, NUTRITION, AND WELLNESS INFORMATION

Newsletter	Approx. Yearly Issues	Annual Cost
Bottom Line /Health BottomLineSecrets.com 800-289-0409	12	$29.95
Consumer Reports on Health www.ConsumerReports.org/health 800-234-2188	12	$24
Environmental Nutrition www.environmentalnutrition.com 800-829-5384	12	$30
Tufts University Health & Nutrition Letter www.healthletter.tufts.edu 800-274-7581	12	$28
University of California Berkeley Wellness Letter www.WellnessLetter.com 386-447-6328	12	$28

Health/Fitness Club Memberships

As you follow a lifetime wellness program, you may want to consider joining a health/fitness facility. Or, if you have mastered the contents of this book and your choice of fitness activity is one you can pursue on your own (walking, jogging, cycling), you may not need to join a health club. Barring injuries, you may continue your exercise program outside the walls of a health club for the rest of your life. You also can conduct strength training and stretching programs within your own home (see Chapters 7 and 8).

To stay up-to-date on fitness and wellness developments, you probably should buy a reputable and updated fitness/wellness book every 4 to 5 years. To stay current, you also might subscribe to a credible health, fitness, nutrition, or wellness newsletter. You can surf the World Wide Web—but be sure that the sites you view are from credible and reliable organizations.

If you are contemplating membership in a fitness facility, do all of the following:

- Make sure the facility complies with the standards established by the American College of Sports Medicine (ACSM) for health and fitness facilities. These standards are given in Figure 11.9.
- Examine all exercise options in your community: health clubs/spas, YMCAs, gyms, colleges, schools, community centers, senior centers, and the like.
- Check to see if the facility's atmosphere is pleasurable and nonthreatening to you. Will you feel comfortable with the instructors and other people who go there? Is it clean and well kept up? If the answer is no, this may not be the right place for you.

FIGURE 11.9 American College of Sports Medicine standards for health and fitness facilities.

1. A facility must have an appropriate emergency plan.
2. A facility must offer each adult member a preactivity screening that is relevant to the activities that will be performed by the member.
3. Each person who has supervisory responsibility must be professionally competent.
4. A facility must post appropriate signs in those areas of a facility that present potential increased risk.
5. A facility that offers services or programs to the youth must provide appropriate supervision.
6. A facility must conform to all relevant laws, regulations, and published standards.

Adapted from ACSM's *Health/Fitness Facility Standards and Guidelines* (Champaign, IL: Human Kinetics, 1997).

- Analyze costs versus facilities, equipment, and programs. Take a look at your personal budget. Will you really use the facility? Will you exercise there regularly? Many people obtain memberships and permit dues to be withdrawn automatically from a local bank account, yet seldom attend the fitness center.
- Find out what types of facilities are available: walking/running track, basketball/tennis/racquetball courts, aerobic exercise room, strength-training room, pool, locker rooms, saunas, hot tubs, handicapped access, and so on.
- Check the aerobic and strength-training equipment available. Does the facility have treadmills, bicycle ergometers, stair climbers, cross-country skiing simulators, free weights, strength-training machines? Make sure the facilities and equipment meet your activity interests.
- Consider the location. Is the facility close, or do you have to travel several miles to get there? Distance often discourages participation.
- Check on times the facility is accessible. Is it open during your preferred exercise time (for example, early morning or late evening)?
- Work out at the facility several times before becoming a member. Are people standing in line to use the equipment, or is it readily available during your exercise time?
- Inquire about the instructors' qualifications. Do the fitness instructors have college degrees or professional certifications from organizations such as the American College of Sports Medicine or the International Dance Exercise Association (IDEA)? These organizations have rigorous standards to ensure professional preparation and quality of instruction.

Quackery/Fraud The conscious promotion of unproven claims for profit.

- Consider the approach to fitness (including all health-related components of fitness). Is it well-rounded? Do the instructors spend time with members, or do members have to seek them out constantly for help and instruction?
- Ask about supplementary services. Does the facility provide or contract out for regular health and fitness assessments (cardiovascular endurance, body composition, blood pressure, blood chemistry analysis)? Are wellness seminars (nutrition, weight control, stress management) offered? Do these have hidden costs?

Personal Trainers

In recent years, **personal trainers** have been in high demand by health and fitness participants. A personal trainer is a health/fitness professional who evaluates, motivates, educates, and trains clients to help them meet individualized healthy lifestyle goals. Rates typically start at $40 an hour and go up from there.

Exercise sessions usually are conducted at a health/fitness facility or at the client's own home. Experience and the ability to design safe and effective programs based on the client's current fitness level, health status, and fitness goals are important. Personal trainers also recognize their limitations and refer clients to other health-care professionals as necessary.

Currently, anyone who prescribes exercise can call himself/herself a personal trainer without proof of education, experience, or certification. Although good trainers should strive to maximize their own health and fitness, a good physique and previous athletic experience do not certify a person as a personal trainer.

Unfortunately, because of the high demands for personal trainers, more than 200 organizations now provide some type of certification to fitness specialists. Thus, for years clients have been confused about how to evaluate the credentials of personal trainers. For one thing, a clear distinction exists between "certification" and a "certificate." A certification implies that the individual has met educational and professional standards of performance and competence that document advanced knowledge. A certificate is typically awarded to individuals who attend a conference or workshop but are not required to meet any professional standards.

Presently, no licensing body is in place to oversee personal trainers. Thus, becoming a personal trainer is easy. At a minimum, personal trainers should have an undergraduate degree and certification from a reputable organization such as ACSM, IDEA Health and Fitness Association, the National Strength and Conditioning Association (NSCA), or the American Council on Exercise (ACE). Undergraduate (and graduate) degrees should be conferred in a fitness-related area such as exercise science, exercise physiology, kinesiology, sports medicine, or physical education.

ACSM offers three certification levels: group exercise leader, health/fitness instructor, and health/fitness director. IDEA offers four levels: professional, advanced, elite, and master. For both ACSM and IDEA, each level of certification is progressively more difficult to obtain. A third organization, the National Strength and Conditioning Association (NSCA), also offers a personal trainer's certification program. When looking for a personal trainer, always inquire about the trainer's education and certification credentials.

A final word of caution: When seeking fitness advice from a health/fitness trainer via the Internet, be aware that certain services cannot be provided over the Internet. An Internet trainer is not able to directly administer fitness tests, motivate, observe exercise limitations, respond effectively in an emergency situation (spotting, administering first-aid or CPR) and, thus, is not able to design the most safe and effective exercise program for you.

Purchasing Exercise Equipment

A final consideration is that of purchasing your own exercise equipment. The first question you need to ask yourself is "Do I really need this piece of equipment?" Most people buy on impulse because of television advertisements or because a salesperson convinced them it is a great piece of equipment that will do wonders for their health and fitness. With some creativity, you can implement an excellent and comprehensive exercise program with little, if any, equipment (see Chapters 6, 7, and 8).

Many people buy expensive equipment only to find that they really do not enjoy that mode of activity. They do not remain regular users. Stationary bicycles (lower body only) and rowing ergometers were among the most popular pieces of equipment in the 1980s. Most of them are seldom used now and have become "fitness furniture" somewhere in the basement.

Exercise equipment does have its value to people who prefer to exercise indoors, especially during the winter months. It supports some people's motivation and adherence to exercise. The convenience of having equipment at home also allows for flexible scheduling. You can exercise before or after work or while you watch your favorite television show.

If you are going to purchase equipment, the best recommendation is to actually try it out several times before buying it. Ask yourself several questions: Did you enjoy the workout? Is the unit comfortable? Are you too short, tall, or heavy for it? Is it stable, sturdy, and strong? Do you have to assemble the machine? If so, how difficult is it to put together? How durable is it? Ask for references—people or clubs that have used the equipment extensively. Are they satisfied? Have they enjoyed using the equipment? Talk with professionals at colleges, sports medicine clinics, or health clubs.

Another consideration is to look at used units for signs of wear and tear. Quality is important. Cheaper brands may not be durable, so your investment would be wasted.

Finally, watch out for expensive gadgets. Monitors that provide exercise heart rate, work output, caloric expenditure, speed, grade, and distance may help motivate you, but they are expensive, frequently need repairs, and do not enhance the actual fitness benefits of the workout. Look at maintenance costs and check for service personnel in your community.

Life Expectancy and Physiological Age

Throughout this book you have studied many factors that affect your health, fitness, and quality of life. The question that you now need to ask yourself is: Are your lifestyle habits accelerating or decelerating the rate at which your body is aging? The Life Expectancy and Physiological Age Questionnaire provided in Lab 11B can help you determine how long and how well you may live. By looking at 46 critical genetic and lifestyle factors, you will be able to estimate your life expectancy and your real physiological age. Of greater importance, most of these factors are under your own control, so you can do something to make them work for you instead of against you.

As you fill out the questionnaire, you must be completely honest with yourself. Your life expectancy and physiological age predictions are based on your present lifestyle habits assuming you continue those habits for life. Using the questionnaire, you will review factors that you can modify or implement in daily living to add years and health to your life. Please note that the questionnaire is not a precise scientific measurement but, rather, an estimated life expectancy analysis based on the impact of lifestyle factors on health and longevity. Also, the questionnaire is not intended to substitute for advice and tests conducted by medical and health-care practitioners.

Unhealthy behaviors precipitate premature aging. For sedentary people, any type of physical activity is seriously impaired by age 40 and productive life ends before age 60. Most of these people hope to live to be age 65 or 70 and often must cope with serious physical ailments. These people *stop living at age 60 but choose to be buried at age 70* (see the theoretical model in Figure 11.10).

Self-Evaluation and Behavioral Goals for the Future

The main goal of this book is to provide the information and experiences necessary to create your personal fitness and wellness program. If you have implemented the programs in this book, including exercise, you should be convinced that a wellness lifestyle is the only way to attain a higher quality of life.

FIGURE 11.10 Relationships between physical work capacity, aging, and lifestyle habits.

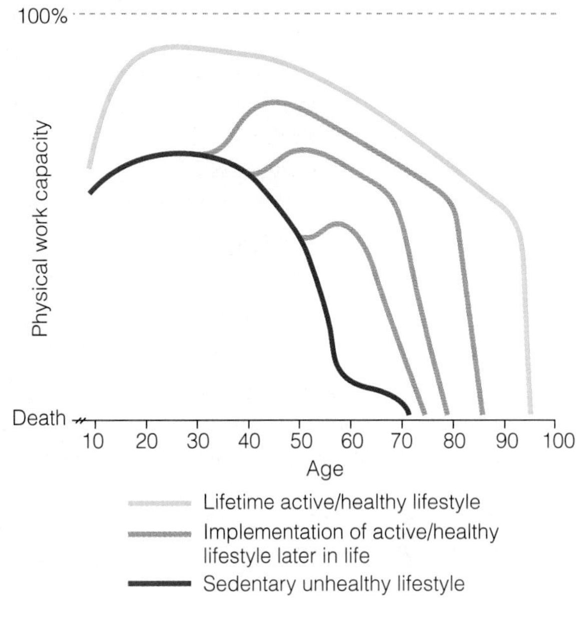

Most people who engage in a personal fitness and wellness program experience this new quality of life after only a few weeks of training and practicing healthy lifestyle patterns. In some instances, however—especially for individuals who have led a poor lifestyle for a long time—a few months may be required to establish positive habits and feelings of well-being. In the end, though, everyone who applies the principles of fitness and wellness will reap the desired benefits.

Throughout this course you have had an opportunity to assess various fitness and wellness components and write goals to improve your quality of life. You now should take the time to evaluate how well you have achieved your own goals. Ideally, if time allows and facilities and technicians are available, reassess the health-related components of physical fitness. If you are unable to reassess these components, determine subjectively how well you accomplished your objectives. You will find a self-evaluation form in part I of Lab 11C.

Critical Thinking

Are there people around you whom you admire and would like to emulate for their wellness lifestyle? Can you identify behaviors these people exhibit that would help you adopt a healthier lifestyle? What keeps you from emulating these behaviors, and how can you overcome these barriers?

Personal trainer An exercise specialist that works one-on-one with an individual and is typically paid by the hour or exercise session.

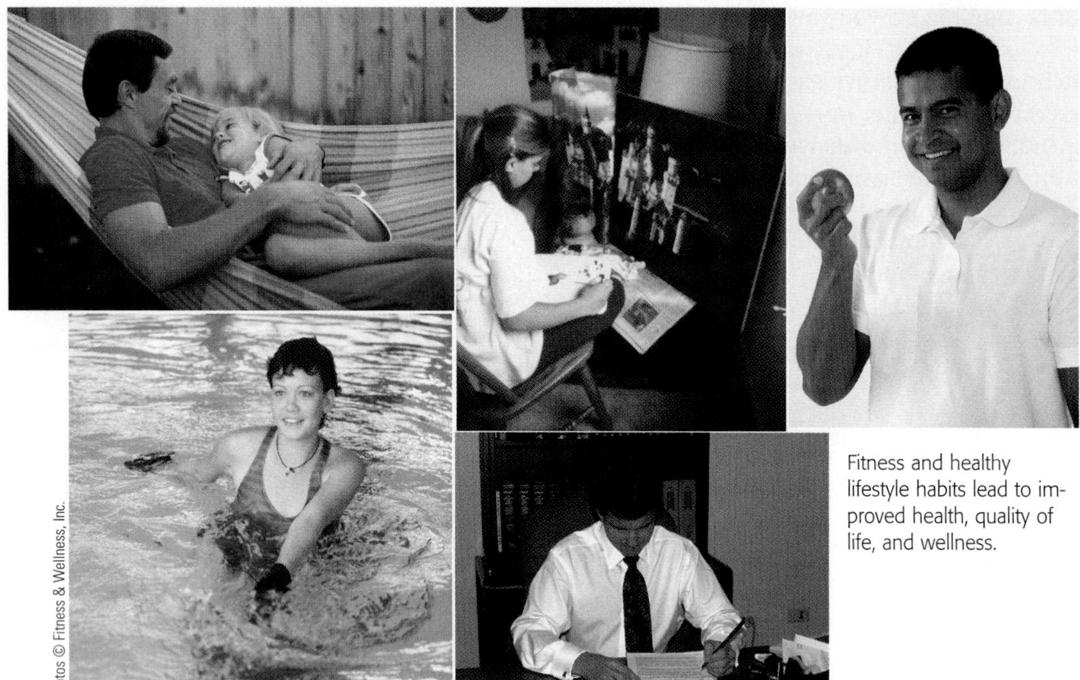

Fitness and healthy lifestyle habits lead to improved health, quality of life, and wellness.

The Fitness Experience and a Challenge for the Future

Patty Neavill is a typical example of someone who often tried to change her life but was unable to do so because she did not know how to implement a sound exercise and weight-control program. At age 24 and at 240 pounds, she was discouraged with her weight, level of fitness, self-image, and quality of life in general. She had struggled with a weight problem most of her life. Like thousands of other people, she had made many unsuccessful attempts to lose weight.

Patty put aside her fears and decided to enroll in a fitness course. As part of the course requirement, a battery of fitness tests was administered at the beginning of the semester. Patty's cardiorespiratory fitness and strength ratings were poor, her flexibility classification was average, and her percent body fat was 41.

Following the initial fitness assessment, Patty met with her course instructor, who prescribed an exercise and nutrition program like the one in this book. Patty committed herself fully to carry out the prescription. She walked/jogged five times a week. She enrolled in a weight-training course that met twice a week. Her daily caloric intake was set in the range of 1,500 to 1,700 calories.

Determined to increase her level of activity further, Patty signed up for recreational volleyball and basketball courses. Besides being fun, these classes provided 4 additional hours of activity per week.

She took care to meet the minimum required servings from the basic food groups each day, which contributed about 1,200 calories to her diet. The remainder of the calories came primarily from complex carbohydrates.

At the end of the 16-week semester, Patty's cardiorespiratory fitness, strength, and flexibility ratings all had improved to the "good" category, she had lost 50 pounds, and her percent body fat had decreased to 22.5!

Patty was tall. Her weight of 190 pounds might be considered too heavy. Her percent body fat, however, was lower than the average for college female physical education major students (about 23 percent body fat).

A thank-you note from Patty to the course instructor at the end of the semester read:

> *Thank you for making me a new person. I truly appreciate the time you spent with me. Without your kindness and motivation, I would have never made it. It is great to be fit and trim. I've never had this feeling before, and I wish everyone could feel like this once in their life.*
>
> *Thank you,*
> *Your trim Patty*

Patty never had been taught the principles governing a sound weight-loss program. In Patty's case, she needed this knowledge but, like most Americans who never have benefited from the process of becoming physically fit, she needed to be in a structured exercise setting to truly feel the joy of fitness.

Even more significant, Patty maintained her aerobic and strength-training programs. A year after ending her calorie-restricted diet, her weight increased by 10 pounds but her body fat decreased from 22.5 to 21.2

percent. As you may recall from Chapter 5, this weight increase is related mostly to changes in lean tissue during the weight-reduction phase.

In spite of only a slight drop in weight during the second year following the calorie-restricted diet, the 2-year follow-up revealed a further decrease in body fat to 19.5 percent. Patty understood the new quality of life reaped through a sound fitness program, and, at the same time, she finally learned how to apply the principles that regulate weight.

If you have read and successfully completed all of the assignments set out in this book, including a regular exercise program, you should be convinced of the value of exercise and healthy lifestyle habits in achieving a new and better quality of life.

Perhaps this new quality of life was explained best by the late Dr. George Sheehan, when he wrote:

> *For every runner who tours the world running marathons, there are thousands who run to hear the leaves and listen to the rain, and look to the day when it is all suddenly as easy as a bird in flight. For them, sport is not a test but a therapy, not a trial but a reward, not a question but an answer.*

The real challenge will come now: a lifetime commitment to fitness and a healthy lifestyle. To make the commitment easier, enjoy yourself and have fun along the way. Implement your program based on your interests and what you enjoy doing most. Then adhering to your new lifestyle will not be difficult.

Your activities over the last few weeks or months may have helped you develop "positive addictions" that will carry on throughout life. If you truly experience the feelings Dr. Sheehan expressed, there will be no looking back. If you don't get there, you won't know what it's like. Fitness is a process, and you will have to put forth constant, deliberate effort to achieve and maintain a higher quality of life. Improving the quality of your life, and most likely your longevity, is in your hands. Only you can take control of your lifestyle and thereby reap the benefits.

Assess Your Behavior

Log on to www.thomsonedu.com/login to determine your risk for heart disease and to modify your Behavior Change Plan to incorporate at least one new activity that is heart-healthy.

1. Do you make a conscious effort to increase daily physical activity and are you able to accumulate at least 30 minutes of moderate-intensity activity on most days of the week?
2. Is your diet fundamentally low in saturated fats, trans fats, processed meats, and do you consume the daily suggested amounts of fruits, vegetables, and fiber?
3. Are you aware of your family history of cardiovascular disease and cancer?
4. Are you familiar with the seven warning signs of cancer and the cancer screening guidelines?
5. Is your life free of addictive behavior? If not, will you commit right now to seek professional help at your institution's counseling center? Addictive behavior destroys health and lives, don't let it end yours.
6. Do you believe in a mutually monogamous sexual relationship as the best way to prevent STIs? If not, do you always take precautions to practice safer sex?
7. Have you carefully considered the consequences of engaging in a sexual relationship, including the risk of STIs, HIV infection, your partner being untruthful about his/her sexual history and STIs, and the potential of an unplanned pregnancy?
8. Are you able to take pride in the lifestyle changes that you have implemented over the last several weeks? Have you rewarded yourself for your accomplishments?

Assess Your Knowledge

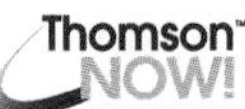

Log on to www.thomsonedu.com/login to assess your understanding of this chapter's topics by taking the Student Practice Test and exploring the modules recommended in your Personalized Study Plan.

1. The constant and deliberate effort to stay healthy and achieve the highest potential for well-being is defined as
   a. health.
   b. physical fitness.
   c. health-related fitness.
   d. wellness.
   e. metabolic fitness.

2. Coronary heart disease
   a. is the single leading cause of death in the United States.
   b. is the leading cause of sudden cardiac deaths.
   c. is a condition in which the arteries that supply the heart muscle with oxygen and nutrients are narrowed by fatty deposits.
   d. accounts for approximately 20 percent of all cardiovascular deaths.
   e. All of the above are correct choices.
3. Regular aerobic activity helps
   a. lower LDL cholesterol.
   b. lower HDL cholesterol.
   c. increase triglycerides.
   d. decrease insulin sensitivity.
   e. accomplish all of the above.
4. Type 1 diabetes is related closely to
   a. overeating.
   b. obesity.
   c. lack of physical activity.
   d. insulin resistance.
   e. All of the above are incorrect choices.
5. Altruism is a
   a. philosophy that the truth must be told at all times.
   b. true concern for and action on behalf of others.
   c. religious doctrine linked to the improvement of humanity's health.
   d. higher state of being that is obtained through meditation.
   e. All are correct choices.
6. Cancer
   a. is primarily a preventable disease.
   b. is often related to tobacco use.
   c. has been linked to dietary habits.
   d. risk increases with obesity.
   e. All are correct choices.
7. A cancer prevention diet should include
   a. ample amounts of fruit and vegetables.
   b. cruciferous vegetables.
   c. phytonutrients.
   d. soy products
   e. All of the above.
8. Cocaine use
   a. causes lung cancer.
   b. leads to atrophy of the brain.
   c. can lead to sudden death.
   d. causes amotivational syndrome.
   e. All are correct choices.
9. HIV
   a. attacks and destroys white blood cells.
   b. readily multiplies in the human body.
   c. breaks down the immune system.
   d. increases the likelihood of developing opportunistic diseases and cancers.
   e. All choices are correct.
10. Your real physiological age is determined by your
   a. birth date.
   b. family's health history.
   c. amount of physical activity.
   d. lifestyle habits.
   e. ability to obtain proper medical care.

Correct answers can be found at the back of the book.

Media Menu

Thomson NOW! *Connections*

- Determine your risk for heart disease.
- Check how well you understand the chapter's concepts.

Internet Connections

- American Heart Association. This comprehensive site is sponsored by the AHA, which provides research, cardiac information for health professionals and the general public, and advocacy. The site features information on a variety of cardiovascular illnesses, healthy lifestyles, and CPR; a searchable encyclopedia on heart and stroke questions, and a ten-question "Healthy Heart Workout" quiz. **http://www.americanheart.org**
- American Cancer Society. This comprehensive site features information on a variety of cancer types and treatment options, including alternative or complementary therapies. It features the popular cancer profiler for personalized cancer treatment information, information about the cancer survivors' network, and a search engine for local resources. **http://www.cancer.org**
- NIDA Drug Pages. This site, from the National Institute of Drug Abuse, features information about a comprehensive list of drugs, including alcohol, nicotine, marijuana, cocaine, ecstasy, amphetamines, steroids, prescription medications, and more. The site also features an excellent chart listing the common drugs of abuse according to category, examples of commercial and street names, as well as intoxication effects and potential health consequences. **http://www.nida.nih.gov/Drugpages**

- American Social Health Association. This site features information on a variety of sexually transmitted infections, a comprehensive frequently asked questions section, as well as information about STI hotlines. It also features a link to iwannaknow.org, the ASHA STI prevention Web site for teens.
http://www.ashastd.org
- Facts On Tap: Alcohol and Your College Experience. This excellent site, geared toward college students, features links to the following topics and more:
- Risky Relationship: Alcohol and Sex
- College Experience: Alcohol and Student Life
- The Naked Truth: Alcohol and Your Body
- When Someone Else's Drinking Gives You a Hangover
http://www.factsontap.org
- Assess Your Risk for HIV and Other Sexually Transmitted Infections. By completing this simple 24-question multiple-choice questionnaire, you will obtain an accurate portrayal of your personal risk for acquiring HIV and other types of sexually transmitted infections.
http://www.thebody.com/surveys/sexsurvey.html

Notes

1. L. Dossey, "Can Spirituality Improve Your Health?" *Bottom Line/Health* 15 (July 2001): 11–13.
2. E. R. Growald and A. Lusks, "Beyond Self," *American Health* (March 1988): 51–53.
3. U.S. Department of Health and Human Services, Centers for Disease Control and Prevention, National Center for Health Statistics, *National Vital Statistics Reports: Deaths Final Data for 2003* 54, no. 13 (April 19, 2006).
4. American Heart Association, *Heart Disease and Stroke Statistics—2006 Update* (Dallas: American Heart Association, 2006).
5. American Heart Association, *1998 Heart and Stroke Facts (Statistical Supplement)* (Dallas: AHA, 1997).
6. See note 3, USDHHS.
7. S. N. Blair, H. W. Kohl III, R. S. Paffenbarger, Jr., D. G. Clark, K. H. Cooper, and L. W. Gibbons, "Physical Fitness and All-Cause Mortality: A Prospective Study of Healthy Men and Women," *Journal of the American Medical Association* 262 (1989): 2395–2401.
8. G. A. Kelley and Z. Tran, "Aerobic Exercise and Normotensive Adults: A Meta-Analysis," *Medicine and Science in Sports and Exercise* 27 (1995): 1371–1377; G. A. Kelley and P. McClellan, "Antihypertensive Effects of Aerobic Exercise: A Brief Meta-Analytic Review of Randomized Controlled Trials," *American Journal of Hypertension* 7 (1994): 115–119.
9. R. Collins et al., "Blood Pressure, Stroke, and Coronary Heart Disease; Part 2, Short-term Reductions in Blood Pressure: Overview of Randomized Drug Trials in Their Epidemiological Context," *Lancet* 335 (1990): 827–838.
10. S. N. Blair et al., "Influences of Cardiorespiratory Fitness and Other Precursors on Cardiovascular Disease and All-cause Mortality in Men and Women," *Journal of the American Medical Association* 276 (1996): 205–210.
11. G. Kelley, "Dynamic Resistance Exercise and Resting Blood Pressure in Adults: A Meta-analysis," *Journal of Applied Physiology* 82 (1997): 1559–1565; G. A. Kelley and K. S. Kelley, "Progressive Resistance Exercise and Resting Blood Pressure: A Meta-Analysis of Randomized Controlled Trials," *Hypertension* 35 (2000): 838–843.
12. "Lipid Research Clinics Program: The Lipid Research Clinic Coronary Primary Prevention Trial Results," *Journal of the American Medical Association* 251 (1984): 351–364.
13. See note 4, AHA.
14. "HDL on the Rise," *HealthNews* (September 10, 1999).
15. A. H. Lichtenstein et al., "Diet and Lifestyle Recommendations Revision 2006: A Scientific Statement From the American Heart Association Nutrition Committee," *Circulation* 114 (2006): 82–96.
16. E. B. Rimm, A. Ascherio, E. Giovannucci, D. Spiegelman, M. J. Stampfer, and W. C. Willett, "Vegetable, Fruit, and Cereal Fiber Intake and Risk of Coronary Heart Disease Among Men," *Journal of the American Medical Association* 275 (1996): 447–451.
17. National Cholesterol Education Program Expert Panel, "Summary of the Third Report of the National Cholesterol Education Program (NCEP) Expert Panel on Detection, Evaluation, and Treatment of High Blood Cholesterol in Adults (Adult Treatment Panel III)," *Journal of the American Medical Association* 285 (2001):2486–2497.
18. A. Jula et al., "Effects of Diet and Simvastatin on Serum Lipids, Insulin, and Antioxidants in Hypercholesterolemic Men," *Journal of the American Medical Association* 287 (2002): 598–605.
19. O. Nygard, J. E. Nordreahaug, H. Refsum, P. M. Ueland, M. Farstad, and S. E. Vollset, "Plasma Homocysteine Levels and Mortality in Patients with Coronary Heart Disease," *New England Journal of Medicine* 337 (1997): 230–236.
20. "The Homocysteine-CVD Connection," *HealthNews* (October 25, 1999).
21. C. J. Boushey, S. A. A. Beresford, G. S. Omenn, and A. G. Motulsky, "A Quantitative Assessment of Plasma Homocysteine as a Risk Factor for Vascular Disease," *Journal of the American Medical Association* 274 (1995): 1049–1057.
22. "Inflammation May Be Key Cause of Heart Disease and More: Diet's Role," *Environmental Nutrition* 27, no. 7 (July 2004): 1, 4.
23. H. R. Superko, "State-of-the Art Heart Tests," *Bottom Line/Health* 19 (February 2005): 3–5.
24. "Predict Heart Disease Better with CRP" *Environmental Nutrition* 28 no. 2 (February 2005): 3.
25. H. K. Choi et al., "Dairy Consumption and Risk of Type 2 Diabetes Mellitus in Men," *Archives of Internal Medicine* 165 (2005): 997–1003.
26. S. A. Glantz and W. W. Parmley, "Passive Smoking and Heart Disease," *Journal of the American Medical Association* 273 (1995): 1047–1053.
27. U.S. Public Health Service, *The Health Consequences of Involuntary Exposure to Tobacco Smoke: A Report of the Surgeon General—Executive Summary* (Rockville, MD: U.S. Department of Health and Human Services, 2006).
28. See note 4, AHA.
29. V. W. Setiawan et al., "Protective Effect of Green Tea on the Risks of Chronic Gastritis and Stomach Cancer," *International Journal of Cancer* 92 (2001): 600–604.
30. L. Mitscher and V. Dolby, *The Green Tea Book—China's Fountain of Youth* (New York: Avery Press, 1997).
31. "Curbing Cancer's Reach: Little Things That Might Make a Big Difference," *Environmental Nutrition* 29, no. 6 (2006): 1, 6.
32. E. E. Calle, C. Rodriguez, K. Walker-Thurmond, and M. J. Thun, "Overweight, Obesity, and Mortality from Cancer in a Prospectively Studied Cohort of U.S. Adults," *New England Journal of Medicine* 348 (2003): 1625–1638.

2. Explain the exercise program that you implemented in this course, indicate your feelings about the outcomes of this program, and evaluate how well you accomplished your fitness goals.

3. List nutritional or dietary changes that you were able to implement this term and the effects of these changes on your body composition and personal wellness.

4. List other lifestyle changes that you were able to make this term that may decrease your risk for disease. In a few sentences, explain how you feel about these changes and their impact on your overall well-being.

Nutritive Value of Selected Foods

APPENDIX A

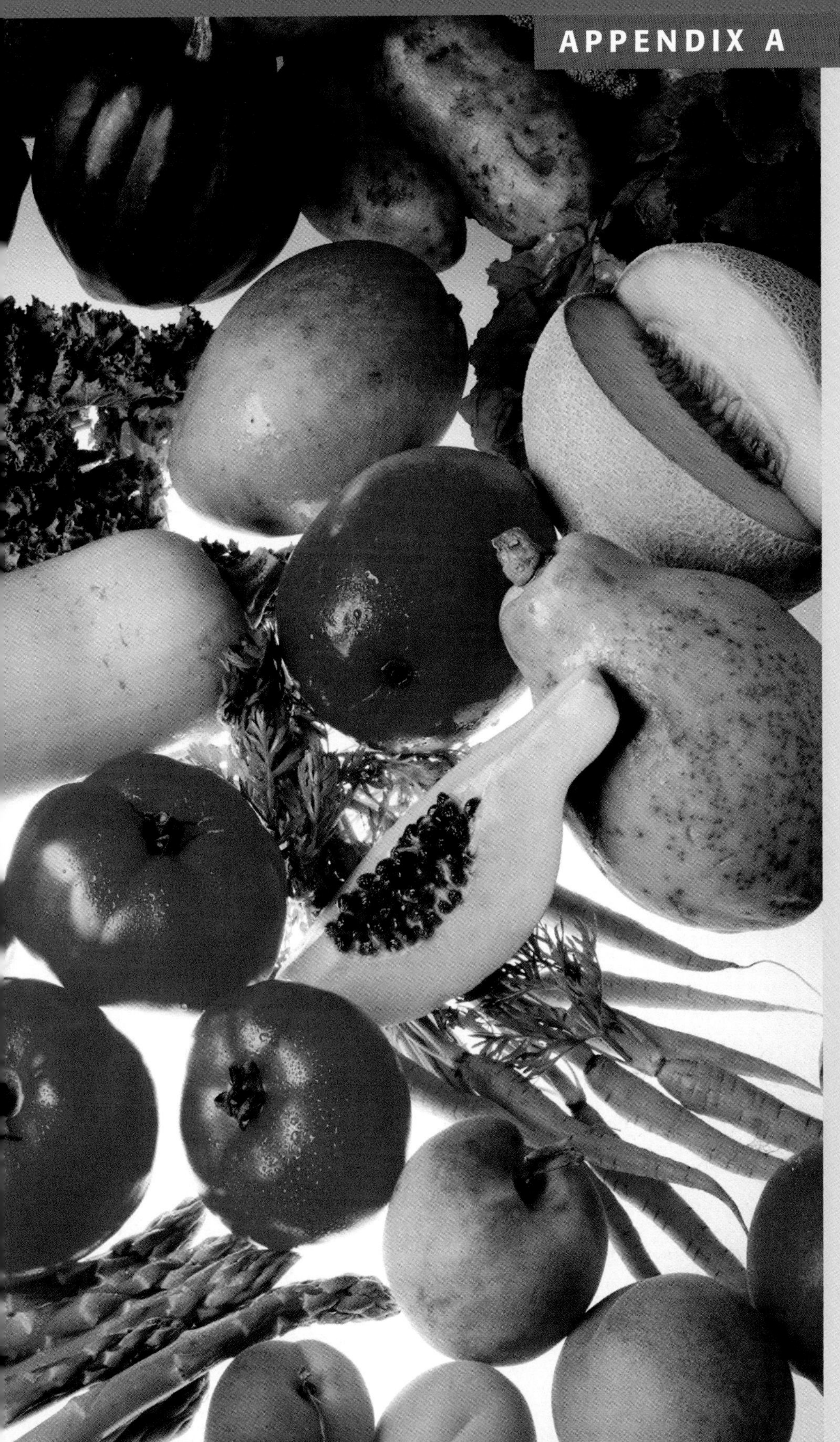

Photo © Eleanor Thompson/CORBIS

Food Description	Qty	Measure	Wt (g)	Ener (cal)	Prot (g)	Carb (g)	Dietary Fiber (g)	Fat (g)	Fat Breakdown (g) Sat	Mono	Poly	Trans	Chol (mg)	Calc (mg)	Iron (mg)	Sodi (mg)	Vit E (mg)	Folate (mcg)	Vit C (mg)	Selenium (mcg)
Almonds, dry roasted, no salt added	¼	cup(s)	35	206	8	7	4	18	1.40	11.61	4.36	—	0	92	1.56	<1	8.97	11	0	1
Apple juice, unsweetened, canned	½	cup(s)	124	58	<1	14	<1	<1	0.02	0.01	0.04	—	0	9	0.46	4	0.01	0	1	<1
Apples, raw medium, w/peel	1	item(s)	138	72	<1	19	3	<1	0.04	0.01	0.07	—	0	8	0.17	1	—	4	6	0
Applesauce, sweetened, canned	½	cup(s)	128	97	<1	25	2	<1	0.04	0.01	0.07	—	0	5	0.45	4	0.27	1	2	<1
Apricot, fresh w/o pits	4	item(s)	140	67	2	16	3	1	0.04	0.24	0.11	—	0	18	0.55	1	1.25	13	14	<1
Apricot, halves w/skin, canned in heavy syrup	½	cup(s)	129	107	1	28	2	<1	0.01	0.04	0.02	—	0	12	0.39	5	0.77	3	4	<1
Asparagus, boiled, drained	½	cup(s)	90	20	2	4	2	0.19	0.06	0	0.12	—	0	20.7	0.81	12.6	1.35	134.1	6.92	5.48
Avocado, California, whole, w/o skin or pit	1	item(s)	170	284	3	15	12	26	3.59	16.61	3.42	—	0	22	1.00	14	3.35	105	15	1
Bacon, cured, broiled, pan fried, or roasted	2	slice(s)	13	68	5	<1	0	5	1.73	2.33	0.57	0	14	1	0.18	291	0.04	<1	0	8
Bagel chips, plain	3	item(s)	29	130	3	19	1	5	0.50	—	—	—	0	0	0.72	70	—	—	0	—
Bagel, plain, enriched, toasted	1	item(s)	66	195	7	38	2	1	0.16	0.09	0.49	0	0	53	2.52	379	0.08	64	0	23
Banana, fresh whole, w/o peel	1	item(s)	118	105	1	27	3	<1	0.13	0.04	0.09	—	0	6	0.31	1	0.12	24	10	1
Beans, black, boiled	½	cup(s)	86	114	8	20	7	<1	0.12	0.04	0.20	—	0	23	1.81	1	—	128	0	1
Beans, Fordhook lima, frozen, boiled, drained	½	cup(s)	85	88	5	16	5	<1	0.07	0.02	0.14	—	0	26	1.55	59	0.25	18	11	1
Beans, mung, sprouted, boiled, drained	½	cup(s)	62	13	1	3	<1	<1	0.02	0.00	0.02	—	0	7	0.40	6	0.04	18	7	<1
Beans, red kidney, canned	½	cup(s)	128	109	7	20	8	<1	0.06	0.03	0.24	—	0	31	1.61	436	0.77	65	1	2
Beans, refried, canned	½	cup(s)	127	119	7	20	7	2	0.60	0.71	0.19	—	10	44	2.10	378	0.00	14	8	2
Beans, yellow snap, string or wax, boiled, drained	½	cup(s)	62	22	1	5	2	<1	0.04	0.00	0.09	—	0	29	0.80	2	0.28	21	6	<1
Beef, chuck, arm pot roast, lean & fat, ¼" fat, braised	3	ounce(s)	85	282	23	0	0	20	7.97	8.68	0.77	—	84	9	2.64	51	0.19	8	0	21
Beef, corned, canned	3	ounce(s)	85	213	23	0	0	13	5.25	5.07	0.54	—	73	10	1.77	855	0.13	8	0	36
Beef, ground, lean, broiled, well	3	ounce(s)	85	238	24	0	0	15	5.89	6.56	0.56	—	86	10	2.08	76	—	9	0	22
Beef, ground, regular, broiled, medium	3	ounce(s)	85	246	20	0	0	18	6.91	7.70	0.65	—	77	9	2.07	71	—	8	0	16
Beef, liver, pan fried	3	ounce(s)	85	149	23	4	0	4	1.27	0.56	0.49	0.17	324	5	5.24	65	0.39	221	1	28
Beef, rib steak, small end, lean, ¼" fat, broiled	3	ounce(s)	85	188	24	0	0	10	3.84	4.01	0.27	—	68	11	2.18	59	0.12	7	0	19
Beef, rib, whole, lean & fat, ¼" fat, roasted	3	ounce(s)	85	320	19	0	0	27	10.71	11.42	0.94	—	72	9	1.96	54	—	6	0	19
Beef, short loin, T-bone steak, lean, ¼" fat, broiled	3	ounce(s)	85	174	23	0	0	9	3.05	4.23	0.26	—	50	5	3.11	65	0.12	7	0	9
Beer	12	fluid ounce(s)	356	118	1	6	<1	<1	0.00	0.00	0.00	0	0	18	0.07	14	0.00	21	0	2
Beer, light	12	fluid ounce(s)	354	99	1	5	0	0	0.00	0.00	0.00	0	0	18	0.14	11	0.00	14	0	2
Beets, sliced, canned, drained	½	cup(s)	85	26	1	6	1	<1	0.02	0.02	0.04	—	0	13	1.55	165	0.03	26	3	<1
Biscuits	1	item(s)	41	121	3	16	1	5	1.40	1.41	1.82	0	<1	33	1.01	205	0.01	26	0	7
Blueberries, raw	½	cup(s)	72	41	1	10	2	<1	0.02	0.03	0.11	—	0	4	0.20	1	0.41	4	7	<1
Bologna, beef	1	slice(s)	28	90	3	1	0	8	3.50	4.26	0.31	—	20	0	0.36	310	—	4	0	—
Bologna, turkey	1	slice(s)	28	50	3	1	0	4	1.00	1.09	0.98	—	20	40	0.36	270	—	—	0	—
Brazil nuts, unblanched, dried	¼	cup(s)	35	230	5	4	3	23	5.30	8.59	7.20	—	0	56	0.85	1	2.01	8	<1	671
Bread, cracked wheat	1	slice(s)	25	65	2	12	1	1	0.23	0.48	0.17	—	0	11	0.70	135	—	15	0	6
Bread, French	1	slice(s)	25	69	2	13	1	1	0.16	0.30	0.17	—	0	19	0.63	152	0.08	37	0	8
Bread, mixed grain	1	slice(s)	26	65	3	12	2	1	0.21	0.40	0.24	—	0	24	0.90	127	0.09	31	<1	8
Bread, pita	1	item(s)	60	165	5	33	1	1	0.10	0.06	0.32	—	0	52	1.57	322	0.18	64	0	16
Bread, pumpernickel	1	slice(s)	32	80	3	15	2	1	0.14	0.30	0.40	—	0	22	0.92	215	0.13	30	0	8
Bread, rye	1	slice(s)	32	83	3	15	2	1	0.20	0.42	0.26	—	0	23	0.91	211	0.11	35	<1	10
Bread, white	1	slice(s)	25	67	2	13	1	1	0.18	0.17	0.34	—	0	38	0.94	170	0.05	28	0	4
Bread, whole wheat	1	slice(s)	46	128	4	24	3	2	0.37	0.53	1.35	—	0	15	1.43	159	0.35	30	0	18
Broccoli, chopped, boiled, drained	½	cup(s)	78	27	2	6	3	<1	0.06	0.03	0.13	—	0	31	0.52	32	1.13	84	51	1
Brownie, prepared from mix	1	item(s)	24	112	1	12	1	7	1.76	2.60	2.26	—	18	14	0.44	82	—	7	<1	3
Brussels sprouts, boiled, drained	½	cup(s)	78	28	2	6	2	<1	0.08	0.03	0.20	—	0	28	0.94	16	0.34	47	48	1
Bulgur, cooked	½	cup(s)	91	76	3	17	4	<1	0.04	0.03	0.09	—	0	9	0.87	5	0.01	16	0	1
Buns, hamburger, plain	1	item(s)	43	120	4	21	1	2	0.47	0.48	0.85	—	0	59	1.43	206	0.03	48	0	8
Butter	1	tablespoon(s)	15	108	<1	<1	0	12	6.13	5.00	0.43	—	32	4	0.00	86	0.35	<1	0	<1
Buttermilk, low fat	1	cup(s)	245	98	8	12	0	2	1.34	0.62	0.08	—	10	284	0.12	257	0.12	12	2	5
Cabbage, boiled, drained, no salt added	1	cup(s)	150	33	2	7	3	1	0.08	0.05	0.29	—	0	47	0.26	12	0.18	30	30	1
Cabbage, raw, shredded	1	cup(s)	70	17	1	4	2	<1	0.01	0.01	0.04	—	0	33	0.41	13	0.10	30	23	1
Cake, angel food, from mix	1	slice(s)	50	129	3	29	<1	<1	0.02	0.01	0.06	—	0	42	0.12	255	0.00	10	0	8
Cake, butter pound, ready to eat, commercially prepared	1	slice(s)	75	291	4	37	<1	15	8.67	4.43	0.80	—	166	26	1.04	299	—	0	<1	—

Cake, carrot, cream cheese frosting, from mix	1	slice(s)	111	484	5	52	1	29	5.43	7.24	15.10	—	60	28	1.39	273	—	13	1	—
Cake, chocolate, chocolate icing, commercially prepared	1	slice(s)	64	235	3	35	2	10	3.05	5.61	1.18	—	27	28	1.41	214	—	11	<1	2
Cake, devil's food cupcake, chocolate frosting	1	item(s)	35	120	2	20	1	4	1.80	1.60	0.60	—	19	21	0.70	92	—	2	0	2
Cake, white, coconut frosting, from mix	1	slice(s)	112	399	5	71	1	12	4.36	4.14	2.42	—	1	101	1.30	318	0.13	35	<1	12
Candy, Almond Joy bar	1	item(s)	49	240	2	29	2	13	9.00	3.63	0.74	0	3	20	0.36	70	—	—	0	—
Candy, Life Savers	1	item(s)	2	8	0	2	0	<1	0.00	—	—	0	0	<1	0.04	1	—	—	0	0
Candy, M & Ms peanut chocolate candy, small bag	1	item(s)	49	250	5	30	2	13	5.00	5.42	2.07	—	5	40	0.36	25	—	17	1	2
Candy, M & Ms plain chocolate candy, small bag	1	item(s)	48	240	2	34	1	10	6.00	3.30	0.30	—	5	40	0.36	30	—	3	1	1
Candy, milk chocolate bar	1	item(s)	91	483	8	53	2	28	16.69	7.20	0.63	—	22	228	0.83	92	—	11	2	—
Candy, Milky Way bar	1	item(s)	58	270	2	41	1	10	5.00	3.50	0.35	—	5	60	0.18	95	—	6	1	3
Candy, Reese's peanut butter cups	2	piece(s)	45	250	5	25	1	14	5.00	6.17	2.34	0	3	20	0.36	140	—	25	0	2
Candy, Special Dark chocolate bar	1	item(s)	41	220	2	24	3	13	8.00	4.59	0.41	0	3	0	0.72	0	—	1	0	1
Candy, Starburst fruit chews, original fruits	1	package	59	240	0	48	0	5	1.00	2.10	1.83	—	0	10	0.18	0	—	0	30	<1
Candy, York peppermint patty	1	item(s)	42	170	1	34	1	3	2.00	1.32	0.12	0	0	0	0.36	10	—	2	0	—
Cantaloupe	½	cup(s)	80	27	1	7	1	<1	0.04	0.00	0.07	—	0	7	0.17	13	0.04	17	30	<1
Carrots, raw	½	cup(s)	61	25	1	6	2	<1	0.02	0.01	0.06	0	0	20	0.18	42	0.40	12	4	<1
Carrots, sliced, boiled, drained	½	cup(s)	78	27.29	0.59	6.41	2.33	0.14	0.02	0	0.08	—	0	23.39	0.26	45.24	0.80	10.92	2.8	0.54
Cashews, dry roasted	¼	cup(s)	34	197	5	11	1	16	3.14	9.36	2.68	—	0	15	2.06	5	0.32	24	0	4
Catsup/ketchup	1	tablespoon(s)	15	14	<1	4	<1	<1	0.01	0.01	0.04	—	0	3	0.08	167	0.22	2	2	<1
Cauliflower, boiled, drained	½	cup(s)	62	14	1	3	2	<1	0.04	0.02	0.13	—	0	10	0.20	9	0.04	27	27	<1
Celery, stalk	2	item(s)	80	11	1	2	1	<1	0.03	0.03	0.06	—	0	32	0.16	64	0.22	29	2	<1
Cereal, All-Bran	1	cup(s)	62	160	8	46	20	2	0.00	0.00	1.00	0	0	300	9.00	160	—	800	12	6
Cereal, All-Bran Buds	1	cup(s)	91	212	6	73	42	3	—	—	—	0	0	0	13.64	606	—	1212	18	26
Cereal, Bran Flakes, Post	1	cup(s)	40	133	4	32	7	1	0.00	0.00	0.71	—	0	0	10.77	293	—	133	0	—
Cereal, Cap'n Crunch	1	cup(s)	36	144	2	30	1	2	0.53	0.39	0.27	—	0	5	6.00	269	—	133	0	7
Cereal, Cheerios	1	cup(s)	30	110	3	22	3	2	0.00	0.50	0.50	—	0	100	8.10	280	—	200	6	11
Cereal, Complete wheat bran flakes	1	cup(s)	39	120	4	31	7	1	—	—	—	0	0	0	23.94	279	—	532	80	4
Cereal, Corn Flakes	1	cup(s)	28	100	2	24	1	0	0.00	0.00	0.00	0	0	0	8.10	200	—	100	6	1
Cereal, Corn Pops	1	cup(s)	31	120	1	28	0	0	0.00	0.00	0.00	0	0	0	1.80	120	—	100	6	2
Cereal, Cracklin' Oat Bran	1	cup(s)	65	266	5	47	7	9	2.70	4.70	1.33	0	0	27	2.38	186	—	218	20	14
Cereal, Cream of Wheat, instant, prepared	½	cup(s)	121	61	2	13	<1	<1	0.01	0.01	0.04	0	0	27	8.60	1	—	357	0	—
Cereal, Frosted Flakes	1	cup(s)	41	160	1	37	1	0	0.00	0.00	0.00	0	0	0	5.99	200	—	133	8	2
Cereal, Frosted Mini-Wheats	5	item(s)	51	180	5	41	5	1	0.00	0.00	0.50	0	0	0	15.30	5	—	100	0	2
Cereal, granola, prepared	½	cup(s)	61	299	9	32	5	15	2.76	4.7	6.53	—	0	48	2.59	13	3.59	51	1	16.95
Cereal, Kashi puffed	1	cup(s)	25	70	3	13	2	1	0.00	—	—	—	0	0	0.72	0	—	—	0	—
Cereal, Life	1	cup(s)	43	160	4	33	3	2	0.35	0.64	0.61	—	0	124	11.92	218	—	142	0	11
Cereal, Multi-Bran Chex	1	cup(s)	58	200	4	49	7	2	0.00	0.00	0.00	0	0	100	16.20	390	—	100	6	5
Cereal, Nutri-Grain golden wheat	1	cup(s)	40	133	4	31	5	1	0.00	0.00	0.67	—	0	0	1.46	279	—	133	20	9
Cereal, oatmeal, cooked w/water	½	cup(s)	117	74	3	13	2	1	0.19	0.37	0.44	—	0	9	0.80	1	0.12	5	0	9
Cereal, Product 19	1	cup(s)	30	100	2	25	1	0	0.00	0.00	0.00	0	0	0	18.00	210	—	400	60	4
Cereal, Raisin Bran	1	cup(s)	59	190	4	47	8	1	0.00	0.10	0.36	—	0	20	10.80	300	—	140	0	—
Cereal, Rice Chex	1	cup(s)	25	96	2	22	<1	0	0.00	0.00	0.00	0	0	80	7.20	232	—	160	5	1
Cereal, Rice Krispies	1	cup(s)	26	96	2	23	0	0	0.00	0.00	0.00	0	0	0	1.44	256	—	80	5	4
Cereal, Shredded Wheat	1	cup(s)	25	88	3	20	3	1	0.04	0.01	0.10	—	0	10	1.08	2	—	12	0	1
Cereal, Smacks	1	cup(s)	36	133	3	32	1	1	0.00	0.00	0.00	—	0	0	0.48	67	—	133	8	17
Cereal, Special K	1	cup(s)	31	110	7	22	1	0	0.00	0.00	0.00	0	0	0	8.70	220	—	400	15	7
Cereal, Total whole grain	1	cup(s)	40	146	3	31	4	1	0.00	0.00	0.00	—	0	1330	23.94	253	31.24	532	80	2
Cereal, Wheaties	1	cup(s)	30	110	3	24	3	1	0.00	0.00	0.00	—	0	0	8.10	220	2.26	200	6	1
Cheese, American, processed	1	ounce(s)	28	106	6	<1	0	9	5.58	2.54	0.28	—	27	156	0.05	422	0.08	2	0	4
Cheese, blue, crumbled	1	ounce(s)	28	100	6	1	0	8	5.29	2.21	0.23	—	21	150	0.09	395	0.07	10	0	4
Cheese, cheddar, shredded	¼	cup(s)	28	114	7	<1	0	9	5.96	2.65	0.27	—	30	204	0.19	175	0.08	5	0	4
Cheese, feta	1	ounce(s)	28	74	4	1	0	6	4.18	1.29	0.17	—	25	138	0.18	312	0.05	9	0	4
Cheese, Monterey jack	1	ounce(s)	28	104	7	<1	0	8	5.34	2.45	0.25	—	25	209	0.20	150	0.07	5	0	4
Cheese, mozzarella, part skim milk	1	ounce(s)	28	71	7	1	0	4	2.83	1.26	0.13	—	18	219	0.06	173	0.04	3	0	4
Cheese, Parmesan, grated	1	tablespoon(s)	5	22	2	<1	0	1	0.87	0.42	0.06	—	4	55	0.05	76	0.01	1	0	1
Cheese, ricotta, part skim milk	¼	cup(s)	62	85	7	3	0	5	3.03	1.42	0.16	—	19	167	0.27	77	0.04	8	0	10
Cheese, Swiss	1	ounce(s)	28	106	8	2	0	8	4.98	2.04	0.27	—	26	221	0.06	54	0.11	2	0	5
Cherries, sweet, raw	½	cup(s)	73	46	1	12	2	<1	0.03	0.03	0.04	—	0	9	0.26	0	0.05	3	5	0
Chicken, broiler breast, meat & skin, flour coated, fried	3	ounce(s)	85	189	27	1	<.1	8	2.08	2.98	1.67	—	76	14	1.01	65	—	5	0	20

Food Description	Qty	Measure	Wt (g)	Ener (cal)	Prot (g)	Carb (g)	Dietary Fiber (g)	Fat (g)	Fat Breakdown (g) Sat	Mono	Poly	Trans	Chol (mg)	Calc (mg)	Iron (mg)	Sodi (mg)	Vit E (mg)	Folate (mcg)	Vit C (mg)	Selenium (mcg)
Chicken, broiler drumstick, meat & skin, flour coated, fried	3	ounce(s)	85	208	23	1	<.1	12	3.11	4.61	2.75	—	77	10	1.14	76	—	9	0	16
Chicken, light meat, roasted	3	ounce(s)	85	130	23	0	0	3	0.92	1.29	0.79	—	64	11	0.92	43	0.23	3	0	22
Chicken, roasted (meat only)	3	ounce(s)	85	142	21	0	0	6	1.54	2.13	1.28	—	64	10	1.03	64	—	4	0	21
Chickpeas or bengal gram, garbanzo beans, boiled	½	cup(s)	82	134	7	22	6	2	0.22	0.48	0.95	—	0	40	2.37	6	0.29	141	1	3
Chocolate milk, low fat	1	cup(s)	250	158	8	26	1	3	1.54	0.75	0.09	—	8	288	0.60	153	0.05	13	2	5
Cilantro	1	teaspoon(s)	2	<1	<.1	<.1	<.1	<.1	0.00	0.00	0.00	—	0	1	0.03	1	—	1	1	<.1
Cocoa, hot, prepared w/milk	1	cup(s)	250	193	9	27	3	6	3.58	1.69	0.09	0.18	20	263	1.20	110	0.08	13	1	7
Coconut, dried, not sweetened	¼	cup(s)	60	393	4	14	10	38	34.06	1.63	0.42	—	0	15	1.98	22	0.26	5	1	11
Cod, Atlantic cod or scrod, baked or broiled	3	ounce(s)	44	46	10	0	0	<1	0.07	0.05	0.13	—	24	6	0.22	35	—	5	<1	17
Coffee, brewed	8	fluid ounce(s)	237	9	<1	0	0	0	0.00	0.00	0.00	0	0	2	0.02	2	0.02	5	0	0
Collard greens, boiled, drained	½	cup(s)	95	25	2	5	3	<1	0.04	0.02	0.16	—	0	133	1.10	15	0.84	88	17	<1
Cookies, animal crackers	12	piece(s)	30	134	2	22	<1	4	1.03	2.29	0.56	—	0	13	0.82	1118	0.04	50	0	—
Cookies, chocolate chip	1	item(s)	30	140	2	16	1	8	2.09	3.26	2.09	0	13	11	0.70	109	0.54	16	<.1	4
Cookies, chocolate sandwich, extra crème filling	1	item(s)	13	65	<1	9	<1	3	0.50	1.39	1.22	1.10	0	3	0.37	64	0.25	6	0	<1
Cookies, Fig Newtons	1	item(s)	16	55	1	10	1	1	0.50	0.50	0.00	0.50	0	5	0.36	60	—	—	<1	—
Cookies, oatmeal	1	item(s)	69	234	6	45	3	4	0.70	1.28	1.85	0	<.1	26	1.94	311	0.23	30	<1	17
Cookies, peanut butter	1	item(s)	35	163	4	17	1	9	1.65	4.72	2.43	0	13	28	0.67	157	0.74	21	<.1	5
Cookies, sugar	1	item(s)	16	61	1	7	<1	3	0.63	1.27	0.87	0	18	5	0.32	50	0.28	8	<.1	3
Corn, yellow sweet, frozen, boiled, drained	½	cup(s)	82	66	2	16	2	1	0.08	0.16	0.26	—	0	2	0.39	1	0.06	29	3	1
Cornbread	1	piece(s)	55	141	5	18	1	5	2.09	1.44	1.50	0	21	88	1.01	209	0.33	36	2	6
Cornmeal, yellow whole grain	½	cup(s)	61	221	5	47	4	2	0.31	0.58	1.00	—	0	4	2.10	21	0.26	15	0	9
Cottage cheese, low fat, 1% fat	½	cup(s)	113	81	14	3	0	1	0.73	0.33	0.04	—	5	69	0.16	459	0.01	14	0	10
Cottage cheese, low fat, 2% fat	½	cup(s)	113	102	16	4	0	2	1.38	0.62	0.07	—	9	78	0.18	459	0.02	15	0	12
Crab, blue, canned	2	ounce(s)	57	56	12	0	0	1	0.14	0.12	0.25	—	50	57	0.48	189	1.04	24	2	18
Crackers, cheese (mini)	30	item(s)	30	151	3	17	1	8	2.81	3.63	0.74	—	4	45	1.43	299	0.66	46	0	3
Crackers, honey graham	4	item(s)	28	118	2	22	1	3	0.43	1.14	1.07	—	0	7	1.04	169	0.09	13	0	3
Crackers, matzo, plain	1	item(s)	28	112	3	24	1	<1	0.06	0.04	0.17	—	0	4	0.90	1	0.02	5	0	10
Crackers, Ritz	5	item(s)	16	80	1	10	1	4	0.50	1.50	0.00	—	0	20	0.72	135	—	10	1	—
Crackers, rye crispbread	1	item(s)	10	37	1	8	2	<1	0.01	0.02	0.06	—	0	3	0.24	26	0.08	5	0	4
Crackers, saltine	5	item(s)	15	65	1	11	<1	2	0.44	0.96	0.25	0.54	0	18	0.81	195	0.15	19	0	2
Crackers, wheat	10	item(s)	30	142	3	19	1	6	1.55	3.43	0.84	—	0	15	1.32	239	0.15	35	0	2
Cranberry juice cocktail	½	cup(s)	127	72	0	18	<1	<1	0.01	0.02	0.06	—	0	4	0.19	3	0.28	0	45	0
Cream cheese	2	tablespoon(s)	29	101	2	1	0	10	6.37	2.85	0.37	—	32	23	0.35	86	0.09	4	0	1
Cream, heavy whipping, liquid	1	tablespoon(s)	15	52	<1	<1	0	6	3.45	1.60	0.21	—	21	10	0.00	6	0.16	1	<.1	<.1
Cream, light whipping, liquid	1	tablespoon(s)	15	44	<1	<1	0	5	2.90	1.36	0.13	—	17	10	0.00	5	0.13	1	<.1	<.1
Croissant, butter	1	item(s)	57	231	5	26	1	12	6.59	3.15	0.62	—	38	21	1.16	424	—	35	<1	13
Cucumber	¼	item(s)	75	11	<1	3	<1	<.1	0.03	0.00	0.04	—	0	12	0.21	2	0.02	5	2	<1
Danish pastry, nut	1	item(s)	65	280	5	30	1	16	3.78	8.90	2.78	—	30	61	1.17	236	0.53	54	1	9
Dates, domestic, whole	¼	cup(s)	44.5	126	1	33	4	<1	0.01	0.01	0	—	0	17	0.45	1	0.02	9	<1	1
Distilled alcohol, 90 proof	1	fluid ounce(s)	28	73	0	0	0	0	0.00	0.00	0.00	0	0	0	0.01	<1	0.00	0	0	0
Doughnut, cake	1	item(s)	47	198	2	23	1	11	1.70	4.37	3.70	—	17	21	0.92	257	—	22	<.1	0
Doughnut, glazed	1	item(s)	60	242	4	27	1	14	3.49	7.72	1.74	—	4	26	0.36	205	—	13	<.1	5
Egg substitute, Egg Beaters	¼	cup(s)	61	30	6	1	0	0	0.00	0.00	0.00	0	0	20	1.08	115	—	60	0	—
Eggs, fried	1	item(s)	46	92	6	<1	0	7	1.98	2.92	1.22	—	210	27	0.91	94	0.56	23	0	16
Eggs, hard boiled	1	item(s)	50	78	6	1	0	5	1.63	2.04	0.71	—	212	25	0.60	62	0.51	22	0	15
Eggs, poached	1	item(s)	50	74	6	<1	0	5	1.54	1.90	0.68	—	211	27	0.92	147	0.48	24	0	16
Eggs, raw, white	1	item(s)	33	17	4	<1	0	<.1	0.00	0.00	0.00	—	0	2	0.03	55	0.00	1	0	7
Eggs, raw, whole	1	item(s)	50	74	6	<1	0	5	1.55	1.91	0.68	—	212	27	0.92	70	0.49	24	0	16
Eggs, raw, yolk	1	item(s)	17	53	3	1	0	4	1.59	1.95	0.70	—	205	21	0.45	8	0.43	24	0	9
Eggs, scrambled, prepared w/milk & butter	2	item(s)	122	203	14	3	0	15	4.49	5.82	2.62	—	429	87	1.46	342	1.04	37	<1	27
Figs, raw, medium	2	item(s)	101	74	1	19	3	<1	0.06	0.07	0.14	—	0	35	0.37	1	0.11	6	2	<1
Fish fillets, batter coated or breaded, fried	3	ounce(s)	85	197.19	12.46	14.42	0.42	10.44	2.39	2.19	5.32	—	28.89	15.3	1.79	452.2	—	17	0	7.73
Flounder, baked	3	ounce(s)	85	114	15	<1	<.1	6	1.15	2.17	1.44	0	44	19	0.35	281	0.41	7	3	34
Flour, all purpose, white, bleached, enriched	½	cup(s)	63	228	6	48	2	1	0.10	0.05	0.26	—	0	9	2.90	1	0.04	114	0	21
Flour, whole wheat	½	cup(s)	60	203	8	44	7	1	0.19	0.14	0.47	—	0	20	2.33	3	0.49	26	0	42

Frankfurter, beef & pork	1	item(s)	57	174	7	1	1	16	6.14	7.79	1.56	—	29	6	0.66	638	0.14	2	0	8
Frankfurter, beef	1	item(s)	45	149	5	2	0	13	5.26	6.44	0.53	—	24	6	0.68	513	0.09	2	0	4
Frankfurter, turkey	1	item(s)	45	102	6	1	0	8	2.65	2.51	2.25	—	48	48	0.83	642	0.28	4	0	7
Frozen yogurt, chocolate, soft serve	½	cup(s)	72	115	3	18	2	4	2.61	1.26	0.16	—	4	106	0.90	71	—	8	<1	2
Frozen yogurt, vanilla, soft serve	½	cup(s)	72	117	3	17	0	4	2.46	1.14	0.15	—	1	103	0.22	63	0.08	4	1	2
Fruit cocktail, canned in heavy syrup	½	cup(s)	124	91	<1	23	1	<.1	0.01	0.02	0.04	—	0	7	0.36	7	0.50	4	2	1
Fruit cocktail, canned in juice	½	cup(s)	119	55	1	14	1	<.1	0.00	0.00	0.00	—	0	9	0.25	5	0.47	4	3	1
Granola bar, plain, hard	1	item(s)	25	115	2	16	1	5	0.58	1.07	2.95	—	0	15	0.72	72	—	6	<1	4
Grape juice, sweetened, added vitamin C, from frozen concentrate	½	cup(s)	125	64	<1	16	<1	<1	0.04	0.01	0.03	—	0	5	0.13	3	0.00	1	30	<1
Grapefruit juice, pink, sweetened, canned	½	cup(s)	125	58	1	14	<1	<1	0.02	0.02	0.03	—	0	10	0.45	3	0.05	13	34	<1
Grapefruit juice, white	½	cup(s)	124	48	1	11	<1	<1	0.02	0.02	0.03	—	0	11	0.25	1	0.27	12	47	<1
Grapefruit, raw, pink or red	½	cup(s)	115	48	1	12	2	<1	0.02	0.02	0.04	—	0	25	0.09	0	0.15	15	36	<1
Grapes, European, red or green, adherent skin	½	cup(s)	80	55	1	14	1	<1	0.04	0.01	0.04	—	0	8	0.29	2	0.15	2	9	<.1
Haddock, baked or broiled	3	ounce(s)	44	50	11	0	0	<1	0.07	0.07	0.14	—	33	19	0.60	39	—	4	0	18
Halibut, Atlantic & Pacific, cooked, dry heat	3	ounce(s)	85	119	23	0	0	2	0.35	0.82	0.80	—	35	51	0.91	59	—	12	0	40
Ham, cured, boneless, 11% fat, roasted	3	ounce(s)	85	151	19	0	0	8	2.65	3.77	1.20	—	50	7	1.14	1275	0.26	3	0	17
Ham, deli sliced, cooked	1	slice(s)	28	30	5	1	0	1	0.50	0.39	0.11	—	15	0	0.00	240	—	—	0	—
Honey	1	tablespoon(s)	21	64	<.1	17	<.1	0	0.00	0.00	0.00	0	0	1	0.09	1	0.00	<1	<1	<1
Honeydew melon	½	cup(s)	89	32	<1	8	1	<1	0.03	0.00	0.05	—	0	5	0.15	16	0.02	17	16	1
Ice cream, chocolate	½	cup(s)	66	143	3	19	1	7	4.49	2.12	0.27	—	22	72	0.61	50	0.20	11	<1	2
Ice cream, chocolate, soft serve	½	cup(s)	87	177	3	24	1	8	5.17	2.43	0.31	—	22	103	0.33	44	0.22	5	1	—
Ice cream, light vanilla	½	cup(s)	66	109	4	18	<1	3	1.71	0.57	0.10	—	17	77	0.05	49	0.08	3	<1	1
Jams, jellies, preserves, all flavors	1	tablespoon(s)	20	56	<.1	14	<1	<.1	0.00	0.01	0.00	—	0	4	0.10	6	0.00	2.20	1.76	—
Jams, jellies, preserves, all flavors, low sugar	1	tablespoon(s)	18	25	<.1	6	<1	<.1	0.00	0.01	0.02	—	0	2	0.05	<1	0.01	—	4.93	—
Kale, frozen, chopped, boiled, drained	½	cup(s)	65	20	2	3	1	<1	0.04	0.02	0.15	—	0	90	0.61	10	0.60	9	16	1
Kiwifruit	1	item(s)	77	53	1	11	3	1	0.02	0.03	0.19	—	0	30	0.38	2	—	<.1	74	—
Lamb, chop, loin, domestic, lean & fat, ¼" fat, broiled	3	ounce(s)	85	269	21	0	0	20	8.36	8.25	1.43	—	85	17	1.54	65	0.11	15	0	23
Lamb, leg, domestic, lean & fat, ¼" fat, cooked	3	ounce(s)	85	250	21	0	0	18	7.51	7.50	1.28	—	82	14	1.60	61	0.12	15	0	22
Lemon juice	1	tablespoon(s)	15	4	<.1	1	<.1	0	0.00	0.00	0.00	—	0	1	0.00	<1	0.02	2	7	<.1
Lemonade, from frozen concentrate	8	fluid ounce(s)	248	131	<1	34	<1	<1	0.02	0.00	0.04	—	0	10	0.52	7	0.02	2	13	<1
Lentils, boiled	½	cup(s)	99	115	9	20	8	<1	0.05	0.06	0.17	—	0	19	3.30	2	0.11	179	1	3
Lentils, sprouted	1	cup(s)	77	82	7	17	0	<1	0.04	0.08	0.17	—	0	19	2.47	8	—	77	13	<1
Lettuce, butterhead, Boston, or bibb	1	cup(s)	55	7	1	1	1	<1	0.02	0.00	0.06	—	0	19	0.69	3	0.10	40	2	<1
Lettuce, romaine, shredded	1	cup(s)	56	10	1	2	1	<1	0.02	0.01	0.09	—	0	19	0.55	5	0.07	77	14	<1
Lobster, northern, cooked, moist heat	3	ounce(s)	85	83	17	1	0	1	0.09	0.14	0.08	—	61	52	0.33	323	0.85	9	0	36
Macadamias, dry roasted, no salt added	¼	cup(s)	34	241	3	4	3	25	4.00	19.86	0.50	—	0	23	0.89	1	0.19	3	<1	1
Mayonnaise w/soybean oil	1	tablespoon(s)	14	99	<1	1	0	11	1.64	2.70	5.89	0.04	5	2	0.07	78	0.72	1	0	<1
Mayonnaise, low calorie	1	tablespoon(s)	16	37	<.1	3	0	3	0.53	0.72	1.70	—	4	<.1	0.00	80	0.32	0	0	—
Milk, fat free, nonfat, or skim	1	cup(s)	245	83	8	12	0	<1	0.29	0.12	0.02	—	5	223	1.23	108	0.02	12	0	8
Milk, fat free, nonfat, or skim, w/nonfat milk solids	1	cup(s)	245	91	9	12	0	1	0.40	0.16	0.02	—	5	316	0.12	130	0.00	12	2	5
Milk, low fat, 1%	1	cup(s)	244	102	8	12	0	2	1.54	0.68	0.09	—	12	264	0.85	122	0.02	12	0	8
Milk, low fat, 1%, w/nonfat milk solids	1	cup(s)	245	105	9	12	0	2	1.48	0.69	0.09	—	10	314	0.12	127	—	12	2	6
Milk, reduced fat, 2%	1	cup(s)	244	122	8	11	0	5	2.35	2.04	0.17	—	20	271	0.24	115	0.07	12	<1	6
Milk, reduced fat, 2%, w/nonfat milk solids	1	cup(s)	245	125	9	12	0	5	2.93	1.36	0.17	—	20	314	0.12	127	—	12	2	6
Milk, whole, 3.3%	1	cup(s)	244	146	8	11	0	8	4.55	1.98	0.48	—	24	246	0.07	105	0.15	12	0	9
Milk, whole, evaporated, canned	2	tablespoon(s)	32	42	2	3	0	2	1.45	0.74	0.08	—	9	82	0.06	33	0.04	3	1	1
Milkshakes, chocolate	1	cup(s)	227	270	7	48	1	6	3.81	1.77	0.23	—	25	299	0.70	252	0.11	11	0	4
Muffin, English, plain, enriched	1	item(s)	57	134	4	26	2	1	0.15	0.17	0.51	—	0	30	1.43	264	—	42	0	—
Muffin, English, wheat	1	item(s)	57	127	5	26	3	1	0.16	0.16	0.48	—	0	101	1.64	218	0.26	36	0	17
Muffins, blueberry	1	item(s)	63	160	3	23	1	6	0.87	1.48	3.25	0	20	50	1.15	288	0.76	29	<1	9
Mushrooms, raw	½	cup(s)	35	8	1	1	<1	<1	0.02	0.00	0.05	—	0	1	0.18	1	0.00	6	1	3
Mustard greens, frozen, boiled, drained	½	cup(s)	75	14	2	2	2	<1	0.01	0.08	0.04	—	0	76	0.84	19	1.01	53	10	<1
Oil, canola	1	tablespoon(s)	14	120	0	0	0	14	0.97	8.01	4.03	—	0	0	0.00	0	2.33	0	0	0
Oil, corn	1	tablespoon(s)	14	120	0	0	0	14	1.73	3.29	7.98	0.04	0	0	0.00	0	1.94	0	0	0
Oil, olive	1	tablespoon(s)	14	119	0	0	0	14	1.82	9.98	1.35	—	0	<1	0.09	<1	1.94	0	0	0
Oil, peanut	1	tablespoon(s)	14	119	0	0	0	14	2.28	6.24	4.32	—	0	0	0.00	0	2.12	0	0	0
Oil, safflower	1	tablespoon(s)	14	120	0	0	0	14	0.84	10.15	1.95	—	0	0	0.00	0	4.64	0	0	0
Oil, soybean w/cottonseed oil	1	tablespoon(s)	14	120	0	0	0	14	2.45	4.01	6.54	—	0	0	0.00	0	1.65	0	0	0

Food Description	Qty	Measure	Wt (g)	Ener (cal)	Prot (g)	Carb (g)	Dietary Fiber (g)	Fat (g)	Fat Breakdown (g) Sat	Mono	Poly	Trans	Chol (mg)	Calc (mg)	Iron (mg)	Sodi (mg)	Vit E (mg)	Folate (mcg)	Vit C (mg)	Sele-nium (mcg)
Okra, sliced, boiled, drained	½	cup(s)	80	18	1	4	2	<1	0.04	0.02	0.04	—	0	62	0.22	5	0.22	37	13	<1
Onions, chopped, boiled, drained	½	cup(s)	106	47	1	11	1	<1	0.03	0.03	0.08	—	0	23	0.26	3	0.02	16	6	1
Orange juice, unsweetened, from frozen concentrate	½	cup(s)	125	56	1	13	<1	<.1	0.01	0.01	0.01	—	0	11	0.12	1	0.25	55	48	<1
Orange, raw	1	item(s)	131	62	1	15	3	<1	0.02	0.03	0.03	—	0	52	0.13	0	0.24	39	70	1
Oysters, eastern, farmed, raw	3	ounce(s)	85	50	4	5	0	1	0.38	0.13	0.50	—	21	37	4.91	151	—	15	4	54
Oysters, eastern, wild, cooked, moist heat	3	ounce(s)	85	116	12	7	0	4	1.31	0.53	1.65	—	89	77	10.19	359	—	12	5	61
Pancakes, blueberry, from recipe	3	item(s)	114	253	7	33	1	10	2.26	2.64	4.74	—	64	235	1.96	470	—	41	3	16
Pancakes, from mix w/egg & milk	3	item(s)	114	249	9	33	2	9	2.33	2.36	3.33	—	81	245	1.48	576	—	105	1	—
Papaya, raw	½	cup(s)	70	27	<1	7	1	<.1	0.03	0.03	0.02	—	0	17	0.07	2	0.51	27	43	<1
Pasta, egg noodles, enriched, cooked	½	cup(s)	80	106	4	20	1	1	0.25	0.34	0.33	0.02	26	10	1.27	6	0.14	51	0	17
Pasta, macaroni, enriched, cooked	½	cup(s)	70	99	3	20	1	<1	0.07	0.06	0.19	—	0	5	0.98	1	0.04	54	0	15
Pasta, spaghetti, al dente, cooked	½	cup(s)	65	95	4	20	1	1	0.05	0.05	0.15	—	0	7	1.00	1	0.04	8	0	40
Pasta, spaghetti, whole wheat, cooked	½	cup(s)	70	87	4	19	3	<1	0.07	0.05	0.15	—	0	11	0.74	2	0.21	4	0	18
Pasta, tricolor vegetable macaroni, enriched, cooked	½	cup(s)	67	86	3	18	3	<.1	0.01	0.01	0.03	—	0	7	0.33	4	0.06	44	0	13
Peach, halves, canned in heavy syrup	½	cup(s)	131	97	1	26	2	<1	0.01	0.05	0.06	—	0	4	0.35	8	0.64	4	4	<1
Peach, halves, canned in water	½	cup(s)	122	29	1	7	2	<.1	0.01	0.03	0.03	—	0	2	0.39	4	0.60	4	4	<1
Peach, raw, medium	1	item(s)	98	38	1	9	1	<1	0.02	0.07	0.08	—	0	6	0.25	0	0.72	4	6	<.1
Peanut butter, smooth	1	tablespoon(s)	16	96	4	3	1	8	1.60	3.96	2.38	—	0	8	0.30	80	1.44	12	0	1
Peanuts, oil roasted, salted	¼	cup(s)	36	216	10	5	3	19	3.12	9.33	5.49	—	0	22	0.54	115	2.50	43	<1	1
Pear, halves, canned in heavy syrup	½	cup(s)	133	98	<1	25	2	<1	0.01	0.04	0.04	—	0	7	0.29	7	0.11	1	1	0
Pear, raw	1	item(s)	166	96	1	26	5	<1	0.01	0.04	0.05	—	0	15	0.28	2	0.20	12	7	<1
Peas, green, canned, drained	½	cup(s)	85	59	4	11	3	<1	0.05	0.03	0.14	—	0	17	0.81	214	0.03	37	8	1
Peas, green, frozen, boiled, drained	½	cup(s)	80	62	4	11	4	<1	0.04	0.02	0.10	—	0	19	1.22	58	0.02	47	8	1
Pecans, dry roasted, no salt added	¼	cup(s)	57	403	5	8	5	42	3.56	24.92	11.66	—	0	41	1.59	1	0.74	9	<1	2
Pepperoni, beef & pork	1	slice(s)	11	55	2	<1	0	5	1.77	2.32	0.48	—	9	1	0.15	224	—	<1	0	—
Peppers, green bell or sweet, raw	½	cup(s)	75	15	1	3	1	<1	0.04	0.01	0.05	—	0	7	0.25	2	0.28	8	60	0
Pickle relish, sweet	1	tablespoon(s)	15	20	<.1	5	<1	<.1	0.01	0.03	0.02	—	0	<1	0.13	122	0.06	<1	<1	0
Pickle, dill	1	ounce(s)	28	5	<1	1	<1	<.1	0.01	0.00	0.02	—	0	3	0.15	363	0.03	<1	1	0
Pie crust, frozen, ready to bake, enriched, baked	1	slice(s)	16	82	1	8	<1	5	1.69	2.51	0.65	—	0	3	0.36	104	0.42	9	0	<1
Pie crust, prepared w/water, baked	1	slice(s)	20	100	1	10	<1	6	1.54	3.46	0.77	—	0	12	0.43	146	—	20	0	—
Pie, apple, from home recipe	1	slice(s)	155	411	4	58	2	19	4.73	8.36	5.17	—	0	11	1.74	327	—	37	3	12
Pie, pecan, from home recipe	1	slice(s)	122	503	6	64	0	27	4.87	13.64	6.97	—	106	39	1.81	320	—	32	<1	15
Pie, pumpkin, from home recipe	1	slice(s)	155	316	7	41	0	14	4.92	5.73	2.81	—	65	146	1.97	349	—	33	3	11
Pineapple, canned in extra heavy syrup	½	cup(s)	130	108	<1	28	1	<1	0.01	0.02	0.05	—	0	18	0.49	1	—	7	9	—
Pineapple, canned in juice	½	cup(s)	125	75	1	20	1	<.1	0.01	0.01	0.04	—	0	17	0.35	1	0.01	6	12	<1
Pineapple, raw, diced	½	cup(s)	78	37	<1	10	1	<.1	0.01	0.01	0.03	—	0	10	0.22	1	0.02	12	28	<.1
Pinto beans, boiled, drained, no salt added	½	cup(s)	114	25	2	5	0	<1	0.04	0.03	0.21	—	0	17	0.75	58	—	146	7	1
Pomegranate	1	item(s)	154	105	1	26	1	<1	0.06	0.07	0.10	—	0	5	0.46	5	0.92	9	9	1
Popcorn, air popped	1	cup(s)	8	31	1	6	1	<1	0.05	0.09	0.15	—	0	1	0.22	<1	0.02	2	0	1
Popcorn, popped in oil	1	cup(s)	33	165	3	19	3	9	1.61	2.70	4.43	—	0	3	0.92	292	—	6	<.1	2
Pork, ribs, loin, country style, lean & fat, roasted	3	ounce(s)	85	279	20	0	0	22	7.83	9.36	1.71	—	78	21	0.90	44	—	4	<1	32
Potato chips, salted	20	item(s)	28	152	2	15	1	10	3.11	2.79	3.46	—	0	7	0.46	169	1.91	13	9	2
Potatoes, au gratin mix, prepared w/water, whole milk, & butter	½	cup(s)	114	106	3	15	1	5	2.94	1.34	0.15	—	17	94	0.36	499	—	8	4	3
Potatoes, baked, flesh & skin	1	item(s)	202	220	5	51	4	<1	0.05	0.00	0.09	—	0	20	2.75	16	—	22	26	2
Potatoes, baked, flesh only	½	cup(s)	61	57	1	13	1	<.1	0.02	0.00	0.03	—	0	3	0.21	3	0.02	5	8	<1
Potatoes, hashed brown	½	cup(s)	78	207	2	27	2	10	1.11	3.13	2.78	—	0	11	0.43	267	0.01	12	10	<1
Potatoes, mashed, from dehydrated granules w/milk, water, & margarine	½	cup(s)	105	122	2	17	1	5	1.27	2.05	1.41	—	2	34	0.22	181	0.54	8	7	6
Pretzels, plain, hard, twists	5	item(s)	30	114	3	24	1	1	0.23	0.41	0.37	—	0	11	1.30	515	—	51	0	2
Prune juice, canned	1	cup(s)	256	182	2	45	3	<.1	0.01	0.05	0.02	—	0	31	3.02	10	0.31	0	10	2
Prunes, dried	2	item(s)	17	40	<1	11	1	<.1	0.01	0.06	0.02	—	0	9	0.42	1	0.00	1	1	<1

Pudding, chocolate	½	cup(s)	144	154	5	23	1	5	2.78	1.94	0.23	0	35	138	1.04	135	0.00	7	<1	5
Pudding, tapioca, ready to eat	1	item(s)	142	169	3	28	<1	5	0.85	2.24	1.93	—	1	119	0.33	226	0.43	4	1	2
Pudding, vanilla	½	cup(s)	136	116	5	17	<.1	3	1.31	1.21	0.16	0	35	133	0.25	134	0.00	6	<1	5
Quinoa, dry	½	cup(s)	85	318	11	59	5	5	0.50	1.30	1.99	—	0	51	7.86	18	—	42	0	—
Raisins, seeded, packed	¼	cup(s)	41	122	1	32	3	<1	0.07	0.01	0.07	—	0	12	1.07	12	—	1	2	<1
Raspberries, raw	½	cup(s)	62	32	1	7	4	<1	0.01	0.04	0.23	—	0	15	0.42	1	0.54	13	16	<1
Raspberries, red, sweetened, frozen	½	cup(s)	125	129	1	33	6	<1	0.01	0.02	0.11	—	0	19	0.81	1	0.90	33	21	<1
Rice, brown, long grain, cooked	½	cup(s)	98	108	3	22	2	1	0.18	0.32	0.31	—	0	10	0.41	5	0.03	4	0	10
Rice, white, long grain, boiled	½	cup(s)	79	103	2	22	<1	<1	0.06	0.07	0.06	—	0	8	0.95	1	0.03	46	0	6
Rice, wild brown, cooked	½	cup(s)	82	82.81	3.27	17.49	1.47	0.27	0.04	0.04	0.17	—	0	2.46	0.49	2.46	—	21.31	0	0.65
Roll, hard	1	item(s)	57	167	6	30	1	2	0.35	0.65	0.98	—	0	54	1.87	310	0.24	54	0	22
Salad dressing, blue cheese	2	tablespoon(s)	31	154	1	2	0	16	3.03	3.76	8.51	—	5	25	0.06	335	1.84	9	1	<1
Salad dressing, French	2	tablespoon(s)	31	143	<1	5	0	14	1.76	2.63	6.56	—	0	7	0.25	261	1.56	0	0	0
Salad dressing, French, low fat	2	tablespoon(s)	33	76	<1	10	<1	4	0.36	1.92	1.64	—	0	4	0.28	262	0.10	1	0	1
Salad dressing, Italian	2	tablespoon(s)	29	86	<1	3	0	8	1.32	1.86	3.80	—	0	2	0.19	486	1.47	0	0	1
Salad dressing, Italian, diet	2	tablespoon(s)	30	23	<1	1	0	2	0.14	0.66	0.51	—	2	3	0.20	410	0.06	0	0	2
Salad dressing, ranch	2	tablespoon(s)	30	146	<1	2	<.1	16	2.32	3.85	8.92	—	1	4	0.03	354	1.85	<1	<.1	—
Salad dressing, thousand island	2	tablespoon(s)	31	115	<1	5	<1	11	1.59	2.46	5.68	—	8	5	0.37	269	1.25	0	0	<1
Salad dressing, thousand island, low calorie	2	tablespoon(s)	31	62	<1	7	<1	4	0.23	1.98	0.82	—	<1	5	0.28	254	0.31	0	0	0
Salami, pork, dry or hard	1	slice(s)	13	52	3	<1	0	4	1.52	2.05	0.48	—	10	2	0.17	289	—	<1	0	3
Salmon, broiled or baked w/butter	3	ounce(s)	85	155	23	0	0	6	1.16	2.29	2.33	—	40	15	1.02	99	1.15	4	2	41
Salmon, smoked chinook (lox)	2	ounce(s)	57	66	10	0	0	2	0.52	1.14	0.56	—	13	6	0.48	1134	—	1	0	22
Salsa	2	tablespoon(s)	16	4	<1	1	<1	<.1	0.00	0.00	0.02	—	0	5	0.16	69	0.19	3	2	<.1
Sardines, Atlantic, with bones, canned in oil	2	item(s)	24	50	6	0	0	3	0.36	0.92	1.23	—	34	108	0.70	121	0.49	3	0	13
Sauerkraut, canned	½	cup(s)	114	22	1	5	3	<1	0.04	0.01	0.07	—	0	34	1.67	751	0.11	27	17	1
Sausage, Italian, pork, cooked	1	item(s)	68	220	14	1	0	17	6.14	8.13	2.23	—	53	16	1.02	627	—	3	1	15
Sausage, smoked, pork link	1	piece(s)	76	295	17	2	—	24	8.58	11.09	2.85	—	52	23	0.88	1137	—	4	0	16
Scallops, mixed species, breaded, fried	3	item(s)	47	100	8	5	0	5	1.24	2.09	1.32	—	28	20	0.38	216	—	23	1	13
Seaweed, spirulina, dried	½	cup(s)	8	22	4	2	<1	1	0.20	0.05	0.16	—	0	9	2.14	79	0.38	7	1	1
Shrimp, mixed species, breaded, fried	3	ounce(s)	85	205.69	18.18	9.74	0.34	10.43	1.77	3.24	4.32	—	150.44	56.95	1.07	292.39	—	20.39	1.27	35.44
Shrimp, mixed species, cooked, moist heat	3	ounce(s)	85	84	18	0	0	1	0.25	0.17	0.37	—	166	33	2.63	190	1.17	3	2	34
Soda, Coca-Cola Classic cola	12	fluid ounce(s)	360	146	0	41	0	0	0.00	0.00	0.00	0	0	—	—	50	—	—	0	—
Soda, Coke diet cola	12	fluid ounce(s)	360	2	0	<1	0	0	0.00	0.00	0.00	0	0	—	—	42	—	—	0	—
Soda, cola	12	fluid ounce(s)	426	179	<1	46	0	0	0.00	0.00	0.00	—	0	13	0.09	17	0.00	0	0	<1
Soda, ginger ale	12	fluid ounce(s)	366	124	0	32	0	0	0.00	0.00	0.00	0	0	11	0.66	26	0.00	0	0	<1
Soda, lemon lime	12	fluid ounce(s)	368	147	0	38	0	0	0.00	0.00	0.00	—	0	7	0.26	41	0.00	0	0	0
Soda, root beer	12	fluid ounce(s)	370	152	0	39	0	0	0.00	0.00	0.00	0	0	18	0.18	48	0.00	0	0	<1
Sour cream	2	tablespoon(s)	24	51	1	1	0	5	3.13	1.45	0.19	—	11	28	0.01	13	0.14	3	<1	1
Sour cream, fat free	2	tablespoon(s)	32	24	1	5	0	0	0.00	0.00	0.00	0	3	40	0.00	45	0.00	4	0	—
Soy sauce	1	tablespoon(s)	18	10	1	2	0	<.1	0.00	0.00	0.01	—	0	3	0.36	1029	0.00	3	0	—
Spinach, canned, drained	½	cup(s)	108	25	3	4	3	1	0.09	0.02	0.23	—	0	138	2.49	29	2.10	106	16	2
Spinach, chopped, boiled, drained	½	cup(s)	90	21	3	3	2	<1	0.04	0.01	0.10	—	0	122	3.21	63	1.87	131	9	1
Spinach, raw, chopped	1	cup(s)	30	7	1	1	1	<1	0.02	0.00	0.05	—	0	30	0.81	24	0.61	58	8	<1
Squash, acorn, baked	½	cup(s)	103	57	1	15	5	<1	0.03	0.01	0.06	—	0	45	0.95	4	—	19	11	1
Squash, summer, all varieties, sliced, boiled, drained	½	cup(s)	90	18	1	4	1	<1	0.06	0.02	0.12	—	0	24	0.32	1	0.13	18	5	<1
Squash, winter, all varieties, baked, mashed	½	cup(s)	103	38	1	9	3	<1	0.13	0.05	0.27	—	0	23	0.45	1	0.12	21	10	<1
Squid, mixed species, fried	3	ounce(s)	85	149	15	7	0	6	1.60	2.34	1.82	—	221	33	0.86	260	—	12	4	44
Strawberries, raw	½	cup(s)	72	23	<1	6	1	<1	0.01	0.03	0.11	—	0	12	0.30	1	0.21	17	42	<1
Strawberries, sweetened, frozen, thawed	½	cup(s)	128	99	1	27	2	<1	0.01	0.02	0.09	—	0	14	0.60	1	0.31	5	50	1
Sugar, brown, packed	1	teaspoon(s)	5	17	0	4	0	0	0.00	0.00	0.00	0	0	4	0.09	2	0.00	<.1	0	<.1
Sugar, white, granulated	1	teaspoon(s)	4	15	0	4	0	0	0.00	0.00	0.00	—	0	<.1	0.00	0	0.00	0	0	<.1
Sweet potatoes, baked, peeled	½	cup(s)	100	90	2	21	3	<1	0.03	0.00	0.06	—	0	38	0.69	36	0.71	6	20	<1
Syrup, maple	¼	cup(s)	80	209	0	54	0	<1	0.03	0.05	0.08	—	0	54	0.96	7	0.00	0	0	<1
Taco shell, hard	1	item(s)	13	62	1	8	1	3	0.43	1.19	1.13	—	0	21	0.33	49	0.22	17	0	2
Tangerine, raw	1	item(s)	84	37	1	9	2	<1	0.02	0.03	0.03	—	0	12	0.08	1	0.17	17	26	<1
Tea, decaffeinated, prepared	8	fluid ounce(s)	237	2	0	1	0	0	0.00	0.00	0.01	0	0	0	0.05	7	0.00	12	0	0
Tea, herbal, prepared	8	fluid ounce(s)	237	2	0	<1	0	0	0.00	0.00	0.01	0	0	5	0.19	2	0.00	2	0	0
Tea, prepared	8	fluid ounce(s)	237	2	0	1	0	0	0.00	0.00	0.01	0	0	0	0.05	7	0.00	12	0	0
Teriyaki sauce	1	tablespoon(s)	18	15	1	3	<.1	0	0.00	0.00	0.00	0	0	5	0.31	690	0.00	4	0	<1
Tofu, firm	3	ounce(s)	79	80	8	2	1	4	0.50	0.87	2.17	—	0	60	1.08	0	—	—	0	—
Tomato juice, canned	½	cup(s)	122	21	1	5	<1	<.1	0.01	0.01	0.03	—	0	12	0.52	328	0.39	24	22	<1

Food Description	Qty	Measure	Wt (g)	Ener (cal)	Prot (g)	Carb (g)	Dietary Fiber (g)	Fat (g)	Fat Breakdown (g) Sat	Mono	Poly	Trans	Chol (mg)	Calc (mg)	Iron (mg)	Sodi (mg)	Vit E (mg)	Folate (mcg)	Vit C (mg)	Selenium (mcg)
Tomato sauce	½	cup(s)	112	46	2	8	2	1	0.18	0.29	0.72	0	0	21	1.08	199	0.39	15	15	1
Tomatoes, fresh, ripe, red	1	item(s)	123	22.13	1.08	4.82	1.47	0.24	0.05	0.06	0.16	—	0	12.3	0.33	6.15	0.66	18.45	15.62	0
Tomatoes, stewed, canned, red	½	cup(s)	128	33	1	8	1	<1	0.03	0.04	0.10	—	0	43	1.70	282	1.06	6	10	1
Tortilla chips, plain	6	item(s)	28	142	2	18	2	7	1.43	4.39	1.03	—	0	44	0.43	150	1	3	0	2
Tortillas, corn, soft	1	item(s)	26	58	1	12	1	1	0.09	0.17	0.29	—	0	46	0.36	42	0.07	26	0	1
Tortillas, flour	1	item(s)	32	104	3	18	1	2	0.56	1.21	0.34	—	0	40	1.06	153	0.06	33	0	7
Tuna, light, canned in oil, drained	2	ounce(s)	57	113	17	0	0	5	0.87	1.68	1.64	—	10	7	0.79	202	0.50	3	0	43
Tuna, light, canned in water, drained	2	ounce(s)	57	66	14	0	0	<1	0.13	0.09	0.19	—	17	6	0.87	192	0.19	2	0	46
Turkey, breast, processed, oven roasted, fat free	1	slice(s)	28	25	4	1	0	0	0.00	0.00	0.00	0	10	0	0.00	330	—	—	0	—
Turkey, breast, processed, traditional carved	2	slice(s)	45	40	9	0	0	1	0.00	0.07	0.14	—	20	0	0.72	540	—	—	0	—
Turkey, roasted, dark meat, meat only	3	ounce(s)	85	159	24	0	0	6	2.06	1.39	1.84	—	72	27	1.98	67	0.54	8	0	35
Turkey, roasted, light meat, meat only	3	ounce(s)	85	133	25	0	0	3	0.88	0.48	0.73	—	59	16	1.15	54	0.08	5	0	27
Turnip greens, chopped, boiled, drained	½	cup(s)	72	14	1	3	3	<1	0.04	0.01	0.07	—	0	99	0.58	21	1.35	85	20	1
Turnips, cubed, boiled, drained	½	cup(s)	78	17	1	4	2	<.1	0.01	0.00	0.03	—	0	26	0.14	12	0.02	7	9	<1
Vegetables, mixed, canned, drained	½	cup(s)	82	40	2	8	2	<1	0.04	0.01	0.10	—	0	22	0.86	121	0.28	20	4	<1
Vinegar, balsamic	1	tablespoon(s)	15	10	0	2	0	0	0.00	0.00	0.00	0	0	0	0.00	0	—	—	0	—
Waffle, plain, frozen, toasted	2	item(s)	66	174	4	27	2	5	0.95	2.12	1.84	—	16	153	2.95	519	0.65	36	0	11
Walnuts, dried black, chopped	¼	cup(s)	31	193	8	3	2	18	1.05	4.69	10.96	—	0	19	0.98	1	0.56	10	1	5
Watermelon	½	cup(s)	77	23	<1	6	<1	<1	0.01	0.03	0.04	—	0	5	0.19	1	0.04	2	6	<1
Wheat germ, crude	2	tablespoon(s)	14	52	3	7	2	1	0.24	0.20	0.86	—	0	6	0.90	2	—	40	0	11
Wine cooler	10	fluid ounce(s)	300	150	<1	18	<.1	<.1	0.01	0.00	0.02	—	0	17	0.81	25	0.02	5	<.1	
Wine, red, California	5	fluid ounce(s)	150	125	<1	4	0	0	0.00	0.00	0.00	0	0	12	1.43	15	0.00	1	0	—
Wine, sparkling, domestic	5	fluid ounce(s)	150	105	<1	4	0	0	0.00	0.00	0.00	0	0	—	—	—	—	—	—	—
Wine, white	5	fluid ounce(s)	148	100	<1	1	0	0	0.00	0.00	0.00	0	0	13	0.47	7	—	0	0	<1
Yogurt, custard style, fruit flavors	6	ounce(s)	170	190	7	32	0	4	2.00	—	—	—	15	200	0.00	90	—	—	0	—
Yogurt, fruit, low fat	1	cup(s)	245	243	10	46	0	3	1.82	0.77	0.08	—	12	338	0.15	130	0.05	22	1	7
Yogurt, fruit, nonfat, sweetened w/low calorie sweetener	1	cup(s)	241	122	11	19	1	<1	0.21	0.10	0.04	—	3	370	0.62	139	0.17	26	1	—
Yogurt, plain, low fat	1	cup(s)	245	154	13	17	0	4	2.45	1.04	0.11	—	15	448	0.20	172	0.05	27	2	8
VEGETARIAN FOODS																				
Prepared																				
Macaroni & cheese (lacto)	8	ounce(s)	226	181	8	17	<1	9	4.37	2.88	0.89	0	22	187	0.77	768	0.29	39	<.1	16
Steamed rice & vegetables (vegan)	8	ounce(s)	228	265	5	40	3	10	1.84	3.91	4.07	0	0	41	1.43	1403	3.05	28	13	8
Vegan spinach enchiladas (vegan)	1	piece(s)	82	93	5	15	2	2	0.34	0.55	1.27	—	0	117	1.13	134	—	46	1	5
Vegetable chow mein (vegan)	8	ounce(s)	227	166	6	22	2	6	0.65	2.66	2.47	0	0	190	3.65	371	0.06	47	7	6
Vegetable lasagna (lacto)	8	ounce(s)	225	177	12	25	2	4	1.92	0.93	0.34	0	10	144	1.91	637	0.05	64	15	19
Vegetarian chili (vegan)	8	ounce(s)	227	116	6	21	7	2	0.24	0.29	0.74	0	<1	68	2.42	383	0.15	58	16	5
Vegetarian vegetable soup (vegan)	8	ounce(s)	226	92	3	14	2	4	0.77	1.67	1.30	0	0	37	1.32	503	0.55	38	24	1
Boca burger																				
All American flamed grilled patty	1	item(s)	71	110	14	6	4	4	1.00	—	—	0	3	150	1.80	370	—	—	0	—
Boca meatless ground burger	½	cup(s)	57	70	11	7	4	1	0.00	—	—	—	0	80	1.44	220	—	—	0	—
Breakfast links	2	item(s)	45	100	10	6	5	4	0.00	—	—	0	0	60	1.44	330	—	—	0	—
Breakfast patties	1	item(s)	38	80	8	5	3	4	0.00	—	—	0	0	60	1.44	260	—	—	0	—
Vegan original patty	1	item(s)	71	90	13	4	0	1	0.00	—	—	0	0	80	1.80	350	—	—	1	—
Gardenburger																				
Black bean burger	1	item(s)	71	80	8	11	4	2	0.00	—	—	0	0	40	1.44	330	—	—	0	—
Chik'n grill	1	item(s)	71	100	13	5	3	3	0.00	—	—	0	0	60	3.60	360	—	—	0	—
Meatless breakfast sausage	1	item(s)	43	50	5	2	2	4	0.00	—	—	0	0	20	0.72	120	—	—	0	—
Meatless meatballs	6	item(s)	85	110	12	8	4	5	1.00	—	—	0	0	60	1.80	400	—	—	0	—
Original	3	ounce(s)	85	132	7	19	4	4	1.80	1.80	0.60	0	24	72	0.00	672	—	12	0	8
Morningstar Farms																				
America's Original Veggie Dog links	1	item(s)	57	80	11	6	1	1	0.00	0.00	0.00	0	0	0	0.72	580	—	—	0	—
Better n Eggs egg substitute	¼	cup(s)	57	20	5	0	0	0	0.00	0.00	0.00	0	0	20	0.63	90	—	24	0	—
Breakfast links	2	item(s)	45	80	9	3	2	3	0.50	0.50	2.00	0	0	0	1.44	320	—	—	0	—
Breakfast strips	2	item(s)	16	60	2	2	1	5	0.50	1.00	3.00	0	0	0	0.27	220	—	—	0	—
Garden veggie patties	1	item(s)	67	100	10	9	4	3	0.50	0.50	1.50	0	0	40	0.72	350	—	—	0	—
Spicy black bean veggie burger	1	item(s)	78	150	11	16	5	5	0.50	1.50	2.50	0	0	40	1.80	470	—	—	0	—

MIXED FOODS, SOUPS, SANDWICHES																				
Mixed Dishes																				
Bean burrito	1	item(s)	149	327	17	33	6	15	8.30	4.73	0.85	0	38	331	2.95	514	0.01	115	4	18
Beef & vegetable fajita	1	item(s)	223	397	23	35	3	18	5.50	7.53	3.45	—	45	84	3.74	757	0.80	23	27	—
Chicken & vegetables w/broccoli, onion, bamboo shoots in soy based sauce	1	cup(s)	162	287	22	6	1	19	5.13	7.65	4.68	—	84	22	1.38	962	1.12	13	8	—
Chicken cacciatore	1	cup(s)	230	266	28	5	1	14	3.98	5.78	3.11	0	103	45	2.21	451	0.00	15	8	22
Chicken waldorf salad	½	cup(s)	100	178	14	6	1	11	1.76	3.18	5.05	0	42	20	0.78	246	0.62	15	2	11
Fettuccine alfredo	1	cup(s)	222	247	11	42	1	3	1.61	0.79	0.43	0	9	153	1.88	386	0.00	103	1	35
Hummus	½	cup(s)	123	218	6	25	5	11	1.38	6.04	2.56	—	0	60	1.93	298	0.92	73	10	3
Lasagna w/ground beef	1	cup(s)	237	288	18	22	2	15	7.47	4.84	0.84	0	68	222	2.33	493	0.22	50	10	22
Macaroni & cheese	1	cup(s)	200	393	15	40	1	19	8.18	6.72	2.66	—	30	323	2.26	800	0.72	12	<1	—
Meat loaf	1	slice(s)	115	244	17	7	<1	16	6.15	6.89	0.83	0	85	54	2.09	423	0.00	20	<1	17
Potato salad	½	cup(s)	125	179	3	14	2	10	1.79	3.10	4.67	—	85	24	0.81	661	—	9	13	5
Spaghetti & meatballs w/tomato sauce, prepared	1	cup(s)	248	330	19	39	3	12	3.90	4.40	2.20	—	89	124	3.70	1009	—	—	22	22
Spicy thai noodles (pad thai)	8	ounce(s)	231	222	9	36	3	6	0.83	3.33	1.83	0	37	32	1.58	598	0.36	44	22	3
Sushi w/vegetables in seaweed	6	piece(s)	156	182	3	41	1	<1	0.10	0.11	0.11	—	0	20	1.54	153	0.12	10	2	—
Tuna salad	½	cup(s)	103	192	16	10	0	9	1.58	2.96	4.23	0	13	17	1.03	412	0.00	8	2	42
Soups																				
Chicken noodle, condensed, prepared w/water	1	cup(s)	241	75	4	9	1	2	0.65	1.11	0.55	—	7	17	0.77	1106	0.10	22	<1	6
Cream of chicken, condensed, prepared w/milk	1	cup(s)	248	191	7	15	<1	11	4.64	4.46	1.64	—	27	181	0.67	1047	—	7	1	8
Cream of mushroom, condensed, prepared w/milk	1	cup(s)	248	203	6	15	<1	14	5.13	2.98	4.61	—	20	179	0.60	918	1.24	10	2	4
Manhattan clam chowder, condensed, prepared w/water	1	cup(s)	244	78	2	12	1	2	0.38	0.38	1.29	—	2	27	1.63	578	0.34	10	4	9
Minestrone, condensed, prepared w/water	1	cup(s)	241	82	4	11	1	3	0.55	0.70	1.11	—	2	34	0.92	911	—	36	1	8
New England clam chowder, condensed, prepared w/milk	1	cup(s)	248	164	9	17	1	7	2.95	2.26	1.09	—	22	186	1.49	992	0.45	10	3	13
Split pea	1	cup(s)	165	85	4	19	2	<1	0.07	0.03	0.18	0	0	30	1.25	608	0.00	61	9	<1
Tomato, condensed, prepared w/milk	1	cup(s)	248	161	6	22	3	6	2.90	1.61	1.12	—	17	159	1.81	744	1.24	17	68	2
Tomato, condensed, prepared w/water	1	cup(s)	244	85	2	17	<1	2	0.37	0.44	0.95	—	0	12	1.76	695	2.32	15	66	<1
Vegetable beef, condensed, prepared w/water	1	cup(s)	244	78	6	10	<1	2	0.85	0.81	0.12	—	5	17	1.12	791	0.37	10	2	4
Vegetarian vegetable, condensed, prepared w/water	1	cup(s)	241	72	2	12	—	2	0.29	0.82	0.72	—	0	22	1.08	822	—	10	1	4
Sandwiches																				
Bacon, lettuce, & tomato w/mayonnaise	1	item(s)	164	349	11	34	2	19	4.54	7.22	6.07	—	20	76	2.54	837	1.16	31	15	—
Cheeseburger, large, plain	1	item(s)	185	609	30	47	0	33	14.84	12.74	2.44	—	96	91	5.46	1589	—	74	0	39
Cheeseburger, large, w/bacon, vegetables, & condiments	1	item(s)	195	608	32	37	2	37	16.24	14.49	2.71	—	111	162	4.74	1043	—	86	2	33
Club w/bacon, chicken, tomato, lettuce, & mayonnaise	1	item(s)	246	555	31	48	3	26	5.94	—	—	—	72	116	4.05	855	1.53	48	9	—
Cold cut submarine w/cheese & vegetables	1	item(s)	228	456	22	51	2	19	6.81	8.23	2.28	—	36	189	2.51	1651	—	87	12	31
Egg salad	1	item(s)	126	278	10	29	1	13	2.96	3.97	4.79	—	217	107	2.60	494	0.13	82	1	24
Hamburger, double patty, large, w/condiments & vegetables	1	item(s)	226	540	34	40	0	27	10.52	10.33	2.80	—	122	102	5.85	791	—	77	1	26
Hamburger, large, plain	1	item(s)	137	426	23	32	2	23	8.38	9.88	2.14	—	71	74	3.58	474	—	60	0	27
Hot dog w/bun, plain	1	item(s)	98	242	10	18	2	15	5.11	6.85	1.71	—	44	24	2.31	670	—	48	<.1	26
Pastrami	1	item(s)	134	331	14	27	2	18	6.18	8.74	1.02	—	51	68	2.64	1335	0.27	21	2	—
Peanut butter & jelly	1	item(s)	93	330	11	42	3	15	3.00	6.87	3.82	—	1	68	2.11	409	2.02	37	<1	—
FAST FOOD																				
Arby's																				
Au jus sauce	1	serving(s)	85	5	<1	1	<.1	<.1	0.02	—	—	—	0	0	0.00	386	—	—	0	—
Beef 'n cheddar sandwich	1	item(s)	198	480	23	43	2	24	8.00	—	—	—	90	100	3.60	1240	—	—	1	—
Curly fries, medium	1	serving(s)	128	400	5	50	4	20	5.00	—	—	—	0	0	1.80	990	—	—	15	—
Market Fresh grilled chicken Caesar salad w/o dressing	1	serving(s)	338	230	33	8	3	8	3.50	—	—	—	80	200	1.80	920	—	—	42	—
Roast beef deluxe sandwich, light	1	item(s)	182	296	18	33	6	10	3.00	5.00	2.00	—	42	130	4.50	826	—	—	8	—
Roast beef sandwich, giant	1	item(s)	228	480	32	41	3	23	10.00	—	—	—	110	60	5.40	1440	—	—	0	—
Roast beef sandwich, regular	1	item(s)	157	350	21	34	2	16	6.00	—	—	—	85	60	3.60	950	—	—	0	—
Roast chicken deluxe sandwich, light	1	item(s)	194	260	23	33	3	5	1.00	—	—	—	40	100	2.70	1010	—	—	2	—

Food Description	Qty	Measure	Wt (g)	Ener (cal)	Prot (g)	Carb (g)	Dietary Fiber (g)	Fat (g)	Fat Breakdown (g) Sat	Mono	Poly	Trans	Chol (mg)	Calc (mg)	Iron (mg)	Sodi (mg)	Vit E (mg)	Folate (mcg)	Vit C (mg)	Selenium (mcg)
FAST FOOD (continued)																				
Burger King																				
BK Broiler chicken sandwich	1	item(s)	258	550	30	52	3	25	5.00	—	—	—	105	60	3.60	1110	—	—	6	—
Croissanwich w/sausage, egg, & cheese	1	item(s)	157	520	19	24	1	39	14.00	—	—	1.93	210	300	4.50	1090	—	—	0	—
Fish Fillet sandwich	1	item(s)	185	520	18	44	2	30	8.00	—	—	1.12	55	150	2.70	840	—	—	1	—
French fries, medium, salted	1	item(s)	117	360	4	46	4	18	5.00	—	—	4.50	0	20	0.72	640	—	—	9	—
Onion rings, medium	1	serving(s)	91	320	4	40	3	16	4.00	—	—	3.50	0	97	0.00	460	—	—	0	—
Whopper	1	item(s)	291	710	31	52	4	43	13.00	—	—	1	85	150	6.30	980	—	—	9	—
Whopper w/cheese	1	item(s)	316	800	36	53	4	50	18.00	—	—	2	110	250	6.30	1420	—	—	9	—
Chick Fil-A																				
Chargrilled chicken garden salad	1	item(s)	275	180	22	9	3	6	3.00	—	—	0	70	150	0.72	660	—	—	30	—
Chargrilled deluxe chicken sandwich	1	item(s)	195	290	27	31	2	7	1.50	—	—	0	70	80	1.80	990	—	—	5	—
Chicken biscuit w/cheese	1	item(s)	151	450	19	43	2	23	7.00	—	—	2.85	45	150	2.70	1430	—	—	0	—
Chicken salad sandwich	1	item(s)	153	350	20	32	5	15	3.00	—	—	0	65	150	1.80	880	—	—	0	—
Chick-n-Strips	4	item(s)	127	290	29	14	1	13	2.50	—	—	0	65	20	0.36	730	—	—	1	—
Coleslaw	1	item(s)	105	210	1	14	2	17	2.50	—	—	0	20	40	0.36	180	—	—	27	—
Dairy Queen																				
Banana split	1	item(s)	369	510	8	96	3	12	8.00	3.00	0.50	0	30	250	1.80	180	—	—	15	—
Chocolate chip cookie dough blizzard, small	1	item(s)	319	720	12	105	0	28	14.00	—	—	2.50	50	350	2.70	370	—	—	1	—
Chocolate malt, small	1	item(s)	418	650	15	111	0	16	10.00	—	—	0.50	55	450	1.80	370	—	—	2	—
Vanilla soft serve	½	cup(s)	94	140	3	22	0	5	3.00	—	—	0	15	150	0.72	70	—	—	0	—
Domino's																				
Classic hand tossed pizza																				
America's favorite feast, 12"	2	slice(s)	205	508	22	57	4	22	9.20	—	—	—	49	202	3.70	1221	—	—	1	—
Pepperoni feast, extra pepperoni & cheese, 12"	2	slice(s)	196	534	24	56	3	25	10.92	—	—	—	57	279	3.36	1349	—	—	<1	—
Vegi feast, 12"	2	slice(s)	203	439	19	57	4	16	7.09	—	—	—	34	279	3.44	987	—	—	1	—
Thin crust pizza																				
Extravaganzza, 12"	¼	item(s)	159	425	20	34	3	24	9.41	—	—	—	53	245	1.95	1408	—	—	1	—
Pepperoni, extra pepperoni & cheese, 12"	¼	item(s)	159	420	20	32	2	24	10.46	—	—	—	54	316	1.34	1362	—	—	<1	—
Vegi, 12"	¼	item(s)	159	338	16	34	3	17	7.08	—	—	—	34	317	1.42	1047	—	—	1	—
Ultimate deep dish pizza																				
America's favorite, 12"	2	slice(s)	235	617	26	59	4	33	12.88	—	—	—	58	334	4.43	1573	—	—	1	—
Pepperoni, extra pepperoni & cheese, 12"	2	slice(s)	235	629	26	57	4	34	13.57	—	—	—	61	332	4.25	1650	—	—	1	—
Vegi, 12"	2	slice(s)	235	547	22	59	4	26	10.19	—	—	—	41	333	4.33	1334	—	—	2	—
In-n-Out Burger																				
Cheeseburger w/mustard & ketchup	1	item(s)	268	400	22	41	3	18	9.00	—	—	—	55	200	3.60	1080	—	—	15	—
Chocolate shake	1	item(s)	425	690	9	83	0	36	24.00	—	—	—	95	300	0.72	350	—	—	0	—
Double-Double cheeseburger w/mustard & ketchup	1	item(s)	328	590	37	42	3	32	17.00	—	—	—	115	350	5.40	1510	—	—	15	—
French fries	1	item(s)	125	400	7	54	2	18	5.00	—	—	—	0	20	1.80	245	—	—	0	—
Hamburger w/mustard & ketchup	1	item(s)	243	310	16	41	3	10	4.00	—	—	—	35	40	3.60	720	—	—	15	—
Jack in the Box																				
Chicken club salad	1	item(s)	535	310	28	15	5	16	6.00	—	—	0	65	300	3.60	890	—	—	54	—
Hamburger	1	item(s)	104	250	12	30	2	9	3.50	—	—	0.88	30	100	3.60	610	—	—	0	—
Jack's Spicy Chicken sandwich	1	item(s)	253	580	24	53	3	31	6.00	—	—	2.81	60	150	1.80	950	—	—	9	—
Jumbo Jack hamburger w/cheese	1	item(s)	294	690	26	60	3	38	16.00	—	—	1.55	75	250	4.50	1360	—	—	9	—
Sourdough Jack	1	item(s)	244	700	30	36	3	49	16.00	—	—	2.98	80	200	4.50	1220	—	—	9	—
Jamba Juice																				
Banana berry smoothie	24	fluid ounce(s)	719	470	5	112	5	2	0.50	—	—	—	5	200	1.08	85	0.32	33	15	0
Chocolate mood smoothie	24	fluid ounce(s)	612	690	16	142	2	8	4.50	—	—	—	25	500	1.08	280	0.00	9	6	4
Jamba powerboost smoothie	24	fluid ounce(s)	730	440	6	103	7	2	0.00	—	—	—	0	1100	1.44	40	17.71	640	294	70
Orange juice, freshly squeezed	16	fluid ounce(s)	496	220	3	52	1	1	0.00	—	—	—	0	60	1.08	0	—	160	246	0
Protein berry pizzaz smoothie	24	fluid ounce(s)	710	440	20	92	6	2	0.00	—	—	—	0	1100	2.62	240	0.31	58	60	4

Kentucky Fried Chicken (KFC)																				
Extra Crispy chicken, breast	1	item(s)	162	470	34	19	0	28	8.00	—	—	4.50	135	19	1.44	1230	—	—	1	—
Hot & spicy chicken, whole wing	1	item(s)	55	180	11	9	0	11	3.00	—	—	0	60	10	0.72	420	—	—	1	—
Original Recipe chicken, drumstick	1	item(s)	59	140	14	4	0	8	2.00	—	—	1	75	10	0.70	440	—	—	1	—
Long John Silver																				
Baked cod	1	serving(s)	101	120	22	1	0	5	1.00	—	—	—	90	20	0.72	240	—	—	0	—
Batter dipped fish sandwich	1	item(s)	177	440	17	48	3	20	5.00	—	—	—	35	60	3.60	1120	—	—	9	—
Clam chowder	1	item(s)	227	220	9	23	0	10	4.00	—	—	—	25	150	0.72	810	—	—	0	—
Crunchy shrimp basket	21	item(s)	114	340	12	32	2	19	5.00	—	—	—	105	500	1.80	720	—	—	1	—
McDonald's																				
Big Mac hamburger	1	item(s)	216	590	24	47	3	34	11.00	—	—	1.48	85	300	4.50	1090	—	—	4	—
Cheeseburger	1	item(s)	121	330	15	36	2	14	6.00	—	—	1.02	45	250	2.70	830	—	—	2	—
Chicken McNuggets	4	item(s)	72	210	10	12	1	13	2.50	—	—	1.13	35	20	0.72	460	—	—	1	—
Egg McMuffin	1	item(s)	138	300	18	29	2	12	4.50	—	—	0.42	235	300	2.70	830	0.72	—	1	—
Filet-o-fish sandwich	1	item(s)	156	470	15	45	1	26	5.00	—	—	1.11	50	200	1.80	890	—	—	1	—
French fries, small	1	serving(s)	68	210	3	26	2	10	1.50	—	—	2.30	0	10	0.36	135	—	—	9	—
Fruit n' yogurt parfait	1	item(s)	338	380	10	76	2	5	2.00	—	—	0.18	15	300	1.80	240	—	—	24	—
Hash browns	1	item(s)	53	130	1	14	1	8	1.50	—	—	2	0	10	0.36	330	—	—	2	—
Honey sauce	1	item(s)	14	45	0	12	0	0	0.00	0.00	0.00	—	0	10	0.18	0	—	—	1	—
McSalad Shaker garden salad	1	item(s)	149	100	7	4	2	6	3.00	—	—	—	75	150	1.08	120	—	—	15	—
McSalad Shaker grilled chicken caesar salad	1	item(s)	163	100	17	3	2	3	1.50	—	—	—	40	100	1.08	240	—	—	12	—
Newman's Own creamy Caesar salad dressing	1	item(s)	59	190	2	4	0	18	3.50	—	—	0.29	20	60	0.18	500	15.40	—	1	—
Plain hotcakes w/syrup & margarine	3	item(s)	228	600	9	104	0	17	3.00	—	—	4	20	100	4.50	770	—	—	1	—
Quarter Pounder hamburger	1	item(s)	172	430	23	37	2	21	8.00	—	—	1.01	70	200	4.50	840	—	—	2	—
Quarter Pounder hamburger w/cheese	1	item(s)	200	530	28	38	2	30	13.00	—	—	1.51	95	350	4.50	1310	—	—	2	—
Sausage McMuffin w/egg	1	item(s)	164	450	20	29	2	28	10.00	—	—	0.59	255	300	2.70	930	0.72	—	1	—
Vanilla milkshake	8	fluid ounce(s)	227	254	9	40	0	7	4.28	1.98	0.26	—	27	331	0.23	215	0.11	16	0	5
Pizza Hut																				
Pepperoni Lovers stuffed crust pizza	1	slice(s)	171	480	23	44	3	24	11.00	—	—	1.05	65	300	2.70	1300	—	—	4	—
Pepperoni Lovers thin 'n crispy pizza	1	slice(s)	94	270	13	22	2	14	7.00	—	—	0.51	40	200	1.44	700	—	—	2	—
Personal Pan supreme pizza	1	slice(s)	73	170	8	19	1	7	3.00	—	—	0.95	15	80	1.86	400	—	—	4	—
Veggie Lovers stuffed crust pizza	1	slice(s)	181	370	17	45	3	14	7.00	—	—	0.53	35	250	2.70	980	—	—	12	—
Veggie Lovers thin 'n crispy pizza	1	slice(s)	110	190	8	23	2	7	3.00	—	—	0.54	15	150	1.44	480	—	—	12	—
Starbucks																				
Cappuccino, tall	12	fluid ounce(s)	360	120	7	10	0	6	4.00	—	—	—	25	250	0.00	95	—	—	1	—
Cinnamon spice mocha, tall nonfat w/o whipped cream	12	fluid ounce(s)	360	170	11	32	0	0	0.50	0.00	0.00	0	5	300	0.72	150	—	—	0	—
Frappuccino, tall chocolate	12	fluid ounce(s)	360	290	13	52	1	5	1.00	—	—	—	3	400	1.80	300	—	—	5	—
Latte, tall w/nonfat milk	12	fluid ounce(s)	360	123	12	17	0	1	0.40	0.16	0.02	0	6	420	0.18	174	—	18	4	—
Latte, tall w/whole milk	12	fluid ounce(s)	360	212	11	17	0	11	6.90	3.24	0.42	—	46	400	0.18	165	—	17	3	—
Macchiato, tall caramel w/whole milk	12	fluid ounce(s)	360	190	6	27	0	7	4.00	—	—	—	25	200	0.36	105	—	—	1	—
Tazo chai black tea, tall nonfat	12	fluid ounce(s)	360	170	6	37	0	0	0.00	0.00	0.00	0	5	200	0.36	95	—	—	0	—
Subway																				
Chocolate chip cookie	1	item(s)	48	209	3	29	1	10	3.50	—	—	1.07	12	0	1.00	135	—	—	0	—
Classic Italian B.M.T. sandwich, 6", white bread	1	item(s)	250	453	21	40	3	24	8.00	—	—	0	56	100	2.70	1740	—	—	24	—
Meatball sandwich, 6", white bread	1	item(s)	284	501	23	46	4	25	10.00	—	—	0.75	56	100	3.60	1350	—	—	24	—
Roast beef sandwich, 6", white bread	1	item(s)	220	264	18	39	3	5	1.00	—	—	0	20	40	3.60	840	—	—	24	—
Roasted chicken breast sandwich, 6", white bread	1	item(s)	234	311	25	40	3	6	1.50	—	—	0	48	60	3.60	880	—	—	24	—
Tuna sandwich, 6", white bread	1	item(s)	252	419	18	39	3	21	5.00	—	—	—	42	100	2.70	1180	—	—	24	—
Turkey breast sandwich, 6", white bread	1	item(s)	220	254	16	39	3	4	1.00	—	—	0	15	40	2.70	1000	—	—	24	—
Taco Bell																				
7-layer burrito	1	item(s)	283	530	18	67	10	22	8.00	—	—	3	25	300	3.59	1360	—	—	5	—
Beef burrito supreme	1	item(s)	248	440	18	51	7	18	8.00	—	—	2	40	200	2.70	1330	—	—	9	—
Grilled chicken burrito	1	item(s)	198	390	19	49	3	13	4.00	—	—	—	40	151	1.44	1240	—	—	2	—
Taco	1	item(s)	78	170	8	13	3	10	4.00	—	—	0.50	25	60	1.08	350	—	—	2	—
Veggie fajita wrap supreme	1	item(s)	255	470	11	55	3	22	7.00	—	—	—	30	150	1.44	990	—	—	6	—

Food Description	Qty	Measure	Wt (g)	Ener (cal)	Prot (g)	Carb (g)	Dietary Fiber (g)	Fat (g)	Fat Breakdown (g) Sat	Mono	Poly	Trans	Chol (mg)	Calc (mg)	Iron (mg)	Sodi (mg)	Vit E (mg)	Folate (mcg)	Vit C (mg)	Selenium (mcg)
CONVENIENCE MEALS																				
Budget Gourmet																				
Cheese manicotti w/meat sauce	1	item(s)	284	420	18	38	4	22	11.00	6.00	1.34	—	85	300	2.70	810	—	31	0	—
Chicken w/fettuccine	1	item(s)	284	380	20	33	3	19	10.00	—	—	—	85	100	2.70	810	—	—	0	—
Light beef stroganoff	1	item(s)	248	290	20	32	3	7	4.00	—	—	—	35	40	1.80	580	—	19	2	—
Light sirloin of beef in herb sauce	1	item(s)	269	260	19	30	5	7	4.00	2.30	0.31	—	30	40	1.80	850	—	38	6	—
Light vegetable lasagna	1	item(s)	298	290	15	36	5	9	1.79	0.89	0.60	—	15	283	3.03	780	—	75	59	—
Healthy Choice																				
Chicken enchilada suprema meal	1	item(s)	320	360	13	59	8	7	3.00	2.00	2.00	—	30	40	1.44	580	—	—	4	—
Lemon pepper fish meal	1	item(s)	303	280	11	49	5	5	2.00	1.00	2.00	—	30	40	0.36	580	—	—	30	—
Traditional salisbury steak meal	1	item(s)	354	360	23	45	5	9	3.50	4.00	1.00	—	45	80	2.70	580	—	—	21	—
Traditional turkey breasts meal	1	item(s)	298	330	21	50	4	5	2.00	1.50	1.50	—	35	40	1.44	600	—	—	0	—
Zucchini lasagna	1	item(s)	383	280	13	47	5	4	2.50	—	—	—	10	200	1.80	310	—	—	0	—
Stouffers																				
Cheese enchiladas with mexican rice	1	serving(s)	276	370	12	48	5	14	5.00	—	—	—	25	200	1.44	890	—	—	12	—
Chicken pot pie	1	item(s)	284	740	23	56	4	47	18.00	12.41	10.48	—	65	150	2.70	1170	—	—	2	—
Homestyle beef pot roast & potatoes	1	item(s)	252	270	16	25	3	12	4.50	—	—	—	35	20	1.80	820	—	—	6	—
Homestyle roast turkey breast w/stuffing & mashed potatoes	1	item(s)	273	300	16	34	2	11	3.00	—	—	—	35	40	0.72	1190	—	—	0	—
Lean Cuisine Everyday Favorites chicken chow mein w/rice	1	item(s)	255	210	12	33	2	3	1.00	1.00	0.50	0	30	20	0.36	620	—	—	0	—
Lean Cuisine Everyday Favorites lasagna w/meat sauce	1	item(s)	291	300	19	41	3	8	4.00	2.00	0.50	0	30	200	1.08	650	—	—	5	—
Weight Watchers																				
Smart Ones chicken enchiladas suiza entree	1	serving(s)	255	270	15	33	2	9	3.50	—	—	—	50	250	1.08	660	—	—	4	—
Smart Ones garden lasagna entree	1	item(s)	312	270	14	36	5	7	3.50	—	—	—	30	350	1.80	610	—	—	6	—
Smart Ones pepperoni pizza	1	item(s)	158	390	23	46	4	12	4.00	—	—	—	45	450	1.80	650	—	—	5	—
Smart Ones spicy penne pasta & ricotta	1	item(s)	289	280	11	45	4	6	2.00	—	—	—	5	150	2.70	400	—	—	6	—
Smart Ones spicy Szechuan style vegetables & chicken	1	item(s)	255	220	11	39	3	2	0.50	—	—	—	10	150	1.80	730	—	—	2	—

Glossary

A

Action stage Stage of change in the transtheoretical model in which the individual is actively changing a negative behavior or adopting a new, healthy behavior.

Acupuncture Chinese medical system that requires body piercing with fine needles during therapy to relieve pain and treat ailments and diseases.

Addiction Compulsive and uncontrollable behavior(s) or use of substance(s).

Adenosine triphosphate (ATP) A high-energy chemical compound that the body uses for immediate energy.

Adequate Intake (AI) The recommended amount of a nutrient intake when sufficient evidence is not available to calculate the EAR and subsequent RDA.

Adipose tissue Fat cells in the body.

Aerobic Describes exercise that requires oxygen to produce the necessary energy (ATP) to carry out the activity.

AIDS (acquired immunodeficiency syndrome) Any of a number of diseases that arise when the body's immune system is compromised by HIV; the final stage of HIV infection.

Air displacement Technique to assess body composition by calculating the body volume from the air replaced by an individual sitting inside a small chamber.

Alcohol (ethyl alcohol) A depressant drug that affects the brain and slows down central nervous system activity; has strong addictive properties.

Alcoholism Disease in which an individual loses control over drinking alcoholic beverages.

Altruism True concern for the welfare of others.

Alveoli Air sacs in the lungs where oxygen is taken up and carbon dioxide (produced by the body) is released from the blood.

Amenorrhea Cessation of regular menstrual flow.

Amino acids Chemical compounds that contain nitrogen, carbon, hydrogen, and oxygen; the basic building blocks the body uses to build different types of protein.

Amotivational syndrome A condition characterized by loss of motivation, dullness, apathy, and no interest in the future.

Amphetamines A class of powerful central nervous system stimulants.

Anaerobic Describes exercise that does not require oxygen to produce the necessary energy (ATP) to carry out the activity.

Anaerobic threshold The highest percentage of the VO_{2max} at which an individual can exercise (maximal steady state) for an extended time without accumulating significant amounts of lactic acid (accumulation of lactic acid forces an individual to slow down the exercise intensity or stop altogether).

Android obesity Obesity pattern seen in individuals who tend to store fat in the trunk or abdominal area.

Angina pectoris Chest pain associated with coronary heart disease.

Angiogenesis Formation of blood vessels (capillaries).

Angioplasty A procedure in which a balloon-tipped catheter is inserted, then inflated, to widen the inner lumen of the artery.

Anorexia nervosa An eating disorder characterized by self-imposed starvation to lose and maintain very low body weight.

Anthropometric measurement Techniques to measure body girths at different sites.

Antibodies Substances produced by the white blood cells in response to an invading agent.

Anticoagulant Any substance that inhibits blood clotting.

Antioxidants Compounds such as vitamins C and E, beta-carotene, and selenium that prevent oxygen from combining with other substances in the body to form harmful compounds.

Aquaphobic Having a fear of water.

Arrhythmias Irregular heart rhythms.

Arterial-venous oxygen difference ($a\text{-}\bar{v}O_2diff$) The amount of oxygen removed from the blood as determined by the difference in oxygen content between arterial and venous blood.

Atherosclerosis Fatty/cholesterol deposits in the walls of the arteries leading to formation of plaque.

Autogenic training A stress management technique using a form of self-suggestion, wherein an individual is able to place himself or herself in an autohypnotic state by repeating and concentrating on feelings of heaviness and warmth in the extremities.

Ayurveda Hindu system of medicine based on herbs, diet, massage, meditation, and yoga to help the body boost its own natural healing.

B

Basal metabolic rate (BMR) The lowest level of oxygen consumption necessary to sustain life.

Behavior modification The process of permanently changing negative behaviors to positive behaviors that will lead to better health and well-being.

Benign Noncancerous.

Binge-eating disorder An eating disorder characterized by uncontrollable episodes of eating excessive amounts of food within a relatively short time.

Bioelectrical impedance Technique to assess body composition by running a weak electrical current through the body.

Biofeedback A stress management technique in which a person learns to influence physiological responses that are not typically under voluntary control or responses that typically are regulated but for which regulation has broken down as a result of injury, trauma, or illness.

Blood lipids (fat) Cholesterol and triglycerides.

Blood pressure A measure of the force exerted against the walls of the vessels by the blood flowing through them.

Bod Pod Commercial name of the equipment used to assess body composition through the air displacement technique.

Body composition The fat and non-fat components of the human body; important in assessing recommended body weight.

Body mass index (BMI) Technique to determine thinness and excessive fatness that incorporates height and weight to estimate critical fat values at which the risk for disease increases.

Bone integrity A component of physiologic fitness used to determine risk for osteoporosis based on bone mineral density.

Bradycardia Slower heart rate than normal.

Breathing exercises A stress management technique wherein the individual concentrates on "breathing away" the tension and inhaling fresh air to the entire body.

Bulimia nervosa An eating disorder characterized by a pattern of binge eating and purging in an attempt to lose weight and maintain low body weight.

C

Calorie The amount of heat necessary to raise the temperature of 1 gram of water 1 degree Centigrade; used to measure the energy value of food and cost (energy expenditure) of physical activity.

Cancer Group of diseases characterized by uncontrolled growth and spread of abnormal cells.

Capillaries Smallest blood vessels carrying oxygenated blood to the tissues in the body.

Carbohydrate loading Increasing intake of carbohydrates during heavy aerobic training or prior to aerobic endurance events that last longer than 90 minutes.

Carbohydrates A classification of a dietary nutrient containing carbon, hydrogen, and oxygen; the major source of energy for the human body.

Carcinogens Substances that contribute to the formation of cancers.

Carcinoma in situ Encapsulated malignant tumor that has not spread.

Cardiac output Amount of blood pumped by the heart in one minute.

Cardiomyopathy A disease affecting the heart muscle.

Cardiorespiratory endurance The ability of the lungs, heart, and blood vessels to deliver adequate amounts of oxygen to the cells to meet the demands of prolonged physical activity.

Cardiorespiratory training zone Recommended training intensity range, in terms of exercise heart rate, to obtain adequate cardiorespiratory endurance development.

Cardiovascular diseases The array of conditions that affect the heart and the blood vessels.

Carotenoids Pigment substances in plants, some of which are precursors to vitamin A. More than 600 carotenoids are found in nature, about 50 of which are precursors to vitamin A, the most potent one being beta-carotene.

Catecholamines "Fight-or-flight" hormones, including epinephrine and norepinephrine.

Cellulite Term frequently used in reference to fat deposits that "bulge out"; these deposits are nothing but enlarged fat cells from excessive accumulation of body fat.

Chiropractics Health-care system that proposes that many diseases and ailments are related to misalignments of the vertebrae and emphasizes the manipulation of the spinal column.

Chlamydia A sexually transmitted disease, caused by a bacterial infection, that can cause significant damage to the reproductive system.

Cholesterol A waxy substance, technically a steroid alcohol, found only in animal fats and oil; used in making cell membranes, as a building block for some hormones, in the fatty sheath around nerve fibers, and other necessary substances.

Chronic diseases Illnesses that develop as a result of an unhealthy lifestyle and last a long time.

Chronological age Calendar age.

Chylomicrons Triglyceride-transporting molecules.

Cirrhosis A disease characterized by scarring of the liver.

Cocaine 2-beta-carbomethoxy-3-betabenozoxytropane, the primary psychoactive ingredient derived from coca plant leaves.

Cold turkey Eliminating a negative behavior all at once.

Complementary and alternative medicine (CAM) A group of diverse medical and health-care systems, practices, and products that are not presently considered to be part of conventional medicine; also called unconventional, nonallopathic, or integrative medicine.

Complex carbohydrates Carbohydrates formed by three or more simple sugar molecules linked together; also referred to as polysaccharides.

Contemplation stage Stage of change in the transtheoretical model in which the individual is considering changing behavior within the next 6 months.

Conventional Western medicine Traditional medical practice based on methods that are tested through rigorous scientific trials; also called allopathic medicine.

Cool-down Tapering off an exercise session slowly.

Coronary heart disease (CHD) Condition in which the arteries that supply the heart muscle with oxygen and nutrients are narrowed by fatty deposits, such as cholesterol and triglycerides.

C-reactive protein (CRP) A protein whose blood levels increase with inflammation, at times hidden deep in the body; elevation of this protein is an indicator of potential cardiovascular events.

Creatine An organic compound derived from meat, fish, and amino acids that combines with inorganic phosphate to form creatine phosphate.

Creatine phosphate (CP) A high-energy compound that the cells use to resynthesize ATP during all-out activities of very short duration.

Cross-training A combination of aerobic activities that contribute to overall fitness.

Cruciferous vegetables Plants that produce cross-shaped leaves (cauliflower, broccoli, cabbage, Brussels sprouts, kohlrabi), which seem to have a protective effect against cancer.

D

Daily Values (DVs) Reference values for nutrients and food components used in food labels.

Dentist Practitioner who specializes in diseases of the teeth, gums, and oral cavity.

Deoxyribonucleic acid (DNA) Genetic substance of which genes are made; molecule that contains cell's genetic code.

Diabetes mellitus A disease in which the body doesn't produce or utilize insulin properly.

Diastolic blood pressure Pressure exerted by blood against walls of arteries during relaxation phase (diastole) of the heart; lower of the two numbers in blood pressure readings.

Dietary fiber A complex carbohydrate in plant foods that is not digested but is essential to digestion.

Dietary Reference Intakes (DRI) A general term that describes four types of nutrient standards that establish adequate amounts and maximum safe nutrient intakes in the diet: Estimated Average Requirements (EAR), Recommended Dietary Allowances (RDA), Adequate Intakes (AI), and Tolerable Upper Intake Levels (UL).

Disaccharides Simple carbohydrates formed by two monosaccharide units linked together, one of which is glucose. The major disaccharides are sucrose, lactose, and maltose.

Distress Negative stress: Unpleasant or harmful stress under which health and performance begin to deteriorate.

Dopamine A neurotransmitter that affects emotional, mental, and motor functions.

Dual energy X-ray absorptiometry (DEXA) Method to assess body composition that uses very low-dose beams of X-ray energy to measure total body fat mass, fat distribution pattern, and bone density.

Dysmenorrhea Painful menstruation.

E

Ecosystem A community of organisms interacting with each other in an environment.

Electrocardiogram (ECG or EKG) A recording of the electrical activity of the heart.

Electrolytes Substances that become ions in solution and are critical for proper muscle and neuron activation (include sodium, potassium, chloride, calcium, magnesium, phosphate, and bicarbonate among others).

Emotional wellness The ability to understand your own feelings, accept your limitations, and achieve emotional stability.

Endorphins Morphine-like substances released from the pituitary gland (in the brain) during prolonged aerobic exercise; thought to induce feelings of euphoria and natural well-being.

Energy-balancing equation A principle holding that as long as caloric input equals caloric output, the person will not gain or lose weight. If caloric intake exceeds output, the person gains weight; when output exceeds input, the person loses weight.

Environmental wellness The capability to live in a clean and safe environment that is not detrimental to health.

Enzymes Catalysts that facilitate chemical reactions in the body.

Essential fat Minimal amount of body fat needed for normal physiological functions; constitutes about 3 percent of total weight in men and 12 percent in women.

Estimated Average Requirement (EAR) The amount of a nutrient that meets the dietary needs of half the people.

Estimated Energy Requirement (EER) The average dietary energy (caloric) intake that is predicted to maintain energy balance in a healthy adult of defined age, gender, weight, height, and level of physical activity, consistent with good health.

Estrogen Female sex hormone essential for bone formation and conservation of bone density.

Eustress Positive stress: Health and performance continue to improve, even as stress increases.

Exercise A type of physical activity that requires planned, structured, and repetitive bodily movement with the intent of improving or maintaining one or more components of physical fitness.

Exercise intolerance Inability to function during exercise because of excessive fatigue or extreme feelings of discomfort.

Explanatory style The way people perceive the events in their lives, from an optimistic or a pessimistic perspective.

F

Fats A classification of nutrients containing carbon, hydrogen, some oxygen, and sometimes other chemical elements.

Ferritin Iron stored in the body.

Fighting spirit Determination; the open expression of emotions, whether negative or positive.

Fight or flight Physiological response of the body to stress that prepares the individual to take action by stimulating the body's vital defense systems.

FITT An acronym used to describe the four cardiorespiratory exercise prescription variables: *F*requency, *I*ntensity, *T*ype (mode), and *T*ime (duration).

Folate One of the B vitamins.

Fortified foods Foods that have been modified by the addition or increase of nutrients that either were not present or were present in insignificant amounts with the intent of preventing nutrient deficiencies.

Frequency Number of times per week a person engages in exercise.

Functional capacity The ability to perform the ordinary and unusual demands of daily living without limitations, excessive fatigue, or injury.

Functional foods Foods or food ingredients containing physiologically active substances that provide specific health benefits beyond those supplied by basic nutrition.

Functional independence Ability to carry out activities of daily living without assistance from other individuals.

G

General adaptation syndrome (GAS) A theoretical model that explains the body's adaptation to sustained stress which includes three stages: Alarm reaction, resistance, and exhaustion/recovery.

Genetically modified foods (GM foods) Foods whose basic genetic material (DNA) is manipulated by inserting genes with desirable traits from one plant, animal, or microorganism into another one either to introduce new traits or to enhance existing ones.

Genital herpes A sexually transmitted disease caused by a viral infection of the herpes simplex virus types 1 and 2. The virus can attack different areas of the body but typically causes blisters on the genitals.

Genital warts A sexually transmitted disease caused by a viral infection.

Girth measurements Technique to assess body composition by measuring circumferences at specific body sites.

Glucose intolerance A condition characterized by slightly elevated blood glucose levels.

Glycemic index An measure that is used to rate the plasma glucose response of carbohydrate-containing foods with the response produced by the same amount of carbohydrate from a standard source, usually glucose or white bread.

Glycogen Form in which glucose is stored in the body.

Goals The ultimate aims toward which effort is directed.

Gonorrhea A sexually transmitted disease caused by a bacterial infection.

Gynoid obesity Obesity pattern seen in people who store fat primarily around the hips and thighs.

H

Hatha yoga A form of yoga that incorporates specific sequences of static-stretching postures to help induce the relaxation response.

Health A state of complete well-being—not just the absence of disease or infirmity.

Health fitness standards The lowest fitness requirements for maintaining good health, decreasing the risk for chronic diseases, and lowering the incidence of muscular-skeletal injuries.

Health promotion The science and art of enabling people to increase control over their lifestyle to move toward a state of wellness.

Health-related fitness Fitness programs that are prescribed to improve the individual's overall health.

Healthy life expectancy (HLE) Number of years a person is expected to live in good health; this number is obtained by subtracting ill-health years from the overall life expectancy.

Heart rate reserve (HRR) The difference between maximal heart rate and resting heart rate.

Heat cramps Muscle spasms caused by heat-induced changes in electrolyte balance in muscle cells.

Heat exhaustion Heat-related fatigue.

Heat stroke Emergency situation resulting from the body being subjected to high atmospheric temperatures.

Hemoglobin Protein-iron compound in red blood cells that transports oxygen in the blood.

Herbal medicine Unconventional system that uses herbs to treat ailments and disease.

Heroin A potent drug that is a derivative of opium.

High-density lipoproteins (HDLs) Cholesterol-transporting molecules in the blood ("good" cholesterol) that help clear cholesterol from the blood.

HIV (human immunodeficiency virus) Virus that leads to acquired immunodeficiency syndrome (AIDS).

Homeopathy System of treatment based on the use of minute quantities of remedies that in large amounts produce effects similar to the disease being treated.

Homeostasis A natural state of equilibrium; the body attempts to maintain this equilibrium by constantly reacting to external forces that attempt to disrupt this fine balance.

Homocysteine An amino acid that, when allowed to accumulate in the blood, may lead to plaque formation and blockage of arteries.

Human papillomavirus (HPV) A group of viruses that can cause sexually transmitted diseases.

Hydrostatic weighing Underwater technique to assess body composition; considered the most accurate of the body composition assessment techniques.

Hypertension Chronically elevated blood pressure.

Hypokinetic diseases "Hypo" denotes "lack of"; therefore, illnesses related to lack of physical activity.

Hyponatremia A low sodium concentration in the blood caused by overhydration with water.

Hypotension Low blood pressure.

Hypothermia A breakdown in the body's ability to generate heat; a drop in body temperature below 95° F.

I

Imagery Mental visualization of relaxing images and scenes to induce body relaxation in times of stress or as an aid in the treatment of certain medical conditions such as cancer, hypertension, asthma, chronic pain, and obesity.

Immunity The function that guards the body from invaders, both internal and external.

Insulin A hormone secreted by the pancreas; essential for proper metabolism of blood glucose (sugar) and maintenance of blood glucose level.

Insulin resistance Inability of the cells to respond appropriately to insulin.

Intensity In cardiorespiratory exercise, how hard a person has to exercise to improve or maintain fitness.

International unit (IU) Measure of nutrients in foods.

Interval training A system of exercise in which a short period of intense effort is followed by a specified recovery period according to a prescribed ratio; for instance, a 1:3 work-to-recovery ratio.

L

Lactic acid End product of anaerobic glycolysis (metabolism).

Lactovegetarians Vegetarians who eat foods from the milk group.

Lapse (v.) To slip or fall back temporarily into unhealthy behavior(s); (n.) short-term failure to maintain healthy behaviors.

Lean body mass Body weight without body fat.

Learning theories Behavioral modification perspective stating that most behaviors are learned and maintained under complex schedules of reinforcement and anticipated outcomes.

Life expectancy Number of years a person is expected to live based on the person's birth year.

Life Experiences Survey A questionnaire used to assess sources of stress in life.

Lipoproteins Lipids covered by proteins, these transport fats in the blood. Types are LDL, HDL, and VLDL.

Locus of control A concept examining the extent to which a person believes he or she can influence the external environment.

Low-density lipoproteins (LDLs) Cholesterol-transporting molecules in the blood ("bad" cholesterol) that tend to increase blood cholesterol.

Lymphocytes Immune system cells responsible for waging war against disease or infection.

M

Magnetic therapy Unconventional treatment that relies on magnetic energy to promote healing.

Maintenance stage Stage of change in the transtheoretical model in which the individual maintains behavioral change for up to 5 years.

Malignant Cancerous.

Mammogram Low-dose X-rays of the breasts used as a screening technique for the early detection of breast cancer.

Marijuana A psychoactive drug prepared from a mixture of crushed leaves, flowers, small branches, stems, and seeds from the hemp plant *cannabis sativa.*

Massage therapy The rubbing or kneading of body parts to treat ailments.

Maximal heart rate (MHR) Highest heart rate for a person, related primarily to age.

Maximal oxygen uptake (VO_{2max}) Maximum amount of oxygen the body is able to utilize per minute of physical activity, commonly expressed in ml/kg/min; the best indicator of cardiorespiratory or aerobic fitness.

MDA A hallucinogenic drug that is structurally similar to amphetamines.

MDMA A synthetic hallucinogen drug with a chemical structure that closely resembles MDA and methamphetamine; also known as Ecstasy.

Meditation A stress management technique used to gain control over one's attention by clearing the mind and blocking out the stressor(s) responsible for the increased tension.

Mediterranean diet Typical diet of people around the Mediterranean region, focusing on olive oil, red wine, grains, legumes, vegetables, and fruits, with limited amounts of meat, fish, milk, and cheese.

Megadoses For most vitamins, 10 times the RDA or more; for vitamins A and D, 5 and 2 times the RDA, respectively.

Melanoma The most virulent, rapidly spreading form of skin cancer.

Mental wellness A state in which your mind is engaged in lively interaction with the world around you.

MET Short for metabolic equivalent, the rate of energy expenditure at rest; 1 MET is the equivalent of a VO_2 of 3.5 ml/kg/min.

Metabolic fitness A component of physiologic fitness that denotes reduction in the risk for diabetes and cardiovascular disease through a moderate-intensity exercise program in spite of little or no improvement in cardiorespiratory fitness.

Metabolic profile A measurement to assess risk for diabetes and cardiovascular disease through plasma insulin, glucose, lipid, and lipoprotein levels.

Metabolic syndrome An array of metabolic abnormalities that contribute to the development of atherosclerosis triggered by insulin resistance. These conditions include low HDL-cholesterol, high triglycerides, high blood pressure, and an increased blood-clotting mechanism.

Metastasis The movement of cells from one part of the body to another.

Methamphetamine A potent form of amphetamine.

Minerals Inorganic nutrients essential for normal body functions; found in the body and in food.

Mitochondria Structures within the cells where energy transformations take place.

Mode Form or type of exercise.

Moderate physical activity Activity that uses 150 calories of energy per day, or 1,000 calories per week.

Monogamous Describes a relationship in which two people have sexual relations only with each other.
Monosaccharides The simplest carbohydrates (sugars), formed by five- or six-carbon skeletons. The three most common monosaccharides are glucose, fructose, and galactose.
Morbidity A condition related to or caused by illness or disease.
Morphologic fitness A component of physiologic fitness used in reference to body composition factors such as percent body fat, body fat distribution, and body circumference.
Motivation The desire and will to do something.
Myocardial infarction Heart attack; damage to or death of an area of the heart muscle as a result of an obstructed artery to that area.
Myocardium Heart muscle.

N

Naturopathic medicine Unconventional system of medicine that relies exclusively on natural remedies to treat disease and ailments.
Neustress Neutral stress; stress that is neither harmful nor helpful.
Nicotine Addictive compound found in tobacco leaves.
Nitrosamines Potentially cancer-causing compounds formed when nitrites and nitrates, which prevent the growth of harmful bacteria in processed meats, combine with other chemicals in the stomach.
Nonmelanoma skin cancer Cancer that spreads or grows at the original site but does not metastasize to other regions of the body.
Nonresponders Individuals who exhibit small or no improvements in fitness, compared with others who undergo the same training program.
Nurse Health-care practitioner who assists in the diagnosis and treatment of health problems and provides many services to patients in a variety of settings.
Nutrient density A measure of the amount of nutrients and calories in various foods.
Nutrients Substances found in food that provide energy, regulate metabolism, and help with growth and repair of body tissues.
Nutrition Science that studies the relationship of foods to optimal health and performance.

O

Obesity An excessive accumulation of body fat, usually at least 30 percent above recommended body weight.
Objectives Steps required to reach a goal.
Occupational wellness The ability to perform your job skillfully and effectively under conditions that provide personal and team satisfaction and adequately reward each individual.
Oligomenorrhea Irregular menstrual cycles.
Omega-3 fatty acids Polyunsaturated fatty acids found primarily in cold-water seafood, flaxseed, and flaxseed oil; thought to lower blood cholesterol and triglycerides.
Omega-6 fatty acids Polyunsaturated fatty acids found primarily in corn and sunflower oils and most oils in processed foods.
Oncogenes Genes that initiate cell division.
Ophthalmologist Medical specialist concerned with diseases of the eye and prescription of corrective lenses.
Opportunistic infections Infections that arise in the absence of a healthy immune system, which would fight them off in healthy people.
Optometrist Health-care practitioner who specializes in the prescription and adaptation of lenses.
Oral surgeon A dentist who specializes in surgical procedures of the oral–facial complex.
Orthodontist A dentist who specializes in the correction and prevention of teeth irregularities.
Osteopath A medical practitioner with specialized training in musculoskeletal problems who uses diagnostic and therapeutic methods of conventional medicine in addition to manipulative measures.
Osteoporosis A condition of softening, deterioration, or loss of bone mineral density that leads to disability, bone fractures, and even death from medical complications.
Overtraining An emotional, behavioral, and physical condition marked by increased fatigue, decreased performance, persistent muscle soreness, mood disturbances, and feelings of "staleness" or "burnout" as a result of excessive physical training.
Overweight An excess amount of weight against a given standard, such as height or recommended percent body fat.
Ovolactovegetarians Vegetarians who include eggs and milk products in their diet.
Ovovegetarians Vegetarians who allow eggs in their diet.
Oxygen free radicals Substances formed during metabolism that attack and damage proteins and lipids, in particular the cell membrane and DNA, leading to diseases such as heart disease, cancer, and emphysema.
Oxygen uptake (VO_2) The amount of oxygen the human body uses.

P

Pedometer An electronic device that senses body motion and counts footsteps. Some pedometers also record distance, calories burned, speeds, "aerobic steps," and time spent being physically active.
Pelvic inflammatory disease (PID) An overall designation referring to the effects of other STIs, primarily chlamydia and gonorrhea.
Percent body fat Proportional amount of fat in the body based on the person's total weight; includes both essential fat and storage fat; also termed fat mass.
Periodization A training approach that divides the season into three cycles (macrocycles, mesocycles, and microcycles) using a systematic variation in intensity and volume of training to enhance fitness and performance.
Peripheral vascular disease Narrowing of the peripheral blood vessels, excluding the cerebral and coronary vessels.
Peristalsis Involuntary muscle contractions of intestinal walls that facilitate excretion of wastes.
Personal trainer A health/fitness professional who evaluates, motivates, educates, and trains clients to help them meet individualized, healthy lifestyle goals.
Physical activity Bodily movement produced by skeletal muscles; requires expenditure of energy and produces progressive health benefits. Examples include walking, taking the stairs, dancing, gardening, yard work, house cleaning, snow shoveling, washing the car, and all forms of structured exercise.
Physical fitness The ability to meet the ordinary as well as the unusual demands of daily life safely and effectively without being overly fatigued and still have energy left for leisure and recreational activities.
Physical fitness standards A fitness level that allows a person to sustain moderate-to-vigorous physical activity without undue fatigue and the ability to closely maintain this level throughout life.
Physical wellness Good physical fitness and confidence in your personal ability to take care of health problems.
Physician assistant Health-care practitioner trained to treat most standard cases of care.
Physiological age The biological and functional capacity of the body in relation to the person's maximal potential at any given age in the lifespan.
Physiological fitness A term used primarily in the field of medicine to mean biological systems affected by physical activity and the role of activity in preventing disease.
Phytonutrients Compounds found in fruits and vegetables that block formation of cancerous tumors and disrupt the progress of cancer.
Prayer Sincere and humble communication with a higher power.
Precontemplation stage Stage of change in the transtheoretical model in which an individual is unwilling to change behavior.
Preparation stage Stage of change in the transtheoretical model in which the individual is getting ready to make a change within the next month.
Primary care physician A medical practitioner who provides routine treatment of ailments; typically, the patient's first contact for health care.
Principle of individuality Training concept holding that genetics plays a major role in individual responses to exercise training and these differences must be considered when designing exercise programs for different people.
Probiotics Healthy bacteria (abundant in yogurt) that help break down foods and prevent disease-causing organisms from settling in the intestines.
Problem solving model Behavioral modification model proposing that many behaviors are the result of making decisions as the individual seeks to solve the problem behavior.
Processes of change Actions that help you achieve change in behavior.
Progressive muscle relaxation A stress management technique that involves sequential contraction and relaxation of muscle groups throughout the body.
Proteins A classification of nutrients consisting of complex organic compounds containing nitrogen and formed by combinations of amino acids; the main substances used in the body to build and repair tissues.

Q

Quackery/fraud The conscious promotion of unproven claims for profit.

R

Rate of perceived exertion (RPE) A perception scale to monitor or interpret the intensity of aerobic exercise.
Recommended body weight Body weight at which there seems to be no harm to human health; healthy weight.
Recommended Dietary Allowance (RDA) The daily amount of a nutrient (statistically determined from the EARs) that is considered adequate to meet the known nutrient needs of almost 98 percent of all healthy people in the United States.
Recovery time Amount of time the body takes to return to resting levels after exercise.
Registered dietitian (RD) A person with a college degree in dietetics who meets all certification and continuing education requirements of the American Dietetic Association or Dietitians of Canada.
Relapse (v.) To slip or fall back into unhealthy behavior(s) over a longer time; (n.) longer-term failure to maintain healthy behaviors.
Relapse prevention model Behavioral modification model based on the principle that high-risk situations can be anticipated through the development of strategies to prevent lapses and relapses.
Repetitions Number of times a given stretching exercise is performed.
Responders Individuals who exhibit improvements in fitness as a result of exercise training.
Resting heart rate (RHR) Heart rate after a person has been sitting quietly for 15–20 minutes.
Resting metabolic rate (RMR) The energy requirement to maintain the body's vital processes in the resting state.
Reverse cholesterol transport A process in which HDL molecules attract cholesterol and carry it to the liver, where it is changed to bile and eventually excreted in the stool.
Ribonucleic acid (RNA) Genetic material that guides the formation of cell proteins.
RICE An acronym used to describe the standard treatment procedure for acute sports injuries: Rest, Ice (cold application), Compression, and Elevation.
Risk factors Lifestyle and genetic variables that may lead to disease.

S

Sedentary Death Syndrome (SeDS) Deaths attributed to a lack of regular physical activity.
Sedentary Describes a person who is relatively inactive and whose lifestyle is characterized by a lot of sitting.
Self-efficacy A belief in one's own ability to perform a given task.
Self-esteem A sense of positive self-regard and self-respect.
Semivegetarians Vegetarians who include milk products, eggs, and fish and poultry in the diet.
Setpoint Weight control theory that the body has an established weight and strongly attempts to maintain that weight.
Sexually transmitted infections (STIs) Communicable diseases spread through sexual contact.
Shin splints Injury to the lower leg characterized by pain and irritation in the shin region of the leg.
Side stitch A sharp pain in the side of the abdomen.
Simple carbohydrates Formed by simple or double sugar units with little nutritive value; divided into monosaccharides and disaccharides.
Skill-related fitness Fitness components important for success in skillful activities and athletic events; encompasses agility, balance, coordination, power, reaction time, and speed.
Skinfold thickness Technique to assess body composition by measuring a double thickness of skin at specific body sites.
SMART An acronym used in reference to Specific, Measurable, Attainable, Realistic, and Time-specific goals.
Social cognitive theory Behavioral modification model holding that behavior change is influenced by the environment, self-efficacy, and characteristics of the behavior itself.
Social wellness The ability to relate well to others, both within and outside the family unit.
Sphygmomanometer Inflatable bladder contained within a cuff and a mercury gravity manometer (or aneroid manometer) from which blood pressure is read.
Spiritual wellness The sense that life is meaningful, that life has purpose, and that some power brings all humanity together; the ethics, values, and morals that guide you and give meaning and direction to life.
Spontaneous remission Inexplicable recovery from incurable disease.
Spot reducing Fallacious theory proposing that exercising a specific body part will result in significant fat reduction in that area.
Step aerobics A form of exercise that combines stepping up and down from a bench accompanied by arm movements.
Sterols Derived fats, of which cholesterol is the best-known example.
Storage fat Body fat in excess of essential fat; stored in adipose tissue.
Stress The mental, emotional, and physiological response of the body to any situation that is new, threatening, frightening, or exciting.
Stress electrocardiogram An exercise test during which the workload is increased gradually until the individual reaches maximal fatigue, with blood pressure and 12-lead electrocardiographic monitoring throughout the test.
Stressor Stress-causing event.

Stroke Condition in which a blood vessel that feeds the brain ruptures or is clogged, leading to blood flow disruption to the brain.
Stroke volume Amount of blood pumped by the heart in one beat.
Structured interview Assessment tool used to determine behavioral patterns that define Type A and B personalities.
Subcutaneous fat Deposits of fat directly under the skin.
Substrates Substances acted upon by an enzyme (examples: carbohydrates, fats).
Sun protection factor (SPF) Degree of protection offered by ingredients in sunscreen lotion; at least SPF 15 is recommended.
Supplements Tablets, pills, capsules, liquids, or powders that contain vitamins, minerals, antioxidants, amino acids, herbs, or fiber that individuals take to increase their intake of these nutrients.
Suppressor genes Genes that deactivate the process of cell division.
Synergistic action The effect of mixing two or more drugs, which can be much greater than the sum of two or more drugs acting by themselves.
Synergy A reaction in which the result is greater than the sum of its two parts.
Syphilis A sexually transmitted disease caused by a bacterial infection.
Systolic blood pressure Pressure exerted by blood against walls of arteries during forceful contraction (systole) of the heart; higher of the two numbers in blood pressure readings.

T

Tachycardia Faster-than-normal heart rate.
Tar Chemical compound that forms during the burning of tobacco leaves.
Techniques of change Methods or procedures used during each process of change.
Telomerase An enzyme that allows cells to reproduce indefinitely.
Telomeres A strand of molecules at both ends of a chromosome.
Termination/adoption stage Stage of change in the transtheoretical model in which the individual has eliminated an undesirable behavior or maintained a positive behavior for more than 5 years.
Thermogenic response Amount of energy required to digest food.
Trans fatty acid Solidified fat formed by adding hydrogen to monounsaturated and polyunsaturated fats to increase shelf life.
Transtheoretical model Behavioral modification model proposing that change is accomplished through a series of progressive stages in keeping with a person's readiness to change.
Triglycerides Fats formed by glycerol and three fatty acids; also called free fatty acids.
Type 1 diabetes Insulin-dependent diabetes mellitus (IDDM), a condition in which the pancreas produces little or no insulin; also known as juvenile diabetes.
Type 2 diabetes Non-insulin-dependent diabetes mellitus (NIDDM), a condition in which insulin is not processed properly; also known as adult-onset diabetes.
Type A Behavior pattern characteristic of a hard-driving, overambitious, aggressive, at times hostile, and overly competitive person.
Type B Behavior pattern characteristic of a calm, casual, relaxed, and easy-going individual.
Type C Behavior pattern of individuals who are just as highly stressed as the Type A but do not seem to be at higher risk for disease than the Type B.

U

Ultraviolet A (UVA) rays Light rays provided by sun lamps and tanning parlors known to damage skin and promote skin cancers.
Ultraviolet B (UVB) rays Portion of sunlight that causes sunburn and encourages skin cancers.
Underweight Extremely low body weight.
Upper Intake Level (UL) The highest level of nutrient intake that seems safe for most healthy people, beyond which exists an increased risk of adverse effects.

V

Vegans Vegetarians who eat no animal products at all.
Vegetarians Individuals whose diet is of vegetable or plant origin.
Very low-calorie diet A diet that allows an energy intake (consumption) of only 800 calories or less per day.
Very low-density lipoproteins (VLDLs) Triglyceride, cholesterol, and phospholipid-transporting molecules in the blood that tend to increase blood cholesterol.
Vigorous activity Any exercise that requires an MET level equal to or greater than 6 METs (21 ml/kg/min). 1 MET is the energy expenditure at rest, 3.5 ml/kg/min, and METs are defined as multiples of this resting metabolic rate (examples of activities that require a 6-MET level include aerobics, walking uphill at 3.5 mph, cycling at 10 to 12 mph, playing doubles in tennis, and vigorous strength training).
Vigorous exercise Cardiorespiratory exercise that requires an intensity level above 60 percent of maximal capacity.
Vitamins Organic nutrients essential for normal metabolism, growth, and development of the body.
Volume (of training) The total amount of training performed in a given work period (day, week, month, or season).

W

Waist circumference (WC) A waist girth measurement to assess potential risk for disease based on intra-abdominal fat content.
Warm-up Starting a workout slowly.
Water The most important classification of essential body nutrients, involved in almost every vital body process.
Weight-regulating mechanism (WRM) A feature of the hypothalamus of the brain that controls how much the body should weigh.
Wellness The constant and deliberate effort to stay healthy and achieve the highest potential for well-being. It encompasses seven dimensions—physical, emotional, mental, social, environmental, occupational, and spiritual—and integrates them all into a quality life.
Workload Load (or intensity) placed on the body during physical activity.

Y

Yoga A school of thought in the Hindu religion that seeks to help the individual attain a higher level of spirituality and peace of mind.
Yo-yo dieting Constantly losing and gaining weight.

Answers to Assess Your Knowledge

1	2	3	4	5	6	7	8	9	10	11
1. a	1. a	1. b	1. e	1. b	1. a	1. c	1. b	1. d	1. a	1. e
2. e	2. a	2. e	2. b	2. c	2. d	2. d	2. e	2. a	2. c	2. b
3. e	3. e	3. c	3. d	3. e	3. c	3. a	3. a	3. b	3. c	3. a
4. c	4. d	4. d	4. a	4. a	4. c	4. b	4. a	4. e	4. e	4. e
5. b	5. c	5. d	5. b	5. b	5. c	5. d	5. b	5. d	5. e	5. e
6. c	6. d	6. a	6. e	6. e	6. e	6. a	6. e	6. b	6. e	6. e
7. a	7. a	7. a	7. b	7. a	7. b	7. c	7. c	7. a	7. a	7. e
8. e	8. b	8. c	8. b	8. c	8. d	8. c	8. b	8. e	8. a	8. e
9. c	9. e	9. a	9. e	9. d	9. c	9. e	9. e	9. a	9. b	9. e
10. b	10. e	10. e	10. e	10. e	10. c	10. e	10. d	10. e	10. c	10. a

Index